Podiatric Dermatology

Podiatric Dermatology

EDITOR

DANIEL J. McCARTHY, D.P.M., Ph.D.

Past President, American Society of Podiatric Dermatology
Chief, Podiatric Section, Surgical Service
Veterans Administration Medical Center
Baltimore, Maryland

ASSOCIATE EDITOR

ROYAL MONTGOMERY, M.D.

Fellow, American Board of Dermatology
Emeritus Staff, Hospital for Special Surgery
New York, New York

WILLIAMS & WILKINS
Baltimore • London • Los Angeles • Sydney

Editor: Jonathan W. Pine, Jr.
Copy Editor: Stephen Siegforth
Design: JoAnne Janowiak
Illustration Planning: Wayne Hubbel
Production: Anne G. Seitz

Accurate indications, adverse reactions, and dosage schedules for drugs are provided in this book, but it is possible that they may change. The reader is urged to review the package information data of the manufacturers of the medications mentioned.

Made in the United States of America

Library of Congress Cataloging in Publication Data

Main entry under title:

Podiatric dermatology.

Includes index.
1. Skin—Diseases. 2. Foot—Diseases. I. McCarthy, Daniel J. (Daniel Joseph), 1929- II. Montgomery, Royal. [DNLM: 1. Foot Dermatoses. 2. Foot Diseases. WE 880 P742]
RL72.P63 1985 616.5 84-21014
ISBN 0-683-05750-2

Composed and printed at the
Waverly Press, Inc.

86 87 88 89 90 10 9 8 7 6 5 4 3 2 1

Preface

Podiatric dermatology, like all other podiatric subspecialties, is characterized by a diversity of emphasis and interests amongst students as well as seasoned practitioners. Consequently, this text represents a variety of subject material and demonstrates a wide range of different emphasis. In some instances, a simplified treatment plan or diagnostic method might be entirely appropriate in dealing with the presenting skin lesion. However, there are other instances in which high technology such as transmission electron microscopy might better be employed to satisfy the need for precise diagnosis.

Dermatology, like all other medical specialties, has experienced significant technological advancement over the past several decades. It is absolutely necessary that podiatric medicine keep abreast of these changes and make contributions to the expanding body of knowledge.

Medicine has long made use of high magnification of tissues made possible by transmission electron microscopy in university as well as hospital settings. However, podiatry has not placed sufficient emphasis upon this critical aspect of study at the collegiate level. For this reason, an introductory emphasis on the nomenclature and diagnostic application of high technology has been included in this text. This material has been organized so as to provide the student with a fundamental understanding of the material in order that he or she be comfortable with ultrastructure as it applies to the skin. It is hoped that this manner of presentation will dispel some of the mystique surrounding the subject.

Podiatry has undergone a startling metamorphosis during the post-World War II era. The profession has emerged as an essentially surgical specialty from its antecedent palliative form. However, this modern emphasis is not to deny the importance of conservative medical care to conditions of the foot and leg. Such care remains an integral part of most podiatric practitioners' technique. Podiatric medicine necessarily interdigitates with other medical specialties, including anesthesiology, internal medicine, pediatrics, pathology, and radiology in its attempts to provide optimal care for podiatric patients. This text is an extension of this eclectic view as it emphasizes podiatric dermatological considerations.

Dermatology and podiatric medicine and surgery are fields of specialization which share much in common since attention to the skin is often a first consideration. In another sense, most of the bone and joint surgery performed by podiatrists is done in order to relieve morbid conditions of the foot such as helomata and intractable plantar keratosis. Therefore, some essential differences exist between the two disciplines.

The pedal extremities are prone to a variety of unique skin conditions by virtue of environmental factors since the foot is most often encased within hostile surroundings. Moisture, darkness, and heat, as well as a variety of man-made materials which clothe the feet, combine to exaccerbate irritating factors. Hygiene, aging and circulatory factors further target the pedal extremities for skin diseases. Therefore, podiatry has a special need for competence and understanding in the diagnosis and treatment of dermatological conditions of the lower extremities.

The field of general dermatology is not wanting for textbooks. Some are encyclopedic while others attempt to briefly distill information. Several such works even deal exclusively with the lower extremities. However, there has not been a dermatological textbook written by and for podiatrists to date. This volume has been prepared in order to address this deficiency.

In preparing this volume, the expertise of faculty members of colleges of podiatric medicine has been enlisted. Indeed, two college Deans have supplied chapters. All contributors are highly qualified to effectively deal with that specialized area of podiatric dermatology to which they have elected to speak. In addition, dermatologists representing such prestigious institutions as the University of Southern Florida and Columbia Presbyterian Hospital of New York City have made significant contributions to this book. The contributions of Royal Montgomery, M.D., as Associate Editor cannot be overstated. It was not possible to extend invitations to contribute to this text to all of the podiatric physicians qualified to do so. Space limitations prevented such comprehensive inclusion, and both the editor and publisher regret this fact.

The senior editor wishes to express his profound thanks to the publisher, Williams & Wilkins, Baltimore, Maryland, for their patient help and assistance during the preparation of this book. Their liberal use of color plates is especially appreciated since this type of illustration is so useful in dermatological presentations.

It is said that physicians never cease to be students. This volume is dedicated to all students of podiatric medicine concerned with the diagnosis and treatment of dermatological conditions of the lower extremities. This appreciation extends to those pursuing their first professional degree as well as to those who have been in practice for many years. Moreover, it is my sincere hope that health care providers representing other disciplines of medicine and surgery and the ancillary sciences will benefit from this textbook.

Daniel J. McCarthy, D.P.M., Ph.D.
Past President and Trustee,
American Society of Podiatric Dermatology
Chief,
Podiatric Section, Surgical Service,
VA Medical Center,
Baltimore, Maryland

Contributors

Carl Abramson, Ph.D.
Professor of Microbiology, Department of Microbiology, Pennsylvania College of Podiatric Medicine, Philadelphia, Pennsylvania

Frederick J. Bartolomei, D.P.M.
Assistant Professor in Podiatric Medicine, Ohio College of Podiatric Medicine, Cleveland, Ohio

Steven J. Berlin, D.P.M.
President, Podiatry Pathology Laboratories, Bel Air, Maryland

James R. Black, D.P.M.
Chief, Podiatric Section, VA Medical Center, Tampa, Florida

Marc A. Brenner, D.P.M.
President, American Society of Podiatric Dermatology, Glendale, New York

Thomas DeLauro, D.P.M.
Academic Dean of the College, New York College of Podiatric Medicine, New York, New York

Gary L. Dockery, D.P.M.
Director, Northwest Podiatric Foundation for Education and Research, Waldo General Hospital, Seattle, Washington; Board of Trustees, American Society of Podiatric Dermatology

Michael Feinstein, D.P.M.
Affiliate Status, Department of Orthopaedic Surgery, Johns Hopkins University Hospital, Baltimore, Maryland

Neil A. Fenske, M.D.
Chairman, Department of Dermatology, University of South Florida, College of Medicine, Tampa, Florida

Arlene F. Hoffman, D.P.M., Ph.D.
Professor, Department of Basic Sciences, Associate Professor of Podiatric Medicine, Chief, General Podiatry Clinic, and Chief, Vascular Clinic, California College of Podiatric Medicine, San Francisco, California

Charles Krausz, D.P.M.
Emeritus Professor of Podiatric Medicine, Pennsylvania College of Podiatric Medicine, Formerly Dean of Temple University School of Chiropody, Philadelphia, Pennsylvania

Wilfred Laine, D.P.M.
Chief, Podiatric Section, VA Medical Center, Clinical Associate Professor, Department of Dermatology, Stanford University School of Medicine, Palo Alto, California

Leonard A. Levy, D.P.M., M.P.H.
Dean, College of Podiatric Medicine and Surgery, University of Osteopathic Medicine and Health Sciences, Des Moines, Iowa

Daniel J. McCarthy, D.P.M., Ph.D.
Past President, American Society of Podiatric Dermatology, Chief, Podiatric Section, Surgical Service, Veterans Administration Medical Center, Baltimore, Maryland

Royal Montgomery, M.D.
Fellow, American Board of Dermatology, Emeritus Staff, Hospital for Special Surgery, New York, New York

Robert G. O'Keefe, D.P.M.
Associate Professor, Department of Surgery, William Scholl College of Podiatric Medicine, Chicago, Illinois

Mary L. Ottinger, D.P.M.
Podiatric Resident, VA Medical Center, Tampa, Florida

Irving Pikscher, D.P.M.
Associate Professor, Department of Podiatric Medicine, Chicago, Illinois

Martin Port, D.P.M.
Trustee, American Society of Podiatric Dermatology, Tampa, Florida

Asher Don Rabinowitz, M.D.
Department of Dermatopathology, Columbia-Presbyterian Hospital, New York, New York

Lee J. Sanders, D.P.M.
Chief, Podiatric Section, VA Medical Center, Lebanon, Pennsylvania

Arthur Steinhart, D.P.M.
Chairman and Associate Professor, Division of Medical Sciences, New York College of Podiatric Medicine, New York, New York

Douglas Taylor, D.P.M.
Resident in Podiatry, VA Medical Center, Battle Creek, Michigan

Damian Turski, D.P.M.
Resident in Podiatry, VA Medical Center, Battle Creek, Michigan

Derrick Whittaker, D.P.M.
Formerly Chief, Podiatric Section, Director of Podiatric Residency Program, VA Medical Center, Battle Creek, Michigan

Contents

COLOR PLATES

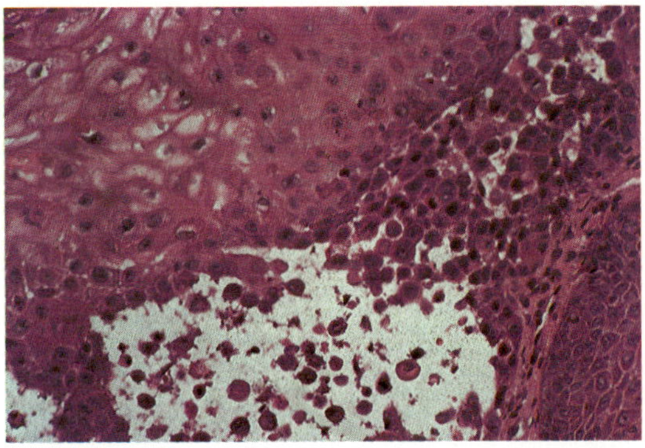

Figure 3.4.

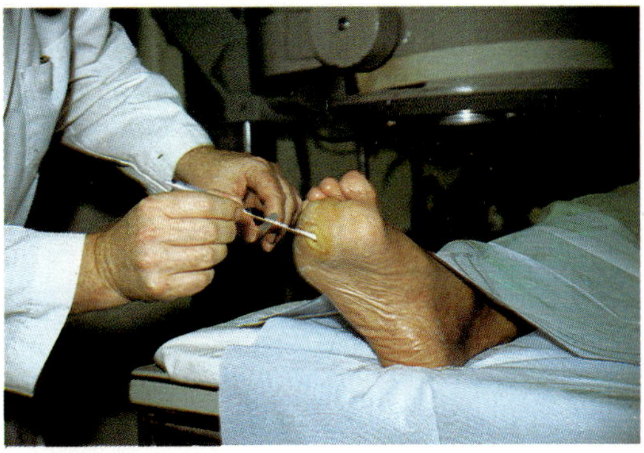

Figure 4.8.

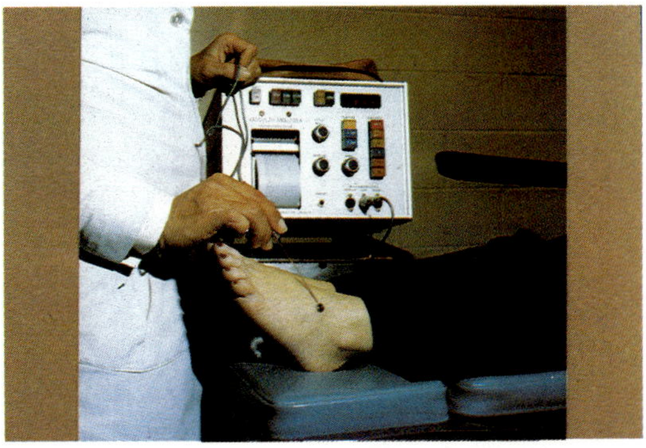

Figure 4.10.

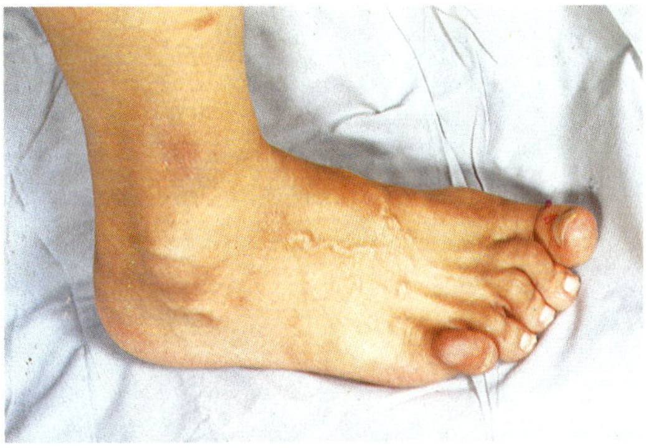

Figure 5.1.

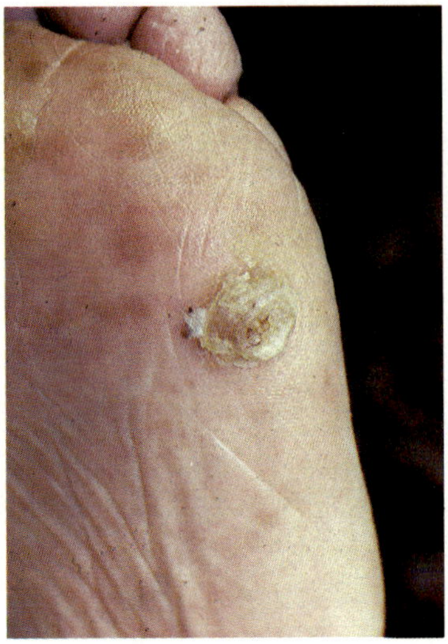

Figure 5.18.

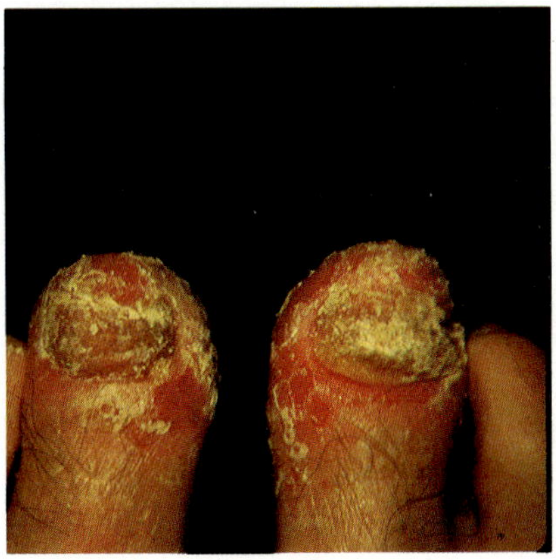

Figure 8.3.

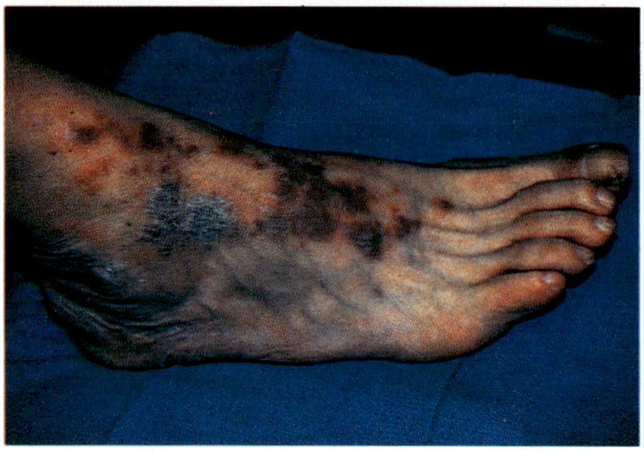

Figure 8.8.

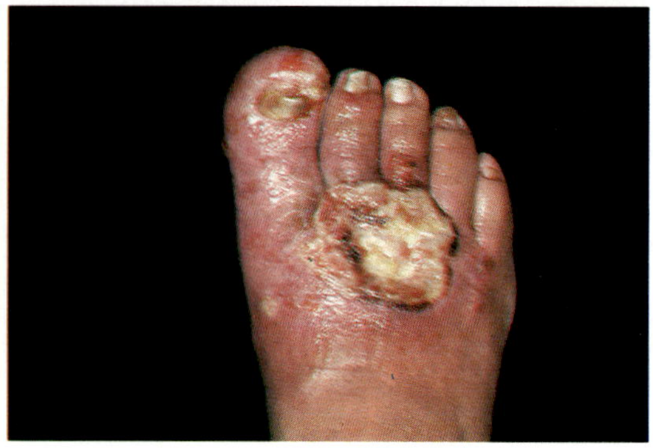

Figure 9.1.

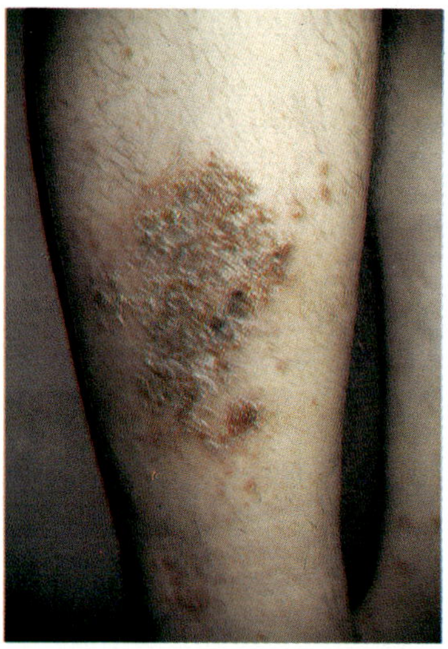

Figure 9.3.

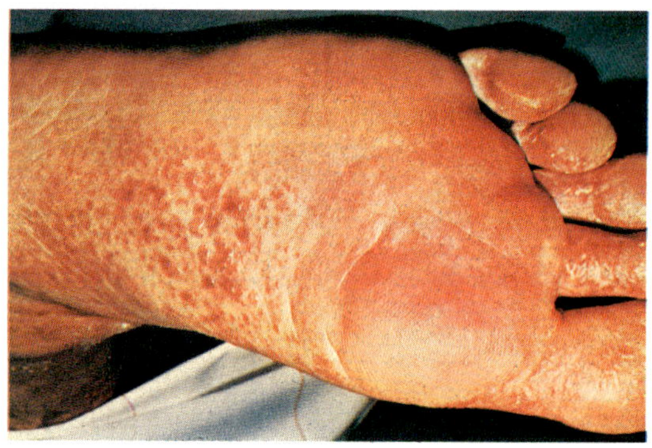

Figure 10.4.

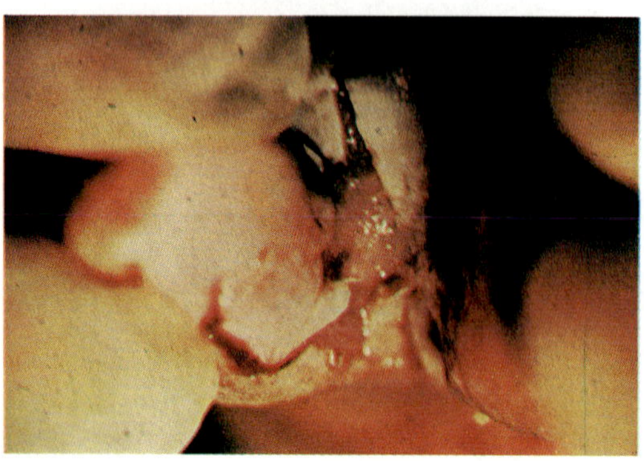

Figure 10.5.

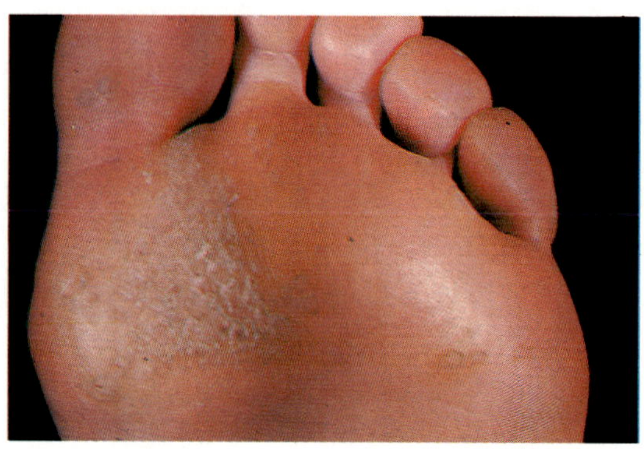

Figure 11.2.

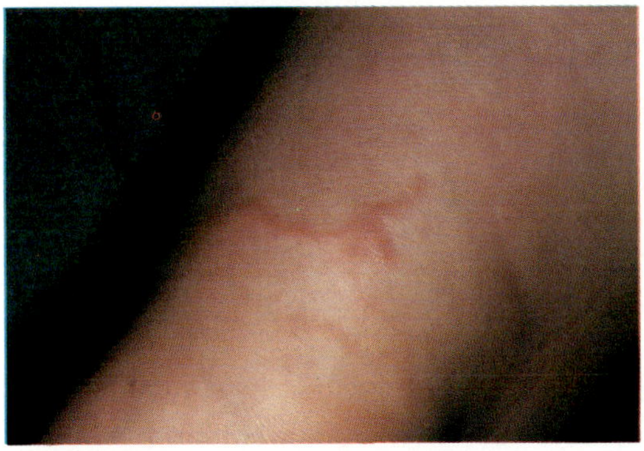

Figure 12.3.

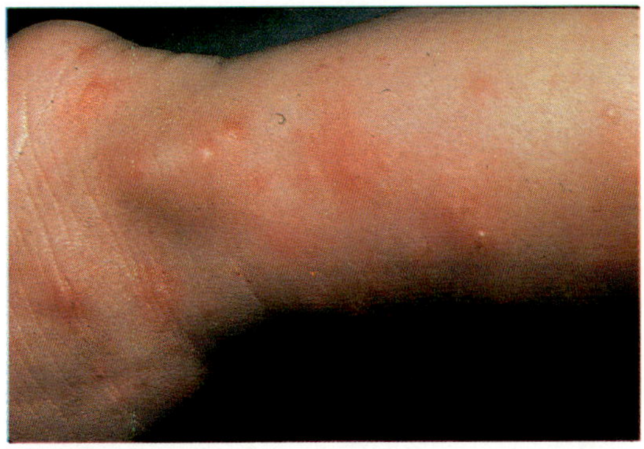

Figure 12.13.

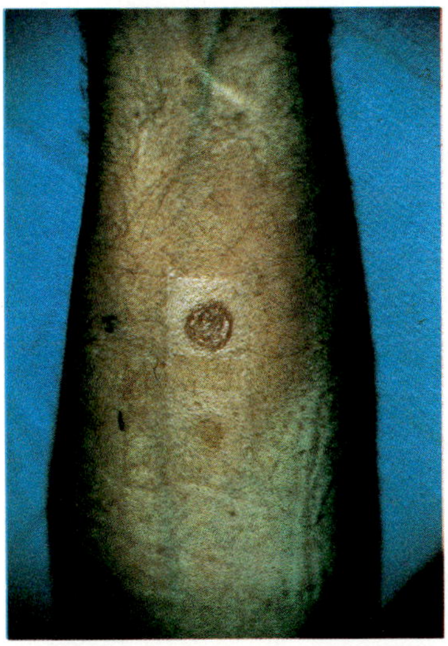

Figure 13.3.

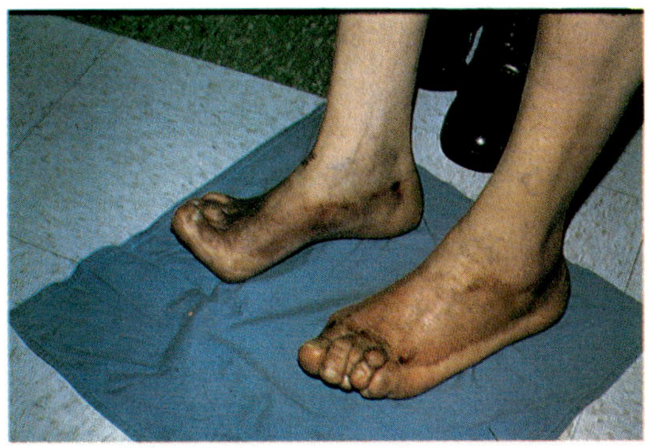

Figure 13.5.

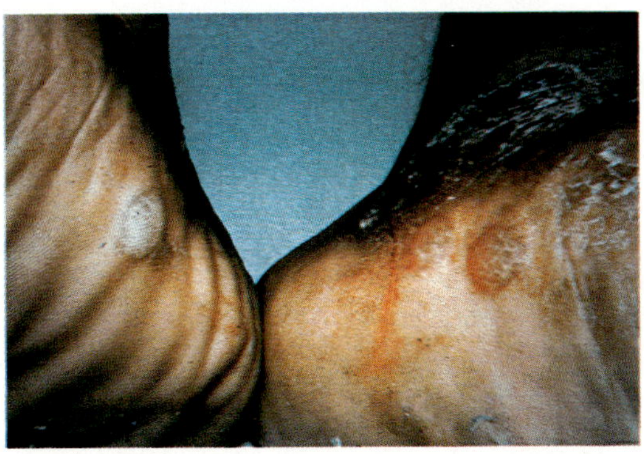

Figure 14.4.

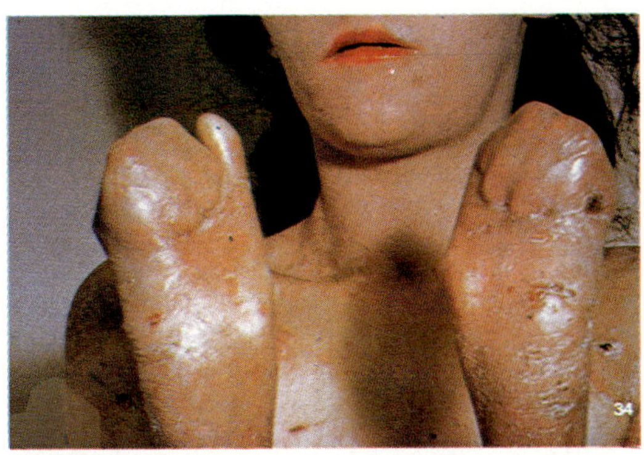

Figure 14.9.

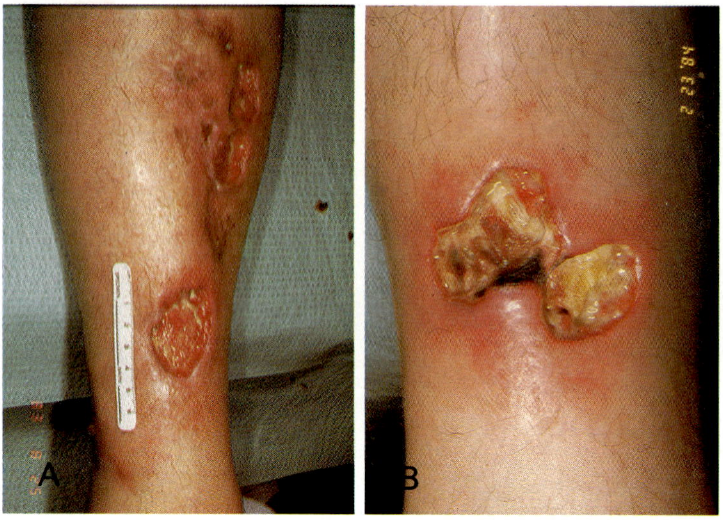

Figure 15.8AB.

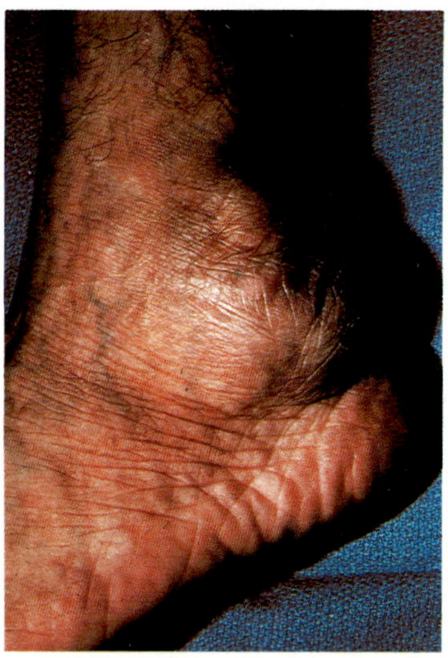

Figure 17.13.

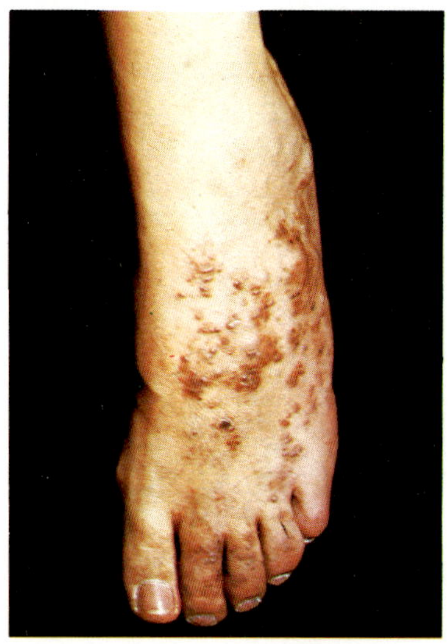

Figure 17.23.

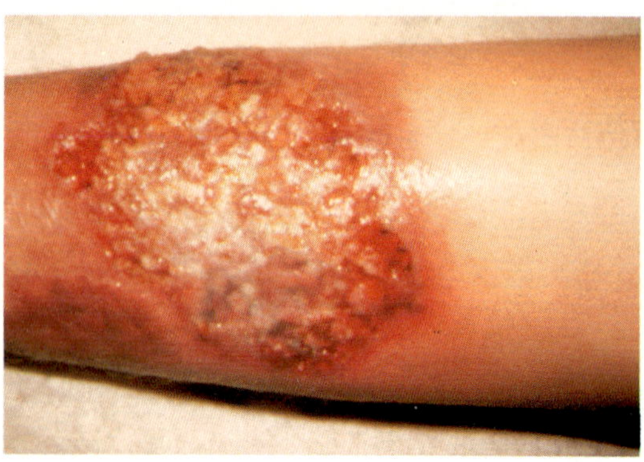

Figure 19.4.

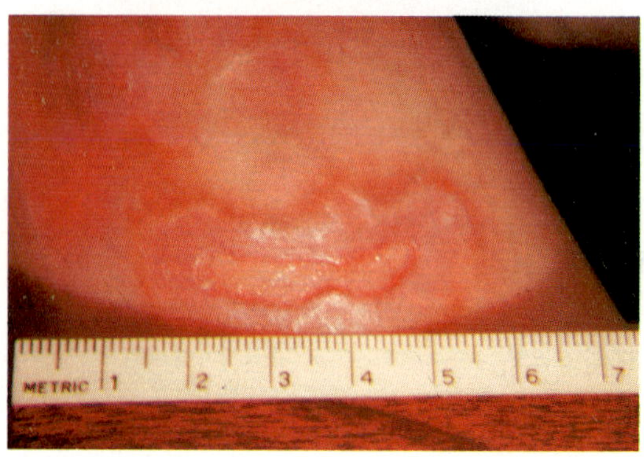

Figure 19.7.

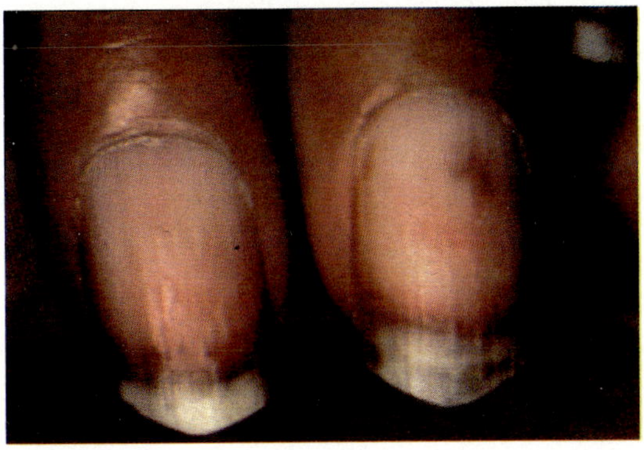

Figure 20.11.

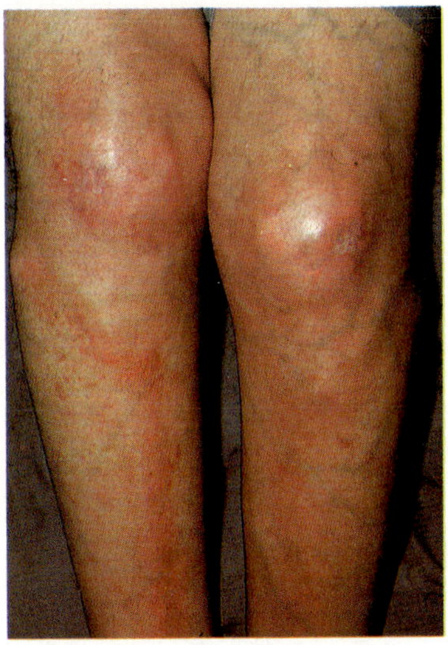

Figure 20.13.

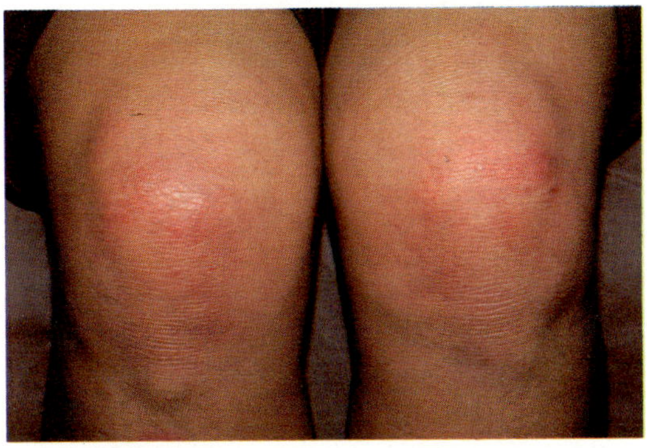

Figure 20.18.

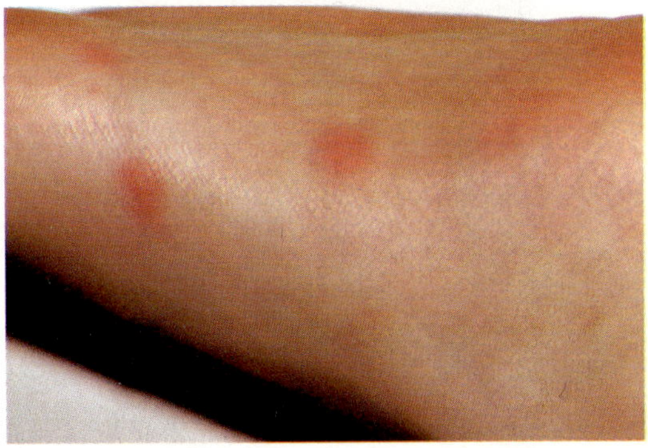

Figure 20.20.

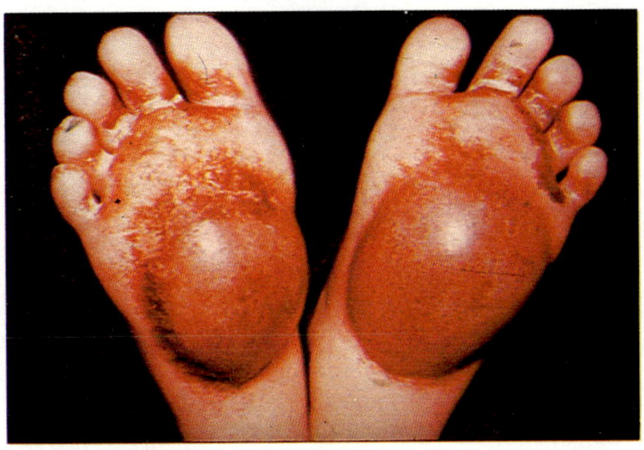

Figure 21.2.

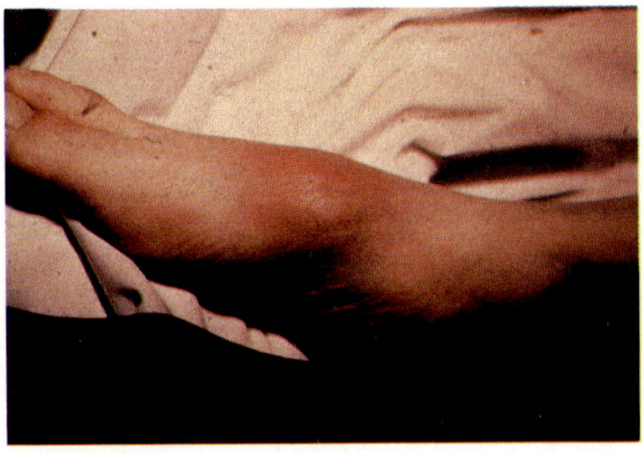

Figure 21.6.

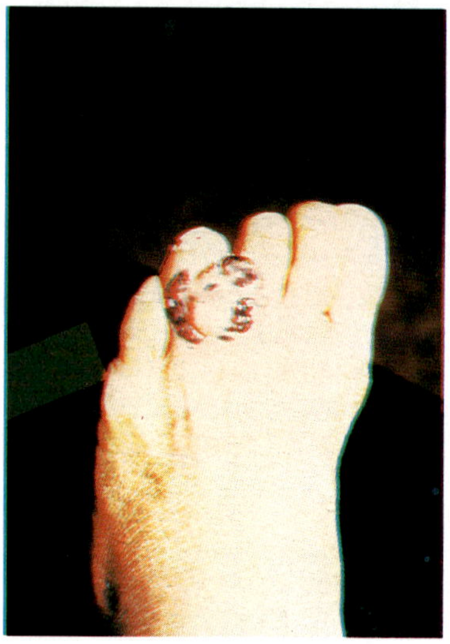

Figure 23.4.

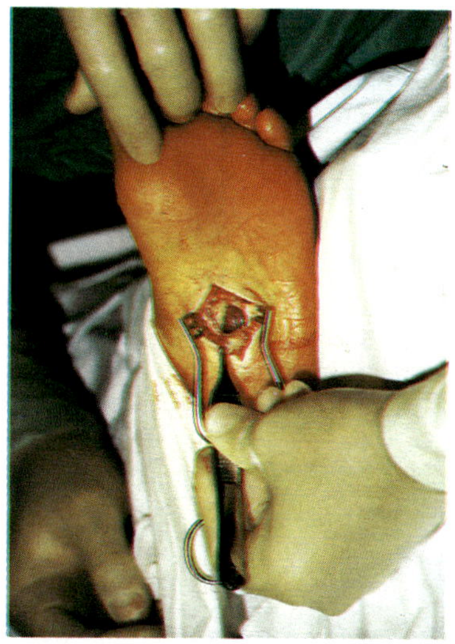

Figure 23.9.

CHAPTER 1

Cutaneous Anatomy

DANIEL J. McCARTHY

The human skin is the largest organ of the body. Its structure varies greatly between different locations and is particularly pleomorphic within the human foot. Consider, for example, the thin skin of the dorsum of the foot with its occasional hairs, as compared with the thick, horny, and hairless skin of the plantar aspect. The skin's structure is further complicated by the presence of adnexa or developmental specializations such as nails and sebaceous and sudoriferous glands, as well as the pilary complexes.

Moreover, the skin is physiologically and biochemically complicated since it is required to serve so many functions. Changes attendant with age, race, and sex further add to the complexities. Consequently, there can be no precise definition of what the skin looks like, except in an abstract sense.

Developmentally, the skin arises from three embryonic sources. The ectoderm provides cells of the epidermis or outer covering. Mesoderm forms the dermis, as well as vascular elements, connective tissue stroma, and the subcutis. Neural ectoderm supplies specialized migratory cells, such as the Langerhans cells and the pigment producing melanocyte (1).

Periderm (epitrichium) is an embryonic specialization of the outer skin of the fetus. This fuzzy layer contains cells with many microvilli which apparently equilibrate with the amnionic fluid. The characteristics of true keratinizing epidermis are assumed early in the secondary trimester, at which time mitosis is generally restricted to the basal cell layer of the epidermis (stratum germinativum or basale).

The dermis has a somewhat metameric organization and develops under the influence of mesenchymal cells, differentiating along the lines of the fibroblast. Elastic, reticular, and collagenic fibers are laid down in a mucopolysaccharide-ground-substance matrix. Blood vessels in distal parts such as the foot may form within mesenchyme as a plexus. Additionally, segmental arteries progressively lay down channels which extend into the extremities (1).

It is an interesting phenomenon that many blood vessels which are important in embryogeny are entirely supplanted by different main stem vessels in the adult. Blood vessel plexuses usually undergo a selective atrophy so that only those vessels most suited for nourishing any given part persist. This type of morphogenesis is usually in response to oxygen gradient responses (2). Such angiogenetic activities are recapitulated during wound healing (Fig. 1.1).

Langer's lines of cleavage, which are characteristic of adult skin, are determined during the fetal period as connective tissue fibers are laid down in response to the prevalent direction of growth of the part.

Adnexa of the skin are derived from the germinativum in response to specific changes of differentiation. The basal cells are modulated along different lines of determination in response to interactions between ectoderm and mesoderm. New and unique biological units are formed as the adnexa develops, and such structures do not arise from "determined" keratinizing epidermis. This distinction is important in considering basal cell carcinoma. Basaliomas do not, in fact, arise from basal cells committed to keratinization but from less determined germinal cells of the integument. Adnexa also maintain less determined reserve cells among the glandular elements. These become important in reconstituting skin defects, in addition to their function of supporting all replacement

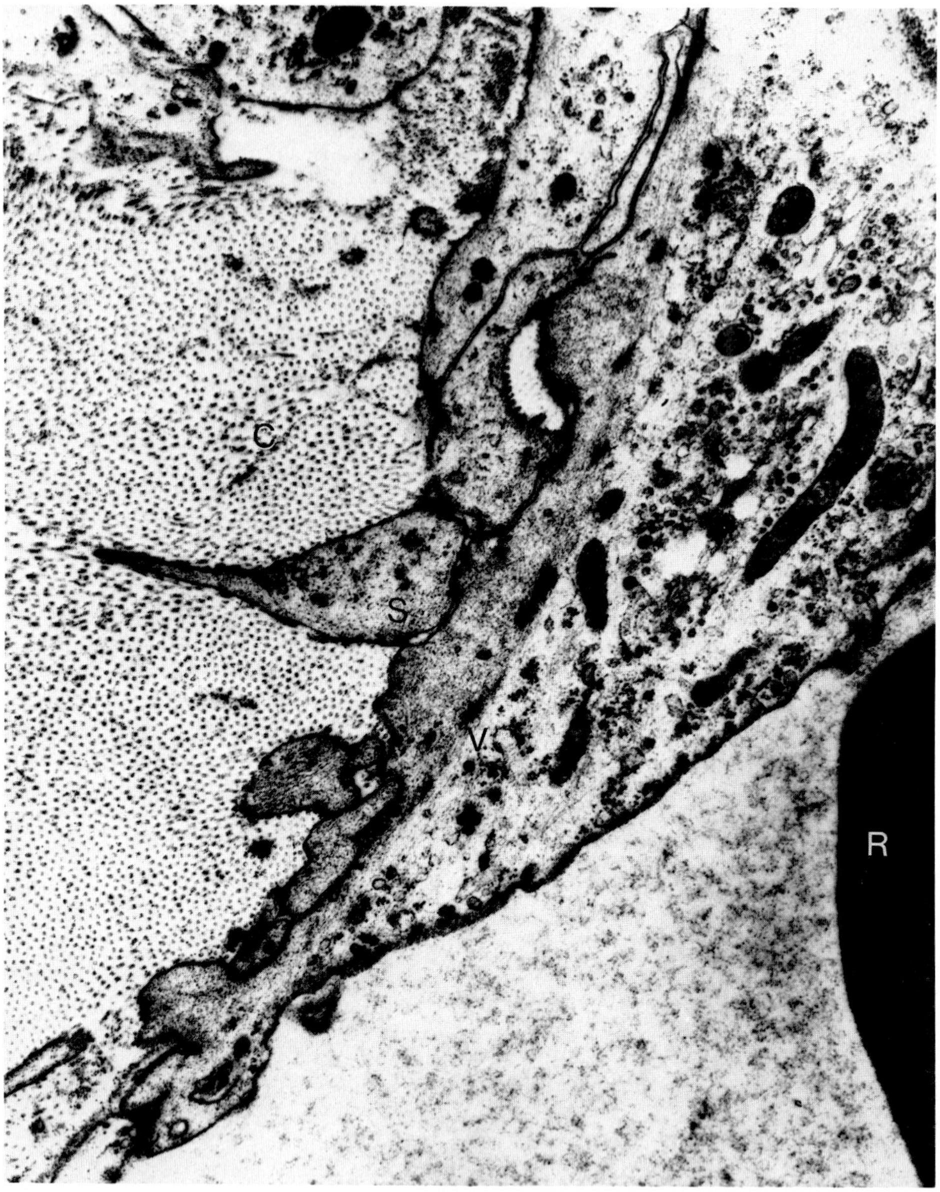

Figure 1.1. Blood vessel sprouting into a dermal collagenic field having low oxygen tension. Transmission electron microscopy. *C,* collagen field; *S*, blood vessel sprout; *V*, blood vessel wall of parent blood vessel; *R*, red blood cell. *Sci Am* 222:40, 1969.

in glands. Such cells retain certain mesenchymal characteristics and may be induced to differentiate and replicate as more determined keratinocytes.

Adult skin has an epidermis composed of four layers or strata (Fig. 1.2). These are the stratum germinativum (basale), stratum spinosum (prickle cell layer), stratum granulosum, and stratum corneum. The stratum lucidum identified by early light microscopists is an artifact of fixation. Before considering the dermis and basement membrane upon which the epidermis is situated, consideration will be given to the characteristics of the cells of the four strata just mentioned.

STRATUM BASALE OR GERMINATIVUM

These cells which rest upon the basement membrane and the dermis are best described as being high cuboidal or low co-

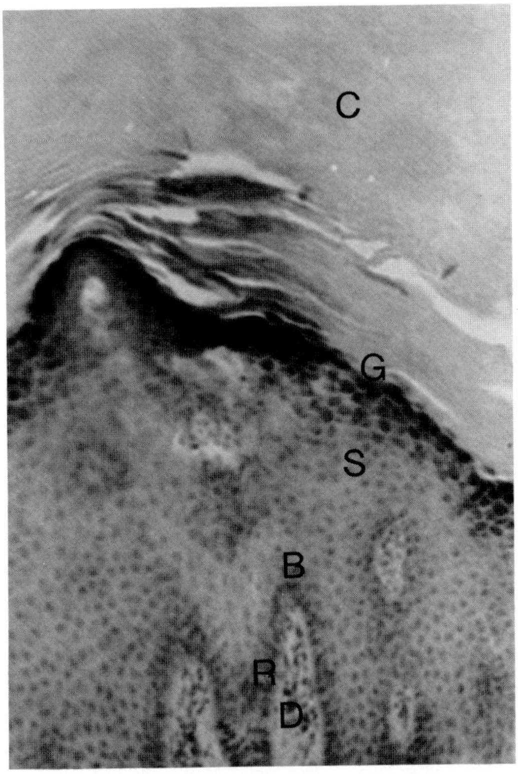

Figure 1.2. Four layers or strata of the human epidermis. Light microscopy. *C,* stratum corneum; *G,* stratum granulosum; *S,* stratum spinosum; *B,* stratum basale; *R,* rete peg of epidermis; *D,* dermis.

lumnar in shape (Fig. 1.3). The cell is dominated by an ovoid, deeply basophilic nucleus, usually without a well-defined nucleolus. Basal cells equilibrate with the dermis beneath, and that surface in contact with the dermis is increased by numerous pedicles which interdigitate with fibrillar and matrix elements of the dermis. In general, cells of the stratum basale are committed toward replication or keratinization. However, under certain inductive influences, they may enter into other pathways of integumentary differentiation (3).

The cytoplasm of basal cells is relatively sparse but dense. Free ribosomes are numerous, as are filaments.

The elements of protein synthesis, rough endoplasmic reticulum, and Golgi apparatus are sparse. The intercellular spaces are normally narrow, and wherever widened, they demonstrate a ribosome-like granular material. Mitochondria are present to a degree.

Hemidesmosomes occur facing upon the basement membrane, and the full desmosome complex can be seen wherever the basal cell abuts upon another or upon a spinosal cell above.

Inclusions such as lipid and glycogen can be identified in some cells of the stratum basale. Vesicles, some of which appear to be pinocytotic, can be seen occasionally, sometimes in association with the much convoluted plasma membrane, which is about 70 Å thick.

Immediately above the basal cell layer is the stratum spinosum. Here, the cells begin to show signs of the specialization called keratinization. This is a commitment toward protein synthesis, which forms keratin.

STRATUM SPINOSUM

Early microscopists incorrectly inferred that cells of the stratum spinosum had intercellular bridges. This phenomenon gave the layer a prickled appearance, hence, the term "prickle cell" (Fig. 1.4). Intercellular spaces among cells of the spinosum are normally narrow and come together as "tight junctions." Here hemi (half) desmosomes come together from each of two contiguous cells to form a full desmosome. No true bridging occurs, however, although this is the impression perceived at the light microscopic level. The filamentous component of cells of the stratum spinosum are significant with respect to the keratinizing process. Tonofilaments pass circumferentially about the nucleus, and some occur as bundles which converge upon the desmosomes. This arrangement constitutes the tonofilament-desmosome complex (TDC). Its appearance is distinctive in healthy cells, but it is frequently severely disrupted in pathologic skin changes.

Cells of the stratum spinosum become progressively flattened and orient parallel to the free surface of the skin as they proceed outward (Fig. 1.2). The cytoplasmic volume increases and is less dense than was the case in the stratum basale. The nucleus becomes more attenuated and flattened as well. Rough endoplasmic reticulum becomes more evident in the spinosum. This subcellular organelle is a tortuous coiled series of tubules lined with ribosomes which provide for the so-called "rough" designation. The structure terminates with bulb-like endings called cisternae. The presence of rough endoplasmic reticulum (RER) is

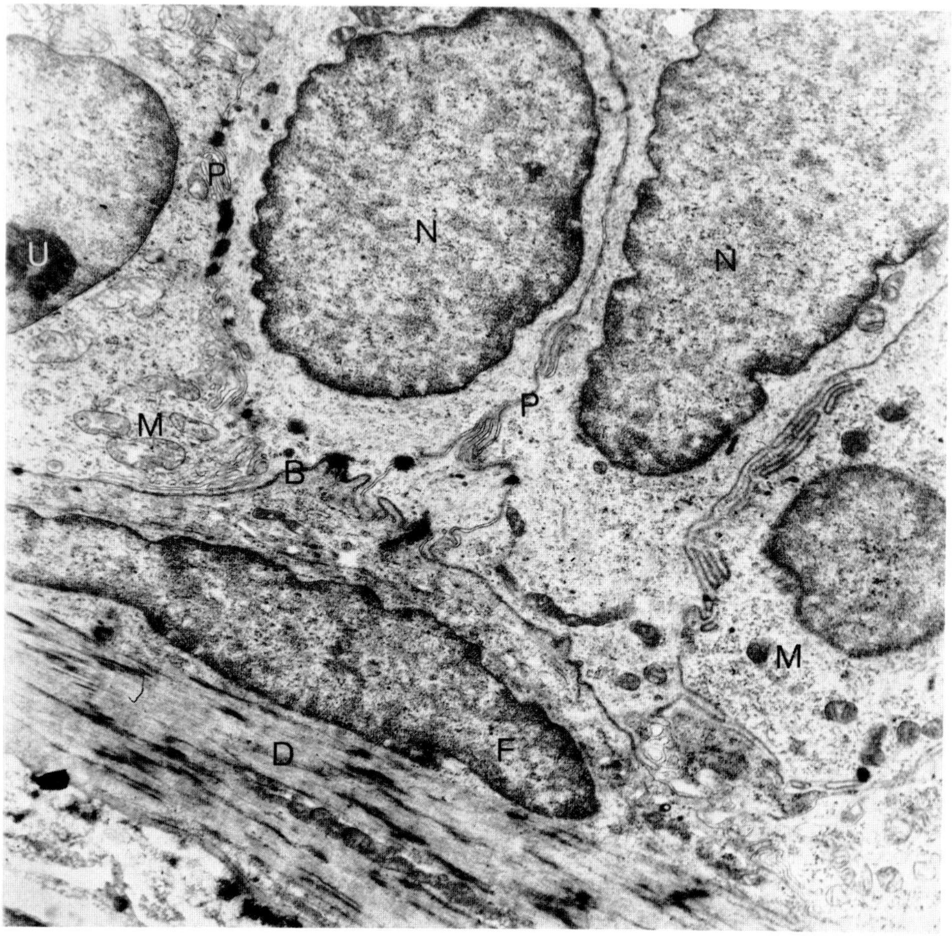

Figure 1.3. Stratum basale of the human skin. Transmission electron microscopy. *D*, dermis; *B*, basement membrane; *P*, plasma membrane; *N*, nucleus of basal cell; *F*, fibroblast; *M*, mitochondria.

indicative of protein synthesis in general and with respect to keratin synthesis in particular in prickle cells.

Golgi vesicles or apparatus give the appearance of stacked tubules which are smooth internally. They are thought to prepare or package or further refine proteinaceous substances. These, too, are more obvious in the stratum spinosum.

Mitochondria are characterized as being the powerhouse of the cell. They are numerous and well formed in the stratum spinosum. These ovoid trilamellar structures have a ladder-like structure centrally. The rungs are the locations of oxidative processes necessary to energize protein synthesis.

A recently identified subcellular organelle important to the function of spinosal cells is the membrane-coating granule (MCG). It is also known as the Odland body or lamellar granule (4). Its general appearance is that of a tiny mitochondria since it, too, has a ladder-like appearance (Fig. 1.5). These organelles originally appear in close proximity to the Golgi apparatus in the lower spinosum, but they move peripherally at higher levels. They appear to ultimately attach to the plasma membrane, as pinocytotic vesicles would, to dump its contents into the intercellular space. It is thought that these lamellar granules contribute a cementing substance which adheres the cells of the upper spinosum and beyond. At these points, the intercellular spaces are widening, and the plasma membranes are far less convoluted and are about 150 Å in thickness.

Prickle cells make their outward passage in about 2 weeks. At the light microscopic

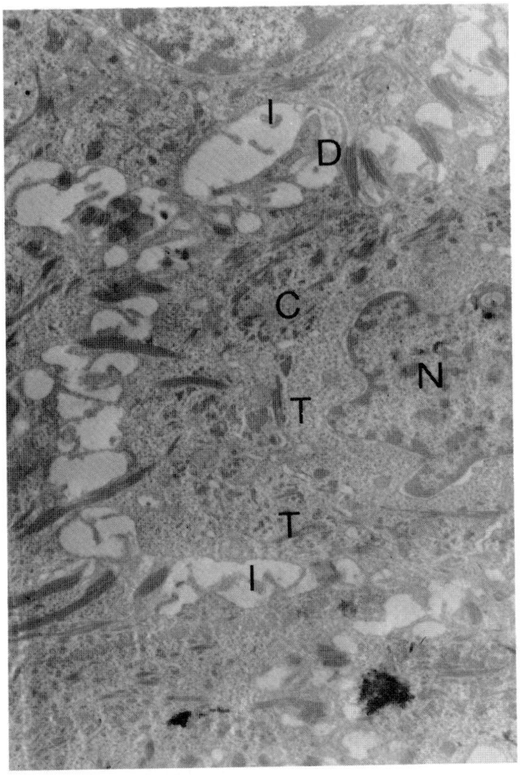

Figure 1.4. Cell of the stratum spinosum. Transmission electron microscopy. *I*, widened intercellular space; *D*, desmosome, *C*, cell cytoplasm; *N*, nucleus; *T*, tonofibril.

level, they demonstrate a vesicular or pyknotic nucleus which may be totally lacking in the upper spinosum. Unlike basal cells, spinosal cells often demonstrate one or more nucleoli. Keratohyaline granules, which are a feature of the stratum granulosum beyond, begin to make their appearance in the outer stratum spinosum.

THE STRATUM GRANULOSUM

The granular layer or stratum granulosum is conspicuous by virtue of its deep and dense basophilic characteristic. Actually, keratohyaline granules have no color in normal living skin. Their refractivity is responsible for the diffusion of colors so that brown or blackish pigments appear blue, as does red blood (1). Cells of the granulosum are quite flat, and the nucleus bulges (Fig. 1.6).

Keratohyaline granules appear to grow or coalesce as an amorphous substance in the granulosum. Tonofilaments are arranged in many directions but remain es-

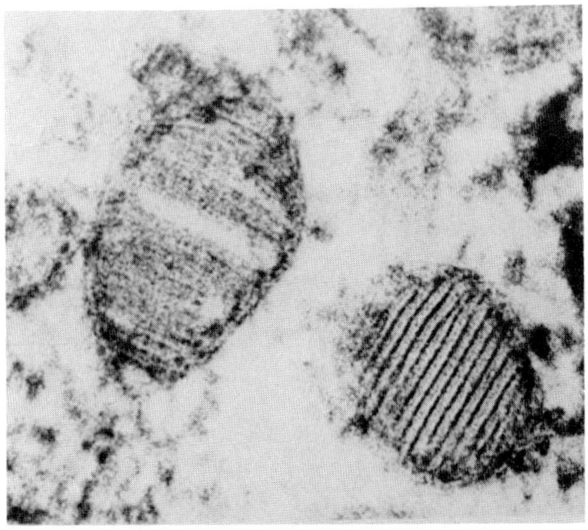

Figure 1.5. Membrane-coating granule (Odland body, lamellar granule). From Zelickson AS: *Ultrastructure of Normal and Abnormal Skin.* Philadelphia, Lea & Febiger, 1969.

sentially parallel to the free surface of the skin. They seem to mesh within the keratohyaline granules. At this time the nucleus, mitochondria, rough endoplasmic reticulum, Golgi apparatus, ribosomes, and keratohyaline granules undergo dissociation, forming a homogeneous or amorphous substance (3). Dehydration occurs, and cells of the granular layer pass outward as stratum corneum.

The processes just described affirm that the stratum Malpighii (strata basale, spinosum, and granulosum collectively) is a living dynamic entity. Each layer is engaged in morphologically identifiable biochemical events. It is, then, totally incorrect to say that cells above the germinativum are in a process of progressive necrosis. The outermost layer, the stratum corneum, is nonliving, however. It represents the culmination of the cellular processes below which lead to the tough, yet resilient and pliable, cornified layer.

THE STRATUM CORNEUM

The stratum corneum is protective against injury and hinders the penetration of microorganisms and harmful solvents into deeper body tissues. The skin provides a barrier between an often hostile external environment to a delicate internal body environment.

Cells of the stratum corneum interdigitate in basket weave-like fashion. Intercellular spaces are relatively wide with an

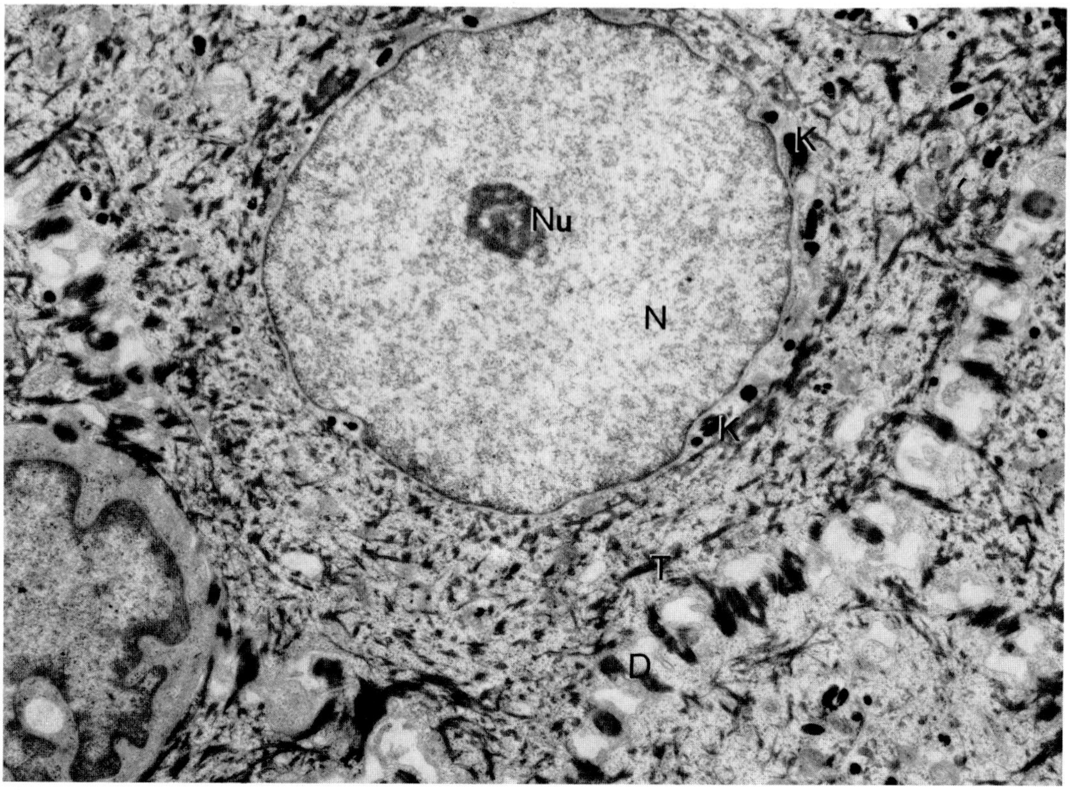

Figure 1.6. Cell of the lower stratum granulosum. Transmission electron microscopy. *K*, keratohyaline granule; *N*, nucleus; *Nu*, nucleolus; *D*, desmosome, *T*, tonofibrils.

amorphous PAS-positive substance intervening. While it is occasionally possible to identify remnants of subcellular organelles in the corneum, it is more often correct to characterize the cell's contents as amorphous (Fig. 1.7). Fibrous elements known to be sulfur-poor traverse the matrix, which is a sulfur-rich protein, along with a lipid moiety. The filamentous fibrous network ensures cohesiveness, flexibility, and elasticity. The cells' proteinaceous contents are biochemically stabilized by sulfur to sulfur bonding.

Mitotic figures are not commonly seen in routine sections of human skin. This is partly due to the fact that the event occurs with relative rapidity. The total life span for keratinocytes is about 4 weeks (1). Mitotic indices ranging from 0.1 to 1 per 1000 epidermal cells are adequate to replace desquamating cells. Moreover, in the economy of nature, four expanded, flattened keratinized corneum cells cover the same area as 100 basal cells. One diminutive basal cell ultimately covers a surface area 25 times its original size by the time it moves up to the free surface of skin. Such cells have a distinctive closely knit polygonal appearance (Fig. 1.8).

Basement Membrane

The dermis and epidermis are separated by a basal lamina or basement membrane which is derived from substances contributed by both sections of the skin. The dermoepidermal junction demonstrates a PAS-positive thin zone of mucopolysaccharide with no evidence of hyaline membrane. The basal cell membrane is paralleled in all its convolutions by a thin adepidermal or dermal membrane. The two lamina are separated by an electron-translucent gap (1).

THE DERMIS

The discussion of the dermis as it underlies the epidermis can be subdivided into papillary (pars papillaris) and reticular (pars reticularis) portions. The hypoderm or subcutaneous fat tissue is sometimes considered part of the dermis.

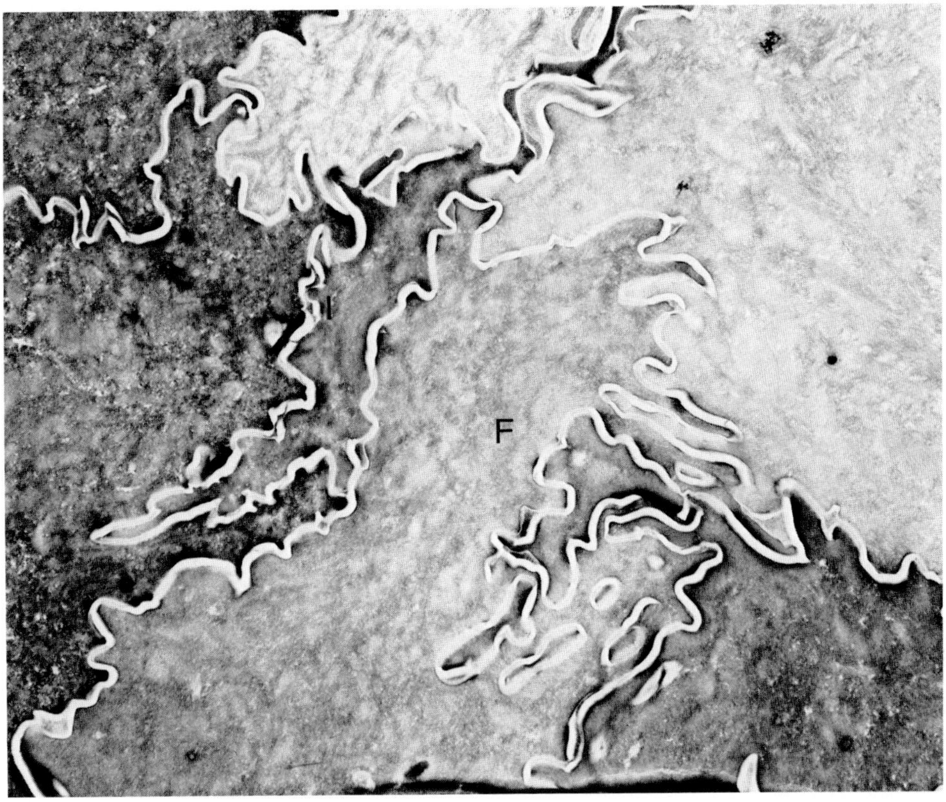

Figure 1.7. Cells of the stratum corneum. Structure of stratum corneum cell. *I*, intercellular space; *F*, fibrillae.

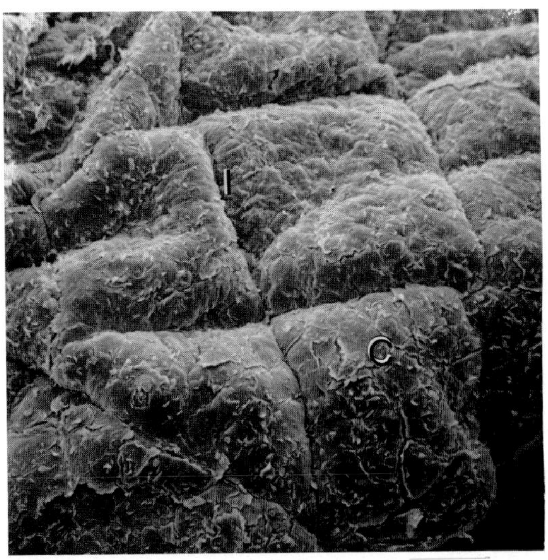

Figure 1.8. Surface appearance of the stratum corneum. Scanning electron microscopy. *I*, intercellular junction; *C*, surface of stratum corneum cell.

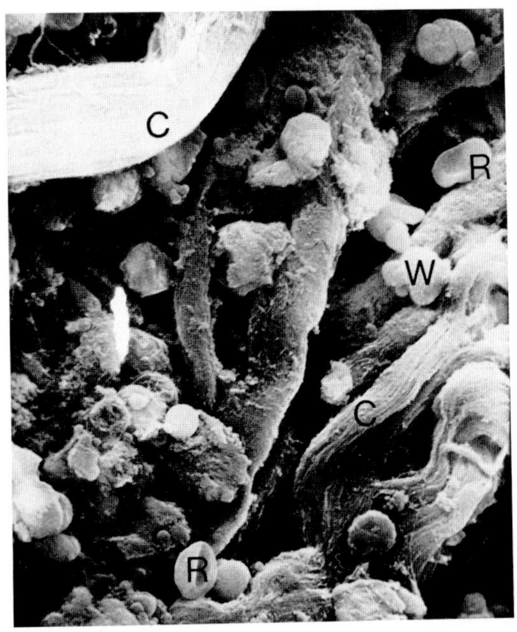

Figure 1.9. Dermis of the skin demonstrating collagenic fibers of various thickness and cellular elements. Scanning electron microscopy. *C*, collagen fiber; *R*, red blood cell; *W*, white blood cell.

The pars papillaris is so named because it is that portion of the dermis which directly interdigitates with the epidermis. This is accomplished by finger-like projec-

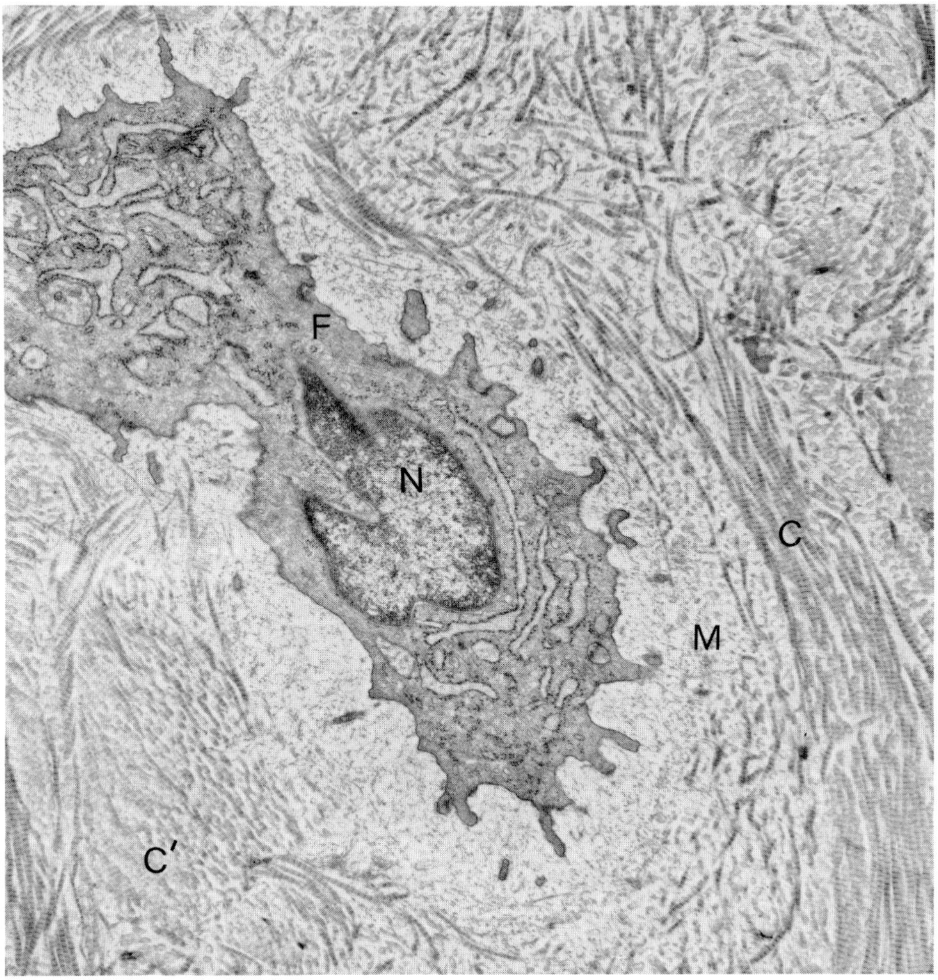

Figure 1.10. Fibroblast surrounded by collagen as viewed by transmission electron microscopy demonstrating its peculiar periodic banding at 2800 Å intervals. *C*, collagen in longitudinal section; *C′*, collagen in cross section; *F*, fibroblast; *N*, nucleus; *M*, ground-substance matrix field. Transmission electron microscopy.

tions or papillae which engage the rete pegs of the epidermis. The papillae and associated superficial dermis immediately contiguous to the epidermis, which forms the pars papillaris, are functionally related to the epidermis (5). It is significant as the site of the inflammatory dermatosis, which is so clinically important. This region is more vascular than the reticularis by virtue of subpapillary plexuses which extend capillary loops into individual papillae.

The papillary dermis contains nerve fibers and lymphatics which may be encased within an elastic fiber stroma. It is more cellular than the reticular portion by virtue of the presence of fibrocytes, histiocytes, and lymphocytes. A "felt" brushwork is formed by elastic fibers which marginates the two dermal regions. Reticular fibers are peculiarly oriented at right angles to the free surface of the skin in a densely organized fashion.

Bundles of collagen intertwined in three-dimensional orientation by elastic fibers characterize the pars reticularis (Fig. 1.9). Collagenic fibers are directed preferentially and relate to the embryogeny and function of the region.

The ground substance or matrix of the dermis is represented by vascular PAS-positive basement membranes (1). Veins, arteries, and nerves occur as triads in the reticular dermis, and the normal cellular population is essentially the same as in the

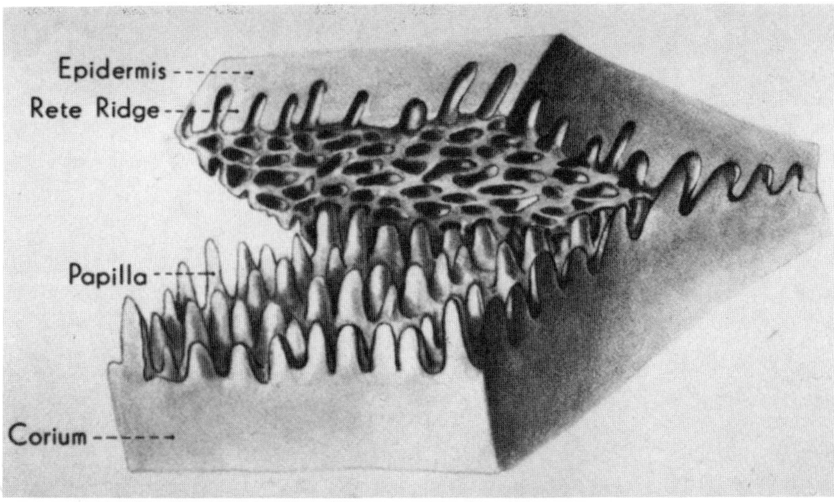

Figure 1.11. Epidermal-dermal interface. From Pinkus H, Mehregan A: *A Guide to Dermatohistopathology*, ed 2. New York, Appleton-Century-Crofts, 1969.

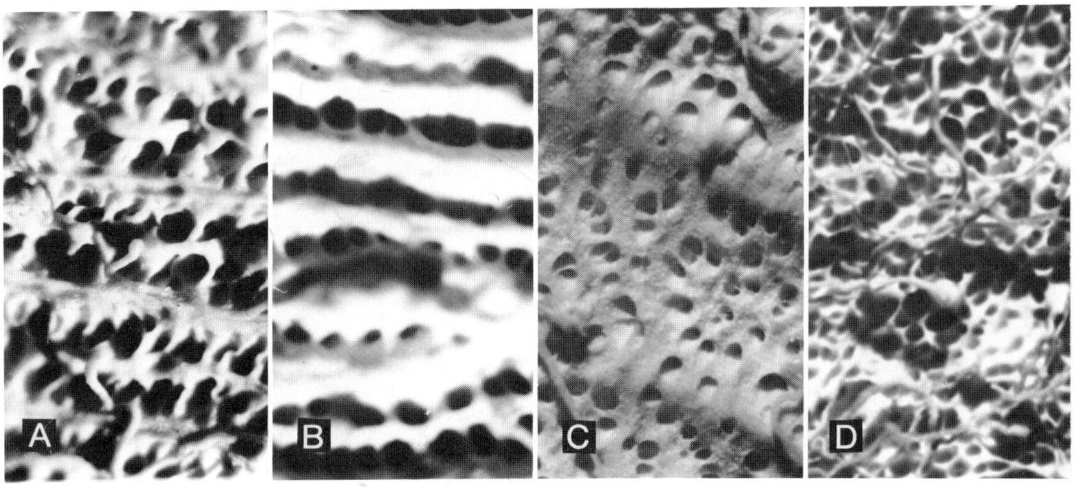

Figure 1.12. Variability of the epidermal-dermal interface within the human foot. Epidermal interface of: *A*, plantar heel; *B*, plantar surface at first metatarsophalangeal joint; *C*, region of insertion of tendo achillis; *D*, surface plantar to the medial longitudinal arch.

pars papillaris. The relative numbers of cells, however, is much reduced.

THE FIBROBLAST

The fibroblast is important to both epidermis and dermis alike. This cell elaborates a substance which influences epidermal cells to undergo mitosis and cell division. Fibroblasts also lay down the mucopolysaccharide matrix of the dermis and the fibrillar elements found therein. Fibroblasts and fibroblast-like cells are found throughout loose and dense connective tissues of the body.

The structural characteristics of fibroblasts reflect its busy role: They have extensive dendritic processes, and the large nucleus is usually oval, faintly staining, and stippled. The light microscope demonstrates it as spindle shaped but the electron microscope reveals the typical thin, flattened branching cytoplasmic processes (Fig. 1.10).

The cytoplasm of fibroblasts is rich in organelles. This is particularly true of rough endoplasmic reticulum, Golgi apparatus, and mitochondria. Dense bodies and vesicles are also common.

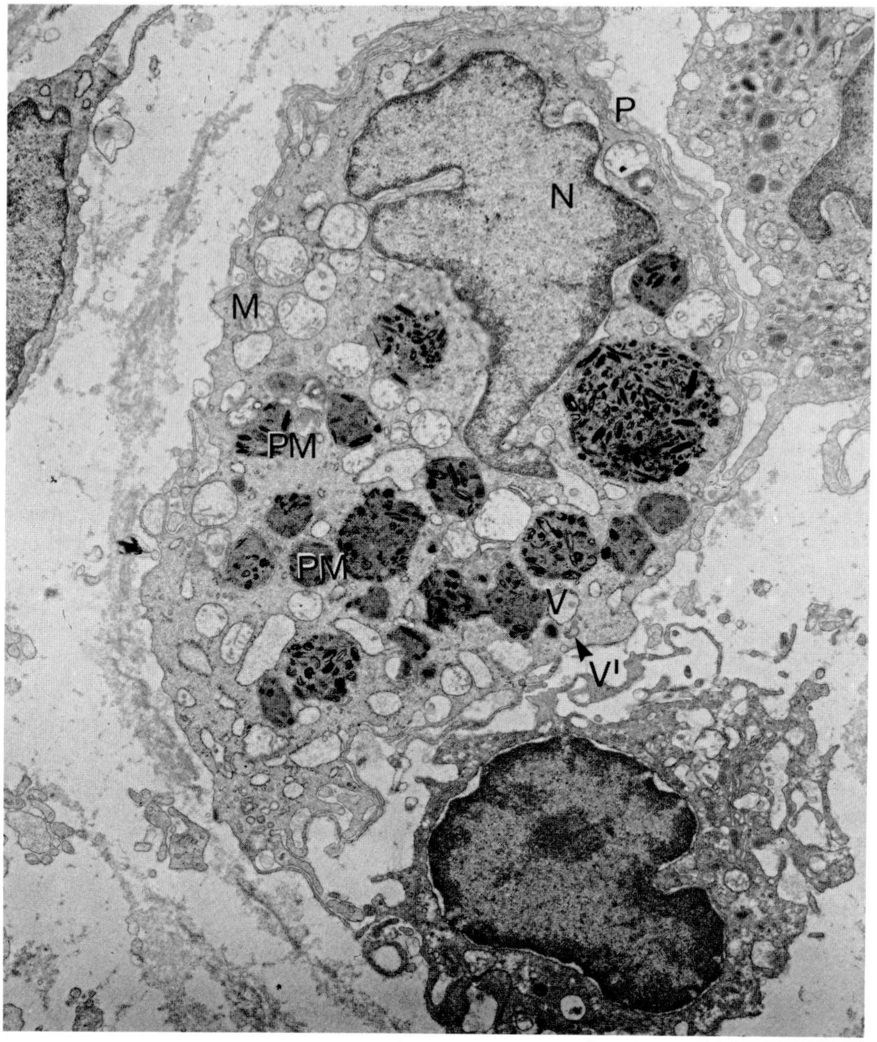

Figure 1.13. Melanophage containing ingested melanosomes and premelanosomes in which tyrosinase-rich melanin granules are identified. Transmission electron microscopy. *P*, plasma membrane; *N*, nucleus of melanophage; *M*, mitochondria, *PM*, premelanosome; *V*, vacuole; *V′*, vesicle.

In the biosynthesis of collagen, proline must be hydroxylated into hydroxyproline. Precursor tropocollagen is synthesized by the rough endoplasmic reticulum. Polysaccharides are then complexed to it in the Golgi apparatus. This substance, as well as other products, is secreted in exocytotic vesicles into the extracellular spaces. Cytoplasmic fibrils observed in the cytoplasm of fibroblasts are not the precursors of collagen but are contractile elements of this migratory cell.

The final aggregation of collagen occurs in the extracellular spaces of the dermis under the influence of the fibroblast. Collagenic fibrils demonstrate cross banding occurring at periodic intervals of 2800 Å. Individual fibrils may aggregate further into bundles of varying size.

Fibroblasts are crucial to the maintenance of the structural integrity of the dermis and to wound healing and scar formation.

The epidermis and dermis exist in functional and morphological relationship and interact in exchanges of inductive biochemical relationships (5). As a result, the skin has the ability to modulate its structural characteristics. Heloma durum is an excellent example of such phenomenon. Dermatoglyphics are special surface configurations of ridges and depressions which re-

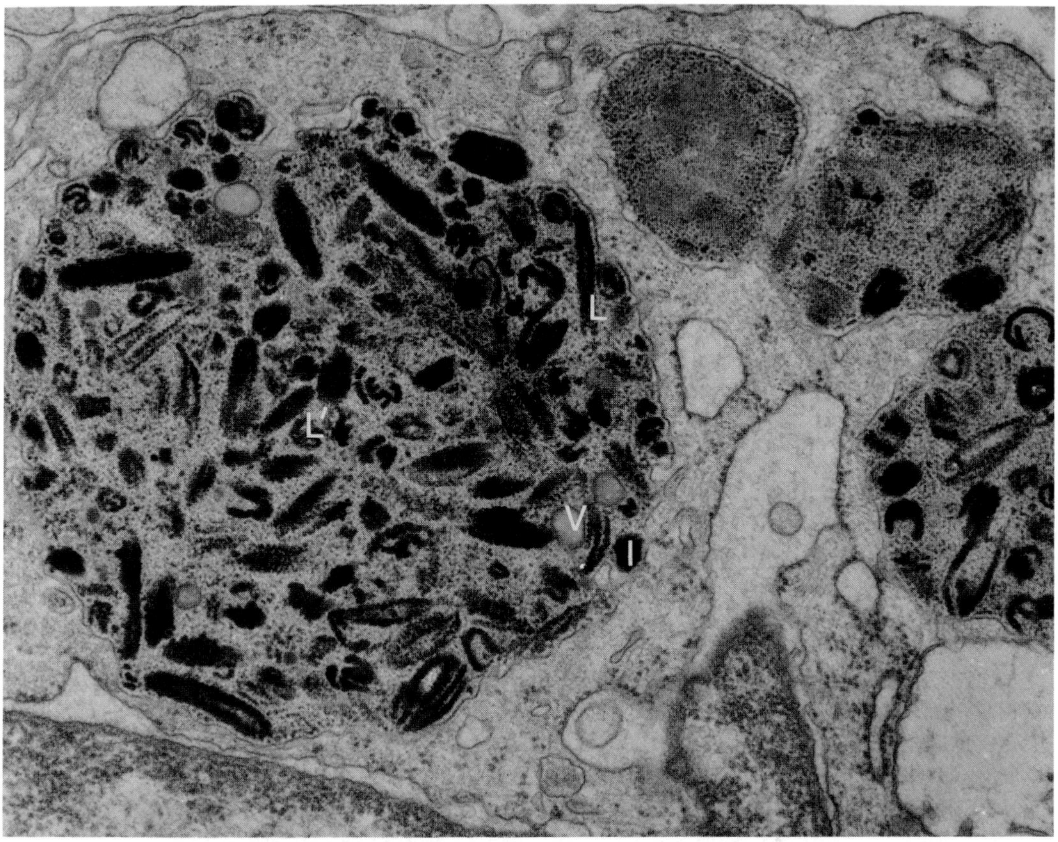

Figure 1.14. Intracytoplasmic detail of melanophage. Note that ingested organelles such as melanosomes and premelanosomes are membrane bound. Transmission electron microscopy. *V,* vacuole; *I*, inclusion body; *L*, premelanosome; *L'*, premelanosome.

flect deep dermal structures. In disease, this feature may become markedly serrated.

THE EPIDERMAL-DERMAL INTERFACE

The epidermodermal interface is a direct reflection of relative thickness of stratum Malpighii and stratum corneum: These measurements correlate directly with the dimensions of rete ridges and the interdigitating dermal papillae (6). Early microscopists defined the epidermodermal interface as having epidermal or rete pegs which interdigitate in glove-like fashion with the dermal papillae. Actually, the epidermis presents a solid mass of cells punctuated by the intrusion of finger-like dermal papillae (Fig. 1.11). It is now incumbent that the epidermis be described as having epidermal ridges. The former "peg" designation reflects error in appraising three-dimensional structures in simple two dimensions. It is interesting to note how varied the epidermodermal interface is at differing locations throughout the human foot (7) (Fig. 1.12*A* to *D*).

The experimental separation of dermis from epidermis is accomplished with difficulty. Cohesion is maintained by means of adepidermal membrane, anchoring fibrils, dermal fibrils, ground substance, hemidesmosomes, and microscopic rootlets (1).

Dendritic Cells

Migratory dendritic cells of neuroectodermal and bone marrow origins are associated with the epidermodermal interface. These migratory cells extend their cytoplasmic dendritic processes between keratinocytes, somehow separating their otherwise tight relationships (8). They represent two cell types: Melanocytes and Langerhans' cells. The melanocyte contains melanin granules which contribute to hair and

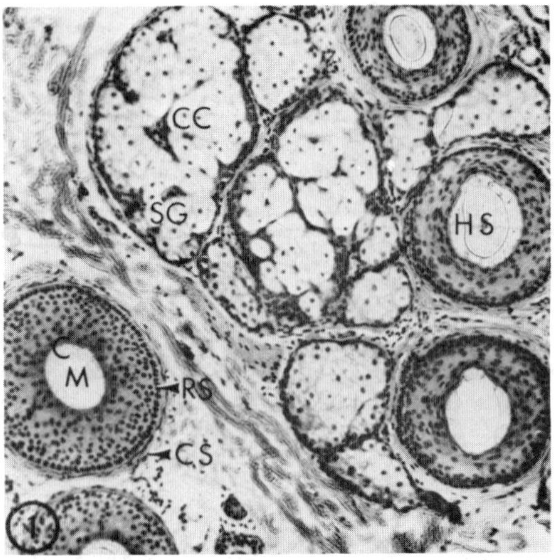

Figure 1.15. Sebaceous glands are usually associated with the follicles and shafts of hair. The central cells of the glandular portions accumulate lipid in their abundant cytoplasm. These cells then disintegrate and become the secretion of the gland. Such processes are of a holocrine mechanism. *SG*, sebaceous gland; *HS*, hair follicle and shaft; *M*, medulla of hair; *C*, hair cortex; *RS*, epithelial root sheath; *CS*, connective tissue root sheath; *CC*, central cells. From Matthews JL, Martin JH: *Atlas of Human Histology and Ultrastructure.* Philadelphia, Lea & Febiger, 1971.

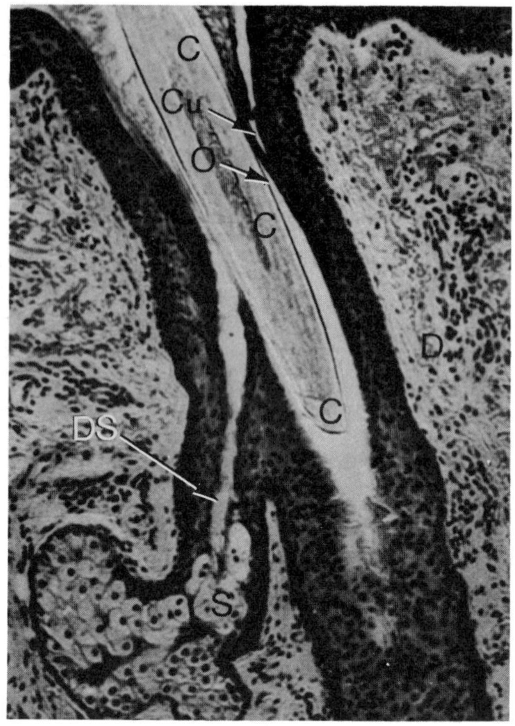

Figure 1.16. Hair structure as observed in the human skin. Note sebaceous gland (*S*) at the lower left. Observe the indicated relationships of cortex (*C*), cuticle (*CU*), outer root sheath (*O*), root sheath and dermis (*D*), and sebaceous gland duct (*DS*).

keratinocytes, thereby providing for the coloration of these structures (9). In dermatitis, the symbiotic relationship between melanocyte and keratinocyte is disturbed. Consequently, inflamed skin of Negroes darken as a result of dispersion and confinement of melanin within the cytoplasm of melanocyte dendrites. Melanophages are cells especially adapted to the phagocytosis of melanocytes and their products (Fig. 1.13).

At least a part of postinflammatory hyperpigmentation may be ascribed to a loss of melanin from the basal layer of the epidermis into the papillary dermis. In the dermis, specialized macrophages (melanophages) ingest or engulf melanin (Fig. 1.13).

Langerhans cells are high level dendritic cells having no melanin (10). They are histologically dopa-negative where melanocytes are positive. Langerhans cellular functions are not completely understood; it is possible they have a phagocytic function. Some authorities believe they have bone marrow origins, and are related to the monocyte series.

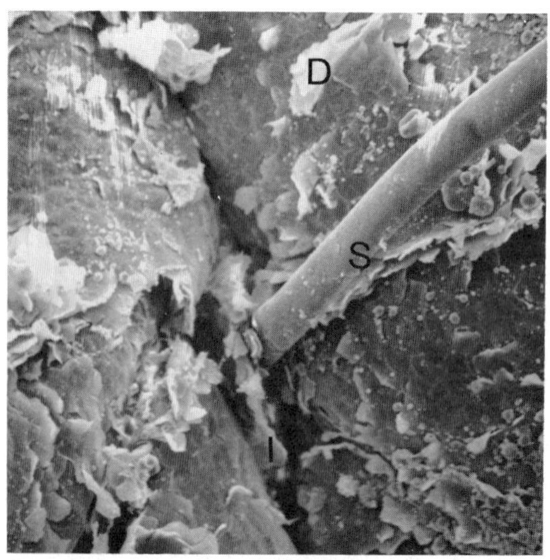

Figure 1.17. Hair shaft emerging from the free surface of skin as revealed by scanning electron microscopy. *D,* surface debris of skin; *S*, hair shaft; *I*, intercellular margin.

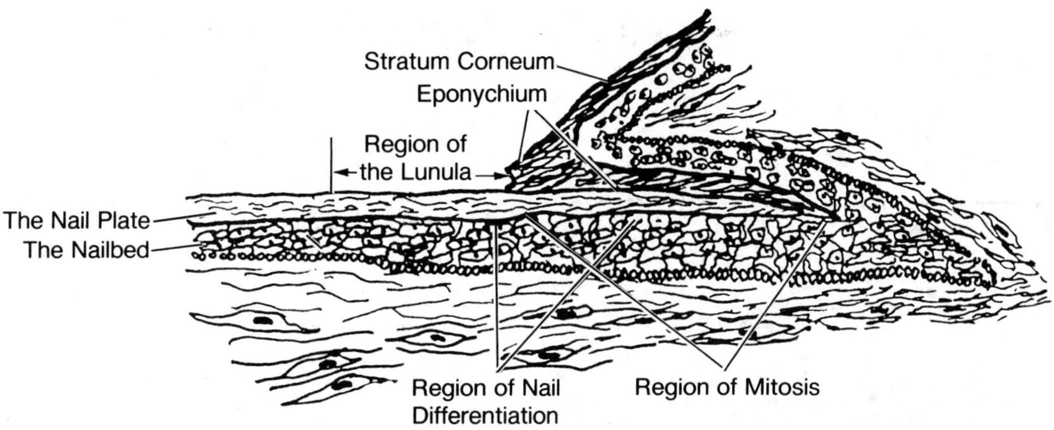

Figure 1.18. Nail matrix tissue. Nail structure as observed in the human foot. Diagrammatic.

A third type of dendritic cell is recognized by some authorities. The so-called indeterminate dendritic cell does not demonstrate either melanosomes or Langerhans granules. However, these cells react with monoclonal antibody OKT6 just as Langerhans cells do (11). Some classifications identify dendritic cells as type I pigment-producing melanocytes; type II as Langerhans cell; and type III as indeterminate (10).

Adnexa

This brief discussion, however limited concerning the basic anatomy of the skin, without mention of the skin's adnexa would be seriously lacking. Such structures include glands, hair, and nails.

Eccrine Glands

Secretory glands such as the sweat apparatus and the pilosebaceous structures are of practical interest to podiatric medicine for its involvements in a number of clinical entities, not the least of which is hyperhidrosis, bromhidrosis, and bromohyperhydrosis of the feet. The structural detail of glands is often tortuous and complicated (Fig. 1.15).

Hair

Hair is a complex structure developed from ectoderm under the inductive influence of the subjacent dermis. Glandular elements and smooth muscle cells are involved in its functional morphology. The structural detail of hair is reviewed in figure 1.16. The surface structure, as demonstrated by scanning electron microscopy, is shown in Figure 1.17.

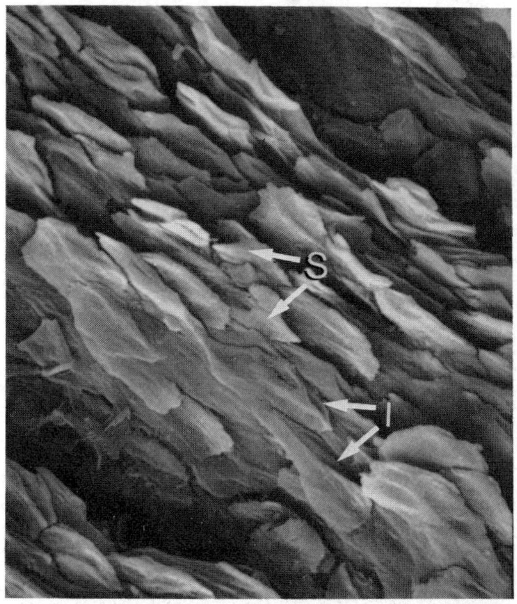

Figure 1.19. Cross sectional detail of nail as revealed by scanning electron microscopy. *S*, surface of cornified cell of nail; *I*, intercellular margin.

Nails

Nails are a distinctive feature of human fingers and toes. They are subject to a great deal of pathology which frequently demands the attention of the podiatric physician and surgeon. The structural detail of human nails is diagrammatically reviewed in figure 1.18. The cross-sectional appearance of the human nail as revealed by scanning electron microscopy is shown in Figure 1.19.

EPIDERMAL REGENERATION

The skin has excellent powers of regeneration (1). The initial event in wound healing is hemorrhage. A clot forms, and a fibrin meshwork is established. A mitotic burst among the germinatival cells occurs at the periphery of the wound. This activity is initiated by depletion of 3′,5′-adenosine monophosphate, the "epidermal chalone" which normally inhibits cell division in the epidermis (12). At the same time, the "epidermal influencing factor," which induces epidermal cell division, is relatively increased (13). Cells of the stratum basale become migratory as mitosis increases the numbers of cells at the germinal layer (Fig. 1.20).

Polymorphonuclear leucocytes followed by lymphocytes invade the wound in a generally predictable and timed sequence (2). Such cells are phagocytic and debride the wound. It is interesting to note that migratory epidermal cells also become phagocytic under certain circumstances as they enter the wound defect (Fig. 1.21).

Migratory basal cells proceed over the contiguous dermis beneath the clot until they meet cells of like type coming from the opposite direction (2). Eventually, the epidermal defect is closed as cells proliferate upward to reconstitute the normal epidermal stratification.

A reserve of relatively undifferentiated epidermal cells can also be recruited from adnexa in the immediate region of the wound. These elements can also assist in epithelializing integumentary defects.

Fibroblasts enter the dermis and synthesize new matrix together with collagenic and reticular fibers. Blood vessels reconsti-

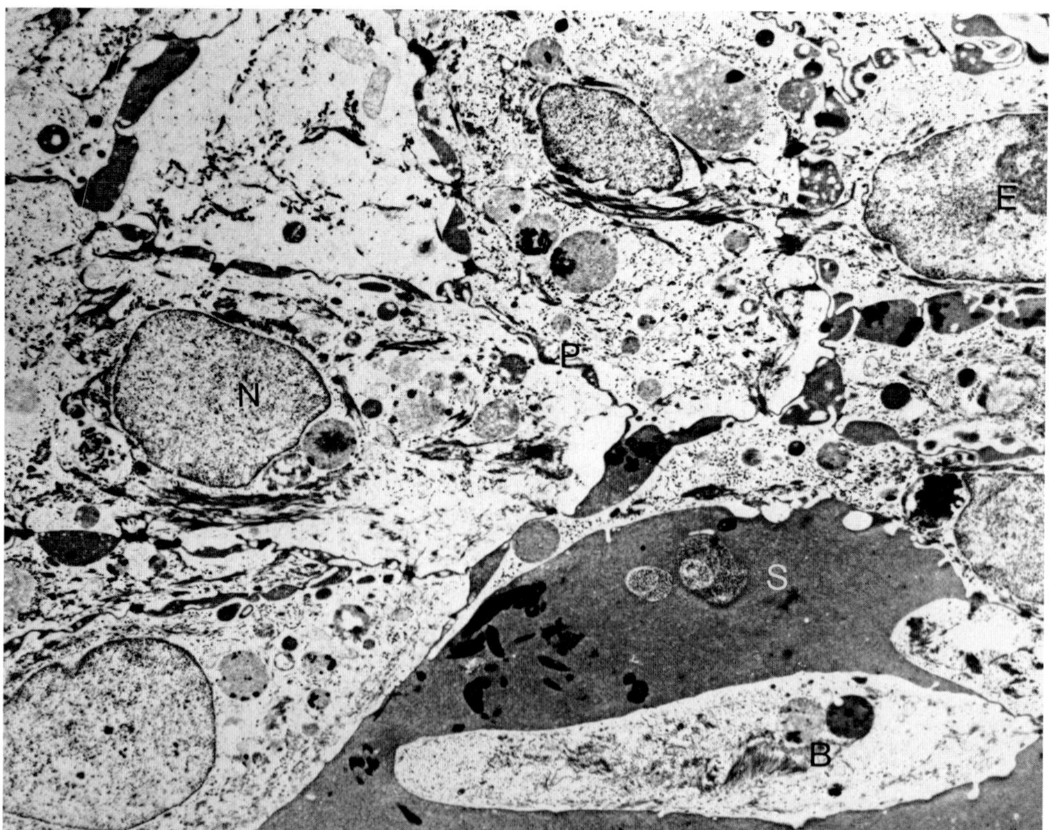

Figure 1.20. Migratory behavior of basal cell during wound healing. *E,* epidermal cell; *P,* plasma membrane; *N,* nucleus; S, wound space; *B,* pseudopod-like extension of basal cell. From Ross R: *Sci Am* 220:40, 1969.

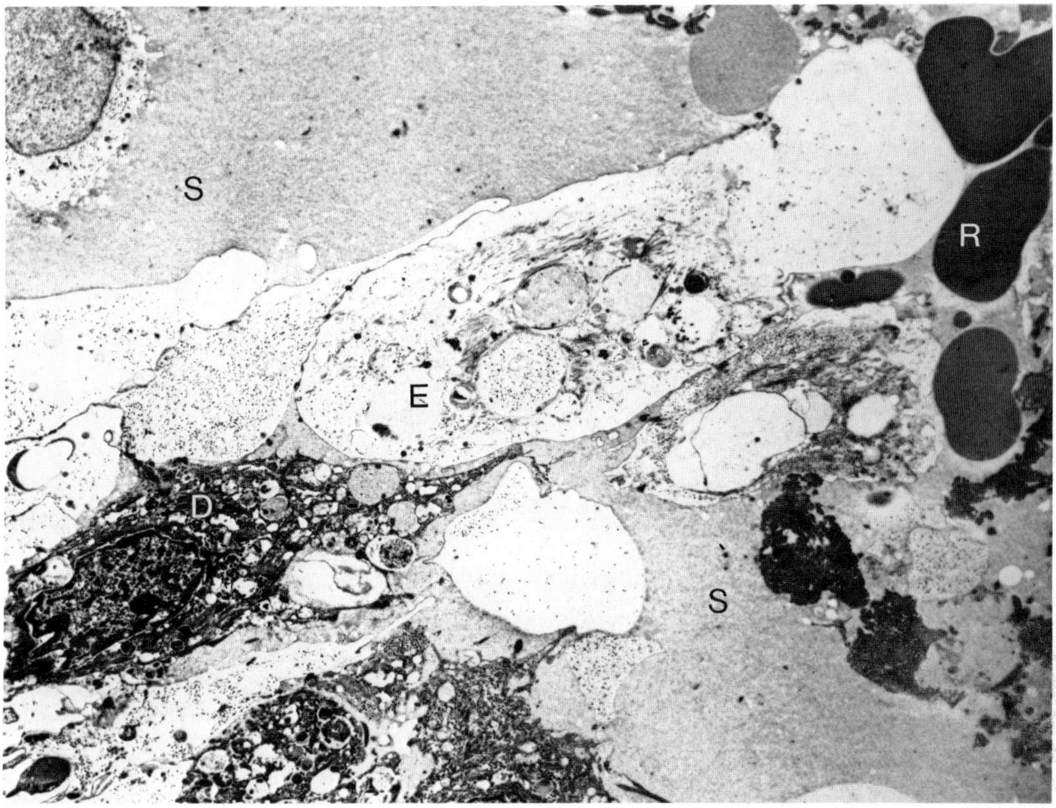

Figure 1.21. Phagocytic behavior of basal cell during wound healing. *D,* wound debris; *E*, epidermal cell acting as phagocyte, *S*, wound space; *R*, red blood cell. From Ross R: *Sci Am* 220:40, 1969.

tute themselves in the dermis by budding into the dermis (Fig. 1.1). Initially, an interlacing network is developed. From this the most useful vessels are selected to continue development while others atrophy.

References

1. Pinkus H, Mehregan A: *A Guide to Dermatohistopathology*, ed. 2. New York, Appleton-Century-Crofts, 1969.
2. Ross R: Wound healing. *Sci Am* 220:40, 1969.
3. Matoltsy AG, Parakkal PF: *Keratinization (in) Ultrastructure of Normal and Abnormal Skin,* Zelickson AS (ed). Philadelphia, Lea & Febiger, 1967.
4. Odland GF: A submicroscopic granular component in the human epidermis. *J Invest Dermatol* 34:11, 1960.
5. McCarthy DJ, Habowsky JEJ: Structural variability of the dermoepidermal interface of the skin of the human foot as related to function. *J Am Podiatry Assoc* 65:450–464, 1975.
6. McCarthy DJ, Habowsky JEJ: Histochemistry and anthropometric analysis of heloma durum. *J Am Podiatry Assoc* 65:4–18, 1975.
7. McCarthy DJ, Habowsky JEJ: The epidermo-dermal interface of the human foot integument as compared with the composite body. In: *Year-Book of Podiatry, 1978/1979.* Mt. Kisco, NY, Futura, 1978.
8. Arey LB: *Human Histology,* ed 4. Philadelphia, W.B. Saunders, 1974.
9. Leeson TS, Leeson CR: *Histology,* ed. 3. Philadelphia, W.B. Saunders, 1976.
10. Ham AW: *Histology,* ed. 7. Philadelphia, J.B. Lippincott, 1974.
11. Chu A, Eisinger M, Lee JS et al: Immunoelectron microscopic identification of the Langerhans cell using a new antigenic marker. *J Invest Dermatol* 78(2):177–180, 1982.
12. Vorhees JJ, Duell EA: Psoriasis as a possible defect in the adenylcyclase, cyclic AMP cascade. *Arch Dermatol* 104:352–358, 1971.
13. Cohen J: Interactions of the skin. *Br J Dermatol* 81(Suppl 3):46–59, 1969.

CHAPTER 2

Physiological Considerations of the Skin

ARLENE F. HOFFMAN

SKIN PHYSIOLOGY

The skin is an interface between the body and the external environment. Although the skin's functions involve a considerable number of essentially independent activities, most of these are related to the skin's unique location and may be classified as being protective in action. These include: shielding the body from external stresses and preventing infections from microorganisms, preventing excessive moisture loss, serving as a clinical and radiant barrier, providing sensation, and providing temperature regulation.

The following chapter will describe these functions and others, including: eccrine gland physiology, skin odor, nail physiology, skin lymph flow, and skin circulatory physiology. Attention has been directed to emphasizing aspects relevant to the foot and the leg. Since this chapter is intended for the clinician rather than the skin physiologist, references cited are mostly review articles and not original papers. Citations have been kept to a minimum. These features, it is hoped, will enable the reader to access a wider range of information.

Mechanical Barrier

The skin serves as a mechanical protective medium shielding the body from external stresses resulting principally from gravity and inertia. The thickness of the skin will vary depending upon the mechanical demand at the location. As an example, the thickness of the stratum corneum is usually 0.015 mm, whereas in the sole of the foot it is 0.6 mm. The protection afforded by the sole of the foot is due mainly to its thickness (1).

To adapt to the numerous and nearly continuous movements of the body, the skin must be a mobile tissue capable of extension and relaxation. The skin's elasticity is due to the mechanical properties of the dermal fibers and their pattern of weave. Elastin fibers (which comprise 5% of fat free dry weight (2) are thought to restore the morphology of the collagen network after deformation (3). Collagen fibers, which comprise 77% fat free dry weight (2), provide resistance to mechanical stress (Fig. 2.1). The ground substance between these fibers is a semifluid and provides resistance to compression and bulk flow. The skin, therefore, can withstand considerable deformation without permanent damage and can resume its previous shape after deformation. When edema is present, this resilience is diminished (4).

Mechanically, the skin can withstand great stress. Yamada quotes experiments to show that the ultimate tensile strength is about 1200 lb/inch^2 (5). When walking barefoot on cement, no part of the foot experiences more than 75 psi, and when walking in a shoe, peak readings are less than 50 psi (6). Consequently, a foot in a regular shoe is subjected to less than one-tenth of that which would cause direct injury or breakdown of the skin.

Since we know that feet do in fact, commonly break down and ulcerate, there seems to be a dichotomy between these findings and what one observes in fact. One of the leading investigators in the field, Paul Brand, has written: "There is no way

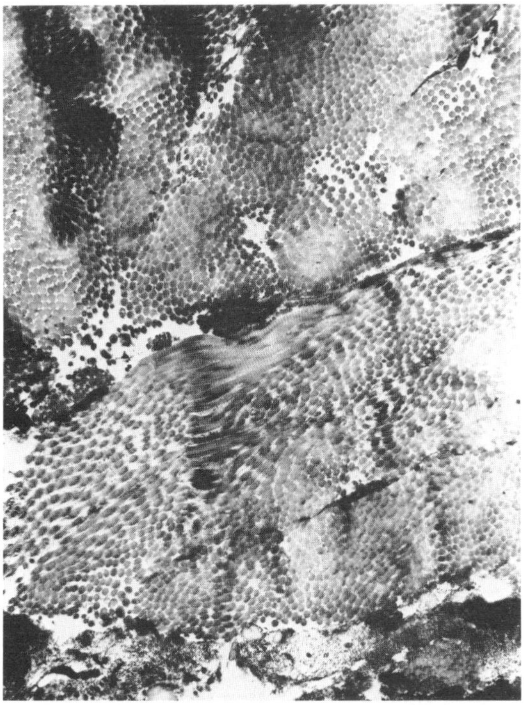

Figure 2.1. Collagen within the dermis provides the skin with resistance to mechanical stress.

(to) account for the ten to one difference between theoretical threshold for damages and the peak pressures of normal walking. At this point there seems to be a gap in our understanding of the cause of tissue breakdown" (7)

Physiologists are quite familiar with the following relationships:

$$\text{Pressure } \alpha \ \frac{\text{Force}}{\text{Area}} = \text{Stress}$$

$$\text{Pressure } \alpha \ \frac{\text{Tension}}{\text{Radius}}$$

Relative to pressures impressing on the foot, the following points can be made: The larger the area of skin exposed to a given force, the lower will be the resultant pressure on that skin. Similarly, the smaller the radius of curvature, the larger will be the resulting pressure. Viewing a transverse plane section of the foot, it may be seen that the radius of curvature of the plantar and dorsal aspect is large and, therefore, the skin will receive minimal pressure from any circumferential pressure. The medial and lateral borders have much smaller radii of curvature, and they will receive much more pressure from the same tension. Therefore, one can see why bony prominences such as bunions and hammertoes have an increased probability for ulceration since their radius of curvature is less than that of a normal foot.

Brand (8) and Thompson (9) delineate three major categories of tissue breakdown to stress, the first being breakdown following exposure to low static pressures (below 1 psi) for extended periods of time. This occurs in shoes, particularly around bony prominences. The cause for this phenomenon is that the resultant pressure becomes high enough to effectively close down arterioles and capillaries which, particularly in the neurotrophic foot, results in frank ischemia and necrosis (Fig. 2.2). The second type of breakdown occurs when the mechanical stress of the tissue is exceeded (increase of 1200 psi). This occurs whenever one encounters a sharp object. Alternately, this can occur if there is loss of subcutaneous tissue. As a result of this loss there will be a decrease in the ability of the foot to spread the load if a specific force is applied. The presence of edema has the same effect. A third mechanism (and one that Brand believes is the most prevalent) is soft tissue destruction resultant from repetitive exertion stress (of 20 psi). Brand and Thompson believe that if stresses are superimposed upon the inflamed response, necrosis and ulceration are inevitable. It is Brand's contention that the process of inflammation greatly lowers the skin's ability to withstand stress and that this process explains why skin will ulcerate before one would predict from laboratory studies.

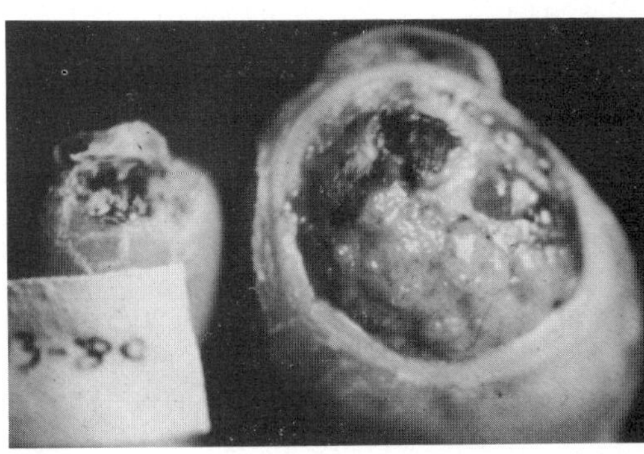

Figure 2.2. Neurotrophic ulcer secondary to burn. (From McCarthy DJ: *Management of Dermal Ulcerations and Wound Complications*. Evanston, IL, Arthur Retlaw, 1981.)

Preventing Skin Infections from Microorganisms

In general, the intact skin presents a formidable and effective barrier to invading microorganisms. When artificially applied on human skin, many pathogenic bacteria (such as β-hemolytic streptococci species and *Staphylococcus aureus*) do not survive for more than a few hours (10)

HUMIDITY

Superficially applied microorganisms survive longer on wet skin (10). Tachibana (11) has noted that the microbial environment of the foot, however, does not increase further following increases in humidity and/or temperature. This is attributed to the foot already supporting a close to maximal bacterial population. She does go on to note that extreme changes in either temperature or humidity are important factors for growth of bacteria on the foot. There are large differences in the environment associated with shoes or with going barefoot. When shoes are worn, the interdigital spaces of the foot are compressed, and evaporation is hindered. The toes are restricted in movement and moisture cannot evaporate. Therefore, those who wear tightly enclosed shoes and have sweaty feet have a higher than normal bacterial count and a greater likelihood of infection than those individuals with drier feet (11). It is, therefore, not surprising that toe interspaces have 100 to 1000 times the bacterial population, compared to that of most other regions of the skin (12).

SKIN SURFACE LIPIDS

Eccrine sweat contains factors that inhibit the growth of *Microsporum gypsium* and *Epidermophyton inguinale*. The fungicidal activity is attributed to acetic, proprionic, caprylic, and lactic acids. Surface lipids of keratinocyte origin have been shown to have antimicrobial effects against many common bacterial pathogens, including *Streptococcus pyogenes*, *Corynebacterium diphtheriae*, *Candida albicans*, and certain strains of *Staphylococcus aureus*. Gram negative rods are not affected by these surface lipids (10, 13).

MICROBIAL POPULATION AND ANTAGONISMS

The largest number of bacteria on the skin is found in sebaceous glands and hair follicles. The skin of the dorsal and plantar aspect of the foot contains no sebaceous glands, and there are normally no hair follicles on the plantar aspect of the foot. On the foot, the bacteria exists principally on the skin surface itself and beneath the superficial cells of the stratum corneum (11).

Tachibana lists the reported frequency of Gram positive and Gram negative bacteria in the normal flora of the foot (11):

Coagulase negative cocci	88–100%
Sarcina	15–17%
Micrococci	95%
S. aureus	1–16%, 56%
Diphtheroids, lipophilic	90%–100%
Diphtheroids, nonlipophilic	13–48%
Enteric bacilli (under age 65)	6–12%
Enteric bacilli (over age 65)	21%
Gram negative coccobacilli	6–10%

It is well known that the resident flora present on the skin surface represents a defense against colonization by potential pathogens. The microbial antagonism is mechanistically complex. Intefering organisms elaborate antimicrobial substances, bacteriocins that inhibit the growth of other bacteria. Bacteriocins produced by Gram positive bacteria are antibacterial only against similar strains or closely related species, while bacteriocins produced by Gram negative bacteria have a wider range (10, 14).

Permeability Barrier

One of the major functions of the stratum corneum is associated with its low permeability properties. It not only effectively retards water loss from the inner hydrated tissue layers but also prevents the entrance of most toxic agents (1). It is now believed that there is not one specific site for the barrier, but rather that the barrier is uniformly present throughout the entire thickness of the stratum corneum (5). The intercellular lipids present in the stratum corneum are known to play an an important part in providing this water barrier (15, 16). Any mechanical or chemical alteration in the stratum corneum impairs the barrier and makes the skin permeable to water and soluble substances (1).

The permeability of the skin rises with hydration of the horny layer (16). It is, therefore, not surprising that intertriginous infections occur frequently. Conversely, when the stratum corneum has less than 10% water, the layer becomes brittle and hard, and skin appears dry and scaley. When this occurs, the interdigitated arrangement and close packing of the overlapping cells are disrupted. The resultant fissures and cracks expose the underlying epidermis to physical and chemical trauma (17).

Radiant Barrier

For skin unprotected by hair or clothing, the only significant defense against the damaging effects of ultraviolet light is the presence of melanin in the epidermis. Without melanin, the epidermis constitutes only a thin membrane which offers little protection against ultraviolet radiation. Within the epidermal cells, melanin provides important protection by scattering and removing free radicals liberated by the incident radiant energy (18).

Closely associated with the protective action of the skin against harmful effects of various portions of the radiant energy spectrum are the cellular changes induced by ultraviolet irradiation. Most of these changes are pathological and are beyond the scope of this chapter. The only healthful result of ultraviolet irradiation on any normal skin is the production of Vitamin D. However, with the current food fortification with vitamins, solar irradiation is no longer necessary. Even if food were not fortified, only very slight amounts of irradiation over very limited areas of skin would be sufficient to produce the required amount of vitamin D (19).

Eccrine Sweat Glands

The soles have large numbers of eccrine sweat glands. Secretion is enhanced by emotional stress and increased temperature. There is some controversy regarding whether the eccrine glands on the sole of the foot respond differently than those of the rest of the body. The consensus of opinion is that the sweat response of a particular part of the body is roughly proportional to the number of sweat glands in the region (20, 21).

Skin Odor

Normally one associates this condition with bromhidrosis. The odors are produced by the microbial production of fatty acids from the surface lipids. Greaves, however, suggests physiological benefits to the odor that skin assumes after puberty (22). This odor results from the action of skin bacteria on keratin and apocrine sweat. He suggests the possibility of pheromone activity resulting in perceived enhanced sexual activity.

Nail Physiology

The nail contains about 18% water. As the diffusion constant of water is about 100 times greater than that of the stratum corneum, the nail plate swells easily and is as porous as hair. If the water content rises to 30% the nail becomes opaque and soft; if it falls below 16% the nail becomes brittle (23). The nail does not contain any sweat glands. Yet the water loss from insensible perspiration per unit surface area of the nail is as high as that of the palms and soles and thus more than most other body regions (24).

Sensation

The skin is richly supplied with nerve endings and provides the body's main access to its environment and an effective sensory defense against harmful agents.

Specific areas of skin are supplied by sensory nerves derived from single dorsal nerve roots, or sensory dermatomes. There is considerable overlap of dermatomes, so that traumatic section of a single dorsal root produces little impairment of sensation.

Sensory nerve fibers can be classified as types A, B, or C, depending on their diameter and action potential. Type A fibers have the largest diameter, the shortest electrical spike potential, and the highest velocity of conduction. Type C fibers are narrower, have a wider-based spike, and conduct more slowly. Mechanoreceptors seem to be largely type A fibers; pain, itch, cold, and warmth sensations seem to be carried by type C fibers. Type B fibers have characteristics between A and C. The specific sensation one experiences appears not to depend on the position of morphological characteristics of the nerve fibers stimulated. Rather, the spatial arrangements of these fibers within tissues, the frequency and sequence of neural volleys fired, and the reception of these volleys by the spinal cord and brain are involved. Sensation of the skin depends on the frequency of impulses, the number of fibers stimulated, and various inhibiting and reinforcing factors in the central nervous system (22, 25).

There are four cutaneous senses: touch-pressure (pressure is sustained touch); cold; warmth; and pain. The skin contains various types of sensory endings. These include naked nerve endings, expanded tips on sensory nerve terminals, and encapsulated endings. The expanded endings include Merkel's disks and Ruffini endings. The encapsulated endings include Vater-Pacinian corpuscles, Meissner's corpuscles, and Krause's end-bulbs. Ruffini endings and Pacinian corpuscles are also found in deep fibrous tissues. In addition, sensory nerves end around hair follicles. However, none of the expanded or encapsulated endings appear to be necessary for cutaneous sensation. Their distribution varies in different regions of the body, and it has been repeatedly demonstrated that all four sensory modalities can be elicited from areas that on histologic examination contain only naked nerve endings. Where they are present, the expanded or encapsulated endings appear to function as mechanoreceptors that respond to tactile stimuli. The nerve endings around hair follicles mediate touch, and movements of hairs initiate tactile sensations. It should be emphasized that although cutaneous sensory receptors lack histologic specificity, they are physiologically specific. Thus, any given ending signals one and only one kind of cutaneous sensation (26).

It is now generally agreed that "itch spots" on the skin have generally no strict anatomical counterpart, being related to a lower threshold of the fine nerve endings in the area. Pain and itch are related protective mechanisms. Pain causes withdrawal from a possibly damaging stimulus, and itch causes scratching. A noxious stimulus of low intensity, perhaps operating over a long period and affecting the outermost skin layer, will be interpreted as itch, while a more penetrating intense stimulus will cause pain (27).

It is interesting to note that one has to lose 50% of the functional free nerve endings before a sensory neuropathy can be detected (28).

Hypodermis

The subcutaneous tissue, or hypodermis, is the deepest and thickest layer of skin. Its function is involved mainly with the metabolism of adipocytes and the biosynthesis and breakdown of lipids. The hypodermis is the chief food storage organ in the body. A well-fed individual would survive many weeks without food.

The hypodermis, at times, has been likened to the insulation surrounding a warm core, functioning much like a "thermos" bottle to keep the body warm. This analogy is not quite correct, since it does not take into account the small amount of heat released during lypolysis of triglycerides to free fatty acids. Instead, the hypodermis should be viewed as being similar to an electric blanket, which is functioning actively to keep the individual warm. The amount of heat produced and the rate of triglyceride lipolysis is under control of the sympathetic nervous system.

A third function of the hypodermis is that of protective padding. The soft, resilient padding provided by fat helps protect the overlying epidermis and underlying muscles from mechanical injury (29). The reader is referred to earlier discussions on mechanical barriers. It should be noted that the hypodermis helps spread the load and increase the radius of curvature, thereby decreasing the probability of ulceration.

Lymph

Review of the literature reveals surprisingly little information about lymph flow through the skin. Greaves, noting this deficit, has written:

> The physiology of the lymph circulation in skin has been neglected. Defective lymph flow may be a significant factor in a wide range of skin diseases, but its role cannot be assessed until more is known of its normal behavior and regulation. Peripheral as well as

central lymphatics are now known to be actively contractile structures, possessing adrenergic and other receptors. Studies on human lymphatics should be done both in vivo and in vitro in order to reveal the factors regulating lymph flow in the skin (22).

Skin Circulatory Physiology

CIRCULATION THROUGH THE SKIN

The anatomy and physiology of cutaneous blood flow is closely correlated with the skin's thermoregulatory function. To illustrate this point, the wide variation in blood flow volume can be noted. The minimum flow that produced during massive cold vasoconstriction is approximately 0.5 ml/min/100 mg tissue. This volume is sufficient to prevent tissue necrosis. The maximal flow produced during vasodilation has been measured at approximately 150 ml/min/100 mg tissue (30, 31). These differences emphasize that cutaneous blood flow is related to heat regulation and is not governed solely by the metabolic requirements of the skin. If metabolic requirements were the controlling factors, one would expect only a two- to threefold increase in blood flow above minimum volume (32).

In my opinion, Margaret Conrad has written one of the best and most carefully researched descriptions of the function of blood vessels found in the skin of the lower extremities (33). She notes that blood vessels of the skin are arranged for ready transfer of heat from the blood to the external environment. The major portion of the microvascular is spread out just under the surface of the skin, and blood heat is readily lost to the environment from the network of venules which hold a larger volume of blood near the surface. Since the heat transfer mechanism serves to regulate the temperature of the body as a whole, the skin vessels are under a high level of central control.

The arteries, filled with warm blood from the core, rise quickly from deep to superficial areas and remain relatively larger (120 μm in diameter) until they penetrate the deep venous plexus, after which they narrow to 12 μm in a space of 3 mm. Resistance is, therefore, kept low in the skin bed, allowing a large volume flow when the arteries are dilated. Most of the flow is directed towards the vascular loop at the surface and then through each of several rich plexuses of veins. Heat is, therefore, brought rapidly from the deep areas to the surfaces where the temperature gradient between the blood and the tissues is steep. Heat is lost from the blood to the surrounding tissues and from there to the external environment (33).

The most efficient heat exchange will occur in the terminal capillary loops which are directed very close to the surface, where the temperature of the adjacent tissues is closest to the environment and where the individual vessel cross sectional area is small and the composite surface area is large. When flow is high and equilibrium between capillary blood and surrounding tissue does not occur, additional heat will be transferred from the blood to the skin by the venous plexus. It is interesting to note that in plantar skin the total blood volume in the plexus is 30 times that of the volume in the capillaries (33).

It is not surprising that arteriovenous (AV) shunts are observed only in plantar skin where the deep venous plexus is present. Were they to occur in other areas, these channels would simply shunt warm blood back to the core. The presence of AV shunts and additional venous plexuses in plantar skin provides this area with a much greater capacity for varying the rate of heat exchange with peripheral tissues. This increased capacity for heat exchange is especially important in the sole of the foot, which may be in direct contact with external surfaces and may rapidly lose or gain heat by conduction. Therefore, in cold weather, one can see that it becomes significantly more difficult for plantar tissue to freeze.

The anatomical arrangement of skin blood vessels suggests that little countercurrent heat exchange would occur since the arteries lie perpendicular rather than parallel to the veins. However, the major deep veins of the extremity do lie in closer association with the arteries, and significant heat should be transferred from the warm arteries to the cold venous blood returning from the surface. This exchange is lessened when the superficial veins are dilated in response to a warm environment and large volumes of blood are returning through veins which have no accompanying arteries. In a cool environment, when superficial veins are constricted, blood will be shunted to deep veins where countercurrent exchange will return blood heat to the core, by-passing the superficial heat exchanges. This conserves body heat (33).

NEURAL CONTROL OF BLOOD FLOW IN THE SKIN

Under steady-state conditions of environmental temperature and metabolic rate, the blood flow in the skin of the lower extremity (and particularly that of the foot and toes) does not follow a steady mean. Rather, it fluctuates widely from one moment to the next. Plethysmographic recorded digital volume varies synchronously in adjacent toes, and in the right and left extremities. This relationship is lost if one of the extremities is sympathectomized. Therefore, it appears that these changes are the result of periodic rhythmic discharges of sympathetic impulses (33). [Author's note: Clinically, using the noninvasive modalities of Doppler, photoplethysmography, and volume plethysymography, I have not noticed the wide fluctuations.] With sympathectomy, digital flow can increase 5- to 10-fold with somewhat less changes recorded in the foot (33).

SKIN COLOR AS RELATED TO THE CIRCULATION

In lightly pigmented skin, a rough approximation of the state of the circulation can be required from a visualization of the skin. The depth of the color supplied by the blood pigments will vary with the quantity of blood held in the venous plexuses just under the surface, and the hue will be determined by the degree of oxygenation of the hemoglobin. In a comfortable environment, where vessels are partially constricted, the normal skin has a light reddish hue, owing to moderate filling of the plexus with blood. It still has a high oxygen content since flow exceeds metabolic requirements. If the vessels are markedly constricted, and the quantity of blood in the plexus is small, the skin will be pale regardless of the state of oxygenation. In venous insufficiency the skin appears bluish because poorly oxygenated blood fills the plexuses. When severely cooled skin is rapidly warmed, the skin color may go from pale to dark blue and then to red (hyperemic skin). Following the release of constriction to cold (pale) skin by rapid warming, the vessels dilate, and the poorly oxygenated blood that was stagnated in the capillaries rushes into the plexuses (dark blue hue). As soon as the oxygen poor blood is washed out, the dilated plexuses become filled with richly oxygenated blood, and the skin remains hyperemic as long as the vessels are dilated and flow exceeds metabolic demands. In conditions where severe organic arterial insufficiency occurs, the hyperemic response may not be observed. The beefy red color that one frequently observes in severely ischemic tissue is caused by ischemic damage to sphincters controlling blood flow (33).

Noninvasive Vascular Testing

TOE PRESSURE SUFFICIENT TO SUSTAIN HEALING

The potential for healing capacity can be determined directly from a pressure-metered doppler or indirectly from a photoplethysymographic sensor placed distal to a digital cuff. Barnes reports that at the pressures between 20 and 30 mm Hg, healing of digital ulcerations is unlikely, while healing is universal at pressures above 80 mm Hg (34).

In my experience obtained from hundreds of ambulatory podiatric patients, healing should be expected at pressures equal to or greater than 50 mm Hg.

References

1. Montagna W, Parakkal PF: *The Structure and Function of the Skin*, ed 3. New York, Academic Press, 1974, p 63.
2. Pearce RH, Grimmer BJ: Age and the chemical constitution of normal human dermis. *J Invest Dermatol* 58:347–361.
3. Pinto J: The dermis. In Montagna W, Parakkal PF (eds): *The Structure and Function of the Skin*, ed 3. New York, Academic Press, 1974, p 130.
4. DeLaney WE, Land WA: *Principles and Practice of Dermatology.* Sydney, Australia, Butterworths, 1978, p 7.
5. Yamada H: *Strength of Biological Materials.* Baltimore, Williams & Wilkins, 1970, pp 224–231.
6. Bauman JH, Girling JP, Brand PW: Plantar pressures and trophic ulcerations: an eval-

uation of foot ware. *J Bone Joint Surg* 45B:652–673, 1963.
7. Brand PW: The insensitive foot. In Jahss MH (ed): *Disorders of the Foot.* Philadelphia, W.B. Saunders, 1982, vol 2, p 1271.
8. Brand PW: The insensitive foot. In Jahss MH (ed): *Disorders of the Foot.* Philadelphia, W.B. Saunders, 1982, vol 2, pp 1268–1286.
9. Thompson D: Pathomechanics of soft tissue damage. In Levin ME, O'Neal LW (eds): *The Diabetic Foot,* ed 3. St. Louis, C.V. Mosby, 1983, pp 148–161.
10. Aly R, Maibach H: Factors controlling skin bacterial flora. In Maibach H, Aly R (eds): *Skin Microbiology: Relevance to Clinical Infection.* New York, Springer-Verlag, 1981, p 29.
11. Tachibana DK: Microbiology of the foot. *Annu Rev Microbiol* 30:351–375, 1976.
12. Noble WC, Somerville DA: *Microbiology of Human Skin.* Philadelphia, W.B. Saunders, 1974, pp 330–331.
13. Aly R, Maibach HI: Susceptibility to skin infection. In Rook AJ, Maibach HI (eds): *Recent Advances in Dermatology.* New York, Churchill Livingstone, 1983, vol 6, p 75.
14. Selwyn S: Microbial interactions and antibiosis. In Maibach HI, Aly R (eds): *Skin Microbiology: Relevance to Clinical Infection.* New York, Springer-Verlag, 1981, pp 63–74.
15. Jarrett A: Introduction: The permeability carrier. In Jarrett A (ed): *The Physiology and Pathophysiology of the Skin.* New York, Academic Press, 1980, vol 6, pp 2111–2114.
16. Potter B: The physiology of the skin. *Annu Rev Physiol* 28:159–177, 1966.
17. Pillsbury, DM, Heaton CL: *A Manual of Dermatology,* ed 2. Philadelphia, W.B. Saunders, 1980, pp 7 and 8.
18. DeLauney WE, Land WA: *Principles of Practice of Dermatology.* Sydney, Australia, Butterworths, 1978, p 8.
19. Nicoll PA, Cortese TA: The physiology of the skin. *Annu Rev Physiol* 34:177–205, 1972.
20. Allen JA, Armstrong JE, Roddie IC: The regional distribution of emotional sweating in man. *J Physiol* 235:749–759, 1975.
21. Kuno Y: *Human Perspiration.* Springfield, IL, Charles C Thomas, 1956, pp 141–156.
22. Greaves MC: Physiology of the skin. *J Invest Dermatol* 67:66–69, 1975.
23. Samman PD: Nail formation and some nail disorders. *J Soc Cosmet Chem* 23:405–413, 1972.
24. Runne U, Orfanos CE: The human nail. Structure, growth and pathological changes. *Curr Probl Dermatol* 9:102–149, 1981.
25. Worobec SM, Solomon LM: Structure and function of the skin. *Major Probl Clin Pediatr* 19:7–27, 1970.
26. Ganong W: *Medical Physiology,* ed 11. Los Altos, CA, Lange 1983, p 85.
27. Savin J: Itching. In Book A, Savin J (eds): *Recent Advances in Dermatology.* New York, Churchill Livingstone, 1980, vol 5, pp 228–230.
28. Brand PW: The insensitive foot. In Jahss MH (ed): *Disorders of the Foot.* Philadelphia, W.B. Saunders, 1982, vol 2, p 1266.
29. Spearman RIC: Structure and function of subcutaneous tissue. In Jarrett A (ed): *The Physiology and Pathophysiology of the Skin.* New York, Academic Press, 1982, vol 7, p 2255.
30. Burton AC: Special features of the circulation of the skin. In Montagna W, Ellis RA (eds): *Advances in the Biology of the Skin, Blood Vessels and Circulation.* Oxford, Pergamon, 1961, vol 2, pp 117–122.
31. Champion RH, Wilkenson DS: Disorders affecting blood vessels. In: Book A, Wilkenson DS, Ebling FJG (eds): *Textbook of Dermatology,* Philadelphia, F.A. Davis, 1968, p 397.
32. Montagna W, Parakkal PF: *Structure and Function of the Skin.* New York, Academic Press, 1974, p 151.
33. Conrad MC: *Functional Anatomy of the Circulation to the Lower Extremities with Color Atlas.* Chicago, Yearbook, 1971, pp 64–95.
34. Barnes RW, Thornhill B, Nix L, Rittgers S, Turley G: Prediction of amputation wound healing. Roles of Doppler ultrasound and digit photoplethysmography. *Arch Surg* 116:80–83, 1981.

CHAPTER 3

Nomenclature of Dermatohistopathology

DANIEL J. McCARTHY

General pathology has developed its own distinctive terminology. As dermatohistopathology developed as a distinct subspecialty, it, too, developed a nomenclature specific unto itself. It will be the intent of this discussion to make known this distinctive vocabulary. In making a pathologic analysis of human skin sections, the examiner should follow an intelligent progression based upon the functional integumentary elements present. The epidermodermal interface presents an especially logical point at which to begin. One can consider the strata basale, spinosum, granulosum, and corneum in order and then examine the pars papillaris and reticularis of the dermis which underlie the epidermis. The exception to this is the overriding presence of a tumor which dominates the field. Many criteria can be employed, but anthropometric anlaysis should be the first considered in evaluating integumentary pathology.

MEASUREMENTS RELATIVE TO THE SUPRAPAPILLARY STRATUM MALPIGHII

Mensuration of the epidermis is a quantitative entity based upon the relative thickness of the spinosal and cornified layers (1). *Acanthosis* is the relative thickening of prickle cells (stratum spinosum) (Fig. 3.1). The stratum granulosum above and the stratum basale below are constant, the latter being but a single row by definition. The term "relative" should be emphasized since the suprapapillary stratum Malpighii is normally less than 10 cell layers thick on the delicate skin of the dorsum of the foot, but averages up to a 10-fold greater thickness on the weight-bearing plantar surfaces of the foot (2).

In general terms acanthosis can be considered simply as epidermal hyperplasia. This needs to be contrasted with pseudoacanthosis, or better, epidermal hypertrophy in which the individual cells of the stratum spinosum have developed much larger than normal. In this instance, the increased dimension is not accomplished by the addition of cells but by the enlargement of relatively fewer prickle cells.

Conversely, hypoplasia or underdevelopment of prickle cells suggests atrophy of the Malpighiian layer. Such alterations are usually accompanied by the reduction of size and shape of rete ridges and the interdigitating dermal papillae.

Hypergranulosis is a multiplicity of cells of the stratum granulosum beyond the usual one or two rows of these deeply basophilic cells (3). Conversely, hypogranulosis is the reduction or even absence of these cells in skin cross sections. Such changes are not infrequently noted about the apex of nucleated tyloma and helomata. Indeed, both hypergranulosis and hypogranulosis can be occasionally related to the same lesion.

Hyperkeratosis characterizes the stratum corneum as being relatively thick. The corneum is usually composed of an amorphous cytoplasm without nuclei (4). This is the normal orthokeratotic condition in which the usual basket weave appearance of cells is maintained. However, if cells of the stratum corneum demonstrate remnants of pyknotic nuclei, the condition is referred to as parakeratosis (Fig. 3.2).

Hyperkeratosis may be expressed by the addition of many highly compressed cor-

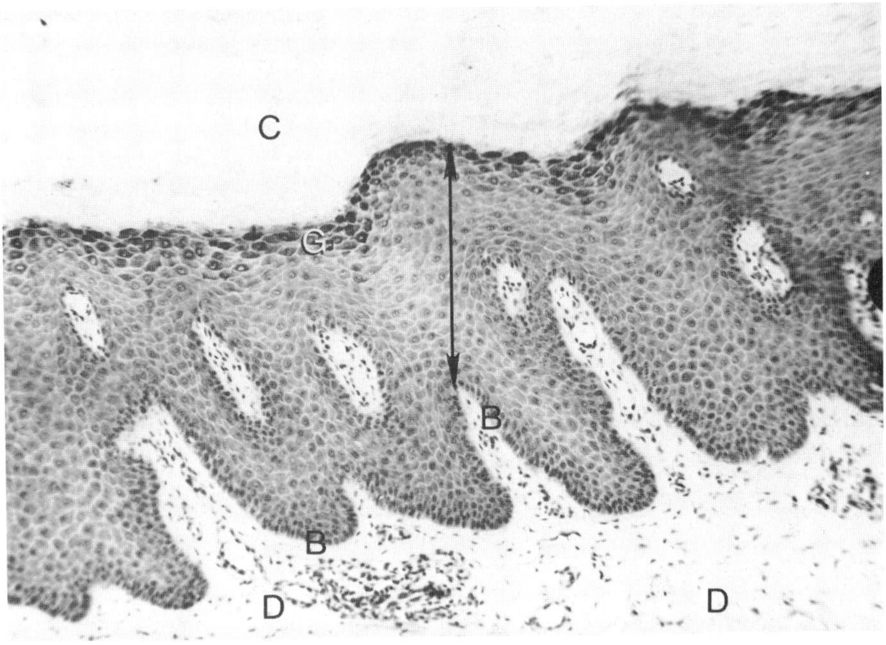

Figure 3.1. Acanthosis, the pathological increase of cells in the suprapapillary stratum Malpighii (*arrow*). Lightmicroscopy. *C*, stratum corneum; *G*, stratum granulosum; *B*, stratum basale; *D*, dermis.

neum cells, or they may be seen as in the normally lamellated condition of the stratum corneum in which individual cells are larger (1).

The quality of staining and differentiation between counterstaining in the processing of tissue slides is a highly variable laboratory process. However, relative judgments often need to be made, such as in determining intracellular edema of prickle cells, which is indicated by reduced stainability. Intracytoplasmic glycogen in spinosal cells also presents a lighter staining condition. Perinuclear halos resulting from retraction of cytoplasm about the nucleus during tissue processing is a fairly reliable indicator of intracellular edema, which is reflected by faint staining characteristics.

Intercellular edema or spongiosis (when extreme conditions exist) is characterized by widened intercellular spaces (Fig. 3.3). Under these conditions, desmosomes become especially apparent, and rupture of contiguous hemidesmosomes can occur. This phenomenon constitutes vesiculation of the stratum spinosum, which may be either diffuse or focal in distribution. Vesiculation and edema of individual cells may advance to form bullae which are gross skin manifestations (5).

The pathologist needs to localize cytological edema as being situated in either the dermis or epidermis. Apparent separation at the epidermodermal junction is most often subepidermal. Vesicles may be suprabasalar or subcorneal: More specifically, they can be characterized as being intragranular or intraspinosal.

Clefts are empty spaces without fluid which may exist either above or below the epidermodermal junction. More often, however, extracellular fluid is present. If masses of intercellular connections are lost or dissolved, or if cells are necrotized with the separation of whole sheets of cells within the spinosum, a condition of *acantholysis* is said to exist (Fig. 3.4). Flat, flaccid vesicles which result from acantholysis are called lacunae (6).

Epidermal exocytosis is the process by which inflammatory infiltrate cells migrate from the dermis into the epidermis through occasional interruptions of the basement membrane. Lymphocytes, neutrophiles, and eosinophiles migrate through the distended intercellular spaces. Polymorphonuclear leucocytes may aggregate as spongiform pustules in the suprapapillary stratum Malpighii or in the stratum corneum (as microabscesses of Munro).

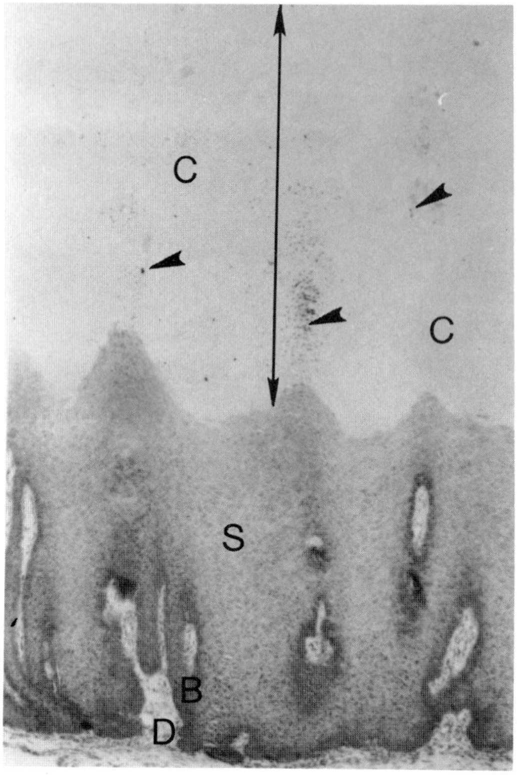

Figure 3.2. Hyperkeratosis is a particularly significant podiatric finding frequently resulting from increased use of the part. In pedal lesions, it is frequently expressed in terms of compression of cells, in addition to being thickened overall. *Arrow* indicates the thickness of the stratum corneum (*C*). *Arrowheads* indicate regions of parakeratosis. *S*, stratum spinosum; *B*, stratum basale; *D*, dermis.

Basal cells are those cells immediately under the inductive influence of the dermis as mediated through the basement membrane. They are committed to self-replication or pass upward as protein synthesizing keratinocytes. The latter will ultimately cornify, dehydrate, and desquamate. This activity, however, must be one in which a regulated biosynthetic process is clearly definable under normal circumstances. Under alternate inductive influences, cells undergo different lines of maturation. The term "basal cell" should be restricted to its occurrence in the epidermis or as the adnexal basal cells. Immature cells or benign tumors are best characterized as basaloid. For this reason, tumor cells of epitheliomas are more correctly called basalioma cells (1).

Basal cells of the epidermis are the usual sites of mitosis. In hyperplastic epidermis, mitosis may be observed above the stratum basale. The term stratum germinativum best describes the expansion or epidermal mitosis beyond the basal layer. In podiatry, such occurrences are common in verrucae plantaris or psoriatic plaques of the lower extremities.

Hyalinization is a pathological state in which contiguous basal cells undergo liquefaction degeneration (7). Subepidermal clefts which parallel the location of the lost basal layer are common. Such occurrences may be diffuse or focal. Basal cells are not identifiable at sites of proliferation and invasion by tumor cells in squamous cell carcinoma. Similarly, they may not be in evidence in lichen planus and discoid lupus erythematosus.

Normal skin demonstrates dendritic elements of melanocytes as they interdigitate among cells of the stratum basale. The subject of melanoma will be dealt with later

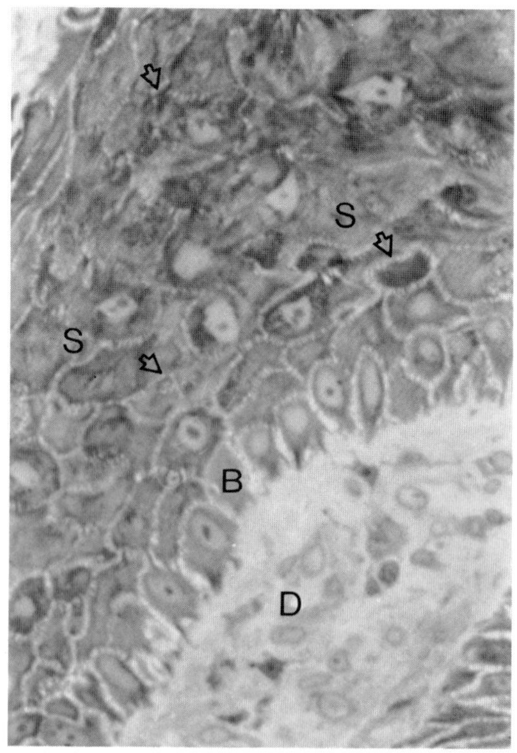

Figure 3.3. Widened intercelluair spaces may be an expression of intercellular edema or spongiosis. Desmosomes (*arrows*) are especially apparent, as they are expanded between cells. *D*, dermis; *S*, stratum spinosum; *B*, stratum basale.

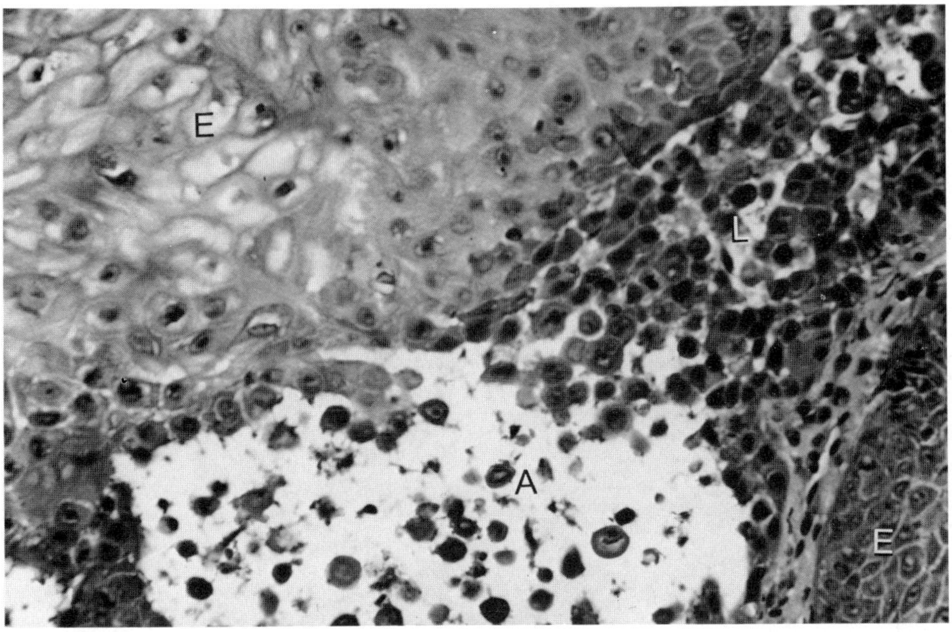

Figure 3.4. Acantholysis may exist between cells or sheets of cells within the stratum spinosum. Lacunae (*L*) are flaccid vesicles which result from acantholysis. *E*, epidermal cells; *A*, region of acantholysis.

in this book. In dermatosis, however, postinflammatory melanization or pigmentation may occur in the subepidermal region. Clumped melanin in a variety of sizes and shapes is most often found phagocytosed by macrophages or melanophages in such instances.

PLEOMORPHISM IN EPIDERMAL CELLS

Normal keratinocytes have predictable morphology and measurement. In disease, these parameters may change, and descriptive terms are needed to identify them. As is often the case, semantics and perception of biological phenomenon change with time, leaving confusion in the wake.

Anaplasia, for example, is meant to convey the notion that malignant cells are a reversion from typical cells to atypical embryonic-like forms. Cancer cells, however, are irregularly formed and are hyperchromatic (8). They have no potential beyond forming other cancer cells and have no relationship to multipotent embryonic cells.

Dysplasia is an appropriate term to designate cells having poor development, hyperchromasia, and irregularities of size and shape. However, the term leaves much to be desired in terms of semantic precision.

Keratinocytes are epidermal cells having clearly defined biosynthetic roles in the production of the protein keratin. These biochemical events are morphologically identifiable. Occasionally, however, one cell (or even groups of cells) may become separated from the normal directive influences and proceed (however incompletely) to undergo a degree of keratinization (Fig. 3.5). Such cells are said to be dyskeratotic. Dyskeratosis has been differentiated by some as being of either benign or malignant nature, but such a differentiation is not helpful.

Basement Membrane

Normal epidemis, glands, and hair follicles have clearly definable basement membranes. Its presence is best demonstrated by periodic acid-Schiff (PAS) stain as a deep pink or reddish line. Transmission electron microscopy clearly defines the structure, which is formed by contributions from both dermis and epidermis. The basement membrane is significant in diagnosis and prognosis in dermatologic oncology (9).

Precancerous keratosis and malignant

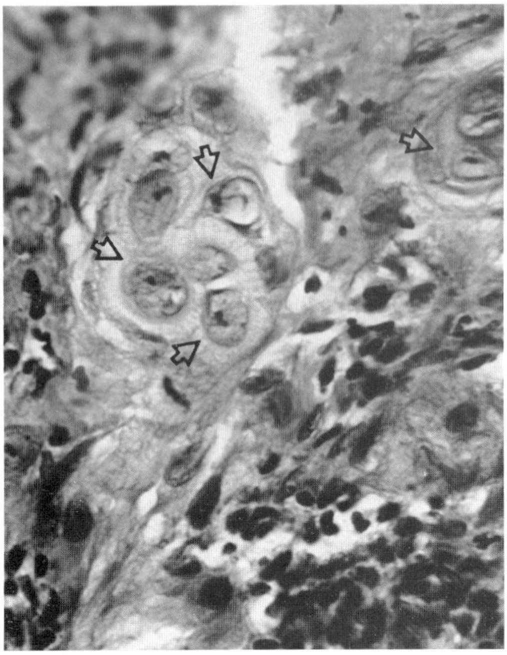

Figure 3.5. Dyskeratosis among keratinocytes of the human skin (*arrows*).

skin diseases such as squamous cell carcinoma demonstrate a loss or breakage away of portions of the basement membrane as the disease process becomes invasive (Fig. 3.6). Often times, this event is accompanied by attemps at reduplication of the lost basement membrane. Squamous cell carcinoma in situ and basal cell carcinomas (which do not metastasize) have intact basement membranes are are not true malignancies.

Basal cell carcinomas, however, often demonstrate locally aggressive behavior, even to the extent of encroaching upon bone. For this reason, this condition is traditionally included among epidermal malignancies.

Papillary Dermis

The pars papillaris of the dermis is more frequently involved in disease than the pars reticularis. Separation of dermis from epidermis best demonstrates the finger-like nature of the dermal papillae. They may be characterized as narrow, wide, long, short, branched, and even totally lacking if the skin is atrophic. Familiarity with the norm is necessary in order to establish the pathological condition when describing tissue sections. Such morphologic characteristics vary from location to location within the same individual.

Papillomatosis is a descriptive term generally designating a condition in which the dermal papillae have become so elongated as to elevate that portion of the skin above the contiguous normal skin (Fig. 3.7).

Light microscopy may reveal abnormal amounts of foreign substances including amyloid, hyaline, and melanin (1). Capillaries within papillae may be characterized as engorged, hyalinized, tufted, or tortuous. The dense region immediately beneath the papillae (subpapillary layer) is highly reflective of disease processes.

Blood vessels may demonstrate puffy endothelia, or they may appear atrophic. Their adventitia may be thickened, and vessel walls can be hyalinized.

The nature and degree of inflammatory infiltrate needs to be recognized. Edema of a perivascular or diffuse nature can be noted (1). Collagen of the subpapillary layer is usually more finely divided than in the reticular dermis. In disease, it may be even

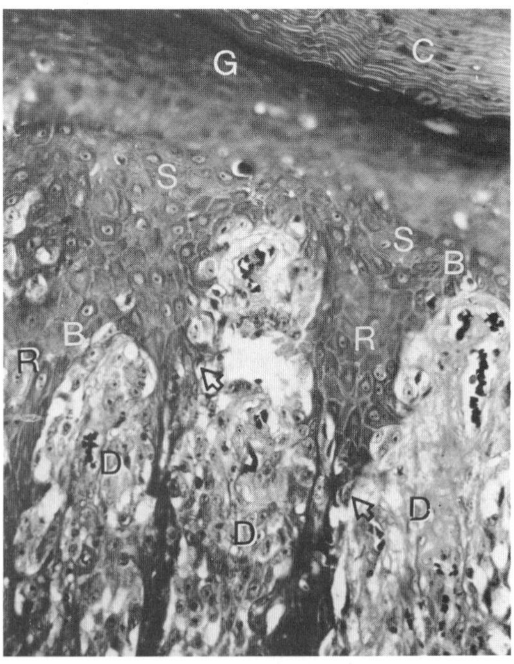

Figure 3.6. Interruption of the basement membrane in human epidermis which occurs as a disease process becomes invasive into the dermis and deeper tissues (*arrows*). *C*, stratum corneum; *G*, stratum granulosum; *B*, stratum basale; *D*, dermis; *R*, rete ridges; *S*, stratum spinosum.

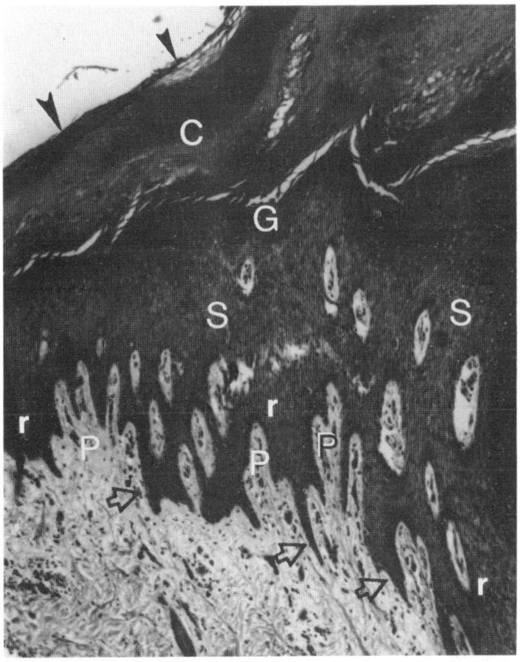

Figure 3.7. Papillomatosis of human skin with elongated dermal papillae (*arrows*). Such hyperkeratotic changes usually elevates the free surface of the skin (*arrowheads*). *C*, stratum corneum; *G*, stratum granulosum; *S*, stratum spinosum; *P*, dermal papillae; *r*, rete ridges.

more finely divided by edema, or it may be more compacted so as to appear sclerosed.

Pigmentary incompetence is a term used to indicate the occurrence of melanophages in the absence of epidermal pigment. Pigments such as hemosiderin and melanin are frequently associated with macrophages. The purpuric condition is identified when disintegrating red blood cells have traumatically extravased through capillary walls and hemosiderin is deposited (11).

Lymphocytes, polymorphonuclear leucocytes, and most other migratory cells in small numbers in the pars papillaris have no particular diagnostic significance. However, in the clinical suspicion of mastocytosis, a small increase in the number of mast cells may confirm the diagnosis.

Reticular Dermis

The pars reticularis is not as commonly affected by dermatoses as the pars papillaris. It is normally more compact and blood vessels are of larger caliber than is the case for the papillary dermis. Collagenic fibers also are broader, more compact and more coarse. A variety of inflammatory infiltrative cells are encountered in diseases involving the reticular dermis, particulary if adnexal glands or hair follicles are involved, or if granulomatous inflammatory changes occur (Fig. 3.8).

Histiocytic Infiltrate

Histiocytes are phagocytic cells which are specifically named for substances they ingest. For example, they are foam cells if fats are engulfed and they have a frothy appearance. If melanin is phagocytosed, they are termed melanophages. The designation of epithelioid cells is given to histiocytes having large, homogeneous cell bodies. Tubercles are nodular aggregates of epithelioid histiocytes (1).

Plasma cells have large eccentrically placed nuclei surrounded by light-staining paranuclear halos. The cytoplasm of the ovoid cell is basophilic and is neither granular nor metachromatic.

Multinucleate giant cells form by the fusion of a number of histiocytes (12). They demonstrate several morphologic variations (Fig. 3.9). If nuclei are arranged in horseshoe configuration, they are of Langhan's type. Foreign body giant cells demonstrate irregularly arranged nuclei. "Touton type" giant cells have circularly arranged nuclei and a foamy cytoplasm.

The normal fibrillar organization of the pars reticularis needs to be understood before pathologic analysis can be made. This

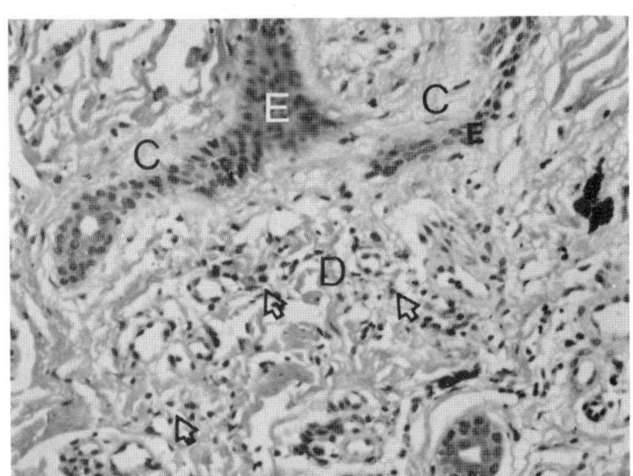

Figure 3.8. Inflammatory infiltrate of the round cell type in the dermis (*D*) of human skin (*arrows*). *E*, epidermis; *C*, collagenic fibers.

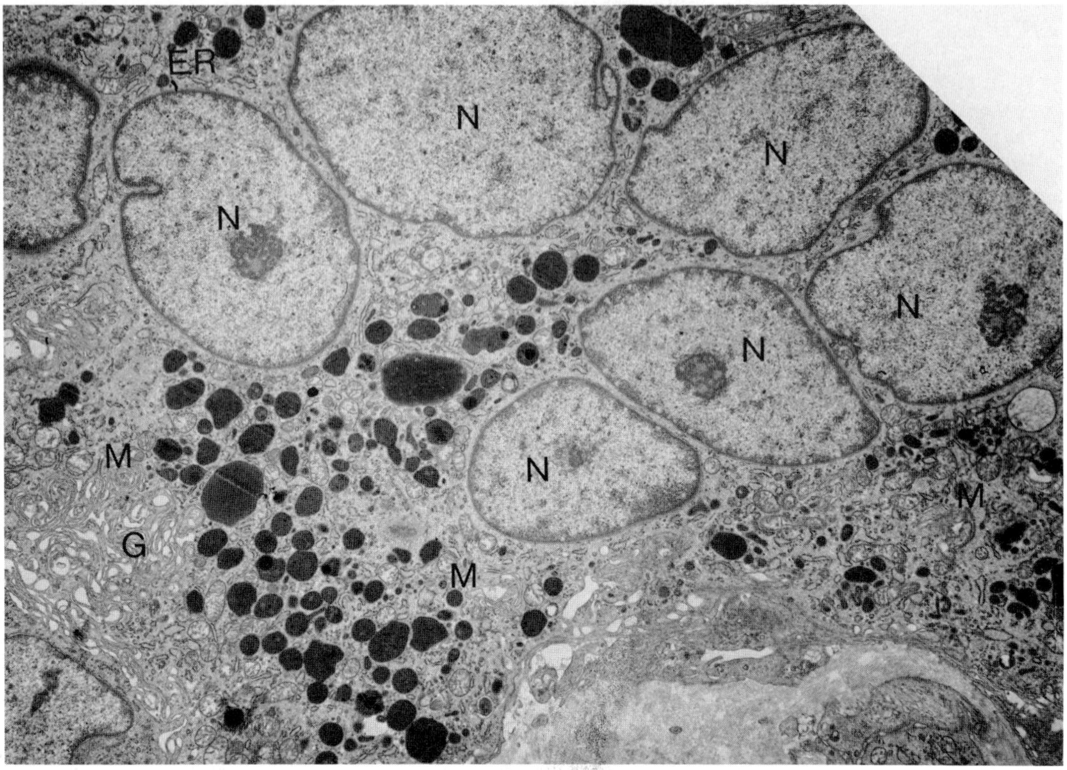

Figure 3.9. Multinucleated giant cells as demonstrated by transmission electron microscopy. Many nuclei (*N*) are situated within a single cell. *G*, Golgi apparatus; *M*, mitochondria; *ER*, rough endoplasmic reticulum.

is difficult since the region varies not only in terms of age, sex, race, and genetic constitution, but also within any given individual (1). Sclerosis is said to occur whenever collagenic fibers become tighlty compacted. Conversely, lymphedema or myxedema may split collagenic fibers and fascicles, leaving many spaces. Elastic fiber fragmentation is also a pathologic finding, but this feature is often mimicked by errors in specimen preparation. Moreover, special stains such as acid-orcein and Giemsa are often needed for the best appreciation of reticular elastic fibers. Acid orcein stains the elastic fibers, while Giemsa is the counterstain. Significance may be attributed to alterations of elastic fiber morphology only if, in addition to fragmentation curling, roughness or uneveness of their structure is encountered.

Complete absence of elastic fibers is a good clue to past granulomatous or inflammatory processes (1). This is true because elastic fibers are not easilly restored by the body's normal reparative processes.

ULTRASTRUCTURAL NOMENCLATURE

The use of traditional light microscopy in pathology will never be replaced, and terms associated with this level of magnification need to be understood in order to comprehend tissue reports from the laboratory. For several decades now, however, transmission electron microscopy has come into increasingly wider use by pathologists. Consequently, medical schools are presently emphasizing ultrastructural anatomy in response to this greater emphasis: Ultrastructure encompasses the subcellular levels of morphology.

The process of cutaneous keratinization is a series of morphologically identifiable biochemical events. To know and understand the involved terminology is to know and understand the process of keratinization of the human skin as well as to have an appreciation of its ultrastructural characteristics.

The dermis contains many structures,

including the secretory portions of glands, hair roots and associated structures, blood vessels, nerves etc. The ultrastructure involved with these structures is extremely detailed and need not be presented in discussions at this level. The reader is referred to such texts as *Atlas of Human Histology and Ultrastructure* (Mathews LL, Martin JH: Philadelphia, Lea & Febiger, 1971) for a basic review of these topics.

A glossary of 40 terms common to cutaneous ultrastructure follows in alphabetical order. An understanding of these terms will assist in understanding ultrastructure as it is revealed by transmission electron microscopy in several of the chapters to follow in this text.

Basal Cell: Those cells situated immediately above the dermis and basement membrane of the epidermis. They are of low columnar type and have a large ovoid nucleus and relatively little cytoplasm, and fewer subcellular organelles.

Basement Membrane: A PAS-positive sheet lining the interface between the dermis below and the basal cells of the epidermis above. It is formed by the basal cells over a fibrillar mat contributed by the dermis.

Chromatin: A granular appearing basophilic material making up the bulk of the nucleus proper. It is rich in DNA, but contains basic protiens and histones, and has a small amount of RNA as well (Fig. 3.10).

Corneum Cell: The most external cell of the epidermis. It is essentially homogeneous and has no nucleus or other evidence of cytopalsmic organelles. Normally such cells are arranged in basket weave order and demonstrate a fine fibrillar matrix.

Cytoplasm: The colloidal contents of the cell, excluding the nucleus: It is made up of a matrix in which formed structures called organelles, along with certain inclusions, can be found.

Dermis: That portion of the skin underlying the epidermis. It is made up of a matrix of ground substance in which collagenic, elastic, and reticular fibers are present. The dermis contains blood vessels, nerves, and secretory portions of glands, and is host to several types of migratory cells.

Desmosomes: Desmosomes are made up of the association of two electron-dense spots or macula. These two bodies occur on either side of "tight junctions" made up of plasma membranes of adjacent keratinocytes. The term "desmos" suggests "fast bonding" of two hemidesmosomes, the term given to the electron-dense spot or macula. There is no actual interconnection between keratinocytes, but conventional light microscopy gave that apperance, and these spinous processes were incorrectly called intercellular bridges in the old histological literature (Fig. 3.11).

Endoplasmic Reticulum (Rough): Rough Endoplasmic Reticulum (RER) are hollow membranous tubules which weave about in the cytoplasm of cells. They have specialized modifications such as bladder-like vesicles, and flattened vesicles or cisternae. Rough endoplasmic reticulum is so called because of the presence of many ribosomes in aggregate along its inner core. Protein synthesis is associated with this organelle (Fig. 3.12).

Endoplasmic Reticulum (Smooth): Smooth endoplasmic reticulum is structurally similar to rough endoplasmic reticulum, except that it is lacking in ribosomal population.

Fibroblast: A fibroblast is the ubiquitous cell of connective tissues and of the dermis of the skin. It is seen as spindle shaped in light microscopy, but transmission electron microscopy reveals it to be stellate with numerous cytoplasmic processes. Its nucleus is pleomorphic (many shaped), and its cytoplasm is rich in organelles. It synthesizes the ground substance of the dermis as well as its fibrillar constituents and is frequently seen surrounded by the typically periodically banded collagenic fibers. This cell is also implicated in the elaboration of the "dermal influencing factor," which is an initiator of epidermal cell mitosis (Fig. 3.12).

Fibrocyte: A more mature form of the fibroblast usually described as having reduced biosynthetic capablilities.

Filaments: A general term for subcellular thread-like cytoplasmic structures. In aggregate, they become known as fibrils, which in turn aggregate to form fibers.

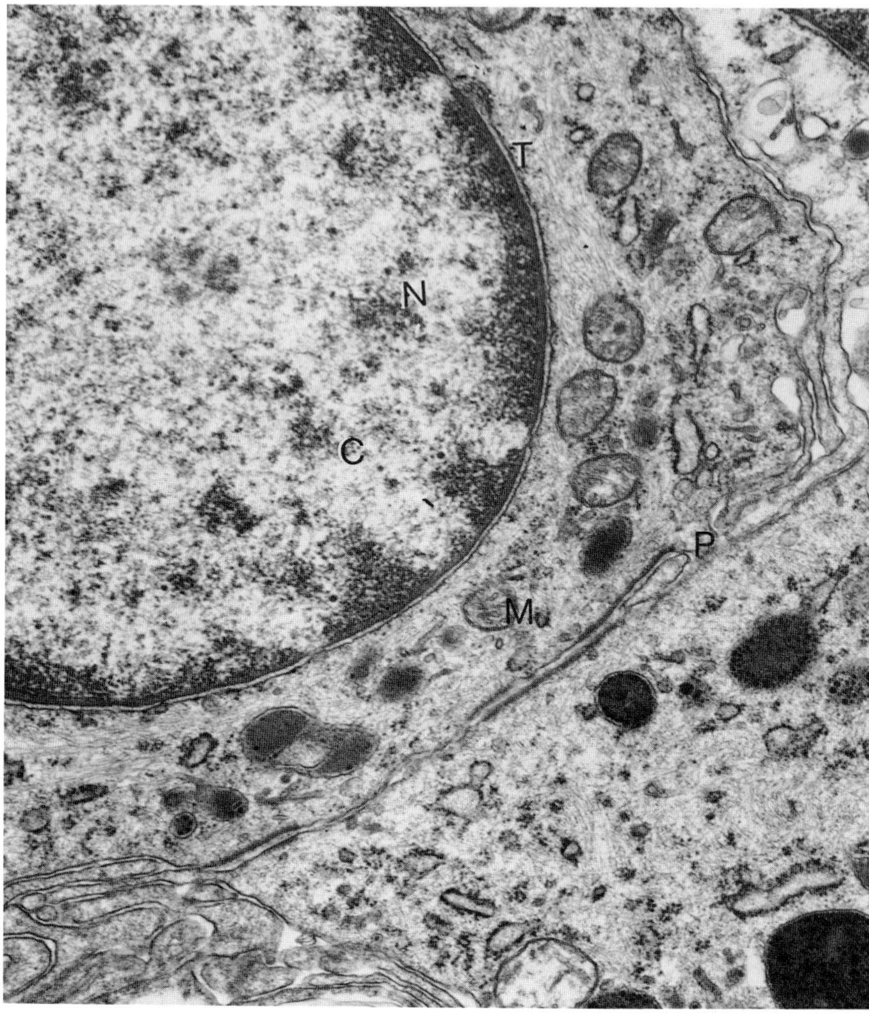

Figure 3.10. Nucleus of cells contains chromatin and is enclosed within a nuclear membrane and may contain an electron-dense nucleolus. Transmission electron microscopy. *T*, trilamellar nuclear membrane; *N*, cell nucleus; *C*, chromatin; *P*, plasma membrane; *M*, mitochondria.

Granulosum Cell: The cell of the stratum granulosum. Such cells are deeply basophilic due to the presence of keratohyaline granules which enmesh with tonofilaments as the process of keratinization is completed and the cells move outward to form the stratum corneum. Much enzymatic activity is associated with granulosum cells.

Golgi Apparatus: Smooth-walled membranous tubules (saccules) which appear to be stacked one upon the other much like hot cakes. They are usually situated between the cell apex and a field of rough endoplasmic reticulum. This organelle modifies proteins synthesized by the rough endoplasmic reticulum, often incorporating carbohydrate materials for subsequent excretion of the substance by means of vesicles (Fig. 3.12).

Ground Substance: PAS-positive mucopolysaccharide material which provides a substrate for collagenic, elastic, and reticular fibers. All of these structures are associated with the biosynthetic activities of the fibroblast (Fig. 3.12).

Hemidesmosome: Those electron-dense spots or maculae occurring at tight junctions of certain cells: In the integumentary system, they occur in the prickle cell layer,

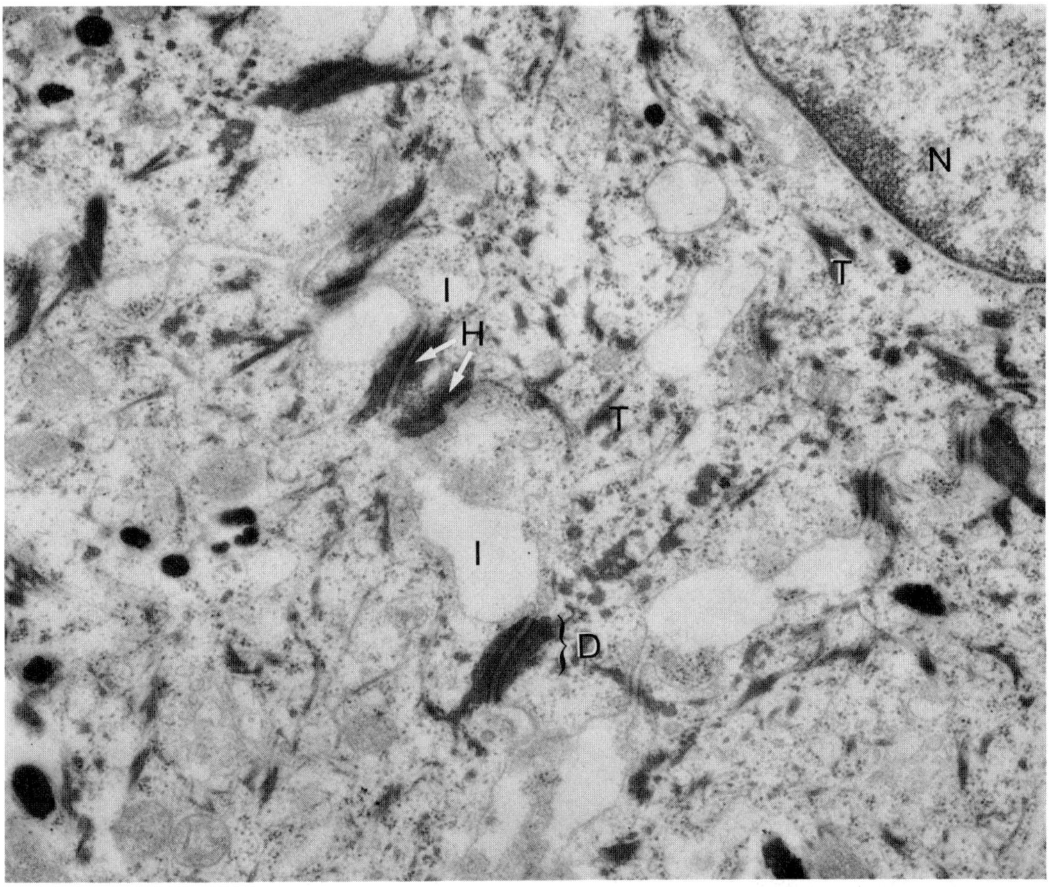

Figure 3.11. Desmosomes are composed of paired hemidesmosomes. In disease they may be dislodged into widened irregular intercellular spaces. Transmission electron microscopy. *N*, cell nucleus; *T*, tonofibril; *I*, intercellular space(s); *H*, hemidesmosomes; *D*, desmosomes.

providing those cells with their spinous appearance. They normally occur in pairs between adjacent keratinocytes at their respective plasma membranes and together constitute the organelle called the desmosome (Fig. 3.11).

Inclusions: Those substances which are found within, but are not part of the cytoplasm of cells. They are usually stored food such as glycogen or pigments (Fig. 3.12).

Intercellular Space: That real or potential space between plasma membranes of adjacent cells. Intercellular spaces are frequently greatly widened and distorted in disease proceses (Fig. 3.11).

Keratin: That tough fibrous protein which is produced as the principal biosynthetic activity of keratinocytes. The stratum corneum represents the highest concentration of keratin and it represents the completion of the process of keratinization (Fig. 3.13).

Keratinocyte: Those epidermal cells committed to the biosynthetic process of keratinization.

Langerhans Cell: A dendritic cell of the monocyte line previusly thought to have been of neural crest origin bearing a general resemblance to a melanocyte. Originally, these cells were thought to have been aged melanocytes. They demonstrate the typical cigar-shaped organelle called the Langerhans granule. Like melanocytes, they become closely associated with the basal cells at the epidermal-dermal junction. Their functions are not well understood at this time, but they may be a type of macrophage.

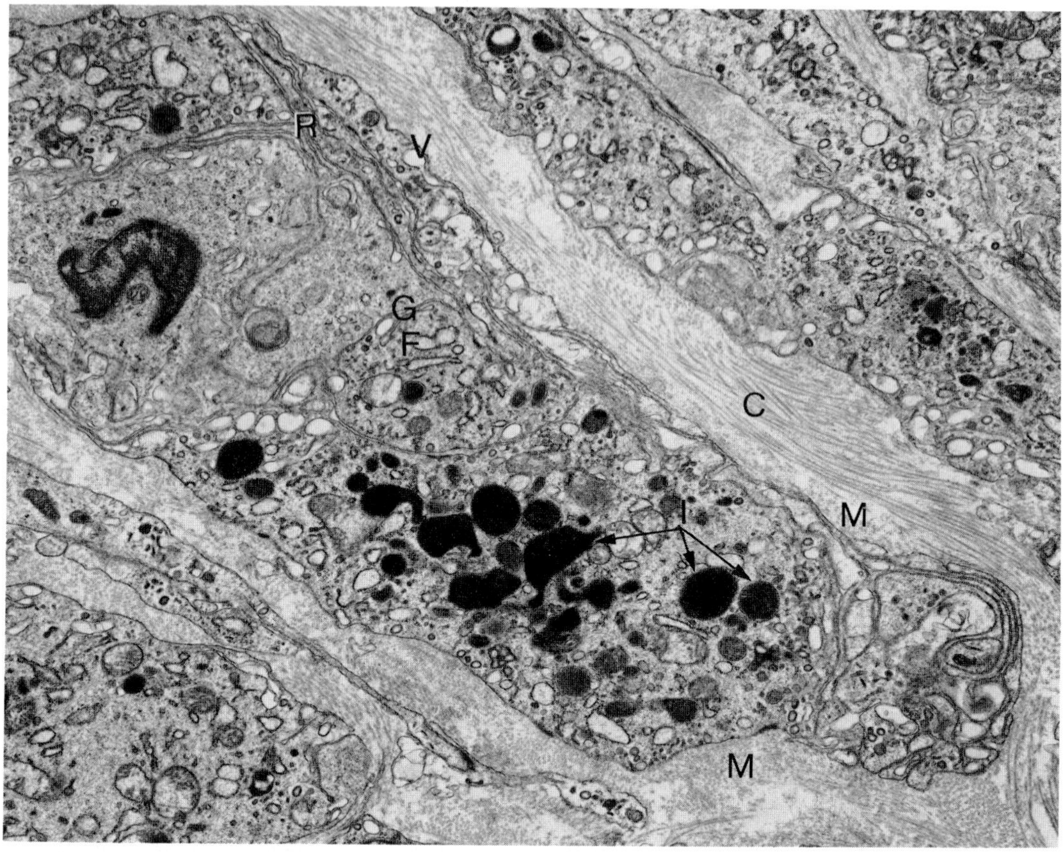

Figure 3.12. Fibroblasts synthesize ground substance to form a dermal matrix as well as collagenic, reticular, and elastic fibers. The cytoplasm of synthesizing cells is rich in endoplasmic reticulum. Inclusion bodies such as glycogen frequently are also found within these cells. Vesicles move synthesized substances into the extracellular environment. Transmission electron microscopy. *R*, rough endoplasmic reticulum; *V*, vesicles; *G*, Golgi apparatus; *F*, fibroblast; *C*, collagenic fibers; *M*, ground substances; *I*, inclusion bodies.

Lysosome: Those membrane-bound organelles which contain hydrolytic enzymes or hydrolases. These structures are usually round or ovoid and measure about 0.5 μm in diameter.

Melanin: That pigment which provides color to the skin and its adnexa. These yellow, brown, and black granules are synthesized by melanocytes which pass the pigment into adjacent epidermal cells through their dendritic processes.

Melanophage: A histiocyte committed to engulfing melanocytes.

Melanosome: Those subcellular organelles of melanocytes which have completed the process of melanin synthesis. Such organelles exist initially as premelanosomes which are ovoid structures having varying degrees or concentrations of tyrosinase-rich electron-dense granules.

Membrane-coating Granules: Those subcellular organelles having a lamellar structure of alternating electron-dense and electron-light bands with diameter or about 2 μm. These organelles are double-membrane bound and form vesicles which extrude their contents into the intercellular spaces of the outer stratum spinosus. This material is PAS-positive and is thought to provide adherence between cells. This organelle is also known as the Odland body and lamellar granule.

Mitochondria: Those trilamellar subcellular organelles which are oval or elongate and which demonstrate ladder-like parallel cristae in the central inner portions. These

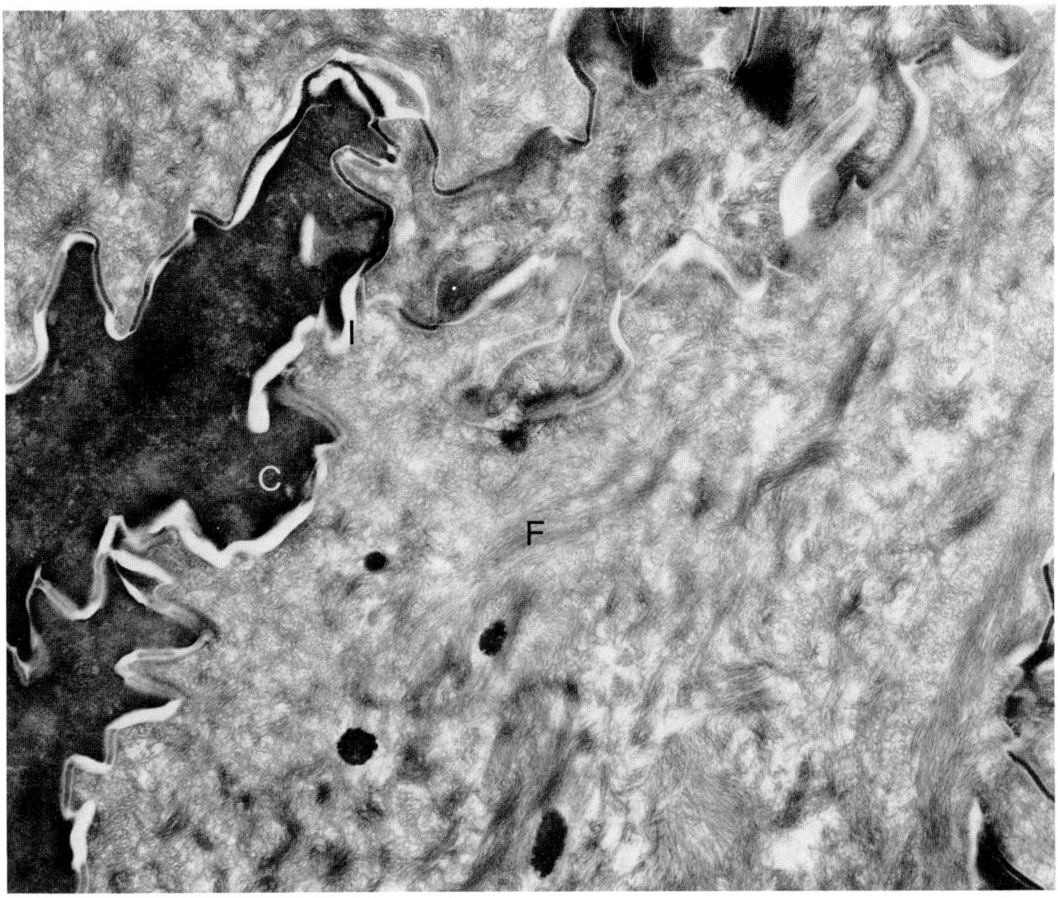

Figure 3.13. The cells of the stratum corneum are somewhat homogeneous but have a sulfur-rich matrix in which are embedded many fine fibrils which are sulfur-poor. Transmission electron microscopy. *I*, intercellular space; *C*, cell of the stratum corneum; *F*, fibrils of the cells of the stratum corneum.

cristae are the locations for processes involving oxidative phosphorylization. This organelle, therefore, is involved in the production of intracellular energy (Fig. 3.14).

Nuclear Membrane: The trilamellar envelope which surrounds the nucleus of all cells. It has an inner electron-dense, a middle electron-light, and an outer electron-dense layer. The nuclear membrane has pores through which directive influences generated within the nucleus are transmitted to the cytoplasm (Fig. 3.10).

Nucleus: The basophilic center of cell life enclosed within the nuclear membrane composed in the main of chromatin. Chemically, it is composed for the most part by deoxyribonucleic acid (DNA), but it also has a smaller amount of ribonucleic acids (RNA). The nucleus governs the replicative and biosynthetic activities of cells (Fig. 3.10).

Odland Body: Synonymous with membrane-coating granule or lamellar granule.

Organelles (Little Organs): Intracytoplasmic subcellualr structures by which essential metabolic functions are accomplished. Included are such membrane bound structures as plasma membranes, mitochondria, rough and smooth endoplasmic reticulum, Golgi apparatus, lysosomes, and coated vesicles. Nonmembrane-bound organelles include free ribosomes, microtubules, centrioles, cilia, flagella, filaments, and fibrils.

Plasma Membrane: The trilamellar outer investment of cells having a thickness

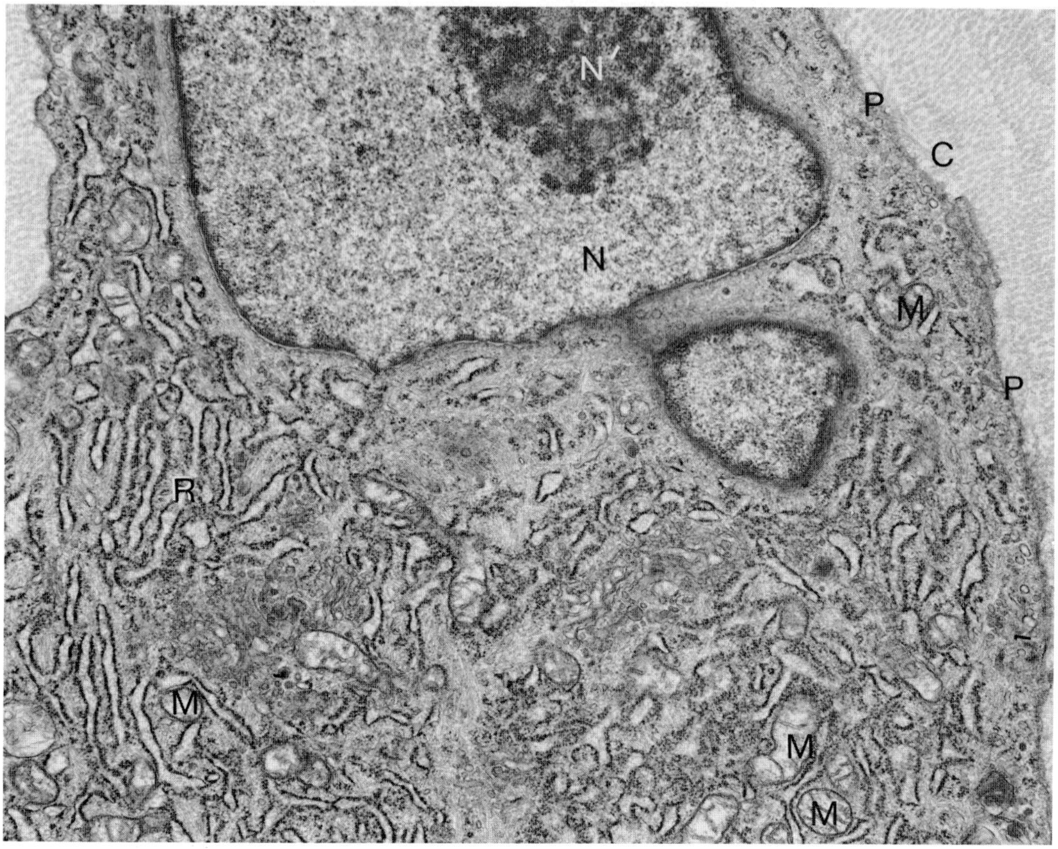

Figure 3.14. Mitochondria are the energy source for intracellular metabolism. Transmission electron microscopy. *N′*, nucleolus; *P*, plasma membrane of the cell; *C*, collagen; *N*, nucleus; *M*, mitochondria; *R*, rough endoplasmic reticulum.

of about 95 Å. Plasma membranes are separated by real or potential intercellular spaces (Fig. 3.14).

Premelanosome: Subcellular organelles of melanocytes which are in some stage of production of the pigment melanin. Premelanosomes represent all particulate stages of maturization of this particular organelle before and after melanin biosynthesis is initiated.

Ribosome (Free): Nonmembrane-bound organelles of cells having a diameter of about 150 Å. They are electron-dense aggregates of ribonucleic acids (RNA). Ribosomes are formed of two subunits in the nucleolus of the nucleus: The organelle is often found free in the cytoplasm, and it also lines the endoplasmic reticulum, giving it its rough appearance.

Spinosal Cell: Cells of the prickle cell layer or stratum spinosum of the epidermis. Desmosomes are placed periodically about the periphery of adjacent cells, giving them a spinous appearance. The nuclei of such cells become progressively smaller as the outer free surface of skin is approached, and their cytoplasm is more extensive than in lower layers. These cells also become more squamous or flattened peripherally.

Tonofilaments: Those nonmembrane bound thread-like and sulfur-poor organelles within the cytoplasm of keratinocytes. They are important in the process of keratinization and enmesh with keratohyaline granules in the stratum granulosum. They swing perinuclearly and converge upon hemidesmosomes to form the tonofilament-desmosome-complex (TDC) (Fig. 3.15).

Vacuoles: Any small space or cavity formed within the protoplasm of cells. In

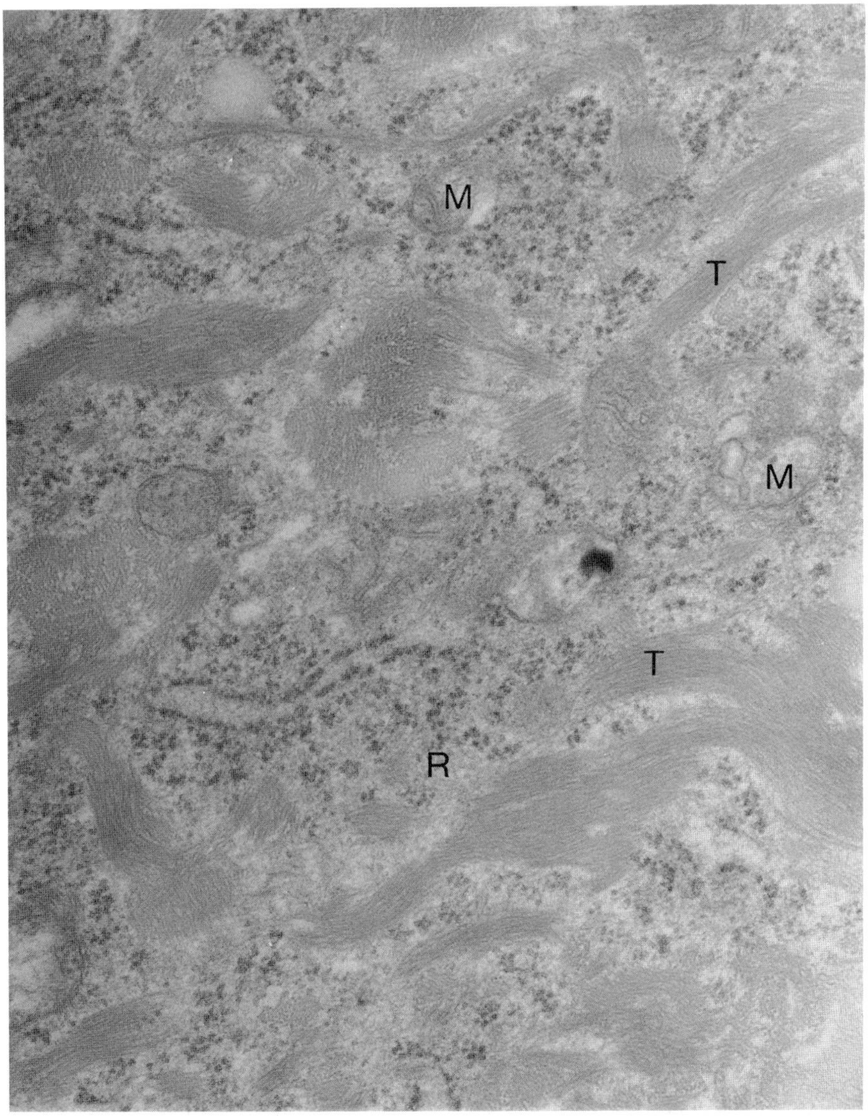

Figure 3.15. Tonofilaments are nonmembrane-bound cytoplasmic organelles important to the process of keratinization. Transmission electron microscopy. *M*, mitochondria; *T*, tonofilament detail; *R*, free ribosomal population.

epidermal cells, they are membrane bound intracytoplasmic spaces of unknown origin and function. It is postulated that they arise from extensive invaginations of the plasma membranes, having engulfed materials from the extracellular spaces.

Vesicles: Small subcellular membrane bound sacs or bladders which may engulf cytoplasmic particles. Vesicles are implicated in the processes of exocytosis and pinocytosis (Fig. 3.12).

References

1. Pinkus H, Mehregan: *A Guide to Dermatohistopathology*, ed 3. New York, Appleton-Century-Crofts, 1984.
2. McCarthy DJ, Habowsky JEJ: Histochemistry and anthropometric analysis of heloma durum. *J Am Podiatry Assoc* 65:4–18, 1975.
3. Van Scott EJ, Edel TM: Kinetics of hyperplasia in psoriasis. *Arch Dermatol* 88:373–379, 1963.
4. Matoltsy AG, Parakkal PF: *Keratinization (in) Ultrastructure of Normal and Abnormal*

Skin, A. S. Zelickson (ed). Philadelphia, Lea & Febiger, 1967.
5. Yale I: *Podiatric Medicine*, ed 2. Baltimore, Williams & Wilkins, 1980.
6. Pearson RW: Studies in the pathogenesis of epidermolysis bullosa. *J Invest Dermatol* 39:551–559, 1962.
7. Sutton RL Jr: *Disease of the Skin*, ed 11. St. Louis, C.V. Mosby, 1956.
8. Ruben P, Bakemeier RF: *Clinical Oncology*. Rochester, NY, University of Rochester Press, 1983.
9. Brody I: Contributions to the histogenesis of basal cell carcinoma. *J Ultrastruct Res* 33:149–156, 1978.
10. Robbins SL: *Pathologic Basis of Disease*. Philadelphia, W.B. Saunders, 1974.
11. Roenick HH: *Office Dermatology*. Baltimore, Williams & Wilkins, 1981.
12. Ham WW: *Histology*, ed 7. Philadelphia, J.B. Lippincott, 1974.

CHAPTER 4

Dermatologic Diagnostic Techniques

DANIEL J. McCARTHY

Accurate diagnosis of dermatological conditions requires that a careful patient history be taken and an adequate physical examination be performed. In this respect, dermatology does not differ from any other medical or surgical specialty.

Systemic diseases may produce dermatological symptoms, and blood chemistry, serology, and blood counts may be required to properly evaluate the condition. These contingencies have been dealt with in other chapters. It is impossible to deal with all possibilities and not become encyclopedic. Rather, it will be the intent of the present discussion to deal with those diagnostic procedures that are commonly involved in the making of diagnoses of localized skin diseases of the lower extremity. These include biopsy, skin testing, potassium hydroxide preparations for the detection of fungal elements, etc. Additionally, brief attention will be given to some newer concepts which have only recently appeared in the literature.

The practice of podiatric medicine has developed a high degree of sophistication in recent years, and the range and complexity of lesions treated by the podiatrist has increased perceptively. This is particularly true of the more unusual neoplastic occurrences of the feet and legs. It follows that the precise diagnosis of many pedal lesions relies heavily upon laboratory identification. Therefore, it will be the intent of this chapter (in part) to present the fundamentals of the techniques of biopsy and to discuss areas having potential for the introduction of misleading artifacts into tissues under examination.

SKIN BIOPSY

Biopsies of skin usually are obtained by excision, curettage, or dermal punch methods. Occasionally, scrapings or smears may be useful in assessing bullous or vesicular lesions.

Excisional biopsies, as they occur in podiatric medicine, are usually part of a planned surgical procedure for which anesthesia and surgical skin preparation are part of the operation.

Punch biopsies may be taken from selected areas in and about the lesion which have been gently cleansed with alcohol sponges, taking care not to disturb crusts or scales which may aid in diagnosis.

If nerve block anesthesia is not convenient, infiltration anesthesia is acceptable using a 26- or 30-gauge needle. Epinephrine (1:100,000) is rarely contraindicated as a hemostatic agent for these purposes. Unfortunately, the various commercially available anesthetic jet devices should not be used in and about the tissues to be biopsied since vacuolization and other artifacts can be introduced into these tissues.

Excisional biopsies, as applied in podiatric practice, usually involve conjoined and elliptical incisions which include the lesion in toto along with a narrow margin of surrounding normal tissue. It should, however, be noted that it is technically more simple and more cosmetically acceptable to enclose the lesion with diamond-shaped or polygonal incisions with sutures coapting the elongate parallel borders (1). Curling of excised tissue may produce a pedunculated or elevated appearance. This can be avoided by placing the specimen dermal side down on a piece of porous cardboard.

Ideally, if curettage is elected, the lesion should be "shelled out" as a single mass if it is at all possible. If this is possible, orientation of the specimen by the technician is more likely to be accurate. Obviously, tissues should be obtained prior to electrodesiccation or the application of other destructive modalities to the lesion.

Tzanck smears of vesiculobullous foot lesions are procedures which should be employed more frequently by podiatric physicians (2). One need only make an incision of the bulla and gently scrape the floor of the lesion, allowing for the collection of materials on the blade of the instrument. The scrapings are then spread evenly over a glass slide. After fixing the slide by dipping it in a 95% aqueous ethanol solution, the smear can be stained for 3 min with a few drops of Giemsa solution. The slide is then rinsed in distilled water, air dried, and cover slipped for microscopic examination.

Dermal punch biopsies have become increasingly popular among podiatrists in recent years. Disposable punches, packaged sterile and ready for immediate use, are presently available in varying diameters. This writer prefers to use 1.0- and 2.0-mm research biopsy tools of high quality stainless steel incorporated into a sterile pack especially prepared for biopsy (Fig. 4.1, *arrow*). For general diagnostic purposes, most practitioners prefer larger punches, however. Such packs are prepared with the intent of accommodating most any eventuality which might require the surgeon to attempt more complex procedures such as wide excision, ligation of bleeders, and primary suture of the wound. However, in most uncomplicated situations, syringe and hypodermic needle, scalpel, scissors, and forceps may be all that will be required.

Some pathologists elect to take several punch biopsies entirely within diseased tissues. Such specimens are less likely to be misoriented by the laboratory as they are prepared for microscopy. Some feel that several areas at the active, progressing borders of relatively new lesions need to be biopsied along with some normal adjacent tissue (3). If lesions appear to be progressively evolving, multiple biopsies of representative lesions may be taken. It is important to realize that deep excoriations often remove most of the epidermis and that such locations should be avoided in taking the biopsies.

The punch biopsy tool is firmly and deftly pressed into the skin using a rotary

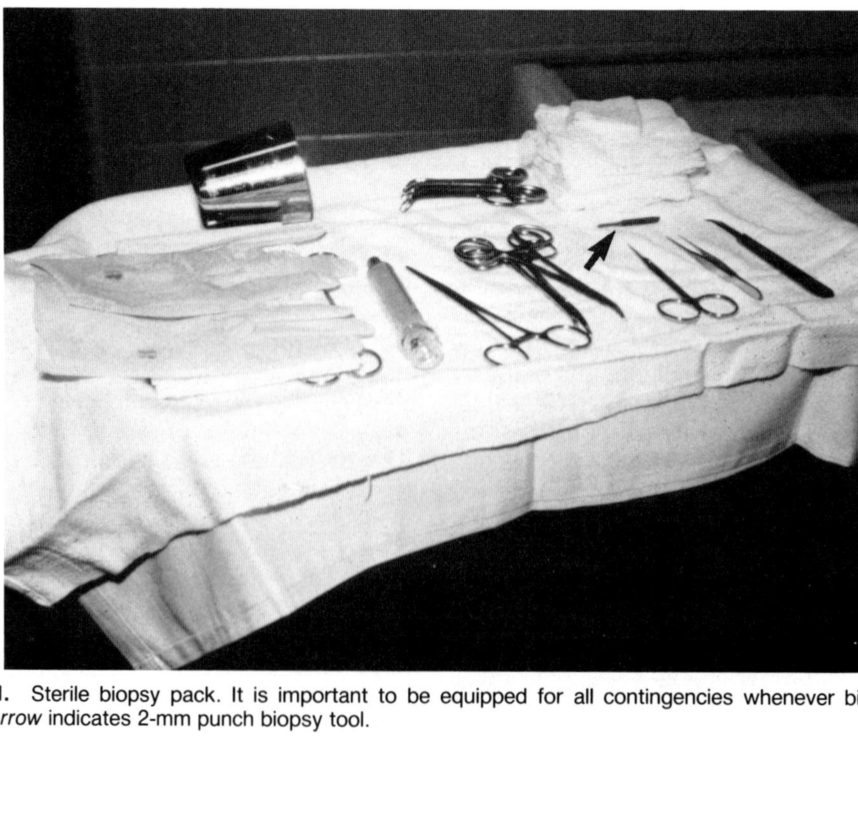

Figure 4.1. Sterile biopsy pack. It is important to be equipped for all contingencies whenever biopsies are planned. *Arrow* indicates 2-mm punch biopsy tool.

motion until the less resistant subcutaneous fatty layer is encountered (Fig. 4.2). Ordinarily, the separated skin plug will pop out of the skin as the instrument is withdrawn (Fig. 4.3). If it is necessary to dissect the plug free, great care not to squeeze too hard should be exercised in delivering it with forceps and freeing its base from the intact skin.

Regardless of whatever biopsy technique is employed, tissues should be immediately placed into an appropriate fixative for transport to the laboratory. For most routine purposes, 10% neutral buffered aqueous formalin is satisfactory. However, podiatrists should be aware of the necessity for alternative fixatives required for special staining techniques (4).

The podiatric surgeon should be familiar with the relative appearance of excisional and punch biopsies as the dermatopathologists views them. Punch biopsies, when viewed microscopically at low power, usually occupy about half of the field (Fig. 4.4). However, all epidermal layers are represented along with the dermis, and the microscopist has a montage of the tissue morphology available. At high power, the cellular morphology, evidence of dyskeratosis, anaplasia, etc., can be seen (Fig. 4.5).

It has been mentioned earlier, but needs restating once again, that several punch biopsies should be taken from any given lesion if at all possible (1). This will allow the microscopist to examine tissue states or reactions from several loci to increase diagnostic accuracy.

Excisional biopsies obviously provide larger masses of tissue which permit a greater opportunity for microscopic examination, both from side to side and through and through the lesions (Fig. 4.6). Each slide fills the microscopic field a number of times even at low magnification and allows for an appreciation of the lesion in toto. Therefore, it is much less likely that alterations of cells as they are in varying degrees of development might be missed during the course of examination. At higher magnifi-

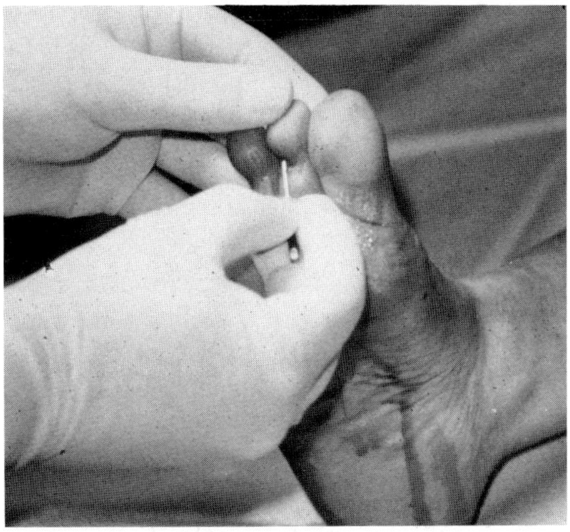

Figure 4.2. Punch biopsies are made with the instrument at right angles to the free surface of skin. Moderate pressure and a deft rotary motion are employed.

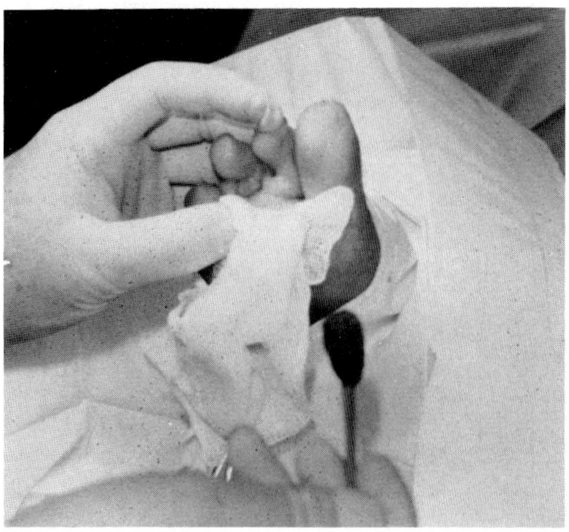

Figure 4.3. Biopsy site following removal of tissue plug. Notice the relative absence of bleeding.

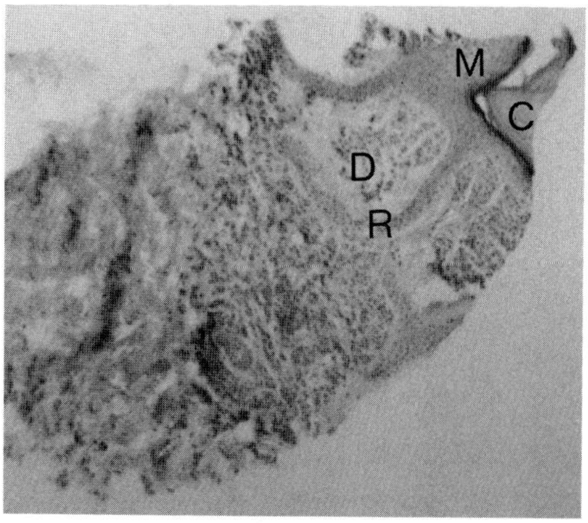

Figure 4.4. Microscopic appearance of 2-mm punch biopsy at low power. *D,* dermis; *R,* rete ridges; *M,* stratum Malpighii; *C,* stratum corneum.

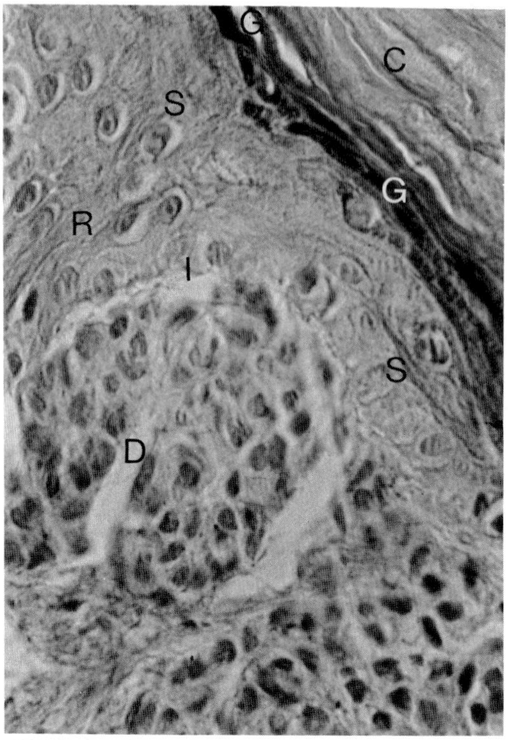

Figure 4.5. Microscopic appearance of 2-mm punch biopsy at high power. *C*, stratum corneum; *G*, stratum granulosum; *S*, stratum spinosum; *R*, rete peg; *I*, dermoepidermal interface; *D*, dermis.

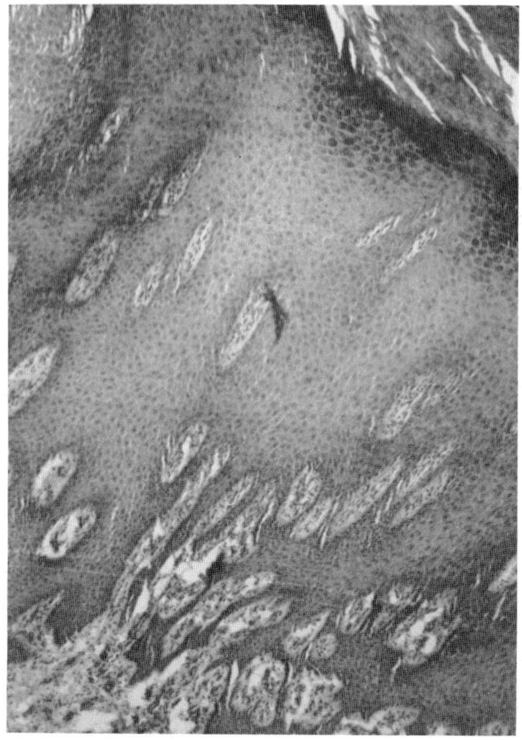

Figure 4.6. Microscopic appearance of excisional biopsy at low power. Many additional fields of examination are available to the microscopist.

cations, an infinitely greater number of fields are available to the microscopists than if the much smaller punch biopsy is used.

The indications for the biopsy of tissues encountered in podiatric medicine are increasing.

The utilization of these techniques have legal as well as medical implications and are performed with the best interests of the patient in mind.

It is possible for otherwise highly qualified pathologists to misinterpret skin specimens from the human foot. This is because tissues are subject to unusual pathomechanical modifications during ambulation. Consequently, mistaken or incomplete diagnosis is a definite possibility, and practitioners need to be aware of such contingencies.

Therefore, it is the responsibility of the podiatric surgeon to supply the pathologist with all pertinent information concerning the lesion to be examined. Not the least of these requirements is to advise as to the age of the patient. Skin changes acceptable with advancing age may be highly questionable at younger periods of life. Location of the lesion, clinical impression, sex, occupation, and any other documentation deemed helpful or contributory by the practitioner will most likely be welcomed by the pathologist.

Most commercial laboratories provide mailing containers which are stamped and self addressed. Fixative solution, usually 10% neutral buffered formaldehyde aqueous, is made available for fixation of tissues destined for routine hematoxylin and eosin studies. Most laboratories involved in dermatohistopathology will wish to examine slides stained by at least two alternative methods.

Acid orcein and Giemsa stain for connective tissue is an excellent adjunct to standard hematoxylin and eosin preparation studies. Podiatric physicians who wish to avail themselves of alternative staining methods to demonstrate specific structures or histochemical features should become acquainted with a range of generally available stains (5, 6) and the specific fixatives required for the proper processing of tissues when a given special stain is to be employed.

The avoidance of introduction of artifacts into biopsy specimens is an important responsibility of the podiatric physician. The high power injection of anesthetic solutions through the skin by special "jet" instruments which may produce deep vacuolization of tissue has already been mentioned. The podatrist should be sure that the laboratory employed adds alcohol to prevent freezing artifact when making specimens in the winter, or whenever specimens must be kept overnight at room temperature to allow fixation before mailing.

In general, delicacy in the handling of all tissues destined for pathologic examination is pivotal for obtaining best results (7). If, for example, the superficial epidermis is squeezed and compressed by excessive forceps pressure upon the biopsy specimen, the tissue superficial to the impingement will appear expanded and pedunculated and may mislead the miscroscopist. Conversely, forceps compression to the deeper dermal structures condenses these tissues and may produce pseudosclerodermatous changes suggestive of scleroderma (8).

The orientation of deep tissues relative to the free surface of the skin can be quantitatively and qualitatively altered significantly by the direction in which the biopsy instrument is positioned. The best preservation of true relationships are obtained when the biopsy is taken at right angles to the free surface of the skin. As the angle of penetration is increased, the relative amounts of stratum corneum, suprapapillary stratum Malpighii, and rete ridges are correspondingly increased, giving the possible appearance of hyperkeratosis and acanthosis (9).

Additionally, pseudosinuses can be artificially introduced into the biopsied tissue by lacerating the free surface and contiguous underlying tissues of the specimen by careless use of forceps or similar instruments (1).

Similarly, pseudocystic structures can be introduced into the deeper structures if they are cleanly perforated by sharp penetrating instruments (5). Furthermore, rough tissue handling can separate epidermis from underlying dermis, giving the microscopic impression of bulla formation.

For all of these reasons and more, it is important that practitioners be aware of, at least to a minimal extent, the essentials of proper microtechnique. Moreover, it is good to understand the alternative histological fixative and stains available to identify chemical alterations in tissues and cells that can greatly aid the pathologist in assisting the podiatric physician in arriving at a final correct diagnosis. Once the diagnosis is in hand, treatment becomes much more simplified and efficacious. A review of special stains is given in Table 4.1.

PATCH TESTING

Modern technology has substantially expanded the choice of materials used in the manufacture of shoes, hosiery, and other apparel covering the lower extremities. Moreover, many medications, new and old, are available for application on the feet and legs. Many of these products have the potential for producing allergic responses which the podiatric physician needs to understand.

Patch tests are employed in an attempt to clinically reproduce allergic contact dermatitis under limited and controlled conditions. Such tests are designed so as to confirm a clinical suspicion or to selectively identify the antigen which is producing the patient's symptoms. Patch testing is a relatively simple podiatric technique. It consists of simply placing the test material(s) under occlusion on the patient's skin, ordinarily, a location on the back or arm where motion is unlikely to occur is selected as the test site. Podiatrists who are not comfortable with these types of tests will find most dermatologists more than willing to lend assistance.

It is important to understand that the methodologies employed are far from being foolproof: Since the environment constantly bombards the population with a great variety of chemical sensitizers, a positive patch test can indicate only prior exposure and may have no relevance to the current complaint of the patient. The possibility exists for cross-allergies or concom-

Table 4.1
Special Stains Available to Identify Specific Substances and Alterations in Tissues and Cells

Tissue constituent	Stain	Appearance of constituent
Amyloid	Crystal violet and orcein-Giemsa	Light blue
Bacteria	Gram stain	Blue (Gram positive)
		Red (Gram negative)
Calcium	von Kossa alizarin	Brown-black (salts of calcium)
		Red
Collagen	Van Gieson	Red (collagen)
		Yellow (muscle and nerve)
	Hematoxylin-eosin	Pink (collagen)
		Blue (nuclei)
Elastin	(Acid) orcein-Giemsa	Dark Brown (elastin fibers)
		Pink (collagen)
		Black (melanin)
		Greenish-yellow (hemosiderin)
		Deep purple (mast cell granules)
Fungi	(Digested) periodic acid-Schiff (PAS)	Red (fungous wall)
	Methenamine silver	Black (fungous wall)
Glycogen	Periodic acid-Schiff	Magenta red (glycogen)
		Red (fungous wall, some mucopolysaccharides)
Iron (hemosiderin pigment)	Prussian blue	Deep blue (tissue iron, ferric and ferrous)
Melanin	Masson's ammoniacal silver nitrate	Black (melanin)
	(Acid) orcein-Giemsa	Greenish-black (melanin)
Mucopolysaccharide (acid) (AMPS)	Alcian blue	Light blue (AMPS)
	colloidal iron	Light blue (AMPS)
	toluidine blue	Purple (metachromatic) (AMPS)
Reticulum	Gomori's and Wilder's	Black (reticulum fibers, melanin and nerves)

itant hypersensitivity with the result that misleading or otherwise confusing results can occur (10).

This is not to say that patch testing has no value whatsoever. However, it is wise to be aware of all contingencies. Still other pitfalls common to patch testing will be added at the close of this brief discussion.

If shoes or hosiery are being tested, an effort should be made to determine the general types of the substance used in footwear. Those substances that are potentially dangerous allergens should be eliminated from the testing plan. Some materials such as emollient creams, cosmetics, and deodorants can be applied directly to the skin. Material from hosiery can also be applied directly. All materials are placed in known order, properly marked and sealed over. Special disc tapes are commercially available which ensure proper masking, placement, and occlusion of the suspected antigens.

Materials from shoes can be cut or curetted out of the foot gear for testing (10). Care must be taken to place these materials in a suitable vehicle. Petrolatum is well suited for such purposes, and commercially available patch test materials are more often than not made up in petrolatum. It is important that solvents such as amyl acetate, chloroform, or turpentine not be used. While they may be excellent solvents, they may themselves produce an eczematous response. The physical state of the material to be tested also needs to be considered; they should not be irritating by virtue of thick, rough surfaces or jagged edges.

Standard patch test antigens prepared in appropriate vehicles in proper concentration are commercially available. Standard test materials, which ordinarily include common medications, preservatives, perfumes, emolients and stabilizers, metals, rubber compounds, epoxies, and plastics, are available. The reader is referred to the following sources for further information:

American Academy of Dermatology
820 Davis Street
Evanston, IL 60201

Hollister-Stier Laboratories
Post Office Box 14957, Department F 74
Atlanta, GA 30325

Trolab
6 B.A.N. Hansens Alle
2900 Hellerup, Denmark

Occasionally, it is necessary to employ patch testing using unusual materials or substances not commonly understood. It is important in such instances to gain all information available concerning these suspected allergens. Totally unknown materials should never be tested since a severe generalized reaction could result (10).

Podiatrists have particular interest in chemicals used in the tanning, dyeing and gluing of both artificial and natural leathers employed in the manufacture of footwear. Such materials can become inducers of allergic contact dermatitis. Additionally, a great number of natural and synthetic materials are used in other items of clothing which come into contact with the foot, and these, too, can become potential sensitizers capable of producing adverse reactions. Commercially available kits are available which can test for allergic reactions. The Hollister-Stier Company lists the following substances as possible sensitizers:

1. Acrylic monomere: methyl methacrylate, one of the most commonly used acrylics, is frequently used in bonding various plastic materials.
2. Bismarck Brown is used in dyeing leather, silk, and wool fabrics.
3. *N*-Cyclohexyl-2 benzothiazole sulfenamide is used as an accelerator in various rubber formulations.
4. Dodecyl mercaptan is employed as a retardant in the polymerization of plastics used in modern footwear.
5. Formaldehyde is employed in manufacturing white leather shoes and in the tanning processes of most leathers.
6. Glutaraldehyde is employed to yield especially soft leathers for use in shoes and gloves as a tanning agent.
7. Hydroquinone monobenzyl ether is employed as an antioxidant in rubber formulations used in footwear.
8. Mercaptobenzothiazole is used in a variety of rubber formulations as an accelerator.
9. *p*-Aminoazobenzene is used in leather dyeing processes.
10. *p*-Phenylenediamine is used in leather dyeing processes.
11. Phenylmercuric acetate and phenylmercuric nitrate are incorporated into the linings of footwear to guard against odor and mildew.
12. *n*-Phenyl-*n*-isopropyl-*p*-phenylenediamine is employed as an antioxidant in rubber formulations used in footwear.
13. Potassium dichromate is employed in dyeing and leather tanning processes required in the manufacture of footwear.
14. Colophony resins are adhesives used in the fabrication of footwear.
15. *p*-tertiary-Butylphenol is a phenol resin constituent in some neoprene resins used in footwear.
16. Tetramethylthiuram is an accelerator in a number of rubber formulations.

Judicious testing of suspected allergens required that they be tested against control substances, and most kits include olive oil and petrolatum for such purposes.

Most chemicals may be tested in concentrations of 0.5 to 1.0% in petrolatum. Cosmetics, perfumes, antibiotics, lanolin, and preservatives are used in concentrations of either 10% or 100%. The reader is referred to *Patch Testing* by Fregert and Bandmann (New York, Springer-Verlag, 1975) for more comprehensive information on the preparation of suspected antigens.

TECHNIQUES FOR APPLICATION OF ALLERGENS IN PATCH TESTING

Antigens can be conveniently applied using commercially available cellulose discs on aluminum strips. These are placed in known concentrations in known quantities in a routine order. They are placed in one or two rows, taped in place with an occlusive airtight tape (Fig. 4.7). Each disc and each row is carefully marked, and the location and type of each test material is recorded on the patient's chart. The tape is usually removed in 48 hours. Interpretation is then made when the tape is removed and at 72 and 96 hr.

It is not difficult to mistake an irritation for allergy in interpreting the results of patch testing. Allergens develop comparatively slowly. It is for this reason that evaluations are made over a 4-day period. Irritant reaction fades relatively quickly after the cellulose test patches are removed.

The proper interpretation of the results of patch testing require some prescribed method for grading reactions. The North American Contact Dermatitis Group has established the following criteria:

1. Relatively weak reactions which are nonvesicular macular erythematous in nature are said to be 1+ reactions.

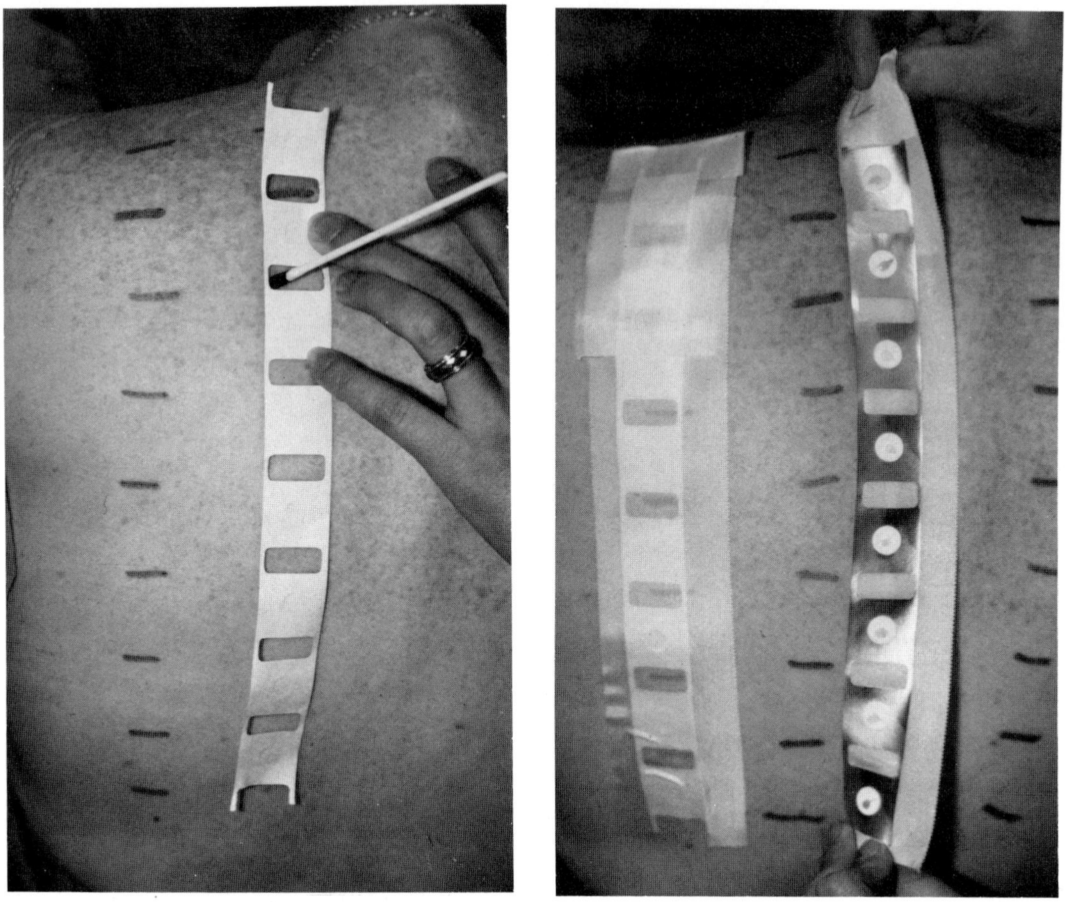

Figure 4.7. (*A* and *B*) Placement of discs in rows for patch testing before placement of occlusive tape. Occlusive tape is removed after 48 hr for the first of several interpretations.

2. Vesicular or strongly edematous reactions are regarded as 2+.
3. Ulcerative or bullous reaction is designated as 3+. Reactions which are doubtful or negative should be duly recorded. Substances which for any reason were not tested may be recorded also.

Another grading system employed by dermatologists employs a scale of one to four: +, erythema; ++, erythema and papules; +++, erythema, papules, and vesicles; ++++, marked edema and vesicles.

False-negative reactions may occur for a variety of reasons. For example, the test material may have been wrongly applied to the wrong part of the body in the wrong concentration and/or in the wrong vehicle. Moreover, the examiner may have made the interpretation at an improper time. Some patients will produce false-negative reactions if they are immunosuppressed or under corticosteroid therapy.

False-positive reactions may be due to pressure effect or may be recorded if they are interpreted at an improper time. Some patients' skin is irritated because they have a low threshold of sensitivity to the substance tested. Some reactions are due to concomitant atopic or acute generalized dermatitis. The presence of an irritating chemical compound, solvent, or vehicle, or improper concentration, also may contribute to false-positive reactions (10).

CULTURE AND SENSITIVITY TESTING

Bacteria and fungi are common contaminants of the human skin, and as such do not evoke pathological responses in their hosts. In podiatric practice, certain microorganisms commonly do, however break free of the ecological niches and invade the tissues of the foot and leg, producing "infection." Implicit to the definition of infection is the concept that tissues are injured and that the body responds by some adverse reactive phenomena.

In the case of pyogenic bacteria, an inflammatory response in and about the skin wound usually ensues with the formation of exudation and pus. Fungi, on the other hand, seldom produce inflammatory responses. Fortunately, a great many antimicrobial agents are available to control these undesirable microscopic intruders. Their intelligent use, however, demands that the offending organisms be identified.

Culture of the offending organisms in the microbiological laboratory and testing for their sensitivity to common antibiotics should be a routine procedure. Individually packaged Culturette (T.M. Marion Scientific, Kansas City, MO) tubes in sterile envelopes are commercially available. One need only swab the skin about the lesion to be tested with an antiseptic to remove surface contaminants and apply the cotton-tipped applicator supplied to the exudate (Fig. 4.8). Ideally, fresh exudate can be expressed for best results in sampling. Using aseptic technique, the swab is returned to the Culturette tube, and the cap is firmly replaced. Stuart's bacterial transport medium is found within the ampule placed within the Culturette tube: it must be crushed within the tube so as to ensure bathing the sample on the swab with the medium. The specimen is then properly labeled with the patient's name, date, specimen source, and any other pertinent data deemed helpful for expeditious handling by the laboratory.

Identification of the offending microorganism(s) and a listing of antibiotics to which it is likely to be susceptible are reported back within several days. Such information is absolutely essential for the effective use of antibiotics and the prevention of development of antibiotic-resistant strains. Certain pathogens, particularly anaerobic bacteria, are fastidious, and more involved subculturing and fermentation testing may have to be employed. Such infections will require more time for laboratory diagnosis.

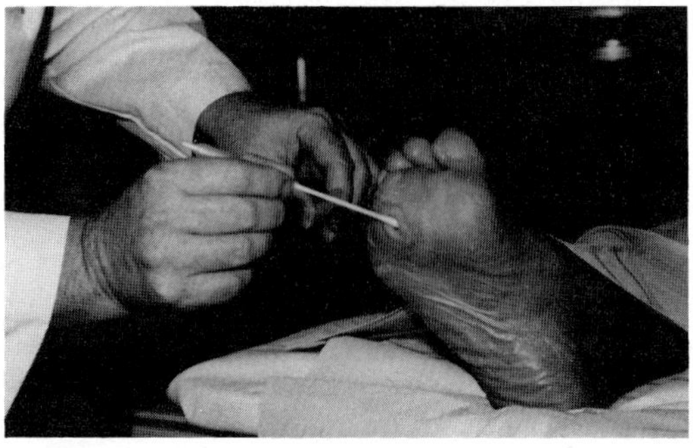

Figure 4.8. Taking specimen for culture and sensitivity testing.

It is often useful to perform a "Gram stain" in the office to determine microbial morphology and its positivity or negativity to the test (11). A heat-fixed smear of the exudate is stained with one of the triphenylmethane dyes (usually crystal violet) and counterstained with a dilute solution of iodine. Alcohol or acetone is then applied as a decolorizing agent. Gram-negative organisms are those which decolorize rapidly. Gram-positive organisms resist decolorization and retain the coloration of the dye employed. Such testing provides for a more intelligent rationale for instituting systemic antibiotics prior to receiving the more definitive results from the culture and sensitivity testing by the laboratory.

The culture of fungal organisms requires special media, and more time for growth is needed than is the case for most bacteria. Sabouraud's agar is the most commonly used media for the growth of fungi, and slanted culture tubes are commercially available to podiatrists for culturing fungi from tissue scrapings or vesicles. Presumptive identification of several common fungi which are frequent etiological agents in dermatophytosis can be made on a colorimetric basis. Tube slants are inoculated and observed over time at room temperature. These kits are commercially available from several sources.

Podiatrists should remember that it is occasionally advantageous to use small portions of biopsied tissues for culture purposes for evidence of deep mycotic or bacterial involvement.

TEST FOR CIRCULATORY INSUFFICIENCY

Poor circulation either on the arterial or venous side may produce untoward skin changes. A wide range of instrumentation is available for the diagnosis of vascular diseases, but a thorough discussion of them is beyond the scope of this study. Practitioners should be aware, however, that their use is fully justified in this classification of dermatologic diagnosis (12).

The use of Doppler ultrasound interprets blood flow by assessing modifications of the sounds of blood coursing through blood vessels. Such sounds can be electronically modified and printed out for analysis.

Plethysmography using pulse volume methods or photoelectric cells measure similar phenomena using different criteria (Fig. 4.9). The relative amplitude of systole, the relaxed phase of diastole, and the recoilability of blood vessels (diacrotic notch) all indicate the health or disease of blood vessels of the lower extremities. Other factors involving the timing of circulatory events may also be diagnostically important and these may be conveniently interpreted along with the other factors on printouts from appropriate instrumentation.

The thermocouple is an ideal device for measuring skin temperature electronically (Fig. 4.10). The experienced practitioner can evaluate skin temperature changes through the rehearsed use of tactile senses of the backs of his or her fingers. However, the use of documented electronic printout information gives best evidence for the patient's progress over time regardless of the modality employed.

WOOD'S LIGHT EXAMINATION

Ultraviolet light filtered to transmit light at a wavelength of 365 mm will produce fluorescence of the skin which can be pa-

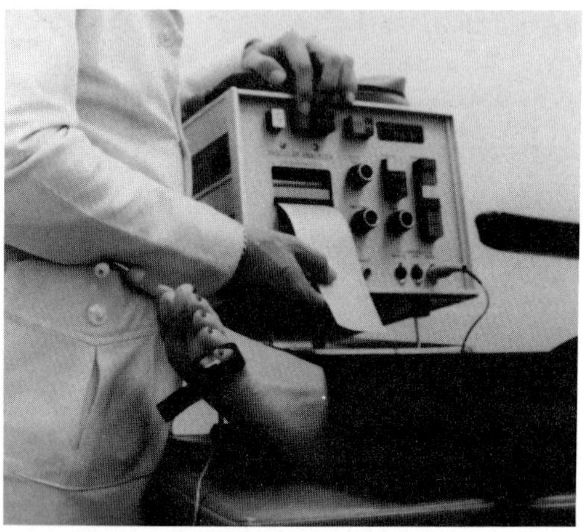

Figure 4.9. Plethysmography for evaluation of the circulatory status in the lower extremities.

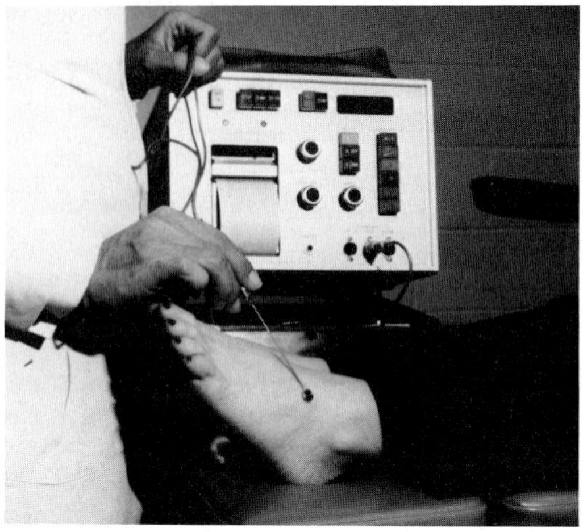

Figure 4.10. Thermocouple for determination of skin temperature of the lower extremities.

thognomonic for several skin conditions. Such devices are commercially available and are known as "Wood's lights" (10. They are relatively inexpensive, simple hand-held devices which are directed at the skin lesion(s) in a darkened room.

Blue-green fluorescence indicates involvement of *Microsporum canis* or *Microsporum audouinni.*

Golden fluorescence is indicative of tinea versicolor.

Reddish fluorescence is produced by bacterial porphyrins associated with *Corynebacterium minutissimum,* which is the etiologic agent of erythrasma.

Yellowish flourescence indicates an optimal tissue concentration for patients taking the antibiotic tetracycline. It is especially evident in the mouth and about hair follicles. Therefore, Wood's light can be an indicator of drug efficacy.

The depigmenting disease vitiligo shows up under Wood's light since the reduction of pigmentation causes reflection of the light.

While the indications for the use of Wood's light are limited, its ease of use and low cost make it appropriate for use in the podiatry office.

DIASCOPY

Some techniques are so simple that they are often overlooked. Such a situation exists with "diascopy," which differentiates erythema secondary to vasodilatation from purpura and is useful in diagnosing vasculitis (10). One simply presses a clear piece of glass, such as a microscope slide, against the skin to be examined. Intact blood vessels will produce blanching of the lesion under the mild pressure of diascopy. Blanching does not occur with purpuretic lesions, however.

POTASSIUM HYDROXIDE MOUNT

Epidermal tissues will undergo lysis in aqueous potassium hydroxide solution. Therefore, the structural elements of fungi, such as hyphae, mycelium, and spores, will stand out under high dry microscopic examination (10). Podiatrists frequently need to differentiate a true mycotic involvement from other skin problems.

Vesicular lesions can be examined by deroofing the lesion and placing the debrided tissue on a microscope slide. Dry, scaly lesions are simply scraped with a scalpel blade onto a slide.

With the tissue to be examined in place on the microscope slide, a drop or two of 10–20% aqueous potassium hydroxide solution is placed over it and coverslipped. Keratinous material is dissolved by gently heating on a hot plate or waving it over a flame. Diagnosis for hyphae, mycelia, and spores will be totally impossible if the tissue is overheated or boiled and these structures are also dissolved. An inexpensive student microscope is all that is needed to identify the characteristic fungal features and to confirm a diagnosis of fungal involvement (Fig. 4.11).

NUCLEAR MEDICINE APPLICATIONS IN PODIATRIC DERMATOLOGY

Traditionally, nuclear medicine employs technetium and gallium scans to identify so-called "hot or cold" spots. The information gained is not pathognomonic for disease but indicates the state of tissue metabolism in or about a part (12). Recently, however, experimental work has been initiated which employs fundamental principles of biochemistry in nuclear medicine to make such testing more specific. Such is the case in the detection of melanotic tumors with special reference to metastasis to distant points.

Tyrosine is the basic precursor substance necessary for the biosynthesis of melanin.

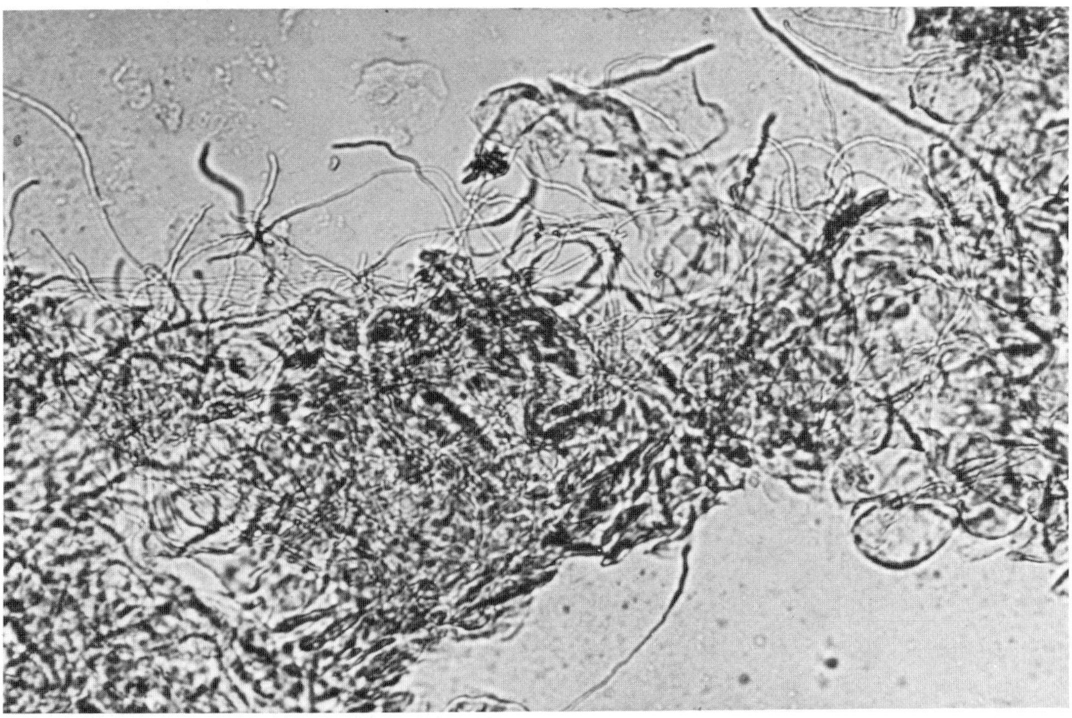

Figure 4.11. Microscopic appearance of potassium hydroxide mount demonstrating fungal morphology.

It has been shown that both amelanotic and melanotic tumors will take up the radioactive analogue of tyrosine ^{123}IMT or ^{123}I-oda-α-methyltyrosine. Such uptake by tumor tissues is more sensitive and specific for the detection of melanoma than is true of ^{67}Gallium (Ga) or ^{203}Lead (Pb) (13).

Gamma scintillation cameras (Fig. 4.12), in line with electronic data and imaging processors, effectively detect radionuclide uptake 60 minutes after injection. Tumor localization is best made after 90 minutes, however, since blood backgrounds are lower. Metastic melanoma as small as 65 mg have been detected using this methodology (13).

Radiolabeled antibodies specific for tumor-associated antigens promise to improve the diagnostic imaging of tumors. External scintigraphy has been used to image human malignancies using antibodies which are specific for carcinoembryonic antigen. Radiolabeled monoclonal antibodies obtained from mouse antisera specific for P 97 has been employed in the diagnostic imaging of melanoma: P 97 is known to be a melanoma-associated antigen which can be safely given to human patients in 1-mg doses. This antigen is localized upon the outer surfaces of tumor cell plasma membranes and is, therefore, quite accessible to the antibody (14).

Undoubtedly this preliminary experimental work holds much promise for both detection and treatment of the potentially deadly melanomas. Present difficulties in its use include a need for better in vivo targeting of antibody to tumor, better in vivo specificity, and the need to limit hepatic uptake of the materials used (14).

ELECTROMETRIC STUDIES

Within the last decade, electrometric studies have been shown to be of value in differentiating benign from malignant neoplasia. The usefulness of such a modality is obvious in diagnosing a lesion suspected of being an amelanotic melanoma, as opposed to some more benign process. This is the kind of knowledge necessary to develop an adequate treatment plan and to establish a prognosis. Additionally, it might well prevent "seeding" tumor cells into the deep tissues in the course of punch biopsy.

A large number of patients with amelanotic and melanotic tumors have been studied electrometrically in Europe over the past two decades (15). In nearly all cases, malignant characteristics could be established on the basis of hypopolarizability or nonpolarizability. Such testing can be performed using a simple potentiometer.

Phase-bound potentials are produced in the skin since the organ is essentially a system of semiconductors and insulators made up of extracellular fluids with interfaces of barrier layers. Differences in electrical potential arise from different mobilities and adsorptions of positive and negative ions on the surface of electronegative

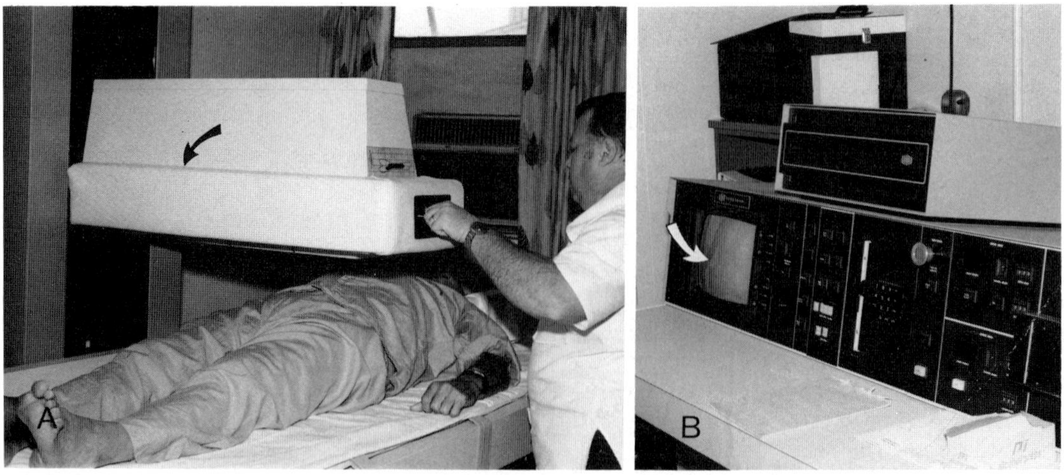

Figure 4.12. Scintillation camera (*arrow*) for imaging in nuclear medicine laboratory is passed over the full length of the patient's body (*A*). Radioactivity is visualized by means of a cathode ray tube (*arrow*) on the console, where photographs can be taken of the image as well (*B*).

and cation-permeable barriers or from the differing penetration ability of these ions to permeate these barriers within the skin (16).

As long as the normal skin barriers remain intact, the active electrical potential and the passive polarizability are unaltered and characteristic. However, in primary skin cancer, and especially in amelanotic melanoma and malignant melanoma, the electronegativity of the integumentary barrier layers decreases. In such instances, measurements of the skin potential yields voltages which are 30–35% lower than those of the normal contiguous normal skin.

Melanoma as well as other primary skin cancers produces an irreversible hysteresis of the tissue barriers at the outset of malignant transformation. Diminution of the charging results, along with the polarizability of the barrier. The tissue barriers demonstrate an increase of ion permeability, while the barrier membranes themselves can become completely nonpolarizable (16).

Electrometric skin studies are more often employed in Europe, but they are still considered experimental here. A number of relatively simple apparatuses for these applications have been developed. Storz et al (17) conducted 2000 electrometric examinations using the electropermeagraph (17). Kiss and Horvath (1969) developed the malignometer which, in addition to a dry cell battery, develops alternating current by means of an oscillator (18). Other devices include the electrodermatometer of Regelsberger and the Whelan apparatus of Midana (19).

Melczer and his co-workers describe methods employing a simple potentiometer, a voltmeter-ammeter method, and a direct reading galvanometer. A nonpolarizable zinc sulfate electrode is employed. Filter paper discs having a surface of about 0.4 cm^2 are soaked in 0.1 N aqueous potassium chloride solution. These are placed on normal skin at several points and upon the lesion to be tested. This procedure is designed to eliminate the possibility of false reading brought about by pressure of the electrode upon the skin.

An indifferent electrode is placed in the palm of the patients' hand. This contact employs filter paper having a diameter of 3 cm which is also saturated with 0.1 N potassium chloride aqueous solution.

The different electrode extends a cotton thread (also soaked with 0.1 N potassium chloride) which is touched to filter paper discs on the normal reference skin. The current from the dry cell batteries attached is switched on, and a zeropoint is established on a direct reading galvanometer. The cotton thread test electrode is then directed to the lesion to be examined, and its polarizability is established (20).

Further refinement of this test can be made by gently scratching the skin of the forearm with a sterile needle until pinpoint bleeding occurs. Such treatment damages the tissue barriers extensively, and most of the polarizability of the skin is lost. The deflection of the needle of the direct reading galvanometer can be regarded as maximal. The apparatus can then be adjusted so that normal intact skin shows minimal deflection while the injured site demonstrates the greatest excursion of the needle. The grade of malignant transformation, then, is roughly proportional to the scale established by the deflection of the ammeter needle at the point of the reference injury site (20).

Using such a test, the practitioner might more confidently and intelligently choose a proper treatment plan. If the skin lesion tests with voltages 30 to 35% lower than normal (as would be the case in high grade malignancies), punch biopsy is contraindicated, and aggressive surgical intervention, including regional lymph node dissection, is probably indicated.

Conversely, more normal electrical potentials indicate that more conservative approaches are permissible. Punch biopsy can then most likely be performed without fear of seeding the deeper tissues with malignant cells. These lesions, then, are benign and are likly to metastasize (16).

It will be interesting to note whether or not electrometric studies, which have gained some popularity in Europe, will be adopted in the United States in the near future.

References

1. Berlin S: Oncology Special Issue (in toto). *J Am Podiatr Assoc* 70:1980.
2. Pinkus H, Mehregan AH: *A Guide to Dermatohistopathology.* New York, Appleton-Century-Crofts, 1969.

3. Mehregan AH, Pinkus H: Selection of site and method for skin biopsy. *Dermatol Dig* 7:49, 1968.
4. Pearse AGE: *Histochemistry, Theoretical and Applied*, ed 2. Boston, Little, Brown, 1960.
5. Pinkus, H, Hunter R: Simplified acid orcein and Giemsa technique for routine staining of skin sections. *Arch Dermatol* 82:699, 1960.
6. Luna LH: *Manual of Histologic Staining Methods of the Armed Forces Institute of Pathology*, ed 3. New York, McGraw-Hill, 1968,
7. Lillie RD: *Histologic Technique and Practical Histochemistry.* New York, McGraw-Hill, 1965.
8. Mehregan AH, Pinkus H: Artifacts in dermal histopathology. *Arch Dermatol* 94:218, 1966.
9. McCarthy DJ: Laboratory considerations in podiatric biopsy techniques. *Curr Podiatr* 8 and 9:9–17, 1981.
10. Roenigk HH: *Office Dermatology.* Baltimore, Williams & Wilkins Co., 1981.
11. Stanier RY, Doudoroff M, Adelberg EA: *The Microbial World.* Englewood Cliffs, NJ, Prentice-Hall, 1961.
12. McCarthy DJ: *Practical Podiatric Medicine: Management of Ulceration and Wounds.* (monogr.). Evanston, IL, Arthur Retlaw & Associates, 1981.
13. Hoffer PB, Gotschalk AP, Zaret BL: *The Yearbook of Nuclear Medicine*, 1983. Chicago, Yearbook Medical Publishers, 1983.
14. Larson SM, Brown JP, Wright PW: Imaging of melanoma with I-^{131}-labeled monoclonal antibodies. *J. Nucl. Med* 24(2):123–129, 1983.
15. Andrade R, Gumport SL, Popkin GL et al: *Cancer of the Skin.* Philadelphia, W.B. Saunders, 1976.
16. Melczer N: Electrometric studies in skin cancer. In: Andrade R, Gumport SL, Popkin GL, Rees TD (eds): *Cancer of the Skin.* Philadelphia, W. B. Saunders, 1976.
17. Storz H, Voelkel A, Krause RA: Zur Auswertung von Gleich-strommessungen an der menschlichen Haut (Elektropermeagramm). *Ärztl Wochenschr* 9:617, 1954.
18. Kiss G, Horvath IL: Elektromas micromodszer es keszulek a bor malignus burjanzasainak a kimutatsara. *Borgyogy Venerol Sz* 45:164, 1969.
19. Regelsberger H: Der bedingte Reflex and die vegetative Rythmik des Menschen dargesteltt an Elektrodermogramm. *Acta. Neuroveg.* Suppl 1: 1950.
20. Melczer N, Kiss J: Zur früzeitigen Erkennung von Melanoblastomen. *Dermatologica* 117:342, 1958.

CHAPTER 5

Helomata and Tylomata

DANIEL J. McCARTHY

The most common of hyperkeratinized lesions of the skin of the human foot are "tylomata" (calluses) and "helomata" (corns). The term helomata represents a variety of expressions such as heloma durum (hard corn), heloma molle (soft corn), heloma milliare (seed corn), heloma neurofibrosum (neurovascular corn), and heloma vascularis (vascular corn). Additionally, there are several lesions which mimic the helomata as they occur on the foot. These include such entities as porokeratosis plantaris discreta, eccrine poroma, arsenical keratosis, epithelial implants, and keratoderma. All of these lesions demonstrate a common characteristic in that they exhibit a degree of cornification of the skin in a localized circumscribed region. This chapter will deal with the etiology, pathogenesis, histopathology, and treatment of these lesions. The occurrences of tylomata as they are found on the human foot will also be discussed in similar terms since these more generalized alterations of the skin develop in response to like stimuli.

The pain and attendant loss of function and productivity to mankind resulting from this group of pedal lesions is incalculable. Most podiatrists would agree that the helomata and tylomata constitute a majority of complaints which patients bring to their attention. An authoritative survey presented in 1960 reviewed 5400 consecutively tabulated podiatric lesions other than nail conditions. Of these, fully 4861 represented some expression of either heloma or tyloma (1). More recently, a survey by the Veterans Administration indicated that helomata and tylomata accounted for the majority of presenting complaints among that essentially male population (2).

HELOMA DURUM

Simply stated, the uncomplicated hard corn can be described as an essentially circumscribed, localized thickening of the epidermis composed of impacted, crenated, distorted, desquamated, compressed dead keratinocytes (3). Such lesions are usually located at sites of pressure and friction such as the interphalangeal joints of the toes (Fig. 5.1).

Grossly, the involved tissues appear as dry horny masses of grayish yellow or white coloration. However, they may present a waxy hyaline appearance or may be reddish to brown in color. Pleomorphism characterizes the common corn. Most lesions are conical in shape, with the apex directed towards the sensitive subepidermal tissues. It should be noted, however, that some lesions of long standing have their deepest dimension and penetration about their periphery. This is assumed to be the result of a central atrophy produced by prolonged pressure from the conical center, which is characteristic of younger lesions. Consequently, growth was retarded in the central regions but was not constrained circumferentially. The pars papillaris is especially evident in such instances (4).

Podiatrists are generally agreed that heloma durum is more a symptom than an actual disease entity. Podiatric surgeons have recognized underlying bony pathology as the direct etiologic factor in the formation of the common hard corn for several decades.

This is not to negate entirely certain environmental factors such as constricting footwear, however (5). There is a disturbing tendency among some practitioners to completely ignore obvious structural imperfec-

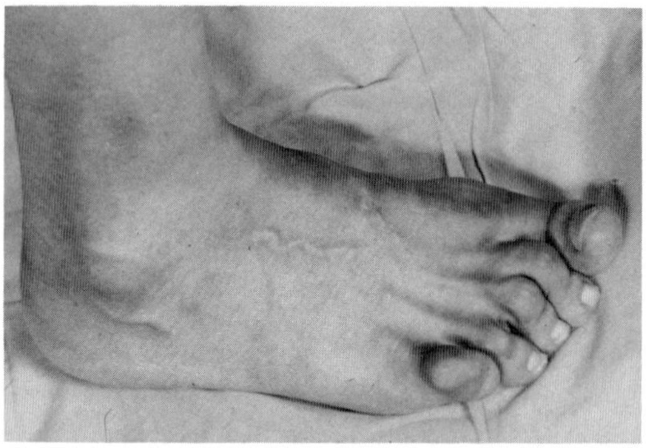

Figure 5.1. Heloma durum of the fifth toe associated with digital contracture and bursitis.

tions of shoes or even hosiery as etiologic in the appearance of unexplainable sudden occurrences of heloma. Podiatrists should not be above questioning the patient as to his or her preferences relative to shoes and hosiery. The simple act of examining the patient's shoe and taking notice of some imperfection at the site of the heloma as it relates to the shoe may avert a surgical procedure which will be costly to the patient both in terms of time and monetary resources.

However, the most common finding relative to the formation of heloma durum is that bone pathology is the direct causative factor in its development (6, 7). Such pathology may relate to hyperplasia of bone, deformity of the digit involved, which together produce a loss of normal joint function. It is usual to identify the head of the proximal phalange or the intermediate phalange as the exciting factor in precipitating those helomata which defy resolution by external conservative measures. Hyperflexure deformities (hammer toes and mallet toes) and rotational alterations of the digital structures have congenital implications. These deformities also predispose to the development of digital helomata. Freed studied the development of the human corn and observed that 85% of all cadavers observed in his research involved some expression of the foot lesion heloma durum (6). Further substantiation of these findings was provided by Bonavilla, Feigenbaum, and Schreiber (8, 9).

Modifications to the epidermis are clinically obvious in heloma durum. It would be logical to assume that these striking changes would be reflected cytologically through transmission electron microscopy. Such is not the case, however. Ultrastructural characteristics of subcellular organelles within individual keratinocytes involved in heloma durum did not differ significantly from those observed in normal skin. This finding suggested that the rather profound tissue changes observed in heloma durum were the result of accretionary changes of the tissues, rather than of intracellular modifications of the individual keratinocytes (7). As a result of the negative results of electron microscopy, my early research was redirected along the more traditional lines of anthropometric analysis, morphology, and histochemistry.

Anthropometric Analysis of Heloma Durum

Epidermal variability, as it was observed between heloma durum and normal interphalangeal skin (Figs. 5.2 and 5.3) was evaluated using parameters implicated in the process of keratinization (10). The Malpighian layer, from stratum germinativum or basale through the stratum spinosum and ending with the stratum granulosum,

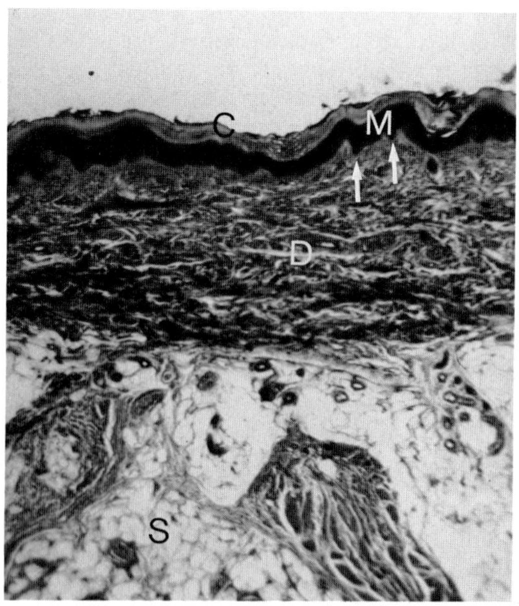

Figure 5.2. Normal interphalangeal skin, light microscopy, hematoxylin and eosin preparation. *Arrows* indicate epidermal rete ridges. *C*, stratum corneum; *M*, suprapapillary stratum Malpighii. *D*, dermis; *S*, subcutaneous tissue.

is representative of the cellular mass implicated in the biochemical events of keratinization. In addition, the number and length of rete pegs provide another parameter, since these structures provide additional cells which may enter into the process of keratinization. Finally, the stratum corneum itself, as representative of the end product of keratinization, is indicative of the efficiency of the process. All of these dimensions lend themselves to direct measurement and comparison.

The acanthosis of the suprapapillary stratum Malpighii is of the order of a sevenfold increase in thickness of the epidermis in heloma durum relative to normal interphalangeal skin (Figs. 5.3 and 5.4). At the same time, the rete pegs extending below the suprapapillary plate in heloma durum increase in length by as much as three times. The greatest increase in thickness of the several parameters measured lies within the stratum corneum of helomatous lesions which demonstrate a 20-fold expansion, as compared to that of the control. Control interphalangeal skin equally divides the stratum Malpighii and stratum corneum in terms of thickness, but in heloma durum the stratum corneum constitutes at least 80% of the total thickness of the epidermis. The number of rete Malpighii decreases in helomatous epidermis, but this finding is more apparent than real since these structures have hypertrophied or coalesced. The length of the rete Malpighii is considerably longer than normal

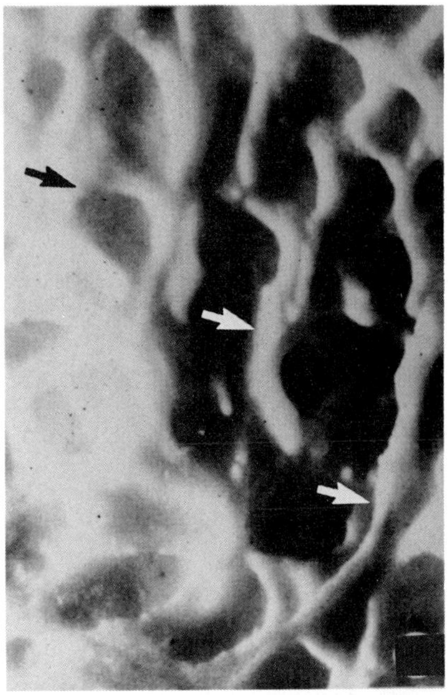

Figure 5.4. Epidermal portion of the epidermal-dermal interface in heloma durum. *Arrows* indicate Hypertrophied and irregular arrangement of the rete Malpighii, which is apparent in this incident light microphotograph.

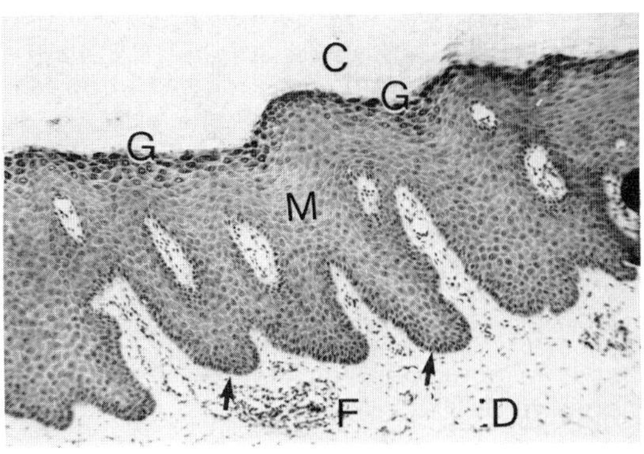

Figure 5.3. Skin of interphalangeal joint region implicated in the formation of heloma durum. *Arrows* indicate elongated hypertrophic rete Malpighii. *D*, dermis; *C*, stratum corneum; *M*, suprapapillary stratum Malpighii; *F*, fibroblasts; *G*, stratum granulosum. Light microscopy and hematoxylin and eosin preparation.

for the region. The variance and standard deviation were computed for the epidermal variations (Table 5.1).

The values determined indicate that the measurement of total epidermis, thickness of stratum corneum and suprapapillary stratum Malpighii, as well as number and length of the rete pegs, tend to be much more homogeneous among the control tissues than in heloma durum; for the latter group these variables are extremely heterogeneous for all parameters. Furthermore, as a given value for an epidermal parameter increases, the standard deviation varies in direct proportion to the degree of change. Therefore, it would seem that all parameters possess a great capacity for structural modulation under the influences of external stimuli.

One might argue that the increased thickness of some of the epidermal variables in heloma durum are attributable to an increase in the individual dimensions of the involved cells. To check this hypothesis, cells of the stratum basale of the epidermis were measured for height and circumference in normal and helomatous tissues (Table 5.2). In applying the Student t test to the differences between mean val-

Table 5.1
Statistical Comparison of Epidermal Components in Normal and Helomatous Interphalangeal Tissue

Epidermal tissue	Computed variables[a]	Total epidermis (mm)	Stratum Malpighii (mm)	Stratum corneum (mm)	Length of rete pegs (mm)
Normal inter-phalangeal	X̄[b]	0.126 (±0.008)	0.050 (±0.003)	0.076 (±0.009)	0.061 (±0.005)
	S^2	0.00137	0.00016	0.00157	0.00018
	S	0.037	0.0125	0.0386	0.0136
Heloma durum	X̄[c]	1.832 (±0.19)	0.370 (±0.03)	1.513 (±0.17)	0.205 (±0.01)
	S^2	0.3756	0.0096	0.3067	0.00145
	S	0.6128	0.0979	0.5538	0.0381

[a] X̄, mean; S^2, variance; S, standard deviation.
[b] Based on 8 specimens.
[c] Based on 10 specimens.

Table 5.2
Statistical Comparison of Height and Circumference of Cells in the Stratum Basale of Normal and Helomatous Interphalangeal Tissue

Stratum basale	X̄[a] (mm)	S^{2}[a]	S[a]	N[a]
Normal skin (cell height)	0.014[b]	5.52	2.35	4
Heloma durum (cell height)	0.015[b]	4.4	2.01	27
Normal skin (cell circumference)	0.035[b]	0.0000250	0.00499	7
Heloma durum (cell circumference)	0.036[b]	0.000776	0.0046	24

[a] X̄, mean; S^2, variance; S, standard deviation; N, number of specimens measured.
[b] Not significant, $P < 0.05$.

ues, no significant difference was noted ($P < 0.05$). Therefore, it is concluded that the increase in thickness is not related to an increase in the mass of individual cells but is the result of accretionary growth of the tissue in heloma durum.

The alterations of structure of the rete Malpighii of the epidermal-dermal interface was studied by the maceration technique to separate the epidermis from dermis. The interfaces between the two elements of skin were demonstrated by photomicrographs utilizing incident light.

Torques and pressure changes applied to the digits result in bony hyperplasia (6). Apparently these same forces evoke tissue responses within the epidermis which are equally capable of epidermal hyperplasia. The dermal papillae of heloma durum show considerable hypertrophy and often seem to coalesce, leaving foot-like projections distally (11). Such structures, when cut tangentially for microscopic examination, appear as islands within the epidermis (Fig. 5.3). Papillae associated with heloma durum also tend to orient in several different directions, as opposed to the smaller, more regularly oriented dermal papillae in normal control interphalangeal skin.

The epidermal portion of the epidermal-dermal interface of heloma durum which is complimentary to the dermal portion reveals a widening of the rete ridges which receive the much hypertrophied and morphologically variable dermal papillae (Fig. 5.4). Additionally, a rather bizarre disorientation of the epidermal ridges is apparent, and there is a noticeable absence of adnexa at the interphalangeal region. This is to be compared with the normal interphalangeal epidermal-dermal interface in which the epidermal portion presents a striking honeycomb regularity of structure. The rete ridges intersect in regular array to receive the finger-like projections of the pars papillaris (Fig. 5.5).

Histochemistry of Heloma Durum

The terms epidermal hyperplasia, acanthosis, hyperkeratosis, and parakeratosis are associated with the tylomata as well as the helomata. I am in agreement with Gibbs

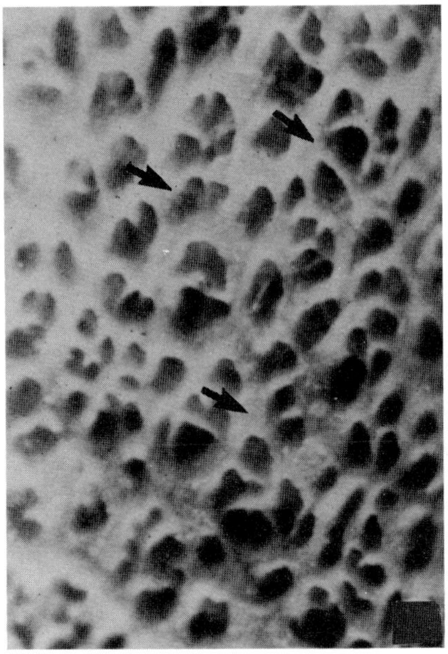

Figure 5.5. Epidermal portion of the epidermal-dermal interface in normal control interphalangeal skin. *Arrows* indicate the regularly arranged structure of the rete Malpighii. Incident light microphotograph.

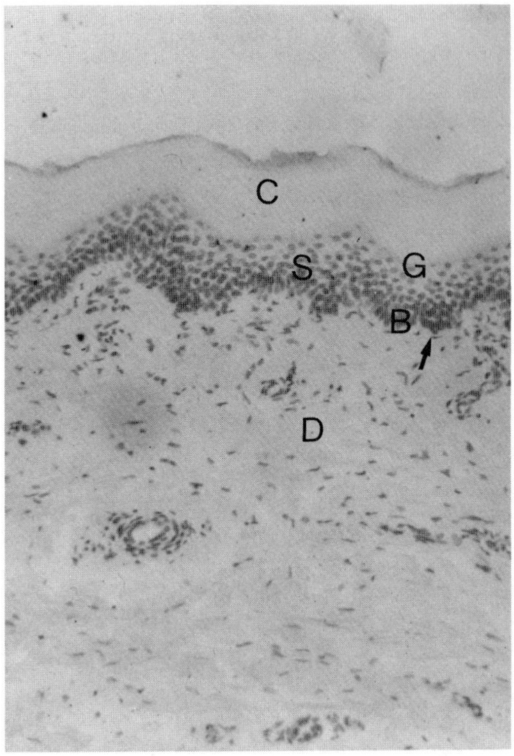

Figure 5.6. Normal interphalangeal skin stained by the Feulgen method for deoxyribonucleic acid (DNA). Light microscopy. Stratum corneum (*C*), stratum granulosum (*G*), stratum spinosum (*S*), stratum basale (*B*), and dermis (*D*) are shown. *Arrow* indicates rete peg.

(12) in that the nontraumatically induced keratodermas should be differentiated from corns and calluses. However, the morphogenesis of heloma and tyloma is essentially the same. The histochemical analysis of interphalangeal skin as it is found in heloma durum is consistent with parakeratosis and acanthosis. DNA is found equally dispersed throughout the stratum Malpighii of both control and heloma durum epidermis, although the quantity in the latter is more due to an increased surface area occasioned by the hypertrophy of the rete pegs and the greater thickness of the suprapapillary stratum Malpighii (Figs. 5.6 and 5.7). On a cell by cell basis, however, and on the basis of staining characteristics, both control and heloma durum demonstrate an equal intensity of DNA. In both types of tissues, the presence of DNA ends abruptly at the stratum granulosum because of the initiation of intense enzymatic activity characteristic to these strata (13) (Figs. 5.8 and 5.9). This finding, however, does not hold true for the most extreme example of parakeratosis, which is the genetically influenced, environmentally controlled condition known as psoriasis (14).

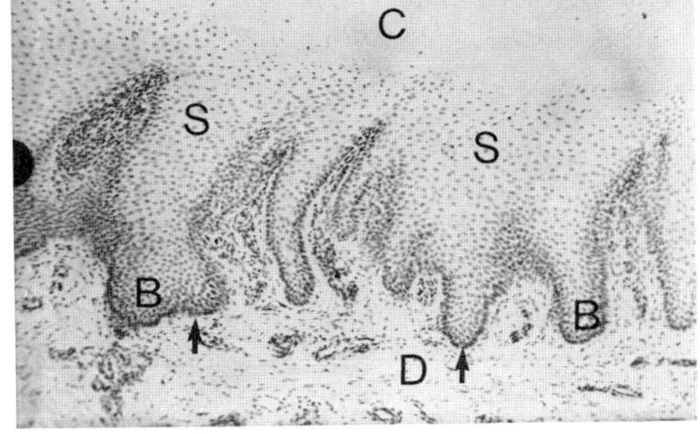

Figure 5.7. Heloma durum at the interphalangeal joint region stained by the Feulgen method for DNA. Light microscopy. *Arrows* indicate rete ridges, stratum corneum (*C*), stratum granulosum (*G*), stratum spinosum (*S*), stratum basale (*B*), and dermis (*D*). Arrow indicates hypertrophied rete Malpighii.

The dermis of heloma durum is remarkable, chiefly for the number and orientation of the fibrocytes. These crowd in large numbers close to the basement membrane

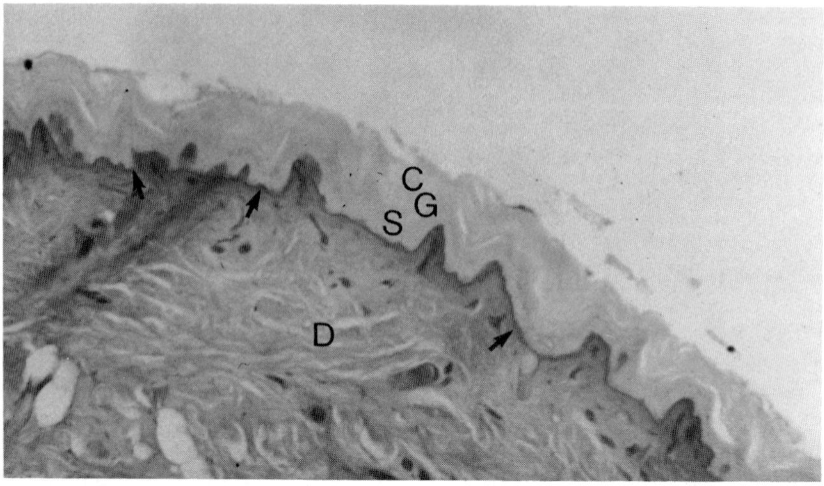

Figure 5.8. PAS (periodic acid-Schiff) stain for mucopolysaccharides in normal interphalangeal skin. *C*, stratum corneum; *G*, stratum granulosum; *S*, stratum spinosum; *D*, dermis. *Arrows* indicate basement membrane.

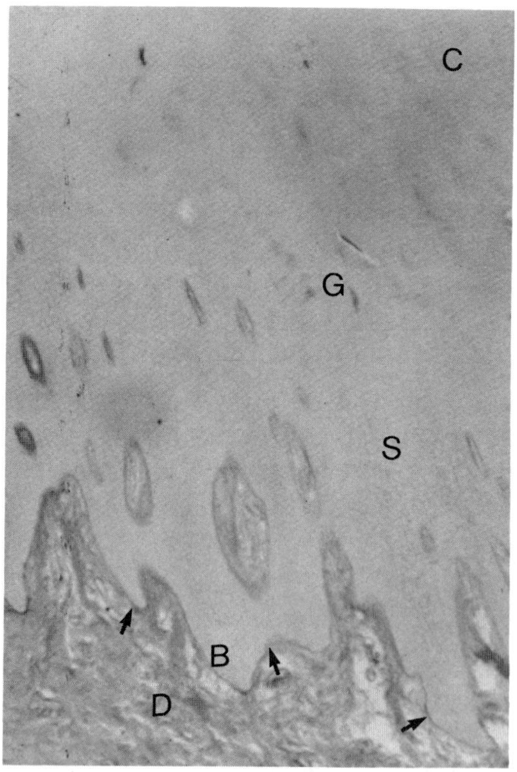

Figure 5.9. PAS (periodic acid-Schiff) stain for mucopolysaccharides in helomatous tissue. *C*, stratum corneum; *G*, stratum granulosum; *S*, stratum spinosum; *B*, stratum basale; *D*, dermis. *Arrow* indicates markedly PAS-positive basement membrane.

of the epidermis, orienting at right angles to the free surface of the skin as if to direct biological messages to the stratum basale.

It is known that a "dermal influencing factor" initiates epidermal cell mitosis and that this undefined substance is a PAS-positive mucopolysaccharide (14). It is also known that extracts of fibrocytes can initiate mitosis of basal cells whereas extracts of the biosynthetic end products of fibrocytes such as collagen and elastic fibers do not have this ability (15). The dermis, ground substance, and fibrous elements are PAS-positive but the region of the basement membrane, particularly in heloma durum, is intensely PAS-positive (Figs. 5.8 and 5.9). I postulate that the fibrocytes are elaborating the substance responsible for increased basal cell mitosis and that their numbers and orientation are in response to inflammatory activities well known to heloma durum (10). This would explain, in part, the occasional remission of helomata following intralesional deposition of corticosteroids: A reduction of the inflammatory response would be expected to decrease the number of fibrocytes responding to external stimuli. Moreover, steroids have a direct effect which suppress synthesis of a variety of substances by fibroblasts. Psoriatic skin, the most extreme case of parakeratosis, is notable also for an increase in PAS-positive substances. Fibroblasts follow closely the invasion of polymorphonuclear leucocytes in wound healing to lay down a network of fibers and ground substance to close wound defects (16). It is my contention that the formation of heloma durum is much like that biosynthetic activity required in wound healing responses.

The fibrous elements of the dermis are increased in heloma durum, and it has been demonstrated that the dermis provides a needed substrate for attachment and orientation of the epidermal basal cells as they form the epidermal-dermal interface (17). The morphologic response of the skin, so sharply altered in heloma durum, depends partly on the mechanical characteristics of the dermal collagenic fiber network (18). Excessive load against the dermis produces annular displacement of collagenous fibers detected by Mallory's acid hematoxylin stain. Load also produces a less oxyphilic and degenerative form of collagenous fibers (19).

The PAS-positive basement membrane at the dermal-epidermal junction is accompanied by a lesser but still noticeably increased reaction in the regions of intercellular boundaries of both stratum Malpighii and stratum corneum. Odland identified an ovoid lamellar subcellular organelle which appears to be displaced peripherally toward the cell boundaries as keratinocytes push towards the free surface of the skin (20). The subcellular organelle has been observed to vesiculate and empty its contents into the intercellular spaces. The extruded substance has been identified as a PAS-positive mucopolysaccharide having cementing qualities. This feature might well account for the tighter adhesion and conservation of the cellular masses which are characteristic of heloma durum.

The RNA and protein concentrations within the stratum Malpighii in both normal and helomatous interphalangeal skin do not appear to differ. Marked alteration in the protein character of the stratum corneum, however, is a striking feature when stained for by the mercury-bromphenol-blue method. All manner of coloration can be seen at the outermost tissue layers in helomata (Fig. 5.10). This feature is indicative of a variety of proteinaceous substances in the corneum. The outermost strata of normal interphalangeal skin, however, reveals an almost homogenous quality of protein.

Parakeratosis results, in part, from the too rapid production of cells, allowing for less time for the enzymes active in the stratum granulosum to effect autolysis of the cytoplasmic elements of epidermal cells (13); this lack of completion of enzyme action produces heterogeneous protein and protein-related compounds in the stratum corneum of heloma durum.

In normal human epidermis, there is an absence of enzymatic activity in the stratum corneum due to complete autolysis in the stratum granulosum as cell constituents, nuclear and cytoplasmic, are rendered

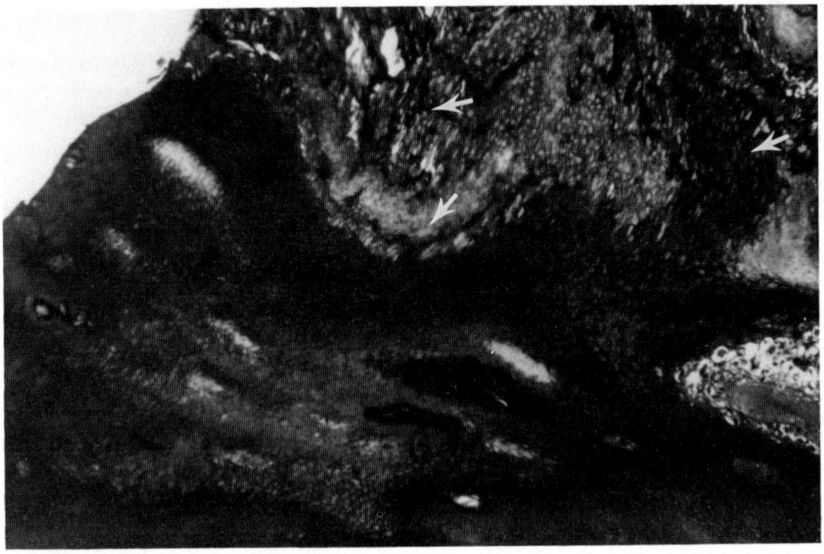

Figure 5.10. Mercury bromphenol blue stain for protein in stratum corneum of heloma durum reveals many colorations, which indicates a variety of protein substances (arrows).

soluble and are dispersed with the removal of enzymes. Jarrett and Spearman have demonstrated the presence of acid phosphatases, nonspecific esterases, lipases, DNA-depolymerase, β-glucuronidase, and ribonuclease, all of which are not found in the keratin of normal skin (14). In the moderately parakeratosed skin of heloma durum, there are few ATPase dendritic cells present. Phospholipids and fats are detectable in the keratin layer (11). Other constituents of parakeratotic stratum corneum include free amino acids, sulfhydryl groups, and nuclear proteins not digested by DNAses. It is not surprising, then, that the parakeratotic stratum corneum typical of heloma durum is so highly metachromatic after testing for proteins.

To review, the histochemical findings of heloma durum are essentially those of parakeratosis resulting from increased proliferation of epidermal basal cells. This increased proliferation results in the acanthosis and hypertrophy of the rete Malpighii as well.

My analysis of the morphogenesis of heloma durum is as follows: The external environment "informs" the dermis as to what (if any) modifications must be made to epidermal morphology (14). In heloma durum, external irritation would evoke an elaboration of histamine on an inflammatory basis, and local vasodilatation of the vascular bed would ensue (21). Inflammatory cell infiltrate may or may not be a concomitant occurrence with the increased blood supply, but fibrocytes do, indeed, respond. The fibrocytes align themselves at right angles to the free surface of the skin and produce additional dermal fibrous structuring upon which the heloma is to be constructed: At the same time these same fibroblasts and fibrocytes elaborate a PAS-positive "dermal influencing factor" which initiates epidermal basal cell mitosis at an advanced rate by reducing the G-1 phase of mitosis (22). This increased proliferative activity would have to counteract the antimitotic activity of the epidermal chalone, a substance identified as similar to, if not identical with, adenosine-3′,5′-monophosphate (23, 24). This substance would be less and less active as the acanthosis is increased (25).

Helomatous keratinocytes would not desquamate in the usual fashion, partly because of external pressure, compaction, and dehydration, and partly because of the presence of an intercellular mucopolysaccharide, as evidenced by PAS-positive reactivity in these spaces. Morphologic changes, then, are the result of proliferation and crowding of cells at the epidermal-dermal junction. This in turn results in hypertrophy of all epidermal structures, including the thickening of the stratum Malpighii and stratum corneum. All of these modifications are in response to biochemical information from the dermis. I do not agree with earlier investigators that the dermal papillae hypertrophy first in the morphogenesis of heloma durum (4). The dermis is more plastic and fluid relative to the firm epidermal cellular mass, and it occupies those spaces created by the proliferative epidermis in a more or less passive fashion (11).

The histochemical alterations of the epidermis are caused mainly by the rapidity of cell transit time, which does not permit complete autolysis at the level of the stratum granulosum (13), which in turn results in the parakeratosis typical of the stratum corneum in heloma durum.

The lesion, heloma durum, presents a most unique example of the extremes of acanthosis, parakeratosis, and alteration of the epidermal-dermal interface morphology. The alterations occur without altering the normal genetic control of epidermal differentiation, as does psoriasis (24).

This discussion of the morphogenetic activities implicit in the development of heloma durum has been detailed and lengthy. However, since similar activities characterize all other helomatous lesions and many of those which mimic heloma, and since tylomata develop along similar lines, lengthy discussion is thought to be both necessary and justified. The treatment of the helomata will be reserved for the concluding section of the general discussion of "corns."

HELOMA MILLIARE

Unlike heloma durum, heloma milliare (seed corns) are more often than not found on nonweight-bearing surfaces of the foot (Fig. 5.11). These lesions are small, circum-

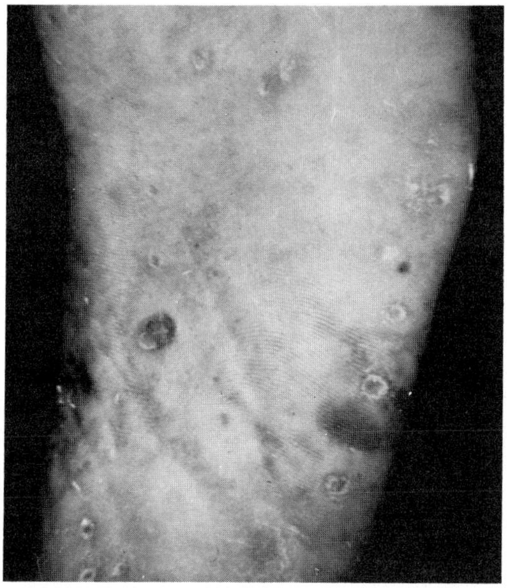

Figure 5.11. Heloma milliare (seed corns) as they are found on the plantar surface of the foot. Courtesy of Drs. I. and J. Yale.

scribed hyperkeratosis which are 3 mm or less in diameter. They occur anywhere on the foot: Moreover, they may be found associated within tyloma, on the heels and balls of the feet as well as in the more thin-skinned areas of the longitudinal arch region.

These lesions seem to be associated with anhydrosis and may be either single or multiple. While heloma milliare are usually pinpoint growths, they may coalesce to form larger lesions which assume a verrucous appearance, and they may fissure.

Small pinpoint lesions resembling heloma milliare are occasionally observed in callous nail grooves. When debriding especially painful callous nail grooves or excising incurvated or impacted nails (usually the great toe), it is good to keep in mind that this contingency may exist.

The pathogenesis of heloma milliare may include avitaminosis, a congenital predisposition involving xerosis or dry skin, as well as localized insults to the epidermis at some point from lasting tacks or other imperfections in the shoes. Improper hosiery can be at fault as well. Trice implicated fungal infections of the feet as etiologic in the formation of some instances of heloma milliare (26).

HELOMA MOLLE

Heloma molle (soft corn) is a circumscribed hyperkeratotic lesion having a tough rubbery consistency because of the accumulation of moisture in the involved epidermal tissues (Fig. 5.12). These lesions occur in the damp, moist, dark interdigital spaces. The fourth interspace is most commonly affected. Here the head of the proximal phalanx of the fifth toe, and the adjacent aspect of the base of the proximal phalanx of the fourth toe, are subject to contact and friction. Usually two closely approximated masses can be identified, in which case they are identified as "kissing lesions." Other common locations for "soft corns" are at the hallucal interphalangeal joint usually associated with hallux abducto valgus, and at the distal interphalangeal joints of the lesser toes.

Uncomplicated heloma molle are usually white, gray, or yellow in coloration. These lesions are especially subject to inflammation and infection which may involve sinus tract formation. Such infections may fulminate to produce generalized cellulitis and lymphadenopathy of the foot and leg, which is especially dangerous when diabetes mellitus or peripheral vascular disease is coexisting.

HELOMA NEUROFIBROSUM

Neurofibrous corns are potentially excruciatingly painful foot lesions. This is due to the plexus of nerve fibers and vascular ele-

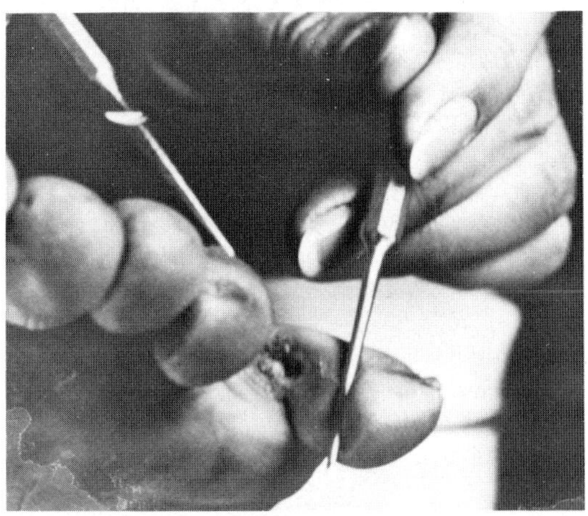

Figure 5.12. Heloma molle of the fourth interspace of the foot with an ulcerating base. Courtesy of Drs. I. and J. Yale.

ments which can be observed superficially. Because of the presence of this plexus, the central core of these lesions present a verrucoid appearance, and their circumferences tend to be more poorly defined than is the case with heloma durum.

The pars papillaris is hypertrophied so as to bring terminal blood vessels and nerves into a superficial relationship with the epidermis. Such tissue modifications are expressions of papillomatosis. The pars reticularis demonstrates fibrotic involvement. Heloma neurofibrosum closely resembles verrucae vulgaris, but viral elements are not present in neurovascular corns, as they are in warty tissues. Subcutaneous changes, including bursal formation and perineural fibromata, may also be associated with these most painful foot lesions.

Like heloma durum but unlike verrucae, heloma neurofibrosum is most likely to occur at points of pinching pressure, including the medial aspect of the hallux, proximal interphalangeal joint of the fifth toe, the fifth metatarsophalangeal joint, and the sesamoid region plantar to the first metatarsal head.

HELOMA VASCULAIRE

Heloma durum may demonstrate hemorrhagic extravasations involving the pars papillaris and suprabasilar regions of the epidermis. Such lesions are referred to as heloma vasculaire: They are also characterized by the presence of capillary loops within the lesion. Depending upon the chemical state of the interstitial bloody coagulum, this type of heloma may exhibit various colorations of brown, red, yellow, and orange (Fig. 5.13).

Heloma vasculaire occur at pressure points where pinching forces may develop. The regions plantar to the first and fifth metatarsal heads, the interphalangeal aspect of the fifth toes, and the distal ends of hyperflexed toes are common locations for its development.

The lesion may be predisposed to by disturbances of circulatory, endocrine, or metabolic functions which lead to capillary fragility. The history often reveals injudicious instrumentation of heloma durum which devitalizes the tissues: minute capillaries may be cut, and pyogenic infection can be introduced into the tissues, all of which can

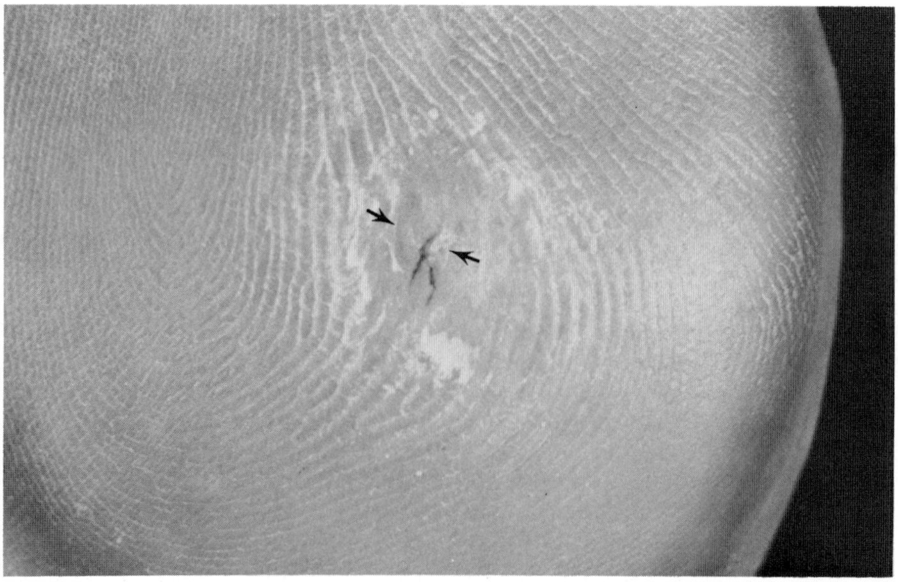

Figure 5.13. Neurovascular corn. Heloma vasculaire occurring on the plantar surface of the foot (*arrows*). Dr. R. Montgomery's case.

lead to the development of heloma vasculaire. As with other forms of helomata, sinus tracts, bursitis, and ulceration may occur, thus further complicating the situation.

TREATMENT OF THE HELOMATA

There is a sense that a discussion of treatment for the usual occurrences of tylomata and helomata is inappropriate to a strictly dermatologic textbook. Such cutaneous lesions are most often symptomatic of some deeper etiology. Bony hyperplasia and skeletal abnormalities are frequently implicated in producing the reactive changes of skin characterized as "corns." Consequently, proper treatment should be directed toward ameliorating the basic underlying cause rather than merely dealing with the external superficial cutaneous symptom.

Recent advances in understanding the biomechanical nature of the human lower extremities and the application of sophisticated podiatric bone and joint surgical procedures have provided satisfactory solutions for many common foot lesions. Functional orthotics and balanced inlays may so control the foot as to correct or accommodate imbalances of the forefoot. Such structural faults may result in a wide range of cutaneous symptomatology, ranging from callous nail grooves to plantar keratosis and digital helomata.

Heloma durum, heloma molle, heloma vasculaire, and heloma neurofibrosum can be effectively and definitively dealt with on a surgical basis. Many procedures and techniques may be employed: Those painful excrescences which involve extensive scarring, bursal involvement, chronic sinus tract formation, fibrosis, perineural fibroma, entrapment of cutaneous nerve, or blood vessel elements, etc., are best excised in toto within conjoined elliptical incisions. Attention should then be directed to the underlying hyperplasia of bone. This may involve resection of the head of the proximal phalanx, excision of part of the intermediate phalanx, or simple resection of an underlying osteophyte or exostosis at whatever level they may occur. One should be aware that there is a tendency for resected phalangeal bones to regenerate, which can produce a surgical failure (Fig. 5.14).

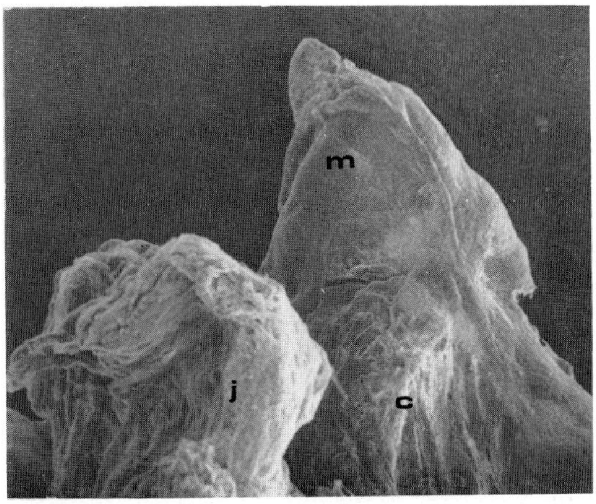

Figure 5.14. Sharp bony exostosis regenerated after resection of the head of the proximal phalanx for correction of heloma durum. The regeneration was responsible for recurrence of a small but painful lesion at the site. *C*, collagenic fibers; *J*, joint capsule; *M*, homogeneous matrix.

In many instances, the podiatric surgeon may elect to bypass the excision of the lesion in less complicated helomata and proceed to correct the bony abnormality through a single incision. In these instances, the skin lesion will resolve in due time since the osseous problem has been corrected. It is interesting to speculate on the modulation of the epidermal-dermal interface and contiguous tissue in this situation. Obviously, profound changes can and do occur within the skin as hyperplastic epidermal structures return to their normal states.

Less enlightened surgeons have been known to simply excise helomata and attempt to close the defect of skin by stretching the margins over the underlying bony problem. Such a simplistic approach is doomed to failure, and the condition will recur worse than before the surgery was performed.

Occasionally, more than one bone is involved in producing helomatous lesions. This is typical for heloma molle in the fourth interspace, where duplicate or "kissing lesions" are in evidence. Experience has proven that resection of the head of the proximal phalanx of the fifth toe as well as of the fibular aspect of the base of the proximal phalanx of the fourth digit is the safest approach to resolve the double legion.

Surgical approaches designed to correct helomata have a rich historical background relative to the evolution of the many operative techniques available. Not all procedures can be recommended, however. It is always essential to clearly understand just what bone is involved in producing any given lesion. If, for example, rotational changes of a digit are a part of the underlying osseous malformation, this problem needs to be resolved along with the correction of the bone abnormality. It is often wise to identify the hyperkeratotic skin lesion with a radiopaque marker such as a fine wire when taking preoperative radiographs. This simple precaution will avoid the error of directing surgical attention to the wrong bony surface, which may result in recurrence of the lesion following surgery. A brief review of digital surgical techniques as they have evolved over the years is recapitulated in Table 5.3.

Bone surgery is not always needed to resolve heloma durum and related lesions. The best example of this is the occasional instance in which hyperflexure deformity at the distal interphalangeal joint produces a "mallet toe" deformity which is manually reduceable. In such cases, tenotomy and capsulotomy at the plantar aspect of the distal interphalangeal joint of the involved digit may suffice. These simple approaches are best implemented by follow up with some type of orthodigital or toe traction device which will maintain the involved toe in a corrected attitude.

Nonsurgical Treatment of Helomata

A substantial percentage of podiatric patients are aged or have systemic problems such as peripheral vascular disease or diabetes mellitus, etc. Such complicating factors can contraindicate surgical intervention for their foot problems. In such instances, a number of palliative, nonsurgical modalities are available. Podiatrists who tend to avoid these mundane activities deny their patients a great deal of relief, temporary though it may be. They also deny themselves the satisfaction of providing a service which is much appreciated. If podiatry were to fail to provide such services, the profession can expect other health care providers to furnish this type of care. Moreover, palliation of chronic foot lesions is necessary to prevent development of potentially serious pedal morbidity.

A variety of techniques and instrumentation are available for the reduction of heloma and tyloma. Scalpels and chisels of several sizes, as well as tissue nippers, are commonly employed for these purposes. Most practitioners become adept at using

Table 5.3
A History of Digital Surgery (1882–1978)

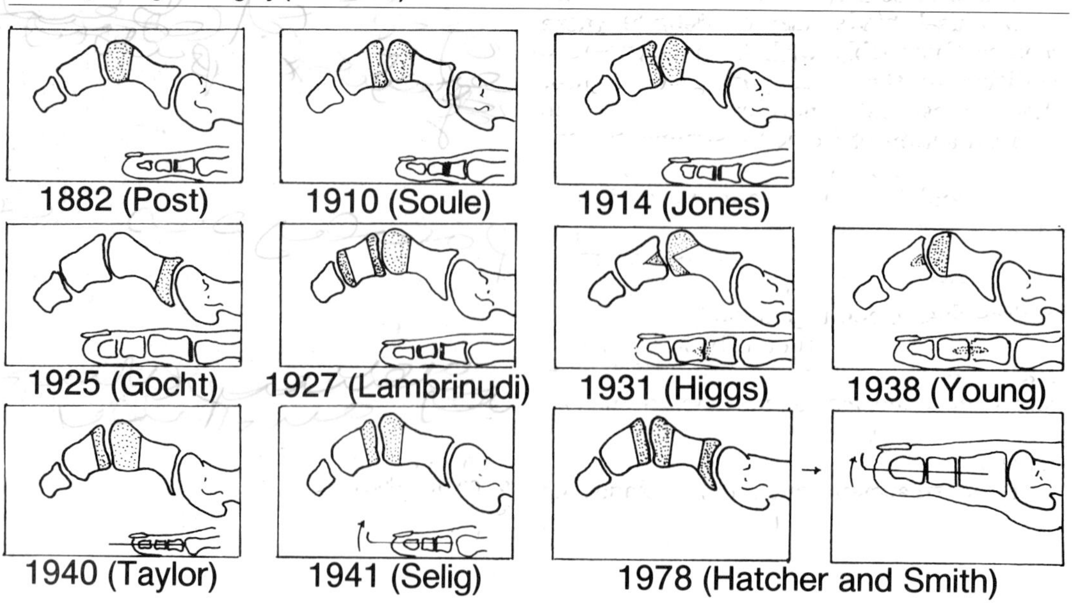

one or two instruments to the exclusion of others.

It is helpful to apply absorbent cotton over hyperkeratotic lesions about to be reduced. Nonsensitizing solutions having keratolytic, antiseptic, or germicidal and analgesic properties are used to saturate the cotton for several minutes prior to instrumentation. Surface active agents, hydrogen peroxide, tincture of green soap solution, and dilute (2–5%) aqueous phenol are commonly employed (3).

Yale states that "The skill of the foot specialist is demonstrated when he (or she) knows how deep to cut and how close to reduce the hyperkeratosis in order to obtain relief of symptoms. The technique requires the sensitivity of a violinist to feel the different textures of the underlying tissues through the operative instrument. Proper wrist motion, finger dexterity and sensory perception are developed only after years of practice" (3).

It is important to remember that helomata and tylomata are pleomorphic and vary considerably in depth. They tend to directly reflect the degree of irritation upon the skin both from within and without. Helomata (corns) have been defined as circumscribed conical accumulations of hyperkeratotic tissues (3–5). The situation in which the periphery of old chronic lesions is the deepest part has already been alluded to. My personal preference is to marginate or isolate these deeper regions with the heel of a chisel blade and to debride these masses thoroughly with tissue nippers in addition to the usual paring techniques. The importance of sharp cutting edges and optimal action of hinged instruments cannot be overemphasized when reducing helomata and tylomata. Some practitioners prefer to reduce excrescences with sandpaper discs or with diamond or steel burrs.

The affinity of cornified epidermis for aniline dyes made it popular in years past to apply dye to hyperkeratotic lesions. This made it possible to better differentiate normal from abnormal tissue and to sharply dissect the lesion in toto with scalpel and forceps.

Home treatment with razor blades or similar paraphernalia or with commercially available corn and callus "cures," usually made up of salicylic acid, frequently produces burning and necrosis of tissue and often initiates secondary infection (Fig. 5.15).

The judicious use of topically applied salicylic acid by professionally trained individuals to selected patients is not contraindicated. Patients whose callosities are too dense for adequate reduction in a single visit, or those who are overly apprehensive for operative reduction of their lesions can benefit from the application of appropriate concentrations of keratolytic agents which are properly shielded from the contiguous normal skin. Those cases involving patients with peripheral vascular disease or diabetes mellitus infections following self-treatment are in especially great danger.

These infections need to be thoroughly debrided, and adequate drainage must be established. Astringent antiseptic soaks and/or wet dressings may be instituted, and a variety of topical medications are available to control infection and to promote healing. Povidone iodine, antibiotics, and proteolytic enzymes are among the most commonly employed substances. When cellulitis, lymphangiitis, and/or lymphadenopathy occurs, it may be necessary to hospitalize patients for best management. This is especially true if patient compliance is a problem—in severe cases, intravenous an-

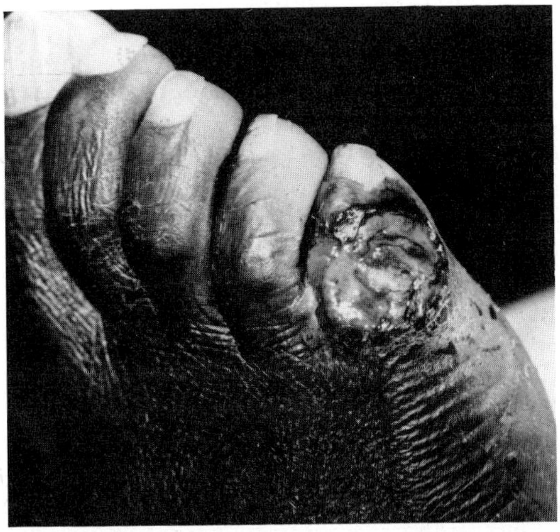

Figure 5.15. Tissue necrosis and secondary infection of heloma durum following the injudicious use of a commercial medication containing salicylic acid. This attempt to "cure" his own corn put this older diabetic patient in the hospital. Intravenous antibiotic therapy was required to prevent serious systemic involvement.

tibiotics may need to be employed. Selection of the antibiotic of choice is made on the basis of culture and sensitivity testing by the laboratory.

Heloma and tyloma which ulcerate are treated similarly according to the severity of the involvement and the patient's state of health.

Once reduced, most hyperkeratotic lesions respond well to protective dressings. This may take the simple form of a generous moleskin patch to disperse pressure locally. The development of pressure absorbing materials as modern technology has advanced plus the ingenuity of podiatrists makes the number and types of shielding seemingly endless. Dr. M. M. Polokoff and others have developed a variety of imaginative pads, shields, and traction devices for both orthodigital correction and for the accommodation of plantar tylomata (27–32).

Permanent devices made precisely to plaster of Paris casts constructed of latex rubber can be very helpful when surgery is not an option. Kits which employ polymers are available for the dynamic fabrication of semipermanent shields on the foot itself. Generally speaking, it is not wise to completely encircle the lesion with the padding material when shielding lesions after palliation. Crescent-shaped pads placed behind the area so as to deflect pressure are preferred.

Temporary dressings applied after palliative treatment of hyperkeratotic foot lesions usually benefit from the application of a suitable topical ointment. The dressing is completed with the application of a small pledget of cotton and a covering of lamb's wool, tape, moleskin, elastoplast, or some similar suitable material. Commercially available cover dressings are especially helpful to the busy practitioner.

During the 1950s and early 1960s a variety of injection techniques became popular for the treatment of heloma durum and related lesions. The simple act of needling the subdermal regions of clavi and instilling a local anesthetic solution can interrupt the underlying fibrous adhesions associated with the lesions and mobilize the skin covering the hypertrophic joint. Austin (33) carried this concept further by placing a small incision through the subhelomatous tissues. Sclerosing solutions and the enzyme hyaluronidase were used as injectibles for a short time. Steinberg developed Keramin solution, a vitamin A product as an injectible for treatment of heloma and verrucae. This material is no longer available, however. Oral vitamin A in water-soluble form has had sporadic popularity for the treatment of hyperkeratosis in general over the years and remains in use to this day.

Corticosteroids and synthetic analogues thereof have been used intra-articularly and periarticularly for more than a quarter of a century. Inflammatory changes in and about the interphalangeal joints are the immediate cause of the external helomatous changes. It is not surprising, then, that corticosteroid injections have been advocated by podiatric authorities in the treatment of helomata (34–38). Their efficacious use over prolonged periods of time is doubtful, however (39). Corticosteroids are best employed in the injection therapy of bursitis associated with helomata. Its usefulness can be augmented by the use of physical modalities such as diathermy and ultrasonic wave (3).

The ability of the podiatrists to determine when surgery is advisable and when a more conservative option is to be preferred is a factor in determining his or her competence. Such good judgment is not only required in the treatment of helomata and tylomata, but in all of the many facets of podiatric medicine and surgery.

Nonoperative Treatment of Heloma Milliare

Seed corns need to be evaluated in the light of the patient's general condition. If avitaminosis is a factor, that contingency should be dealt with. Dry skin may or may not have a congenital basis. Regardless of the cause, dry skin needs to be moisturized by one of the many commercially available emollient products. If fungal etiology is suspected, proper diagnostic evaluation should be made and treated accordingly. The management of the dermatophytes have been dealt with elsewhere in this text.

Sharp dissection or curettage, followed by application of silver nitrate in strength, is usually helpful.

Nonoperative Treatment of Heloma Molle

Soft corns are frequently associated with infections and sinus tract formation. In such instances, adequate drainage and debridement of the associated hyperkeratotic tissues should be accomplished. Antiseptic astringent soaks or wet dressings may be instituted. Topical antibiotics or antiseptic or germicidal preparations can be used to advantage as the indications warrant. It is important not to institute any treatment which might tend to further devitalize the already tender tissues.

In uncomplicated heloma molle, thorough reduction of the lesion, followed by the application of silver nitrate in strength and repeated at appropriate intervals, can be of great help. Lesions which are treated early may resolve without operative intervention. The indications for bone resection have already been mentioned. Adequate separation of the involved toes should be accomplished by any one of many means available. It is important to inspect the patient's footwear to ensure that these external factors are not involved in producing excess compression, heat, and perspiration which are associated with the formation of heloma molle.

Nonoperative Treatment of Heloma Neurofibrosum

Neurofibrous corns frequently require excision of the offending tissue, together with surgical correction of the underlying bony abnormality.

Conservative care begins with proper shielding of the lesion and dealing with whatever biomechanical foot problem has predisposed to the condition.

Careful atraumatic reduction of the lesion, along with the application of silver nitrate in strength, may be of benefit. Other palliative measures directed at eliminating or reducing the fibrotic involvement of heloma neurofibrosum include the judicious application of salicylic acid, vesicants, and cantharides (3). Electrodesiccation and cryosurgery in the form of carbon dioxide ice or liquid nitrogen have been recommended in selected cases of neurofibrous helomata (3) (Fig. 5.16).

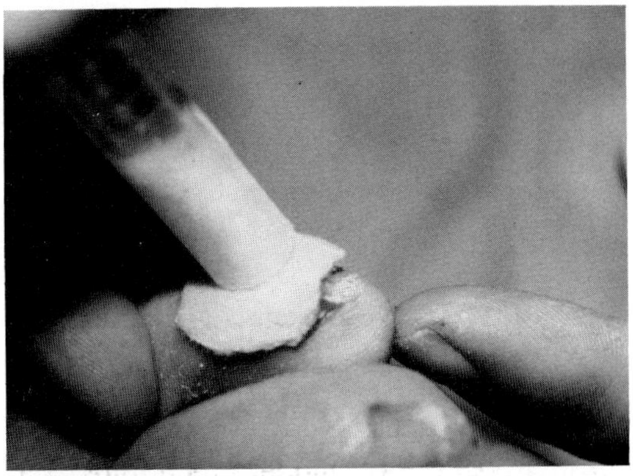

Figure 5.16. The application of carbon dioxide ice in the treatment of heloma neurofibrosum. The normal tissue surrounding the lesion is shielded by a ring of moleskin. Hyperkeratotic tissue should be atraumatically debrided prior to cryocautery, and a suitable ointment should be applied to the properly shielded lesion after treatment.

Nonoperative Treatment of Heloma Vasculaire

The surgical and conservative treatment of vascular corns is essentially similar to that of heloma neurofibrosum. Coexisting infection should be appropriately treated. The possibility of avitaminosis-C should be considered since capillary fragility can predispose to these types of lesions.

LESIONS WHICH MIMIC HELOMA

Several lesions of the human foot appear much like some of the expressions of the helomata. Verrucae plantaris may appear much like heloma neurofibrosum or heloma vasculaire, but verrucae has been dealt with elsewhere in this text. A brief review discussing arsenical keratosis, eccrine poroma, epithelial implants, keratoderma, and porokeratosis plantaris discreta will be presented at this point.

Arsenical Keratosis

Arsenical keratosis are associated with exposure to arsenic either from the environment or in medications. The palms and soles are predisposed to the development of these lesions (40). In years past, inorganic trivalent arsenic was commonly employed in the treatment of syphilis. Since the advent of antibiotics, patients are no longer subjected to the medical use of arsenical compounds. Environmental concerns have further reduced exposure of the population to arsenic. Consequently, the incidence of the arsenical keratosis is expected to become rare indeed.

Arsenical keratosis may be psoriasiform or eczematoid but more often appears as discrete amber-hued papules. The nails may demonstrate Mee's lines (transverse white streaks), and the palms and soles can be generally thick and leathery (3).

Systemic symptoms frequently accompany the appearance of arsenical keratosis on the feet. Hypoproteinemia, sodium depletion secondary to severe diarrhea, thrombocytopenic anemia, eosinophilia, and the appearance of stippled basophiles are characteristic blood findings. Fatigue, pruritis, arthritis, loss of appetite, nausea, and vomiting reflect arsenical toxemia.

Treatment for the arsenical keratosis is first directed toward removal of the offending substance and any other local irritants present. The reader is referred to Chapter 19 for additional information on arsenical keratosis. Reduction of the lesions by the instrumentation of choice and/or the judicious application of keratolytics such as salicylic acid is indicated. There is some evidence that ultraviolet irradiation in proper dosage helps in establishing normal keratinization of the involved areas. Corticosteroids incorporated in tape or ointment form are useful in reducing inflammatory reactions. The therapeutic qualities of vitamin A creams and ointment of ammoniated mercury, or the emollient application of lanolin, cocoa butter, and/or mineral oil can be of further assistance in normalizing the involved integument.

Eccrine Poroma

Eccrine poromas are essentially flattened, smooth-surfaced lesions with a pedunculated base which are usually located interdigitally (41). They have been reported elsewhere on the toes as well as on the palms and soles as nodules. Generally, the lesion appears after the fourth decade of life.

Histologically, the mass may resemble amelanotic melanoma, cicatrix, dermatofibroma, and granuloma pyogenicum. The clinical picture, however, is more typical. The involved cells are of basaloid appearance. Some are of nevoid type with hyperchromatic nuclei. The small benign tumor cells aggregate into intertwined bundles which extend from the epidermis into the pars reticularis of the dermis as anastomosing strands (3).

The treatment of eccrine poroma (which has been implicated with the intraepidermal sweat duct unit) (42) is essentially the same as for porokeratosis plantaris discreta, which will be discussed subsequently.

Epithelial Implants

Horny plaques or plugs of cornified tissue, referred to as epithelial implants, are usually developed as postoperative complications (3). These growths originate in the subcutaneous tissues which have been seeded by epidermal cells carried deep during some phase of surgery. Faulty suturing, needle penetration, and poor apposition of skin margins during closure have all been implicated in the development of epithelial implants.

Dry skin especially predisposes to this condition (3). Highly melanized skin, especially that of negroes, is prone to develop these undesirable skin growths. Avitaminosis may be involved when the skin tone is poor.

The treatment of epithelial implants is directed towards enucleation of the lesions by the instrumentation of choice. Sharp dissection is preferred, although sanding discs and diamond burrs can be useful in reduction of the keratotic plug. Curettage followed by gentle electrocoagulation or electrodesiccation and fulguration can be useful. Prevention of further inflammation by shielding and padding the part is a valuable adjunct in treatment. Topical application of water-soluble vitamin A cream and corticosteroids in tape or ointment form may assist in establishing normal keratinization of the involved tissues.

Keratoderma

Keratoderma plantaris is a circumscribed lesion which is morphologically similar to arsenical keratosis. Many of these lesions are known to be an heredofamilial condition transmitted as a Mendelian dominant trait (43). Localized friction and pressure can also be an etiologic factor. In general, keratoderma plantaris appears as relatively small discrete papules having a diameter of 1 to 3 mm. A central translucent center is commonly present. While these lesions are typically found on the palms and soles, similar lesions have been observed throughout all body surfaces. These occurrences result from systemic pathology, including infection and the ingestion of gold compounds (3, 40).

Obviously, drug-induced keratoderma is treated initially by the avoidance of the involved systemically administered medication.

The local treatment of keratoderma involves the debridement or reduction of the individual lesions with the instrumentation of choice. Keratolytics such as salicylic acid, judiciously applied, can be useful. As is true for most hyperkeratotic situations, the topical application of vitamin A (0.3% concentrations), and emollients such as cocoa butter, lanolin, or mineral oil, can be of benefit. Topical corticosteroids in ointments or incorporated in tape can be of help in establishing normal keratinization patterns. Ultraviolet irradiation in proper dosages can also be of assistance in this regard.

Porokeratosis Plantaris Discreta

Porokeratosis plantaris discreta is a sharply demarcated hyperkeratotic lesion of the foot first described by Drs. Steinberg and Taub in 1969. It is capable of producing sharp, excruciating constant pain. The lesion is thought to develop its lamellated horny plug from direct pressure upon the plantar surface of the foot, which obstructs the ducts of sweat glands. Dr. Steinberg tells of the great debate which arose concerning porokeratosis at the New York Academy of Medicine when it was first identified. This type of debate continues to the present day. However, porokeratosis plantaris discreta is listed and defined by the Armed Forces Institute of Pathology as a specific entity.

The growth is characterized as a hyperkeratosis of the epidermal sweat duct with formation of a cornoid lamella. The epidermis is acanthotic, and agranulosis is observed at some locations. The sudiferous apparatus of the deeper portion of the dermis exhibits dilatory changes (Fig. 5.17).

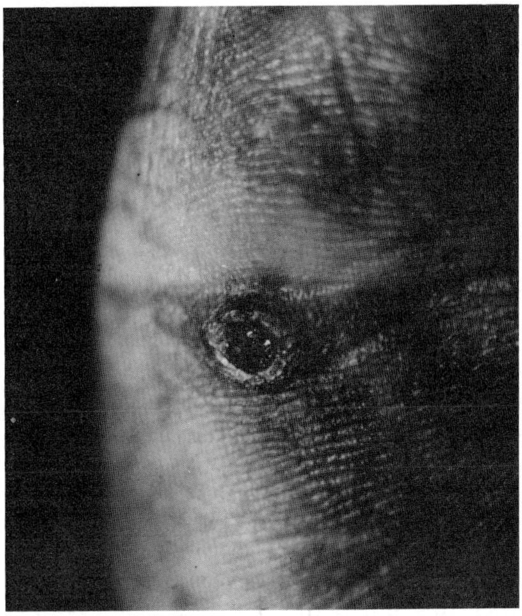

Figure 5.17. Clinical appearance of porokeratosis plantaris discreta (*Arrows*).

Porokeratotic lesions appear as white, gray, or yellowish-white lesions which are most painful when palpated from side to side. Unlike verrucae, there are no vascular elements within the growth. Lesions may extend to a depth of as much as 1.5 cm, and they occur most commonly in the age group 22 to 55. Podiatric pathology laboratories of Baltimore, MD, currently classifies porokeratosis plantaris discreta in three categories. Grade 1 lesions are those which are morphologically concave and do not penetrate the dermis. Grade 2 porokeratosis is a slightly nippled growth which pierces the dermis. Grade 3 lesions are also characterized as being nippled, but these growths invade the dermis and subcutaneous fatty tissues.

The treatment of porokeratosis plantaris discreta may be directed toward destruction or excision of the lesion. Cryosurgery utilizing probe temperatures of −30 to −50°F may be effective (3).

Surgical excision of the mass under local anesthetic using aseptic technique is most commonly used. The excision should be wide and deep enough to include all of the supposed glandular elements of the lesion. Electrodesiccation of the base to effect hemostasis and to provide additional tissue destruction may follow excision. As an alternative to electrodesiccation, Yale advises packing the surgical defect with Gelfoam which is left in situ under compression for 5 days (3).

Postoperative debris can be effectively dealt with using proteolytic enzymes. As always with plantar foot lesions, irritation and friction to the part should be minimized with some type of shielding or foot orthotic.

TYLOMATA

Tylomata (calluses) are generalized thickenings of the epidermis which have a gray or yellowish coloration and are most commonly associated with weight-bearing areas of the foot (3). Most of these lesions are mechanically induced. The use of balanced inlays and functional foot orthosis have been briefly dealt with in connection with the control of forces developing in the rear foot and expressing themselves in the forefoot as helomata. A full and proper discussion of this type of treatment falls into the area of foot orthopedics and is beyond the scope of a dermatological textbook. A good working knowledge of foot orthopedics is, however, implicit in the training of the modern podiatric practitioner and is assumed to be well understood. Histologic modifications of skin involved in the development of tylomata demonstrate alterations of structure involving the subcutaneous tissues as well as the dermis and epidermis.

Most definitions of callosities suggest that the thickening of the epidermis is generalized or diffuse at the area of irritation and that it gradually shades off into the contiguous normal skin (5). It has been my experience that a most painful burning type of tyloma is that which is deeply hyperkeratotic and which terminates abruptly as the sulcus of the toes is approached. This deep sharp line of demarcation is broad and may extend as much as 5 cm across. Upon careful reduction, the bases of such lesions characteristically demonstrate a rather glistening white appearance arranged in streaks consistent with the pattern of the epidermodermal interface. The area distal to the line of hyperkeratotic demarcation in the sulcus of the toes is often intensely hyperemic.

In examining tylomata of the plantar surface of the forefoot, it is not uncommon to find a conical shaped lesion at points of great pressure. These can be referred to as intractable plantar keratosis since they defy all attempts to deal with them by conservative means (Fig. 5.18).

Intractable plantar keratosis has been dealt with in a variety of surgical plans. It is beyond the scope of dermatology to address all of the surgical options available since most of them involve bone and joint revisions. They need to be briefly reviewed, however, to reinforce the concept that tylomata with and without conical nuclei known as intractable plantar keratosis are symptoms of musculoskeletal abnormalities.

Intractable plantar keratosis associated with the plantar surface of the fifth metatarsal head may respond to plantar condylectomy or metatarsal head resection. In addition, several osteotomies have been devised which alter the fifth metatarsal head position so as to minimize mechanical insults to this region. The principle of osteotomy involving the metatarsal neck or head has been applied to the second, third,

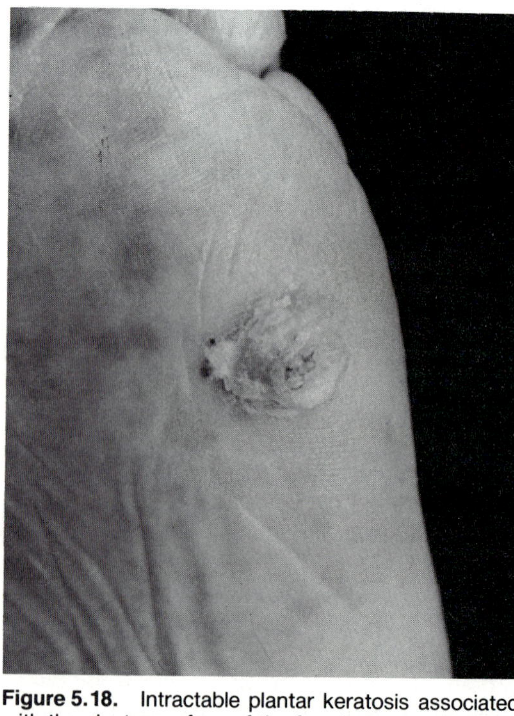

Figure 5.18. Intractable plantar keratosis associated with the plantar surface of the foot in the region of the fifth metatarsal head.

and fourth metatarsals as well. Osteotomies at the base of the involved metatarsal can also be utilized to elevate the distal end of the bone away from the plantar skin lesion. Step down osteotomies of the chevron type can be employed to establish an acceptable parabola configuration of the metatarsal pattern if a congenital fault has altered function so as to produce a painful plantar lesion.

Lesions under the first metatarsal head may be due to a plantarflexed first ray: This contingency may be surgically addressed using a procedure such as Jones' suspension operation. Hypertrophy and/or displacement of the sesamoids beneath the head of the first metatarsal may produce plantar-nucleating tylomas, and these offending ossicles can be excised. Similarly, other offending supernumerary bones such as the os vesaleanum or os tibiale externum may require excision in order to relieve pain from hyperkeratotic lesions which develop at these pressure points.

Interphalangeal sesamoids, ossified and otherwise, may produce a heloma like lesion on the plantar aspect of the digits. Such lesions are most common under the hallux, and these may also be excised to the patient's advantage. It is interesting to review some of the surgical procedures employed from a historical perspective. Not all of them are to be recommended, however (Table 5.4). The reader is referred to the podiatric literature of the last several decades for an in-depth appreciation of all of the techniques available. This material is encyclopedic and certainly beyond the scope of this chapter.

One of the great problems existing when treating all manner of tylomata is the loss of adequate fat pad to protect the underlying skeletal structures. Attempts to find the ideal material to provide an external cushion to accommodate this problem have been partially successful. Commercially available products such as Molo and Spenco have wide usage for these and other pur-

Table 5.4
A History of Metatarsal Surgery (1916–1973)

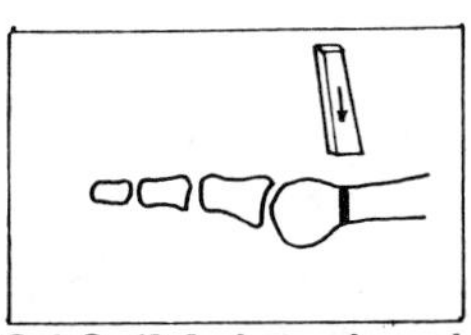
1916 (Meisenbach)

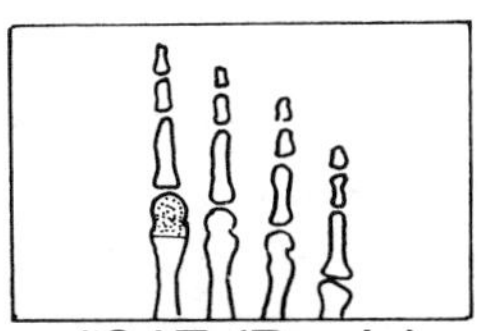
1917 (Davis)

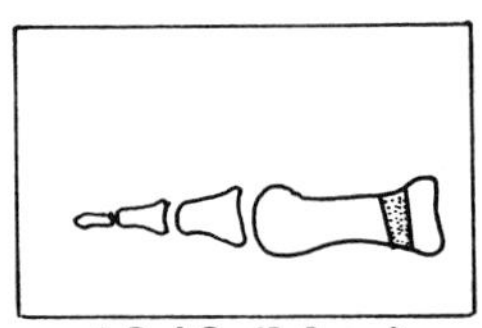
1940 (Mau)

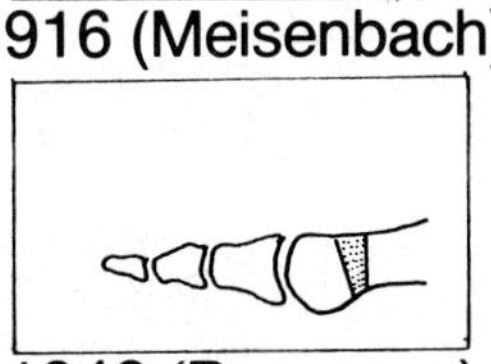
1948 (Borggeve)

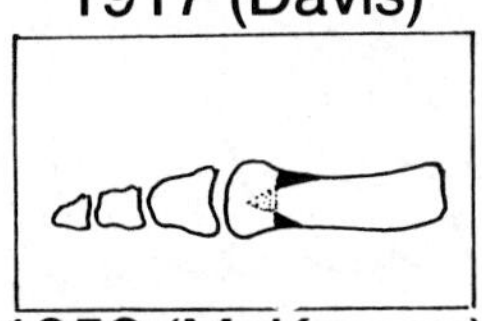
1952 (McKeever)

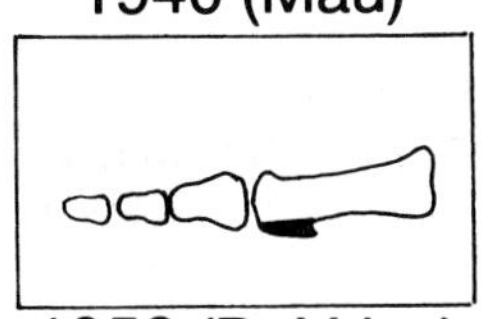
1953 (DuVries)

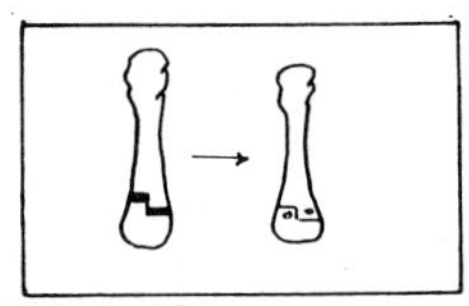
1954 (Giannestras)

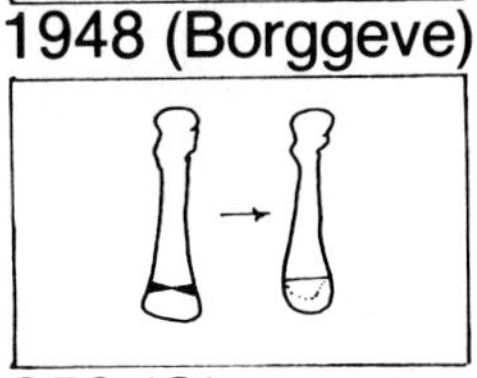
1958 (Giannestras)

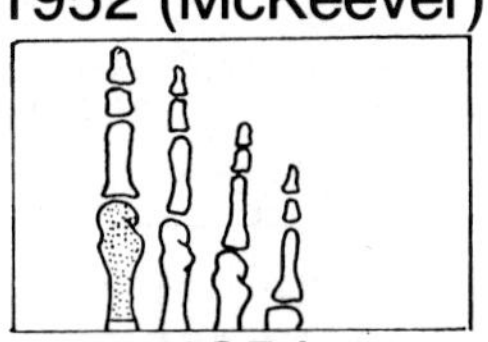
1954 (Rutledge-Green)

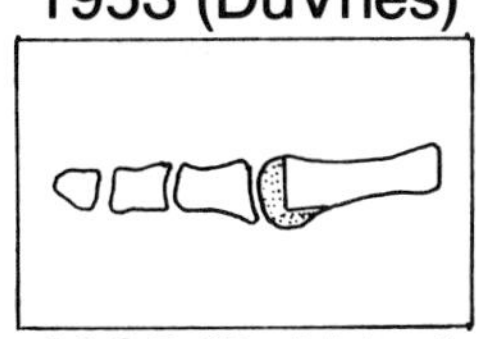
1965 (DuVries)

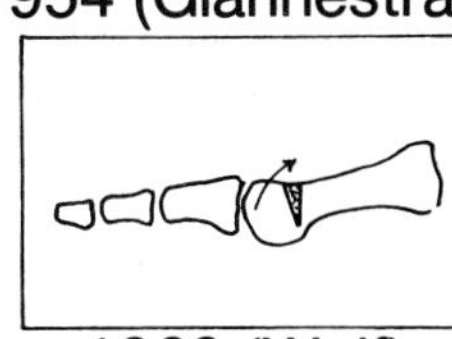
1969 (Wolf)

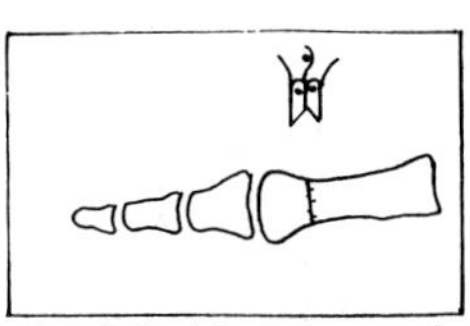
1969 (Addante)

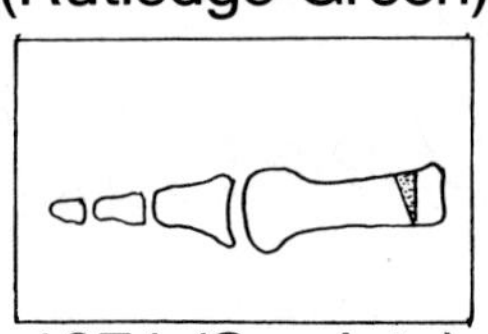
1971 (Scarlato)

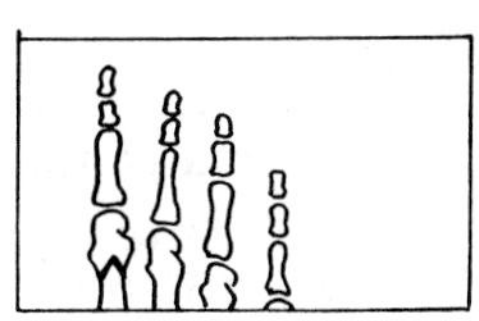
1973 (Jacoby)

poses. New polymers are constantly being developed in the hope of finding still better materials.

Interest in surgically implanting a material such as silastic beneath bony points of pressure has been a matter of research for some time. Unfortunately, an acceptable methodology has thus far eluded the profession, but experimentation is presently continuing.

The burning, throbbing discomfort of tylomata can be further complicated by the presence of adventitious bursae, sinus tract formation, and entrapment of perineural fibroma in the tissues plantar to bony prominences. Such contingencies are often overlooked during the course of bone and joint surgery designed to correct plantar hyperkeratotic foot lesions.

Just as was true for the helomata, the tylomata are subject to cracking and fissuring which may lead to secondary infection which needs to be treated locally, systemically, or in combination in the usual manner.

The plantar surface of the forefoot is only one location where tyloma may be found. Other common sites for the development of pedal calluses include the medial aspect of the foot where the head of the talus is prominent, the tuberosity of the navicular, the dorsal surface of the first cuneometatarsal articulation, the medial or dorsal aspect of the first metatarsal head in hallux abducto valgus or hallux rigidus or limitus, and the fibular aspect of the fifth metatarsal head in tailor's bunion deformity. Still another particularly troublesome area is the perimeter of the heel, with which problems frequently occur with the wearing of open-heeled shoes and obesity. It has been postulated that the quality and quantity of the fat covering the plantar aspects of the tuberosities of the calcaneus is diminished with age and compacts in a squared-off fashion. This degenerative change is reflected in the skin of the heel, which becomes hyperkeratotic and is subject to cracks and fissuring.

The reader is referred to the pathogenesis of heloma durum for an accounting of the morphological and biochemical events leading to hyperkeratinization as presented in this chapter. They are essentially the same in both heloma and tyloma. Lemont points out one area of difference in that mechanical and shear forces directed at the plantar surface of the skin of the foot produce a break and disruption of the stratum granulosum (44). This phenomenon is to be differentiated from agranulosis (the failure of the stratum granulosum to develop focally).

The palliative care of tylomata is similar to that given for the helomata, except that much larger areas of the skin are involved. The instrumentation and principles of dressing and padding these lesions are also the same for all practical purposes.

References

1. Adam J: American Board of Chiropodical Dermatology Report on Skin. Annual Meeting, National Association of Chiropodists, Chicago, 1960.
2. McCarthy DJ, Port M, Chu S: Characteristics of podiatric care in the Veterans Administration. *J Am Podiatry Assoc* 70(8):385–396, 1980.
3. Yale I: *Podiatric Medicine.* Baltimore, Williams & Wilkins, 1980.
4. Krausz CE, Rowe CG: Chiropodical classification and treatment of epidermal excrescences. *Am J Surg* 44(1):328–335, 1939.
5. Montgomery RM: Painful cutaneous lesions of the foot. *South Med J* 63:615–619, 1970.
6. Freed JD: Histologic post mortem evaluation of bone hyperplasia acompanying digital clavus. *J Am Podiatry Assoc* 59:467, 1969.
7. McCarthy DJ, Habowsky JEJ: A cytological survey of skin in heloma durum using electron microscopy. *J Am Podiatry Assoc* 62(7):239–249, 1972.
8. Bonavilla CJ: Histopathology of heloma durum: some significant features and their implications. *J Am Podiatry Assoc* 58:423, 1968.
9. Feigenbaum A, Schreiber LF: A compend of helomata. *Curr Podiatry* 13:1, 1964.
10. McCarthy DJ, Habowsky JEJ: Alterations in epidermal and dermal histo-differentiation in normal and hyperkeratinizing skin interpreted through histochemistry and anthropometric analysis. *J Am Podiatry Assoc* 65(1):2, 1975.
11. McCarthy DJ, Habowsky JEJ: Alterations in skin morphology in heloma durum utilizing maceration technique for examination of epidermal-dermal interface. *J Am Podiatry Assoc* 62(8):303–308, 1972.
12. Gibbs RC: Skin and nail changes in the elderly foot. *J Am Podiatry Assoc* 65:471–

474, 1975.
13. Pinkus H, Mehregan A: *A Guide to Dermatohistopathology.* New York, Appleton-Century-Crofts, 1969.
14. Jarrett A, Spearman RIC: *Histochemistry of the Skin in Psoriasis.* Princeton, NY, D. Van Nostrand, 1964.
15. Briggaman RA, Wheeler CE: Epidermal-dermal interactions in adult human skin. II. The nature of the dermal influence. *J Invest Dermatol* 56:18, 1971.
16. Ross R: Wound healing. *Sci Am* 220:40, 1968.
17. Wessels NK: Differentiation of epidermis and epidermal derivatives. *N Engl J Med* 277:21, 1967.
18. Carr EE, Millington PF: Load consequent changes in microstructure of human skin. *J Physiol (Lond)* 203:7, 1969.
19. Evan JH, Siesenhop WW: *Proceedings of the Seventh International Conference of Medical Electro- and Bioengineering*, Stockholm, 1967.
20. Odland GF: A submicroscopic granular component in human epidermis. *J Invest Dermatol* 34:111, 1960.
21. Feldberg W: *Histamine.* Ciba Symposium. Boston, Little, Brown, 1956.
22. Malkinson F: Epidermal cell kinetics. In *Yearbook of Dermatology.* Chicago, Yearbook Medical Publishers, 1972.
23. Bullough AD, Laurence GG: The control of epidermal mitotic activity in the mouse. *Proc R Soc Lond (Biol)* 15:517, 1968.
24. Vorhees JJ, Duel EA: Psoriasis as a possible defect of the adenyl cyclase, cyclic AMP cascade. *Arch Dermatol* 104:352, 1971.
25. Le Blond EP, Walker EE: Renewal of cell populations. *Physiol Rev* 36:255, 1956.
26. Trice EW: A new hypothesis on the etiology of heloma milliare. *J Natl Assoc Chirop* 45:28–29, 1955.
27. Polokoff MM: Lesser toe latex shield made with tubular gauze. *J Am Podiatry Assoc* 48:432–433, 1958.
28. Polokoff MM: Removable shield for lesions about the head of the fifth metatarsal. *J Am Podiatry Assoc* 57:566–568, 1967.
29. Polokoff MM: Removable felt appliances to protect multiple deformities of the same foot. *J Am Podiatry Assoc* 64:890–896, 1974.
30. Polokoff MM: Traction appliance for the third toe. *J Am Podiatry Assoc* 65:1011–1012, 1975.
31. Polokoff MM: Double ring toe traction device. *J Am Podiatry Assoc* 66:35–37, 1976a.
32. Polokoff MM: Buttress appliance. *J Am Podiatry Assoc* 66:261–263, 1976b.
33. Austin DW: New concepts in the treatment of helomata. *J Natl Assoc Chirop* 40:1927, 1950.
34. Locke RK: Arthridities and allied disorders as factors in everyday chiropody practice and their treatment. *J Natl Assoc Chirop* 46:756–777, 1956.
35. Locke RK: Corticosteroid injection therapy in the foot. *J Am Podiatry Assoc* 48:505–511, 1958.
36. Ashur M, Farrar R: Griseofulvin in the treatment of tinea pedis. *J Am Podiatry Assoc* 51:103–108, 1961.
37. Cameron DJ: A new rapid and prolonged acting steroid for intraarticular inflammatory disorders. *J Am Podiatry Assoc* 56:317–319, 1966.
38. Prentice H: Sublesional administration of corticosteroids: a new technique with broad implications in podiatry. *J Am Podiatry Assoc* 51:791–800, 1961.
39. Levy SE: A controlled evaluation of subdermal corticosteroid injections. *J Am Podiatry Assoc* 48:403–407, 1958.
40. Vance EE, Levy L: Recognizing arsenical keratosis. *J Am Podiatry Assoc* 66:91–94, 1976.
41. Gibbs RC: Differential diagnosis of plantar verrucae. *J Am Podiatry Assoc* 59(3):90–92, 1969.
42. Kipping H: A case of eccrine poroma. *J Bull Millard Fillmore Hospital, Buffalo,* NY 9:95–97. 1962.
43. Fred HL, Giesler RG, Berry W et al: Keratosis palmaris et plantaris. *Arch Intern Med* 113:866–871, 1964.
44. Lemont H: Comments on the histologic differentiation of genetic and mechanically induced keratosis. *J Am Podiatry Assoc* 66(4):259–260, 1976.

CHAPTER 6

Onychopathy

CHARLES KRAUSZ

Onychopathy is defined as any disease or abnormality found in the nail area. The latter not only includes the nail plate but also the nail grooves, nailbed, nail matrix, and eponychium. Next to epidermal excrescences, nail lesions are the most common problem observed in podiatric practice. Sixty-one percent of all patients who consult a foot doctor will present some ungual disturbance. This statement is based on a survey which I have conducted in both my private and clinical practices. During a 41-year period, I have examined 12,500 patients. Of that number, 7670 have displayed one or more nail disorders. This survey extends from October 28, 1942, to July 13, 1984. The following tabulation (Table 6.1) indicates the economic importance and wide range of nail disorders (1).

The need to conduct a podiatric nail survey was inspired by statistics recorded in Pardo-Castello's treatise on nail diseases (2). In a 6-month period, he reported seeing 192 nail abnormalities on the fingers and toes of 464 patients. His observations were made in the Dermatological Service of the University Hospital, Havana. As could be expected, a large percentage of these cases were ungual manifestations of cutaneous disorders. A search of the literature indicated that C.J. White published a somewhat similar survey in 1902 (3). White was a founding member of the American Dermatology Association and the first professor of Dermatology at Harvard University. Of the 485 nail cases that he reported, 63% were associated with a skin disease. In our survey it has been determined that 71% of the nail problems observed in podiatric practice are traumatic in origin. This is understandable because the location of the foot makes it vulnerable to many athletic, household, and occupational injuries.

The above surveys indicate that an abnormal condition of one or more nails is a common occurrence. These ungual abnormalities may result from traumatism, chemical irritants, bacteria, or fungi. They may also be associated with a number of cutaneous affections, or with various general diseases. In cases of onychocryptosis and onychoschizia the nail plate is involved primarily. In most of the other lesions mentioned in our survey, the nail plate is implicated secondarily as a result of morbid changes in the matrix, nail bed, or surrounding soft tissues. From the appearance of the diseased nail, it is sometimes difficult to come to a definite conclusion with regard to the underlying cause, since similar appearances may be produced by totally different agents. It is, therefore, necessary to obtain a history of injury or local irritation, or to look for other causative factors such as some cutaneous or general disease. When only one nail is involved, the presumption is that some local cause is responsible. When nails on both feet are affected more or less symmetrically, it points to some general disturbance.

Nail disorders may be classified under the following divisions:

1. Traumatic nail disorders: As the main function of the toenail is to protect the distal phalanx from injury, it is only natural that the most common nail lesions seen by the podiatrist-chiropodist are found in this group. Onychocryptosis, onychauxis, and onychophosis are examples of traumatic nail disorders.
2. Neoplasia of nails.
3. Nail dystrophies: any changes which occur in the texture or color of the nail due to interference with function of the nail matrix are known as nail dystrophies. Included in this category is onychatrophia, onychorrhexis, leukonychia, Beau's lines, onycholysis, and onychomadesis.
4. Ungual manifestations of cutaneous diseases: As

Table 6.1
Survey of Nail Disorders

No. of podiatric patients observed	12,500
No. of nail disorders	7670
Percentage of nail disorders	61%
Survey	
Onychocryptosis	1982
Onychauxis and onychogryphosis	1724
Onychophosis	1457
Onychomycosis	624
Onychatrophia	337
Onychorrhexis	293
Subungual heloma	202
Leukonychia	193
Onychia and paronychia	183
Beau's lines	171
Onycholysis	169
Onychomadesis	119
Traumatic onychophyma	84
Onychoschizia	24
Psoriasis	17
Subungual exostosis	17
Periungual fibroma	16
Anonychia	9
Polyonychia	7
Melanonychia striata	7
Macronychia	5
Periungual verruca	5
Subungual verruca	5
Hapalonychia	5
Koilonychia	5
Pachyonychia	3
Chondroma	2
Onychophagia	2
Syphilis	1
Avitaminosis	1
Ichthyosis	1

the nail is an appendage of the skin, almost any skin disease may present nail symptoms. Onychomycosis, or ringworm of the nail, is the most common lesion in this group, followed by psoriasis and eczema.

5. Ungual manifestations of systemic diseases: Syphilis, tuberculosis, arthritis, arteriosclerosis, diabetes, and other systemic diseases sometimes affect the function of the matrix, with resultant changes in the nail plate.
6. Congenital nail disorders: Errors of development produce anomalies of the nail which are the same as occur in other systems of the body. Anonychia, polyonychia, macronychia, and pachyonychia are examples of this group.

TRAUMATIC NAIL DISORDERS

Onychocryptosis

Synonyms: ingrown nail, onyxis, unguis incarnatus, Nagelzwang (Ger.), una encarnada (Span.).

Definition: Onychocryptosis is a condition in which the lateral, or free edge, of the nail has penetrated the epidermic layers and has become embedded in the adjacent soft tissues, either laterally or anteriorly.

Etiology: Traumatism is the exciting cause in the production of an ingrown nail. The most common traumatic factors are:

1. Faulty footgear: Tight shoes or stockings cause the soft structures of the nail groove to press against the lateral edge of the nail plate. The forward thrust of the foot in walking increases the pressure and forces the lateral border of the nail to penetrate the nail groove.
2. Improper nail care: the patient may experience some discomfort on the side of the nail. In order to overcome this, he cuts a corner out of the nail plate, leaving a small spur. This spur pierces the nail groove as the nail grows forward.
3. Injury: Occasionally, ingrown nail is caused by an injury such as stubbing the toe or dropping some heavy object on it. Certain anatomical peculiarities found on the distal aspect of the toe are predisposing causes of onychocryptosis. An example of this is the so-called inverted nail (Fig. 6.1). This is a nail in which the lateral border curves inward toward the center line of the toe. It is also known as an incurvated nail or involuted nail. Another anatomical development which can result in onychocryptosis is hypertrophy of the unguilabia. This is a fat, chubby lateral nail fold often found in the obese patient.

Pathology: The ingrowing portion of the nail has penetrated the soft tissues of the nail groove, causing an inflammatory reaction to be set up within the involved area. The break in the skin continuity allows pyogenic bacteria to enter the wound, with resultant pus formation. If untreated for a period of time, periungual granulations

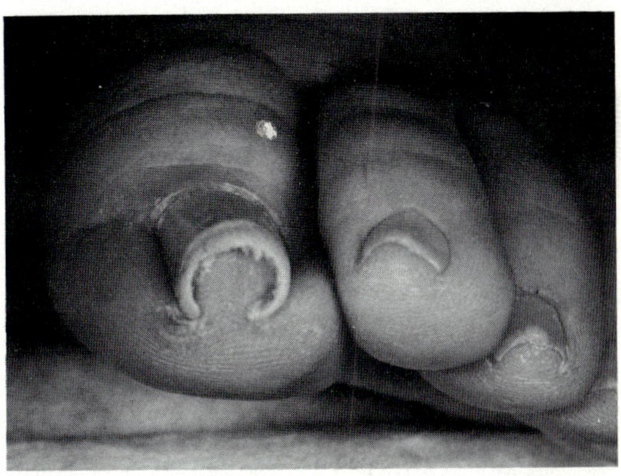

Figure 6.1. Onychocryptosis of the great toenail secondary to inversion.

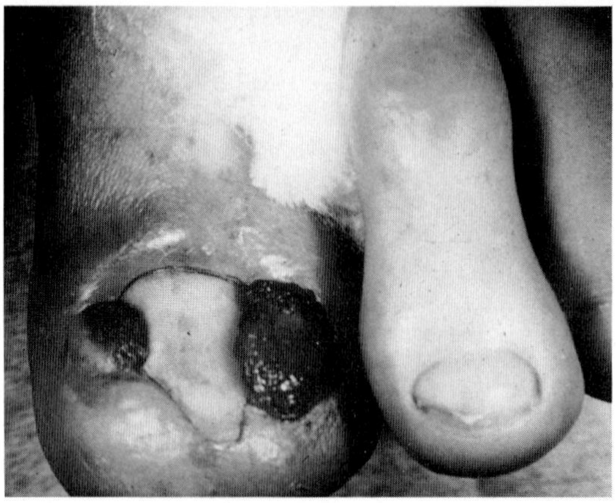

Figure 6.2. Granulation tissue associated with chronic onychocryptosis.

(proud flesh) may form (4). The ingrown portion of the nail acts as a foreign body, and this prevents the granulating edges of the wound from uniting. The proud flesh becomes excessive and projects from the nail groove (Fig. 6.2). These periungual granulations consist of a network of newly formed capillaries.

Symptoms: The lateral side of the toe is red and swollen, and the patient suffers pain, especially when pressure is exerted either against the soft tissue or downward on the nail plate. If infected, pus will exude from the wound. When proud flesh is found projecting from the nail groove, it has the appearance of a mass of raw tissue which bleeds freely upon the slightest provocation. It may be no larger than a pinhead or may, in advanced cases, pile up a mass which covers half the plate. There is usually a bloody, purulent, fetid discharge present.

Treatment

Authors are in general agreement that a spur of nail is the exciting agent in the dynamics of this disease. It is obvious that its elimination should relieve the problem. However, the mechanics of partial or complete nail removal has resulted in a wide variety of clinical approaches. C.J. Heifetz made a search of medical literature appearing from 1814 to 1934 (5). He uncovered 87 separate articles dealing with treatment. These writers believed that their method was best. In the hands of each individual, this was probably true. The treatment which follows was developed within the podiatric profession and has been used routinely for more than 80 years. In 1982 cases of ingrown nail reported in my survey, this technique proved to be 91% successful.

Partial Onychectomy

After sterilization of hands, instruments, and field of operation, the operator should locate the exact position of the ingrown portion of the nail, using for this purpose a blunt probe, or a round excavator. This preoperative examination of nail and groove is of utmost importance in the success of the treatment (6). Failure to give the patient the necessary relief is usually due to hasty and careless examination. Having definitely located the offending portion of the nail, the thumb and forefinger of the operator are used to grasp the toe firmly along the sides at about the region of the first joint. This serves three purposes: (*a*) locks the toe; (*b*) aids in cutting off sensation; and (*c*) helps in drawing the soft structures of the lateral nail fold away from the nail plate. Using a nail splitter, a small nick is made on the anterior free edge of the nail plate. This split is made as close to the affected side as possible. It should be made on an angle in the direction of the lateral edge so as to clear the ingrown portion. A narrow onychotome is then placed in this slit. Pressure is exerted on the onychotome, which cuts through and splits the nail back to the lateral edge just behind the spur. After the offending portion of the nail is free, a slight rolling motion of the onychotome downward and outward toward the lateral nail fold will lift the fragment from the nail groove. If the nail fragment is attached to a small portion of the nail bed, it is grasped with tweezers or hemostat and dissected loose from the soft structures with the onychotome. The groove should be cleaned out with alcohol or peroxide and should again be examined to make sure that no spur of nail remains to further irritate the soft structures. A small packing of gauze or cotton is placed in the affected nail groove. Using a nail probe, the packing is forced down and under the lateral edge of the nail plate.

A wet dressing of Burow's solution (one part of Burow's in two parts of water) is used if the condition is mildly inflamed. If proud flesh is present, it should be touched up with 50% silver nitrate (7). After the wound has healed, the nail groove must be packed at regular intervals until the nail has grown completely out of the lateral fold. This part of the treatment is very important as it forces the soft tissues back to their normal position. Any pressure caused by pointed or narrow shoes, or high heels, should be corrected by prescribing more conservative footgear. Patients should be advised to cut their nails straight across, rather than cut them rounded, and should be cautioned against cutting down the corners of the nail.

Nine percent of the ingrown nail patients recorded in my survey did not respond to the treatment outlined above. These individuals all presented severely inverted nails. It must be kept in mind that the transverse contour of the nail is in exact ratio to the convexity of the matrix. Therefore, the correction must be directed to the incurvation of both plate and matrix. The use of the following procedure will rectify the problem.

Nail Matrix Phenolization

After complete sterilization, anesthesia is induced by the injection of lidocaine around the base of the toe. A tourniquet is applied to control hemorrhage. The lower jaw of a nail forceps is inserted under the free edge of the nail. This is forced posteriorly and under the nail wall, splitting the plate. An onychotome is used to separate the underside of the posterior nail fold from the dorsal surface of the nail root. The semidetached portion of the nail is grasped with a hemostat. Holding the hemostat in one hand, the onychotome is utilized to dissect the nail fragment free from the underlying bed and matrix. The resulting cavity is examined to ensure the removal of all nail tissue. The area is mopped as dry as possible with a gauze sponge. Pure liquified phenol is applied with a cotton-tipped applicator. The applicator is worked under the nail wall and left in place for no longer than 2 min (8). The area is then flushed out with alcohol. The wound is packed with gauze, and a bandage is applied. The toe should be redressed in 48 hour.

Total Nail Avulsion

As mentioned earlier in this article, most cases of onychocryptosis respond favorably to partial removal of the affected nail. There are some circumstances in which a complete nail avulsion may be indicated. In removing the entire plate, both C.J. Heifetz (1938) and L. Frost (1958) recommended the use of a spatula-shaped elevator (9). This instrument has a slightly convex rounded head on its superior surface with a handle approximately 4 inches long. After complete sterilization, anesthesia is achieved by the injection of lidocaine. The ungual elevator is forced under the free edge of the nail. The instrument is grasped so that the thumb rests just behind the convex head. The undersurface of the elevator rests on the flexed index finger of the operator. Once the elevator has passed under the entire length of the nail, it is moved in a semicircular arc to loosen the plate from the underlying tissue. With the elevator still under the nail, the thumb is moved forward to the dorsum of the plate, and the entire nail is lifted from the bed. Any superfluous tissue in the bed or grooves is removed. A Telfa dressing is placed over the bed, and a gauze dressing is applied.

ONYCHAUXIS AND ONYCHOGRYPHOSIS

Synonyms

Onychauxis is also known as club nail. Onychogryphosis has two synonyms, ram's horn nail and Hostler's toe (Fig. 6.3). The latter term was coined by our British colleagues. In the early part of this century, local transportation was largely dependent on horse-drawn vehicles. A person who

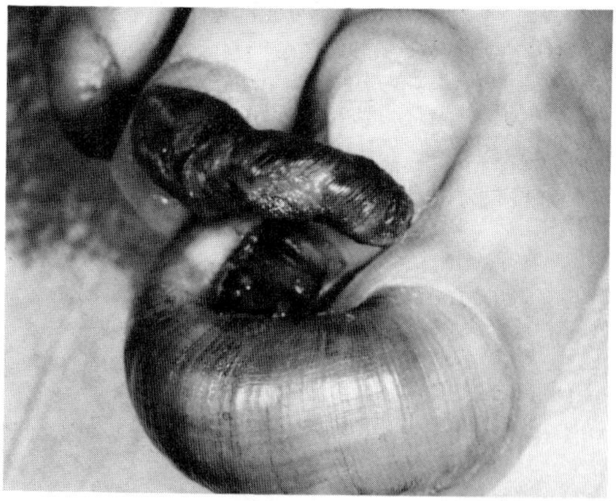

Figure 6.3. Club nail of onychgryphosis.

groomed a horse was known as a hostler. Having one's toe stepped on by a horse was a common occupational injury. It is not surprising that a club nail became somewhat of a symbol of their trade.

Definition

Onychauxis is a hypertrophy of the nail in any or all of its dimensions. Onychogryphosis is a hypertrophy of the nail of long standing in which the plate is curved or hooked in form. The etiology, pathology, and treatment are the same as in onychauxis.

Etiology

The most common cause of this condition is trauma to the matrix. It also may follow a previous attack of onychia. It is sometimes observed as an ungual symptom of certain skin diseases such as ringworm or psoriasis (7). Club nail may eventually develop following an attack of arthritis of the interphalangeal joint of the great toe.

Pathology

The papillae of the matrix become enlarged as a result of one of the above etiological factors. The enlarged papillae cause an increase in the number of nail cells. This results in nail hypertrophy.

Symptoms

Onychauxis appears thicker and harder than a normal nail (10). If treatment is neglected for a long period of time, the nail becomes deformed (onychogryphosis). The plate is usually brittle and may present a roughened, wavy surface. The color varies from gray to brown or black. Nail hypertrophy tends to increase with the age of the individual. In other words, as one grows older, the pedal nails grow slower but thicker.

Treatment

A cotton pad is saturated in 1% compound solution of cresol (U.S.P.). This is applied to the thickened nail for 2 min. The solution serves both as an antiseptic and a softening agent. The reduction of a club nail should be a painless podiatric procedure (11). If nail reduction causes pain, it is due to the torsion of the nail at its base. This can be easily avoided by grasping the toe firmly between the thumb and index finger at the interphalangeal joint. A heavy nail forceps is used to remove small sections of the plate. Care should be exercised so that only one jaw of the forceps is out of sight at one time. Knowing that the jaws must meet, the underlying tissue will not be pinched or cut if this plan is followed. Following the reduction of the thickened nail, any rough edges are smoothed off with burr and electric drill. A probe is used to remove corneous cells remaining in the bed or grooves. The most satisfactory postoperative application following the reduction of a club nail is a cocoon dressing. The area is covered with absorbent cotton. The edges of the cotton must be packed into all the crevices of the posterior and lateral nail folds. After the cotton is smoothed in the longitudinal axis of the toe, flexible collodion is applied over the entire surface. This is worked back under the lateral and posterior grooves. This provides a comfortable dressing which will remain in place for 1 to 3 weeks. For those patients who desire a complete removal of club nail for cosmetic or other reasons, consult the section Total Nail Avulsion.

Bizarre deformity will occur to the club nail in which the patient neglects podiatric care. One such case was observed in a 68-year-old white female. Her great toenail extended around the end of the second toe and pressed into the lateral side of this digit. The second nail curved under the distal end of the second toe. The third nail grew medialward over the dorsum of the second toe. The fourth and fifth toes were slightly hypertrophied. The patient admitted that she had not visited a chiropodist for at least 12 years.

ONYCHOPHOSIS

Synonym

Callous nail groove.

Definition

Onychophosis is a condition in which there is a thickening of the epidermis in the lateral nail groove with or without the formation of heloma (Fig. 6.4).

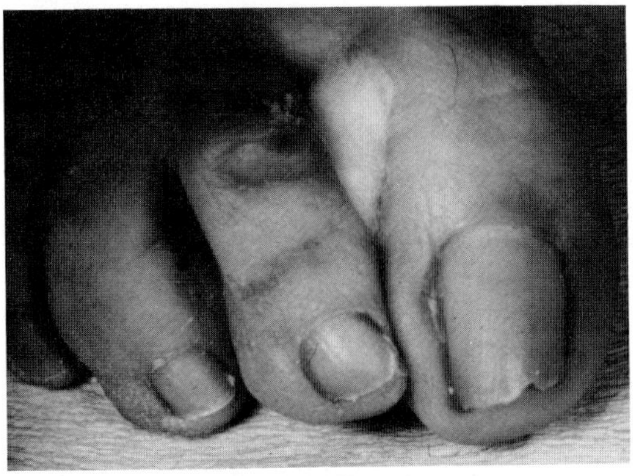

Figure 6.4. Onychophosis of the great toe.

Etiology

The majority of these cases are caused by either a short stocking or a shoe with insufficient toe room. Among shoes, the high heeled pump is by far the greatest offender (12). Improper footgear, whether it be a shoe or stocking, causes the soft tissues of the nail fold to be forced against the lateral edge of the nail. The callus forms as a protection to prevent the nail from penetrating these tissues. When a heloma is present, it may be caused by the localized pressure of a roughened edge of nail. This is often induced by the patient who persists in probing the groove with scissors or nail file.

Symptoms

The patient complains of pain on slight pressure, and in advanced cases the lateral nail fold may be red and swollen. Examination will disclose a callosity or heloma in the nail groove. Onychophosis is more common in women than in men.

Treatment

The affected nail groove is examined to determine the location of the callous tissue. A pledget of cotton is saturated in a 1% compound solution of cresol. This is packed into the sulcus and left in place for 2 min. If the examination indicated that there is insufficient space to debride the groove, a wedge-shaped section of nail is removed. This will allow greater access to the involved area. The callous tissue is then removed with an onychotome. A small amount of 10% salicylic acid ointment is inserted in the groove and held in place with gauze or cotton packing. If severe inflammation is present, it can be controlled by a wet dressing of Burow's solution. Most cases of onychophosis are caused by faulty footgear. If a pump is the culprit, it must be eliminated, and a more conservative shoe must be prescribed with a moderate height heel.

The acrylic resins used in dentistry are sometimes employed to correct a callus nail groove (13). S.C. Sivitz (1953) and P. Mogull (1954) have authored separate articles in which methyl methacrylate is recommended for this purpose. In a number of selected cases, I have used this technique successfully. The materials which are needed include: methyl methacrylate monomer (liquid), methyl methacrylate polymer (powder), fine camel hair brush (artist type), and a glass pallet with two wells (dapping dish).

In this procedure the groove is cleared of callus as described above. Use an eyedropper to place a small quantity of monomer in one well of the dapping dish. A small amount of the polymer is placed in the other well. The toe is grasped between the thumb and forefinger of the operator. The thumb is used to draw the soft structure of the nail lip away from the plate. The brush is dipped into the monomer, and the liquid is stroked into the groove. With the moist tip of the brush, a small amount of the polymer is picked up from the other well. This bead of powder is transferred to the groove and smoothed out with the brush. Three or four more applications of polymer are worked into the groove. The moist material will dry in about 3 minutes. These acrylic dressings can be replaced about every 3 weeks until correction is attained (14).

SUBUNGUAL HELOMA

Definition

A subungual heloma is a circumscribed overgrowth of epidermis found under the nail plate of a toe (Fig. 6.5).

Etiology

The cause of this condition is always traumatic. A shoe box, which is not high enough or too narrow across the toes, will press on the nail plate (12). The intermit-

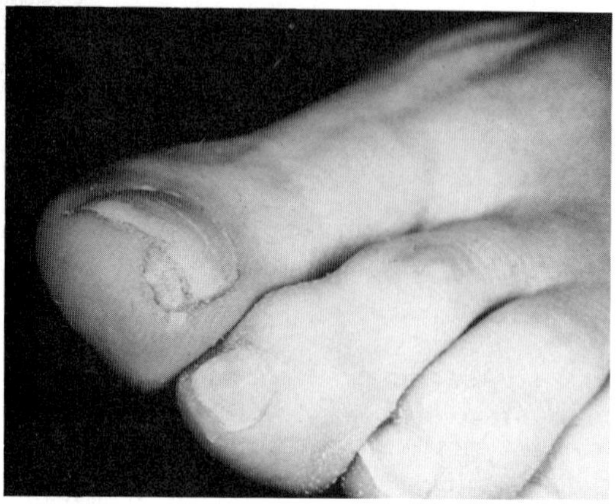

Figure 6.5. Subungual heloma of the great toe.

tent pressure causes a localized corneous hypertrophy. The majority of subungual helomata will be found in young adults. Occasionally I have observed this condition in an elderly arthritic patient. The individual had developed a small exostotic growth on the dorsum of the distal phalanx. Counter pressure from the shoe on the osteophyte was responsible for the lesion.

Symptoms

Pain on pressure is present, and the heloma may be large enough to cause the nail to separate from its bed and be forced upward over the affected area. This particular symptom is more noticeable in the lesser toes because the great toenail is attached to a more extensive surface and is stronger in structure and, therefore, more resistant to pressure.

A cornified area is readily seen under the nail as its darker color makes it sharply defined in the nail bed. The patient may give a history of pain at night from the pressure of the bed covering. Subungual heloma often exists simultaneously with onychophosis.

Treatment

In most instances, subungual helomata are curable. This is possible because the causative pressure usually comes from only one pair of shoes. The guilty shoe should be singled out and discarded. Those growths occurring at the distal or lateral borders of the nail are easily exposed for treatment by means of a nail nipper and onychotome. A piece of nail the size of the heloma is removed in order to permit free access to the entire growth so that it can be removed in its entirety. Once exposed the heloma is dissected out with an onychotome or pointed scalpel (15).

ONYCHIA AND PARONYCHIA

Synonyms

Onychia is also known as onychitis (Fig. 6.6). Paronychia has several synonyms: panaris, panaritium, paronychitis, runaround, whitlow.

Definition

Onychia is an inflammation of the nail matrix, often resulting in suppuration and shedding of the nail (16). Paronychia is an inflammation of the matrix in which the surrounding and deeper structures are involved. From the above definitions, it can readily be seen that paronychia is simply advanced onychia. It is often difficult to distinguish between the two conditions, as the etiology and symptoms may be identical.

Etiology

It is possible to find onychia associated with either cutaneous or systemic diseases. However, the vast majority of onychial lesions observed in podiatric practice are of traumatic origin. The most common cause cited in our literature is the ill-fitting shoe. The dropping of a metal tool on the toe is an everyday occupational hazard. Stubbing the foot against a heavy object is a fairly common household injury. The infection from a neglected ingrown nail often extends

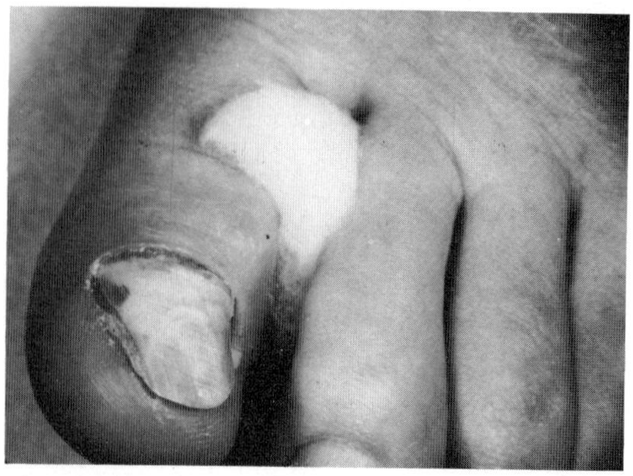

Figure 6.6. Onychitis or onychia of the great toe.

to the matrix, creating an onychia. During the summer season foreign bodies may be the exciting cause of this disorder in children. Running barefoot on the boardwalk may allow a splinter to enter the periungual tissues, and in a like manner, a thorn may be encountered at the country day camp.

The morbid habit of nail biting (onychophagia) may be seen in children. I have observed two cases of low grade onychia caused by nail biting of the great toe. A somewhat similar nervous affliction seen in adults is the habit of picking or tearing the periungual tissues and nail (onychotillomania). Severe paronychia caused by this habit has been encountered in the clinic of a mental hospital. On rare occasions, parasites, such as the itch mite, sand flea, and housefly, may be the causative factor in onychia (17). In the skin disease called scabies, the female itch mite (acarus scabiei) burrows under the epidermis and deposits her eggs. If the site of the burrow is in the posterior nail fold, an inflammation of the matrix will result (18). The seashore beaches are the habitat of the sand flea (pulex penetrans). The female extends her proboscis into the skin of the host to obtain nourishment. According to Macleod, the favorite areas of attack on the foot, are the sole, interdigital cleft, and nail fold (19). Any abrasion in the latter will permit the entrance of infective material. The housefly sometimes deposits eggs in the skin. In a day or two, these eggs hatch, producing a small nest of larvae (maggots). This condition is called myiasis. A case of onychial inflammation caused by maggots has been reported by Bates (20). The patient presented a great toe which was inflamed. The plate was loosened from its bed. Coiled up in a nest close to the lunular area were six larvae. Subsequent laboratory examination proved them to be maggots, and the case was diagnosed as onychomyiasis.

Pathology

Any of the above factors will cause the matrix to become inflamed. If the inflammation is not arrested, suppuration will result. With the production of pus, tissue destruction occurs, and the mechanical union of the nail and matrix is lost. The nail may be partially loosened or may fall off entirely, depending on the area of the matrix involved. If the matrix is completely destroyed, the nail will not be replaced. Partial destruction of the matrix will result in a malformation of the new nail (onychauxis). In paronychia, tissue destruction may extend until the bone is involved, producing an osteitis.

Symptoms

Inflammation will be present with all its clinical signs. There may be a retraction of the posterior nail fold from the nail plate. Pus is usually present in either the posterior or lateral nail folds. The nail may be loosened from the bed and be shed (onychomadesis).

Treatment

If seen early, the case may simply present swelling and redness of the nail wall without suppuration. Insert a small gauze packing in the groove and apply a wet dressing of Burow's solution. The patient is advised to cut the front end of the shoe to relieve pressure. If infection is present, the pus must be drained. In order to accomplish drainage, the nail must be removed in part or entirely, depending on the size and location of the suppurative tract. The wound is packed with gauze, taking care to keep the soft tissue separated from the nails. A wet dressing of either Burow's solution or betadine solution is prescribed. The patient is instructed to elevate the foot and to apply the prescribed solution on returning home. The toe is dressed in 24 hr.

ONYCHYPHEMIA

Definition

Onychyphemia is defined as bleeding under the nail (Fig. 6.7).

Etiology

Trauma is the most common cause of subungual hemorrhage. Contusion of the toe is a frequent industrial injury. Many claims are paid every year by insurance companies for accidents of this type. The dropping of heavy objects, stubbing the toe against pieces of furniture, and forcefully pulling vacuum sweepers against the foot are common household injuries. According

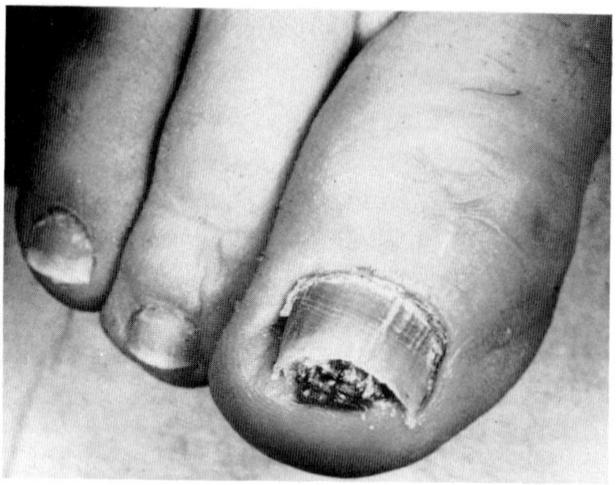

Figure 6.7. Onychyphemia of the great toe.

to Pardo-Castello and Pardo, subungual hemorrhage is occasionally observed in scruvy, hemophilia, and bacterial endocarditis (16).

Pathology

The force of the trauma causes an effusion of blood under the nail. If the plate has not been torn loose, the blood cannot escape to the surface. This collection of blood is known as a hematoma. When the force of the blow is not great enough to cause a complete avulsion, a partial fracture may be manifested in the plate (21). The coagulated blood will adhere to this fracture as a small dark spot (petechia) or a transverse streak (vibex) on the underside of the nail. As the nail grows forward, these bruised areas will finally be eliminated at the free edge. In those cases in which the nail is partially or completely torn off, pathogenic organisms may gain entrance, causing an abscess under the posterior nail fold. The trauma may be great enough to injure the distal phalanx, resulting in a localized periostosis on the dorsal surface of the distal phalanx. This will develop into a subungual exostosis in 6 months to 1 year following the original accident.

Symptoms

In the case of profuse hemorrhage of the nail bed, the pain will be intense for a few hours after the injury. The nail appears to be stained red by the suffused blood. The red color will turn black after coagulation (ecchymosis). As a rule, the nail becomes loose and is shed (onychomadesis) after a few weeks. The new nail usually becomes thicker (22).

Treatment

The severity and type of the traumatism is the guide to the treatment along with routine x-ray examination. If seen immediately after the injury, cold compresses should be applied for the first 12 h. This will minimize the amount of swelling. Following this, our first consideration is to relieve the pressure of the extravasated blood. This blood cannot escape because it is trapped by the nail plate above and the nail bed beneath. After careful cleansing of the entire toe, several small holes are bored through the nail plate with a 1/16-inch round dental burr and electric drill. This allows the blood under the nail plate to escape. A gauze pad is applied to the toe, and a wet dressing is prescribed for the patient's use on returning home. The case should be redressed in 48 hr.

NEOPLASMS

Subungual Exostosis

DEFINITION

Subungual exostosis is a bony overgrowth arising from the dorsal surface of the distal phalanx of a digit (Fig. 6.8).

ETIOLOGY

The exostosis is usually the aftermath of an injury such as stubbing the toe or dropping some heavy object on it.

PATHOLOGY

As a result of the injury, an acute periostitis occurs on the dorsal, lateral, or medial surface of the distal phalanx. The acute

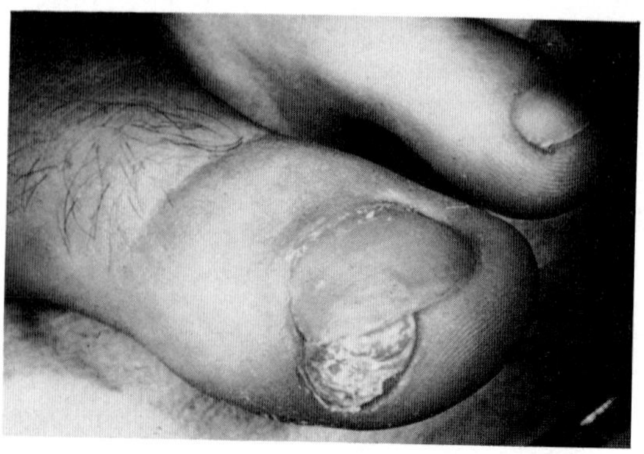

Figure 6.8. Subungual exostosis of the great toe.

stage passes into the subacute, productive stage, and cartilage develops at the site of the injury (23). As time does on, this cartilaginous growth becomes calcified. The upward growth of this bony mass often raises the nail from its bed.

SYMPTOMS

The patient complains of acute pain immediately following injury. This is followed by an indefinite tenderness under the nail plate. The free edge of the nail begins to change color to either a yellow or gray. Eventually, the nail is raised from its bed. Beneath the nail plate is found a rounded firm tumor-like elevation. A positive identification of this lesion is confirmed by x-ray.

TREATMENT

Anesthesia is induced by the injection of lidocaine. A tourniquet is applied to control hemorrhage. The overlying nail plate is cut away to expose the tumor-like mass. The amount of nail removed will be dependent on the size and location of the exostosis. Sometimes a small wedge-shaped section from the anterior free edge will be sufficient. When the exostosis is more proximal, the entire center of the nail may have to be removed. A ¼-inch mastoid gouge is then inserted under the distoplantar margin of the growth. The handle of the gouge is held high, meeting the skin at about a 45° angle. With a rolling motion of the gouge, it is pushed firmly downward and backward until the posterior limit of the exostosis is reached. The handle of the gouge is then lowered, and with a little leverage the entire mass is lifted from its bed. A definite cavity on the phalanx should result. Any rough edge is removed with a bone rasp. A compression bandage of gauze is applied. The toe is redressed in 48 hr. The patient is permitted full functional weightbearing in a cut-out shoe after the first redressing. Healing usually occurs in 10 to 20 days.

CHONDROMA

Chondroma is a tumor of cartilaginous tissue. According to G.T. Pack, there are two types, enchondroma and ecchondroma (24). The former arises from a small preexisting island of cartilage in an abnormal location such as the shaft of a phalanx or a metatarsal. One such case was observed by J.T. Sharp in a 40-year-old Caucasian janitress. She displayed a rounded semifirm enlargement on the lateral aspect of the great toe. No inflammation was present. The nail was normal in size and shape. This enlargement had first appeared about 2 years before and had slowly increased in size. It was assumed that intermittent trauma had stimulated the development of cartilaginous cells. The growth was removed surgically, and there has been no recurrence after 3 years.

An ecchondroma is an overgrowth arising where cartilage is normally found. One case was reported by C.G. Rowe in a 17-year-old black girl. She presented a cauliflower-like growth which extended from the posterior nail fold (Fig. 6.9). Subsequent surgical removal showed that the growth was connected to the cartilage at the base of the first phalanx. The laboratory report disclosed that the growth was composed of cartilaginous tissue.

During a 21-year period, there were 573 tumors of the hands and feet treated at the Memorial Hospital for Cancer and Allied Diseases of New York. Of that number, only two cases of chondroma were found on the toes.

PERIUNGUAL FIBROMA

Periungual fibroma is a benign tumor composed of fully developed connective tissue and is found in the lateral or posterior nail folds (23). Most of these growths extend distalward from under the nail wall. The pressure on the matrix may create a longitudinal canal in the convex nail plate.

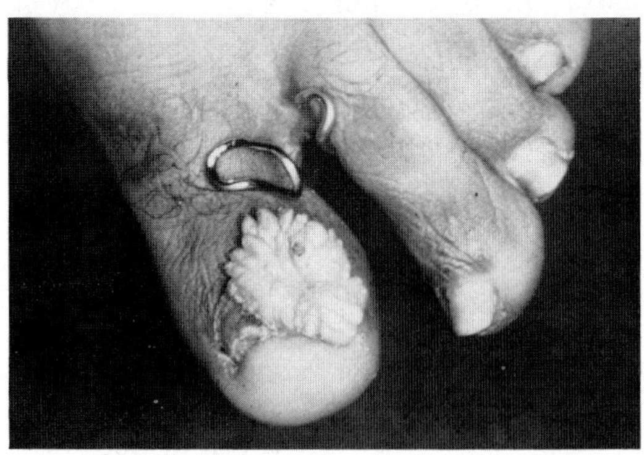

Figure 6.9. Ecchondroma of the great toe.

Subungual fibromas seldom caused discomfort. Surgical removal is only indicated in those cases in which pain is a factor.

VERRUCA

Two types of this growth are found in the nail area, subungual verruca and periungual verruca (23). The latter is present in either the lateral or posterior nail grooves (Fig. 6.10). These are commonly found on the fingers of children. They are rare on the toes. The subungual type are more common on the lower extremity. A.J. Firth reported an unusual case in a 14-year-old caucasian youth. A single verruca covered the nailbed and had forced the nail to grow vertically from the posterior nail fold. The plate had lost its horny character and was dull gray in color. Four weekly applications of 50% salicylic acid ointment resulted in a complete cure. Eleven months later, the old nail had been replaced by a normal one. In either type of verruca, a moleskin shield containing an aperture the size of the growth is placed on the toe. The escharotic is placed in the aperture, and the dressing is replaced at weekly intervals.

GRANULOMA PYOGENICUM

Granuloma pyogenicum is a fungating growth composed of a network of newly formed capillaries which appear at a site of trauma (23). In podiatric practice, this lesion is usually referred to as proud flesh or exuberant granulations. It is commonly associated with ingrown nail and appears as a cherry-like nodule extending from the nail groove. Being highly vascular, it bleeds at the slightest provocation. Granuloma pyogenicum may also occur under the nail plate in onychia. The plate overlying the growth should be removed with a nail splitter. One or two applications of 50% silver nitrate will eliminate the granuloma.

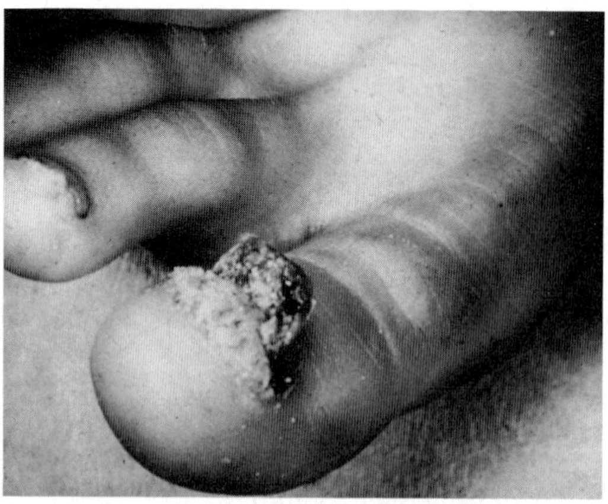

Figure 6.10. Subungual verruca vulgaris.

GLOMUS TUMOR

Glomus tumor is a rare neoplasm which may develop in the corium of the nailbed (24, 25). It shows through the nail plate as a small bluish discoloration. Trauma may cause a hypertrophy of the glomus body. This presses on the nervous plexus and causes intense pain. Glomi are minute vascular-muscular formations found in the tips of the digits and nailbed. They apparently serve as a shunt between the arterial and venous systems in regulating temperature control of the digits. Glomus tumor was reported by J.V. Ganley in a 30-year-old school teacher following trauma to the great toe. She complained of excruciating pain and displayed a bluish discoloration under the plate. Upon surgical exposure, the lesion appeared as a small granulomatous mass. The report of the pathologist confirmed the diagnosis.

MELANOMA

Melanoma is a tumor which is made up of melanin-pigmented cells. These pigmented areas may exist for years as harmless moles. If activated by trauma, chemicals, or radiant energy, it may develop into a malignancy (26). The color may be brown, slate-blue, or black. Melanoma metastasize by way of the lymph channels. In the lower extremity, melanomic emboli usually skip the popliteal space to lodge in the inguinal lymph nodes. Melanomas in the ungual area have been reported by B. Bornstein, J. Bates, W. Ignatoff, and P. Quintavalle. The initial symptom in three of these cases was a longitudinal pigmented band in the nail plate (Fig. 6.11). Later, granulation tissue developed under the edge of the nail. These lesions are radioresistant, so that either surgical saucerization or amputation is the choice of treatment. Prognosis is good if diagnosis is established early, and theapy is instituted without delay.

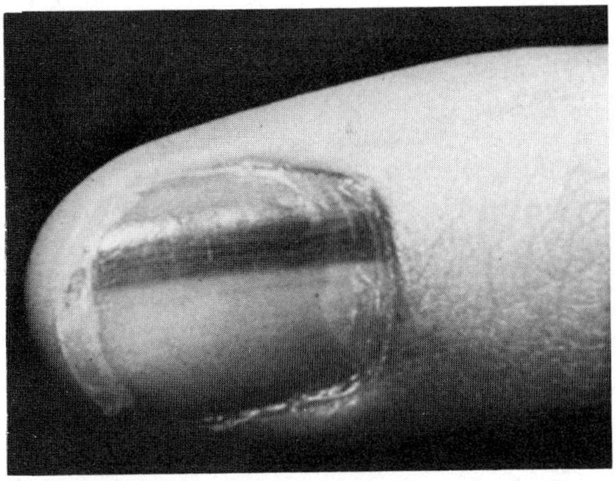

Figure 6.11. Early acral lentiginous melanoma involving the nail plate.

ONYCHODYSTROPHIES

Onychatrophia

Onychatrophia is a diminution in the normal development of the nail in size, thickness, or texture (Fig. 6.12). Atrophic nails sometimes do not grow to form a free edge. They may appear as small stumps or irregular pieces of epidermal filament. This condition is more common on the lesser toes, especially the fifth toe. Atrophic nails are usually congenital in origin. Pardo-Castello states that onychatrophia is frequently observed in leprosy (16).

ONYCHORRHEXIS

Onychorrhexis is a condition in which longitudinal striations occur in the nail plate, with or without the formation of fissures (Fig. 6.13). The undersurface of the nail plate presents longitudinal ridges and depressions parallel to each other. These correspond to similar longitudinal depressions and ridges in the nailbed. If the nail becomes thinned, these ridges are visible on the outer surface of the nail. Onychorrhexis may be associated with: excessive dryness of the nail, advanced age, and nutritional disorders.

LEUKONYCHIA

Leukonychia is a condition which is characterized by the presence of white spots or streaks in the nail plate. It is classified as follows:

Leukonychia punctata—white spots
Leukonychia striata—white streaks
Leukonychia totalis—completely white

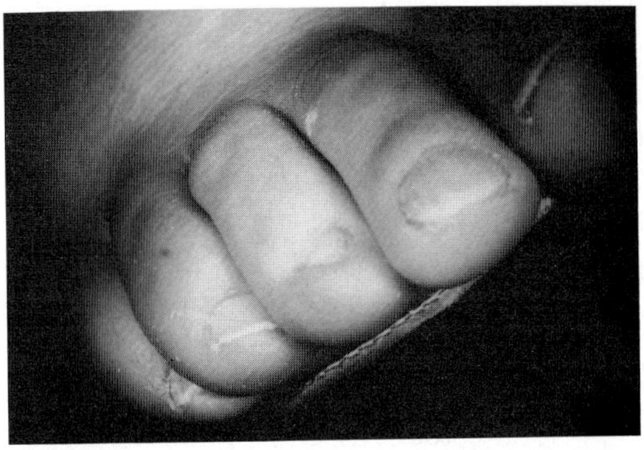

Figure 6.12. Onychotrophia involving the third toe.

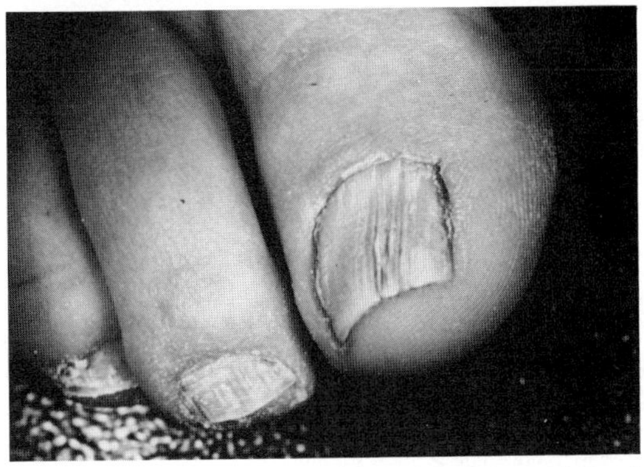

Figure 6.13. Longitudinal striations characteristic of onychorrexis.

Leukonychia is more common on the fingers than on the toes. The exact cause is unknown.

BEAU'S LINES

This is a condition which was first described by a French physician, J.H.S. Beau (1806–1865). It is defined as transverse furrows found in the nail plate which are the aftermath of some pathological disturbance in the matrix (Fig. 6.14). These lines appear in the lunular area and progress forward with the growth of the nail until they are eliminated at the free edge. As a general rule, this transverse furrow is rather superficial, but occasionally the transverse linear depression affects the entire thickness of the nail, dividing it into an anterior discolored deciduous portion and a posterior normally growing nail (27). The anterior part of the nail separates from the bed and is shed. The great toenail is the one most commonly affected. Beau's lines are caused

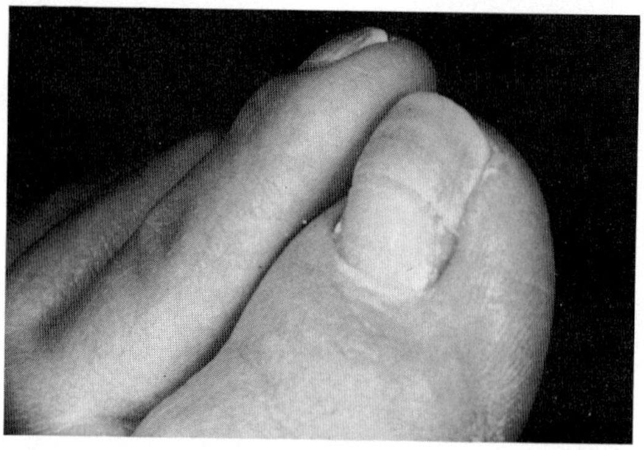

Figure 6.14. Transverse furrows typical of "Beau's lines."

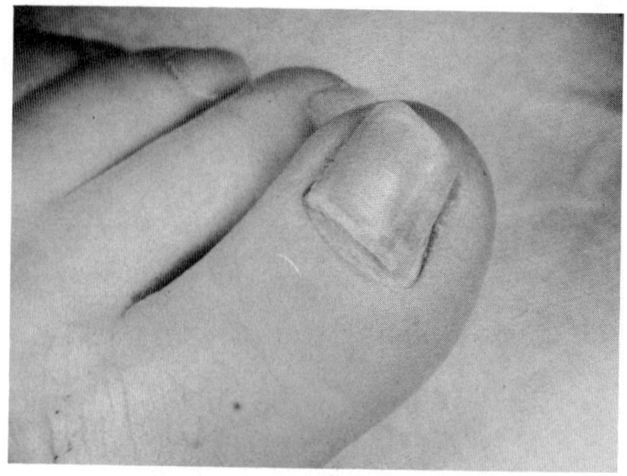

Figure 6.15. Onychomadesis of the great toe.

by a sudden arrest of the production of normal nail cells. This produces a gap in the continuity of the nail plate. The presence of Beau's lines may serve to ascertain the approximate date of the occurrence of the disturbance. The nail plate takes about 180 days to grow from the matrix to the free edge. The location of the defect will tell with some certainty the time at which the arrest of the function took place. Beau's lines may follow trauma, onychia, nervous shocks, and acute inflammatory diseases.

ONYCHOLYSIS AND ONYCHOMADESIS

Onycholysis is the gradual separation of the nail plate from its bed, beginning at the free edge and progressing slowly toward the root. Onychomadesis is the separation of the nail plate from its bed, beginning at the proximal end and progressing distally until the nail plate is shed (Figs. 6.15 and 6.16). These two conditions may be differentiated as follows:

Onycholysis	Onychomadesis
Separation of nail from its bed beginning at free edge	Separation of nail from its bed, beginning at proximal end
Slow process	Rapid process
Slight inflammatory changes or none at all	Usually follows acute inflammation in posterior nail fold
Associated with:	Associated with:
Slight trauma	Severe trauma
Psoriasis of nail	Dermatitis exfoliativa
Onychomycosis	Scarlet fever and other eruptive fevers
Onychauxis	Acute onychia

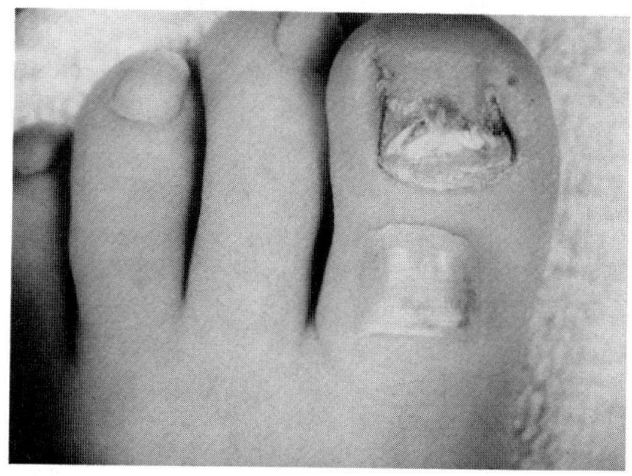

Figure 6.16. Onychomadesis (same case showing shed nail).

ONYCHOSCHIZIA

This is a condition in which the nail separates into two layers and, often, the uppermost layer flakes off (27). In those cases which we observed, the nail grows normally until nearing the free edge, where it unfolds and scales off. The cause is unknown.

HAPALONYCHIA

Hapalonychia or onychomalacia is a condition in which the nail plate is softened and bends easily. Instead of being horny and resistant to pressure, it is pliable like a sheet of latex rubber. According to Pardo-Castello it may be caused by hyperhidrosis, endocrine disorders, and exposure to caustic chemicals (16).

MELANONYCHIA STRIATA

Melanonychia striata is the presence of a congenital longitudinal pigmented band in the nail. It is brown or black in color. It is caused by a small pigmented nevus in the matrix. This pigmentation is uniform in width and extends from the posterior nail fold forward to the distal end. The pigmented band involves the entire thickness of the nail (Fig. 6.17).

UNGUAL MANIFESTATIONS OF CUTANEOUS DISEASES

Onychomycosis

INTRODUCTION

Onychomycosis, also known as tinea unguium or ringworm of the nail, is defined as a localized infection of the nail or nailbed caused by pathogenic fungi (Fig. 6.18). Robert Hooke (1635–1703) was the first person to describe fungi. He was able to demonstrate that these organisms were capable of producing disease on plant life. The first fungus disease in humans was not discovered until 1839. This was the skin disease known as favus which, incidentally, may show symptoms in the nail. With the discovery of the anthrax bacillus by Pollender in 1849, the efforts of biologists were directed toward the search for disease-producing bacteria. As they looked for germs, their interest in fungi was more or less pushed into the background. By 1890 it was known that some fungi were capable of causing disease in humans. However, the full impact of fungi as pathogens was not realized until the World War I era. In 1906, Raymond Sabouraud (1864–1938), an outstanding French dermatologist, stated: "The onychomycoses are rare in the toes." (28). In 1927, Albert Strickler, founder of the Philadelphia Skin & Cancer Hospital, wrote: "Ringworm of the nails is uncommon" (29). In 1936, Pardo-Castello published the first edition of his book on nail diseases (2). He pointed out that onychomycosis was one of the most common of nail disorders. He stated that 18% of the patients attending his service at the University of Havana presented some degree of mycotic involvement of the ungual area. This stimulated a new wave of interest in the problem of onychomycosis. Pardo-Castello listed a number of widely divergent fungi as causative organisms of fungal nail

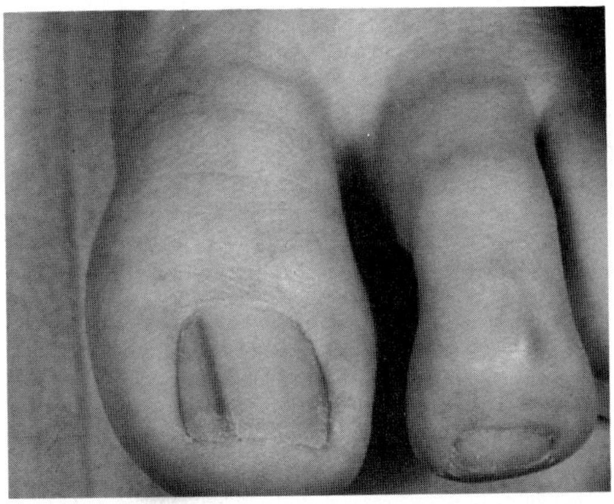

Figure 6.17. Melanonychia striata of the great toe.

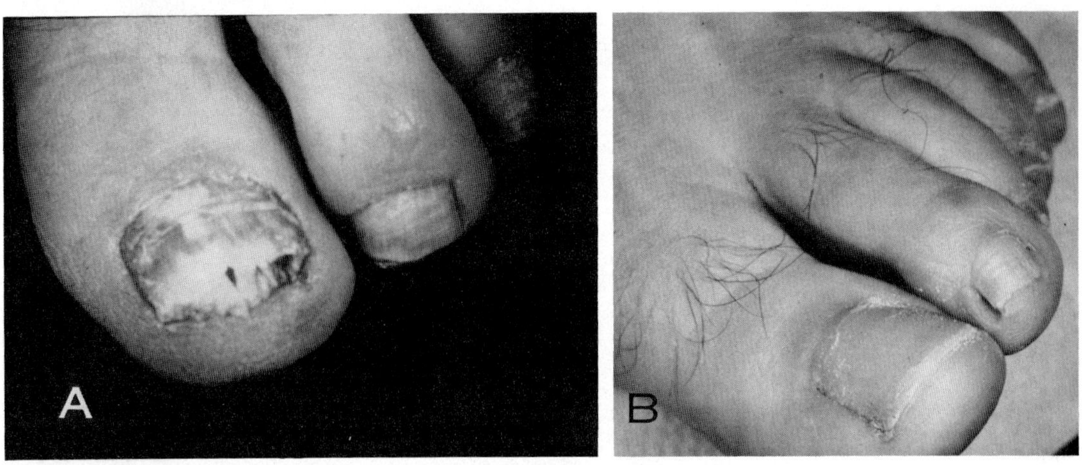

Figure 6.18. Onychomycosis involving the distal subungual region (*A*). Same case is shown following periodic debridement and application of undecylinic acid solution (*B*).

disturbances. In the last 40 years, many improvements have been made in diagnostic laboratory technics, so that today we can be more definitive in detecting the causes of mycotic diseases. It can now be said with a reasonable degree of certainty that the two most common fungi responsible for onychomycosis are *trichophyton rubrum* and *Trichophyton mentagrophytes*. Since the advent of Dermatophyte Test Media, I found only one case of mycotic nail which was not caused by either of the above organisms. The exception was *Candida albicans* (30).

TRICHOPHYTOSIS UNGUIUM

Definition

This is a localized nail disease caused by *Trichophyton* and is characterized by keratoid degeneration of the involved tissue with disfiguration of the nail (30).

Etiology

The most common causative organisms are *T. rubrum* and *T. mentagrophytes*.

Pathology

The fungi enter beneath the distal or lateral edge of the nail. It attacks the undersurface of the plate and the nailbed. This causes the formation of degenerated epithelial cells, which raises the nail from its bed.

Symptoms

This is primarily a dry lesion. The infection may involve the entire nail or may appear as irregularly shaped striations. The affected area usually presents a yellow or brown pigmentation. It is rare to find the infection on all of the nails. Some degree of onycholysis is present, and the plate may be hypertrophied.

Treatment

Apply a soak of 1% compound solution of cresol to the area for 2 min. Remove as much diseased nail as possible with heavy nail forceps and onychotome. All rough edges of nail are reduced with burr and electric drill. Any subungual debris is cleared from the area with a probe and dental polishing brush. An antifungal solution is applied to the denuded nailbed. There are a number of these solutions on the market. Among those in most common use are Desenex (Pharmacraft), Fungoid Tincture (Pedinol), Lotrimin (Delbay), Synergine (Olan), and Tinactin (Schering). The patient is instructed to apply the solution twice per day. In addition, 125-mg tablets of griseofulvin are prescribed q.i.d. The patient should be checked every 6 weeks. At that time, any diseased nail is eliminated with burr or onychotome.

The failures reported in private practice are usually observed in those patients who will not cooperate with the above routine. From 1966 to 1976, we maintained a foot clinic in a denominational home for senior citizens. In this home we obtained good results with periodic nail debridement and the local application of a fungal solution. In this instance, we had what might be termed a captive audience. A registered nurse was responsible for the daily applications of the medication between visits to the foot clinic. Successive appointments in the clinic were maintained on schedule due to the vigilance of our volunteer assistants.

One must keep in mind that the average nail growth on a toe is about 2 mm per week. Therefore a cure cannot be attained in less than 8 months. The practitioner should never promise the patient that the new nail will return to normal thickness as a result of the therapy. Permanent ungual hypertrophy of some degree is a common aftermath of a mycotic infection. This is due to the action of the fungus on the cells of the matrix. These cells are often altered in character and produce nail thickening.

If the mycotic nail causes the patient constant pain, surgical avulsion is indicated (Fig. 6.19). However, as a routine procedure, avulsion is frowned upon by Cleveland White, Pardo-Castello, and many other authors. A dermatological symposium was held in Scottsdale in 1965 (31). At that meeting, the chairmen of the dermatology departments of six major universities declared that nail avulsion is recommended only when considerable pain is present. Postoperative pain is one of the objections to surgical intervention, along with delayed healing. Regrowth of the nail may take at least 6 months. Recurrence of the infection in the new nail is always a possibility.

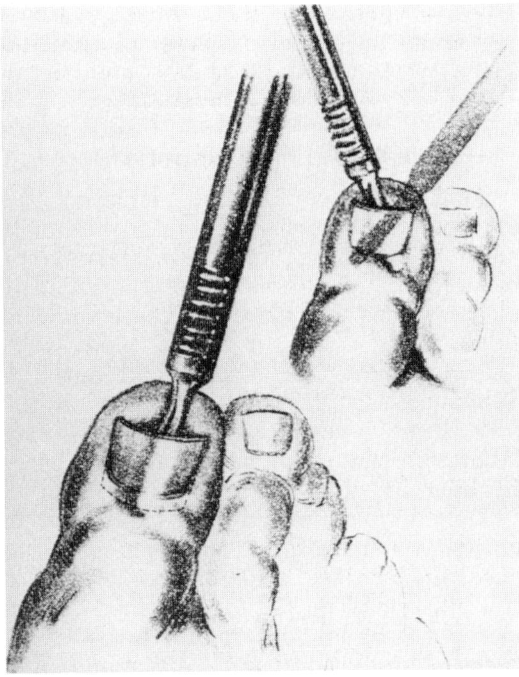

Figure 6.19. Use of the Frost elevator for surgical avulsion of the nail.

CANDIDIASIS OF THE NAIL

Synonym

Moniliasis of the nail.

Definition

This is a type of onychomycosis caused by *Candida albicans* with resultant inflammation of the periungual tissues (Fig. 6.20).

Pathology

The *Candida* gains entrance at either the distal or lateral edges of the nail. The organism may progress proximally into the matrix area, causing an onychia.

Symptoms

A monilial infection of the nails is more common on the fingers than on the toes. Of the 625 cases of onychomycosis observed in our survey, only six were diagnosed as candidiasis. In reviewing the podiatric literature over a 25-year period, we found only one article on the subject. Goldman and Unger reported seeing seven cases in the clinics of the New York College (32).

Unlike trichophytosis unguium, which is a dry lesion, candidiasis is more or less moist in the acute stage. It is characterized

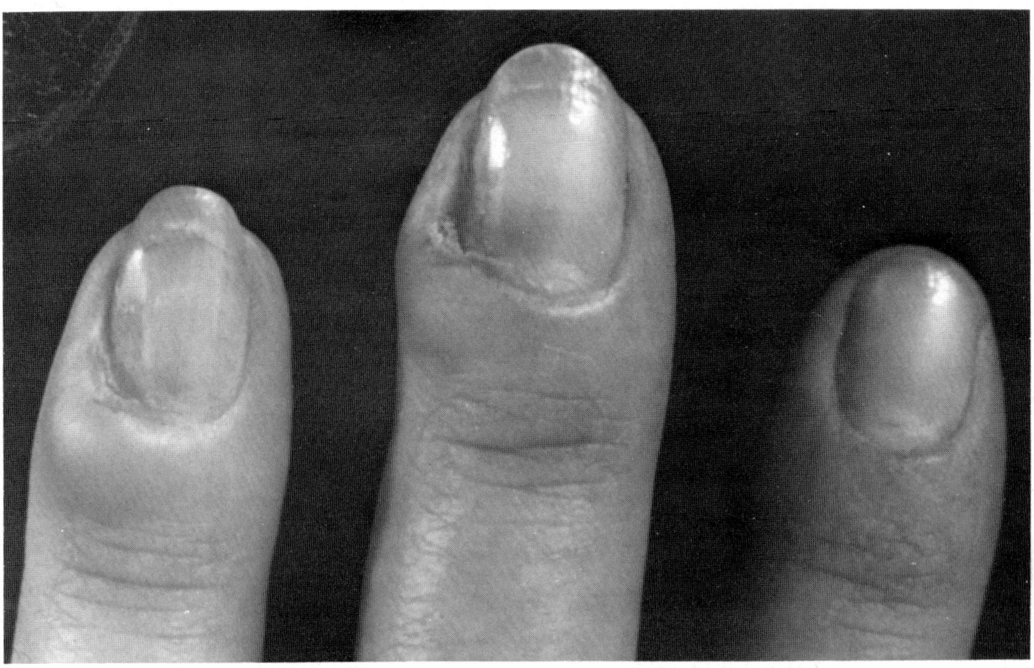

Figure 6.20. Onychomyosis of the nail plate involving *Candida* species.

by a typical onychial swelling in the posterior nail fold. A thin exudate may be present in the nail grooves. This exudation contains the parasite in almost pure culture, although *Staphylococcus albus* is a common contaminator. The nail may become loosened and shed. The new nail will usually show some degree of hypertrophy.

Treatment

If seen during the acute stage, all loosened nail is removed with nail forceps or onychotome to facilitate drainage. Any exudate is cleaned out from the denuded area. Small gauze packs are placed in the nail grooves and a gauze dressing is applied. On returning home, the patient is instructed to use wet soaks of Betadine. When the active infection has subsided, applications of Fungizone cream (Squibb) or 5% gentian violet are prescribed twice per day.

Onychomycosis is not a disease which will result in a fatal outcome. However, it is often the focus for extensive ringworm infections on other areas of the body (33). As in any other infection, professional care should be instituted as early as possible and should be continued until the problem is contained.

PSORIASIS

This is a chronic inflammatory skin disease of unknown origin, characterized by reddish, dry, sharply defined patches covered by overlapping silvery scales. This is one of the most common of the dermatoses. According to Macleod, 7% of patients seeking treatment for skin diseases are afflicted with psoriasis (19). The condition may be present on any surface of the body. It seems to have a predilection for the extensor surface of the extremities, especially the elbows and knees. Forcible removal of an overlapping psoriatic scale will result in a minute bleeding point. This is pathognomonic of psoriasis and is known as Auspritz's sign (H. Auspritz, 1835–1886). Pardo-Castello, Pillsbury, and others estimate that 15% of psoriatic patients will have nail involvement. Any or all of the following may be ungual symptoms of psoriasis (2): (*a*) onycholysis with a mild degree of nail hypertrophy; (*b*) multiple Beau's lines with loss of luster; (*c*) grayish areas in the plate with underlying hyperkeratosis; and (*d*) pitting of the nail (punctiform depressions) (34). Most of these nails are refractory to therapy. The periodic reduction of the nail with burr and electric drill will control the hypertrophy.

CONTACT DERMATITIS

This is an acquired skin sensitivity to external contact with vegetable, mineral or animal substances (35). The primary symptoms in the epidermis are erythema, papules, vesicles, or pustules. These may be followed by scales or crusts, along with varying degrees of itching and burning. When contact dermatitis appears on the toes, it may involve the nail area. This may be manifested in the acute stage as a paronychia with abundant exudation, followed by shedding (onychomadesis). In the chronic type, scaling of the periungual tissues will be present. The dorsal surface of the plate may be mildly deformed with a grayish color and loss of luster. In acute cases of contact dermatitis of the nail area, soothing lotions or a soak of a mild antiseptic solution is indicated. However, in any variety of contact dermatitis, the causative agent must be eliminated in order to resolve the problem.

DERMATITIS EXFOLIATIVA

This is a chronic inflammatory skin disease involving the entire body surface and characterized by deep redness and continuous flaky desquamation. The exact cause is unknown. It sometimes follows an acute toxemia or local irritation. The nail symptoms are: (*a*) scaly, red nail grooves; (*b*) loss of color in the plate; and (*c*) shedding of the nail (onychomadesis).

ICHTHYOSIS

Ichthyosis or fish skin disease is a congenital hypertrophic disorder marked by dryness or scaliness plus a variable amount of papillary hypertrophy. When this is present on the lower extremity, it is usually accompanied by multiple onychauxis.

RADIODERMATITIS

The nail matrix is extremely sensitive to the exposure of roentgen rays and radium. If overexposure occurs from either of the above, we may expect to find the following changes: onychorrhexis; discoloration and deformity of the plate; atrophy and pigmentation in the periungual tissues; and formation of telangiectasis.

UNGUAL MANIFESTATIONS OF SYSTEMIC DISEASES

Syphilis is a contagious venereal disease leading to many cutaneous and structural lesions due to the organism *Treponema pallidum*. The nail symptoms will vary according to the stage of the disease. In the primary stage, syphilis will manifest itself at the point of entrance of the organism in the form of a hard, indurated ulcer called a chancre. In the nail area, the chancre will appear as a periungual ulcer which may become secondarily infected with pyogenic bacteria, with resultant onychia (16). Later, the nail is shed (onychomadesis), followed by a new deformed nail. In the secondary phase of syphilis, we find widespread pustular lesions, which will often be followed by abundant scaling. Multiple onychia is the usual nail lesion. In the tertiary stage, nutritional changes occurring in the matrix often result in a thickened nail (onychauxis). This nail is usually detached to some extent from the nailbed. Slight inflammatory changes occur in the posterior nail fold, and the nail is shed. The new nail is hypertrophied and raised from the bed. Often this cycle is repeated about every 10 or 12 months.

Syphilologists have described many divergent nail lesions associated with congenital syphilis. However, there is no one nail disorder which can be found consistently in this type of disease.

Hippocratic nail is one in which there is an increase in the convexity of the nail plate in both its longitudinal and transverse axes, with a reduction in size of the lateral nail folds. There is clubbing of the ends of the digits so that they appear like the end of a drumstick. This condition is more common on the fingers than on the toes. It may be observed in pulmonary tuberculosis, in tumors of the lungs, and in chronic heart disturbances.

Leprosy is a chronic infectious disease characterized by lesions of the skin, mucous membranes, peripheral nerves, and various organs due to *Mycobacterium leprae* (Hansen's bacillus). In the neural type, anesthesia of the hands and feet is a frequent development. When nerve destruction develops, the reparative process is retarded or terminated. Slight injuries of the extremities fail to heal. Slow ulceration and absorption takes place until the distal portions of fingers and toes disappear. Ulceration and gangrene of the ends of toes and fingers will involve the nail matrix. The nail plate becomes atrophied as the matrix is destroyed. If the gangrenous process continues to total destruction of the matrix, no nail will be present.

Peripheral vascular disorders include arteriosclerosis, thromboangiitis obliterans, and Raynaud's disease. Arteriosclerosis is a loss of elasticity and thickening of the coats of the arteries with inflammatory changes which may be degenerative or productive. It is one of the most common contributing factors to foot problems in the elderly. The author served in the foot clinic of a denominational retirement home for 10 years. A survey of the medical records of that period indicated that 52% of the guests were under treatment for arteriosclerosis of the lower extremities (36). Thromboangiitis obliterans (Buerger's disease) is an inflammation of the intima of the blood vessels with clot formation, particularly in the larger arteries of the leg. In both of these diseases, onychatrophy is observed in the early stage. The late nail symptoms are cyanosis, ulceration, and gangrene. Raynaud's disease is a vasomotor neurosis characterized by arterial ischemia. The early nail symptoms are atrophy, onychorrhexis, thinning of the posterior nail fold, and pterygium (hypertrophy of the eponychium). A late ungual symptom is ulceration of the periungual tissues. Gangrene is rare in Raynaud's disease.

Diabetes is a disturbance of carbohydrate metabolism caused by a deficiency of insulin (37). Although mild cases of this disease may be controlled with diet, most patients require treatment with insulin or some oral hypoglycemic agent. Therefore, it is imperative that the family physician be consulted at regular intervals. Our observations indicate that, once these patients pass 55-year-old milestone, they become more prone to nail problems. At this stage, home nail care becomes more difficult. Many of these individuals are limited in bending forward due to arthritic changes in the back, pelvis, or knees. Faulty vision is another handicap to proper nail hygiene. The expert handling of forceps and drill by the podiatrist-chiropodist will avoid the possible trauma or infection of self-care.

When infection does occur in the ungual area (Fig. 6.21), drainage followed by wet dressings and the application of topical antibiotics is our plan of attack. The patient is instructed in the use of wet soaks of saline solution. These soaks should be made at least twice per day for a period of 5 min. Following the wet dressing, the patient should dress the area with an antibiotic cream. Choice of the latter is determined by antibiotic sensitivity studies. In our opinion, podiatric care should be administered at least every 6 weeks in order to maintain the foot health of the adult diabetic.

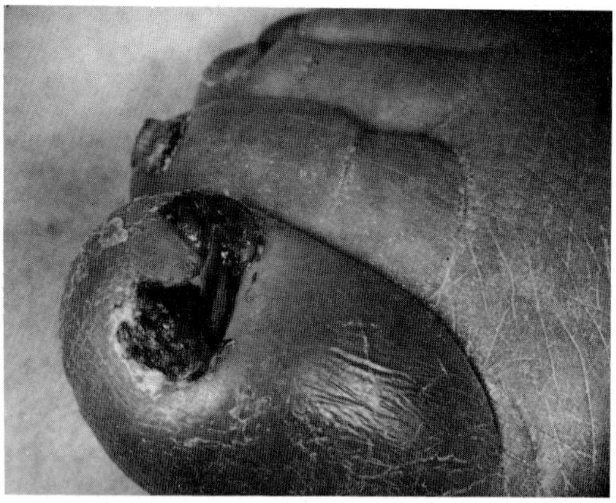

Figure 6.21. Infection produced by self-treatment in a diabetic patient.

Arthritis is defined as an inflammation of a joint. One must bear in mind that the nail matrix is in close proximity to the interphalangeal articulation of the great toe. Inflammation of this joint will also involve the matrix during the acute stage of the disease. As a result, the matrix cells become altered in character. As new cells develop and the nail grows forward, it will be hypertrophied (onychauxis).

Koilonychia or spoon nail is a concavity of the plate in both its transverse and longitudinal axes (38) (Fig. 6.22). It is a rare nail lesion and has been observed in several types of anemia and in certain thyroid disturbances (39). I practiced for 25 years before I saw my first case of koilonychia. This patient was a 36-year-old white male with microcytic anemia. Both great toes presented the classical picture of spoon nail. The lateral and distal edges of the plate were curved upward. There were practically no lateral nail folds. The dorsal surface of the nail was smooth and slightly pink in color. The lesser toenails were normal, except for slight longitudinal striations. Unlike the great toes, all the fingernails were flat and not cupped. They were pale gray in color and displayed lateral and distal edges rising above the body of the nail.

Avitaminosis is any disease due to a deficiency of vitamins. I have observed only one case of avitaminosis. This was in a 3-year-old white girl with multiple longitudinal striations (onychorrhexis) on all nails of both fingers and toes. The youngster was referred to a pediatrician, who adminis-

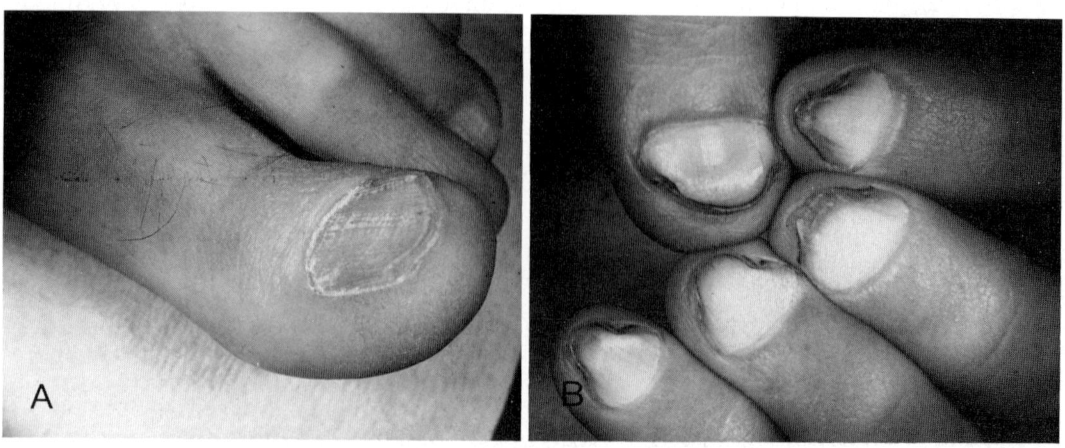

Figure 6.22. Koilonychia of great toe (*A*). Fingernails of same patient (*B*).

tered massive doses of vitamin B complex. The girl was observed again when she was 5 years old. At that time, there was considerable improvement, with limited striations present in the great and second toes. Three years later, the second toes displayed a single onychorrhexis. The great toes were normal, exept for a slight degree of onycholysis.

CONGENITAL NAIL DISORDERS

Anonychia is a congenital absence of a nail. In these cases the distal phalanx is either underdeveloped or absent. Dr. P.F. Grove reported a case of unilateral anonychia in the great toe of a 45-year-old male (Fig. 6.23). The x-ray disclosed the presence of a rudimentary distal phalanx. Although the digit was slightly shorter than the other toe, it functioned in a normal manner. Dr. L.I. Silverman observed a 5-year-old boy who had no nails on either foot. The toes were somewhat shorter than normal, but this did not interfere with locomotion. The fingernails were normal.

Macronychia is a congenital problem in which the nail is normal in shape and texture but is excessively large (Fig. 6.24). It is usually associated with macrodactylia. Dr. D.G. Stelmach described a case in a 30-year-old white male. Both great toes were excellent samples of localized giantism with nails that were abnormally large. The x-ray presented an unusual bony structure. The distal phalanx had two separate heads which were fused into a single broad base. Two irregularly shaped proximal phalanges articulated with the distal phalanx. These were parallel and articulated with the head of the first metatarsal. The first metatarsal was perfectly formed, except that it was about twice the size of the second metatarsal. This anomaly did not handicap the patient in his daily activities. Dr. G.E. Harford has observed macronychia in three generations of one family. It occurred unilaterally. The x-ray revealed a distal and proximal phalanx fused into a single bone with dual heads. The first metatarsal was normal in size and shape.

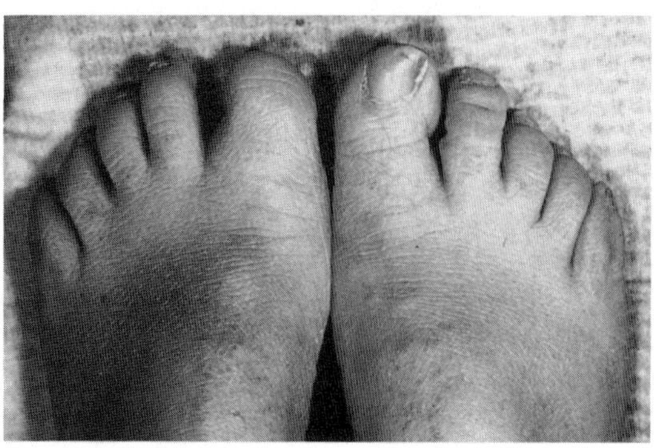

Figure 6.23. Anonychia of the left hallux.

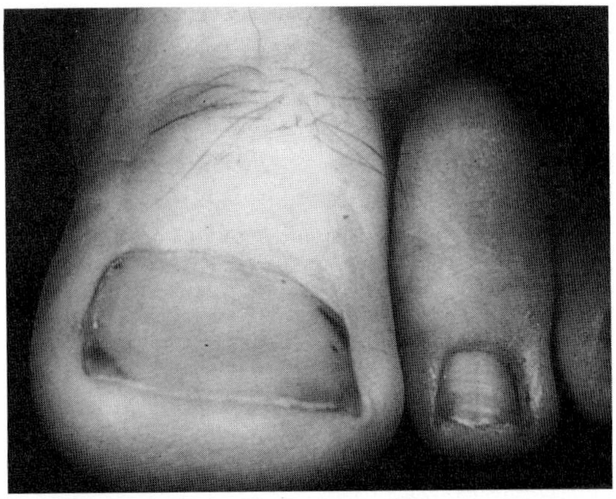

Figure 6.24. Macronychia of the great toe.

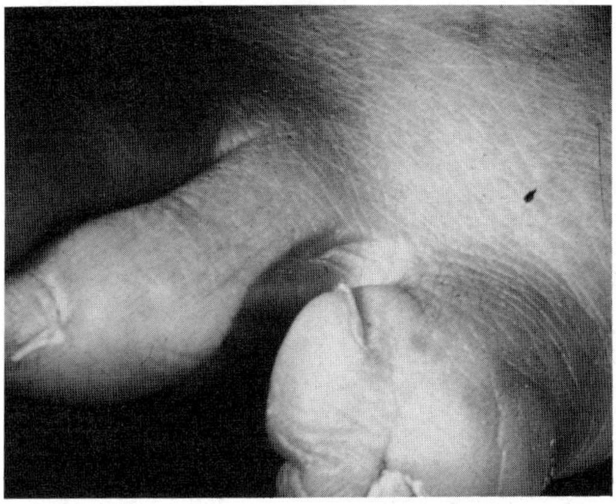

Figure 6.25. Polyonychia involving the fifth toe.

Polyonychia is the presence of more than one nail on a digit (Fig. 6.25). Dr. G.V. Feldman presented a case of polyonychia in a 20-year-old white female. Her right 5th toe was fan shaped and was twice as wide as the neighboring 4th toe. In most cases of polyonychia, the nails are equal in size and lie parallel on the dorsal aspect of the toe. In Dr. Feldman's case, the nail on the dorsum was small in size and had a tendency to grow vertically. The second nail appeared on the lateral side of the 5th toe

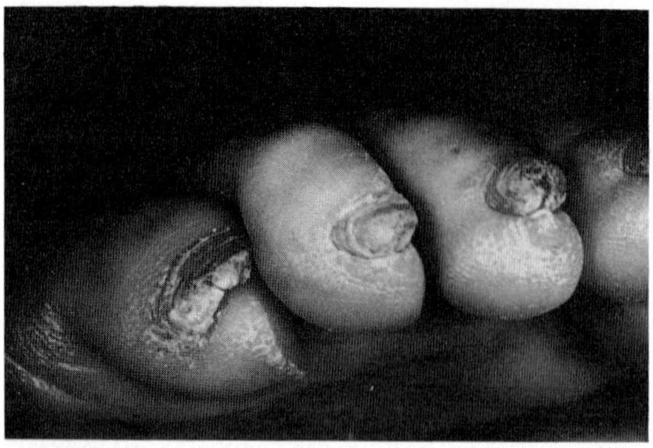

Figure 6.26. Pachyonychia or congenital hypertrophy of the nail plate and nailbed.

and was slightly hypertrophied. The x-ray displayed two separate distal phalanges. These articulated with an abnormally large proximal phalanx (40). A similar enlargement was present in the 5th metatarsal. There was a congenital osseous bridge (synostosis) connecting the shafts of the 4th and 5th metatarsals.

Pachyonychia is a congenital hypertrophy of nail plate and nailbed (Fig. 6.26). The following is a differentiation between this lesion and club nail:

Pachyonychia	*Onychauxis*
Hypertrophy of plate and bed	Hypertrophy of nail only
Congenital	Usually traumatic
All nails are affected on both fingers and toes	Usually one nail is affected—rarely, all
Surface is smooth	Surface is often rough
Nail is adherent to bed	Nail is often detached from bed (onycholysis)
Subungual hyperkeratosis never present	Subungual hyperkeratosis often present

Dr. W.B. Ignatoff reported a case in a 23-year-old white male. Hypertrophy of the nail and bed was present on all nails of both hands and feet. The plate was light brown in color, and the surface was smooth. The patient displayed leukokeratosis of the tongue. A small area of follicular keratosis was present on the dorsum of both feet. Periodic reduction of the nails allowed the patient to lead a normal life. He plays golf regularly and enjoys daily walking.

References

1. Krausz CE: Nail survey of 12,500 patients. *Br J Chirop* 48(9):239, 1983.
2. Pardo-Castello V: *Diseases of the Nails.* Springfield, IL, Charles C Thomas, 1936.
3. White CJ: Clinical study of 485 cases of nail disease. *Boston Med Surg J:* 1902.
4. Boyd W: *Textbook of Pathology,* ed 7. Philadelphia, Lea & Febiger, 1961, p 1340.
5. Heifetz CJ: Ingrown toe nail. *Am J Surg* 39(2):298, 1938.
6. Krausz CE, Mueller JJ: *Chiropody Quiz Compend,* ed 3. New York, Harriman Printing Co., 1939, p 104.
7. Anderson ISC: *Onychocryptosis and Allied Conditions.* London, Actinic Press, 1952, p 21.
8. Dagnall JC: History, development and current status of nail phenolization. *Chiropodist* 36(9):315, 1981.
9. Frost L: Atraumatic nail avulsion with a novel ungual elevator. *J Am Podiatry Assoc* 48(2):52, 1958.
10. Jablon VA: Onychauxis. *Chirop Rec* 16(7): 21, 1933.
11. Krausz CE: Traumatic nail disorders. *Chiropodist,* 6(5):165, 1951.
12. Carleton FJ: *Shoes & Feet.* West Chester, PA, C.H. Andress, 1940, pp 147 and 190.
13. Sanders SC: Acrylic nail groove protector. *J Natl Assoc Chirop* 456(7):23, 1955.
14. Sivitz SC: Acrylic resins. *J Natl Assoc Chirop* 43(7):34, 1953.
15. Gross RH: *Modern Foot Therapy.* New York, Modern Foot Therapy Publishing Co., 1948, p 174.
16. Pardo-Castello V, Pardo OA: *Diseases of the Nail.* Springfield, IL, Charles C Thomas, 1960, p 27.
17. Romoser WS: *Science of Entomology.* New York, Macmillan, 1973.
18. Friedman R: *Story of Scabies.* New York, Froben Press, 1947, pp 343–363.
19. Macleod JMH: *Diseases of the Skin.* New York, Paul B. Hoeber, 1926, p 1245.
20. Bates JE: Onychomyiasis. *J Natl Assoc Chirop* 37(10):47, 1947.
21. Roditi B: Nails as an illustration of the principles of pathology. *Chiropodist* 21(11):288, 1947.
22. Rowe CG, Krausz CE: Traumatic inflammation of the nail bed. *JCS Chirop Soc Pennsylvania* 1(2):6, 1939.
23. Samman PD: *The Nails in Disease,* ed 2. London, W. Heinemann, 1972, p 146.
24. Pack GT: *Tumors of Hands and Feet.* St. Louis, C.V. Mosby, 1939, pp 28, 73, and 129.
25. Kurtz AD: *Cyclopedia of Medicine,* vol 9. Philadelphia, F.A. Davis, 1937, p 15.
26. Bornstein B: Melanoma. *J Am Podiatry Assoc* 57(8):377, 1967.
27. Heller J: *Die Krankheiten der Nagel,* ed 2. Berlin, Springer, 1927, p 119.

28. Sabouraud R: *Topographical Dermatology.* New York, Rebman Company, 1906, p 409.
29. Strickler A: *Diseases of the Skin and Syphilis.* Philadelphia, F.A. Davis, 1927, p 438.
30. Krausz CE: Onychomycosis. *Austr Podiatrist* 12(1):5, 1976.
31. Schering Corp: Appraisal of a Significant Advance in Topical Antifungal Therapy, Scottsdale, AR, 1965, p 167.
32. Goldman L, Unger L: A comprehensive treatment of monilial infection of skin and nails. *Am Podiatry Assoc* 48(8):371, 1958.
33. Stickel WJ: Ringworm. *Chirop Rec* 13(2):7, 1930.
34. Sidi E et al: *Psoriasis.* Springfield, IL, Charles C Thomas, 1968, p 69.
35. Fisher AA: *Contact Dermatitis,* chap 9. Philadelphia, Lea & Febiger, 1967.
36. Krausz CE: Foot problems of the senior citizen. *Curr Podiatry* 23(7):15, 1974.
37. Sindoni AM Jr: *The Diabetic's Handbook,* ed 2. New York, Ronald Press, 1959, p 199.
38. DeNicola P et al: *Nail Diseases in Internal Medicine.* Charles C Thomas, Springfield, IL, 1974, p 39.
39. Pierre M: *The Nail.* Edinburgh, Churchill Livingstone, 1981.
40. Gamble FO, Yale I: *Clinical Foot Roentgenology.* Huntington, NY, R.E. Krieger, 1975.

CHAPTER 7

Disorders of Keratinization

ARTHUR STEINHART

Disorders of keratinization represent a significant portion of the foot conditions treated by the podiatrist. The hyperkeratinizing lesions referred to as the helomata and tylomata have been discussed in a previous chapter. Psoriasiform disorders will be discussed in the chapters to follow, along with pityriasis rubra pilaris, and will, therefore, not be dealt with at this point. These several distinctions have been made because of their special podiatric relevance and biological significance.

The present study will emphasize those skin conditions characterized by varying degrees of dry scaling skin known as ichthyoses. Many of these diseases exhibit some degree of hereditary influence. Ichthyosis vulgaris, sex-linked ichthyosis, lamellar ichthyosis, and bullous ichthyosiform erythroderma are included in this particular grouping. Several keratinizing disorders of the adnexa will also be reviewed. Brief discussions on Darier's disease, keratosis pilaris, Kyrle's disease, keratosis pilaris atrophicus, lichen spinulosis, phrynoderma plantar-palmar keratoderma, Unna-Thost disease, Greither's syndrome, keratoderma hereditarium mutilans, Howel-Evans syndrome, pachyonychia congenita, disseminated palmoplantar keratoderma, porokeratosis mibelli, mal de Meleda, Papillon-Lefèvre syndrome, and Richnar-Hanhart syndrome will be provided in this chapter. Clearly, there is considerable complexity associated with the more rarely occurring disorders of keratinization.

The anatomy and physiology of the skin in general and that of the lower extremities in particular have been discussed in Chapters 1 and 2. An understanding of normal structure and function of the human skin is a prerequisite to understanding disorders of the skin: The reader is referred to these earlier chapters to review such matters.

The biosynthesis of keratin has been studied in some depth, but the process is still not fully understood. Keratin is a protein composed of several polypeptide chains. It is normally insoluble in water, dilute acid, and alkali solutions. It is keratin which provides the tough resilient covering of the body. Its greatest concentration is to be found in the outermost layer of the epidermis, the stratum corneum. The cells constituting this layer are normally hexagonal and are about 30 μm wide. This is to be compared with cells of the stratum basale which are low columnar cells which measure only 6 μm. However, in dyskeratotic diseases, morphology and chemistry of the epidermal cells can vary considerably.

Most of the normal activities associated with keratinization occur at the level of the stratum spinosum. The role of the tonofilament-desmosome complex has already been mentioned (Chapter 1). "T"-cell activity and membrane-coating granules are also implicated in this biochemical process.

Under normal circumstances, the stratum corneum demonstrates a brick wall-like arrangement of cells. Nonliving cornified keratinocytes constitute the bricks, while the widened intercellular spaces contain a mortar-like material.

Keratin polypeptides in many disorders of keratinization, such as pityriasis rubra pilaris and the ichthyoses, have been found to be different in proportion and type from those of normal skin (2–5).

Matrix, which is histidine rich, is formed in the T-cells through mixing of the keratohyaline granules with other cytoplasmic constituents. The density of the cell membrane is increased through the deposition of material at its inner aspect. It is this thickened membrane of protein and carbohydrate which provides resistance to the action of keratinolytic agents.

Membrane-coating granules have been found to contain parallel lipid-containing lamellae 20Å thick. Migration of these granules to the keratinocyte's apex occurs in the T-cells. This is followed by release of the lipid lamellae to the extracellular space.

Cells which are normally cornified are described as being "orthokeratotic." The palms and soles normally exhibit compact orthokeratosis while other body areas demonstrate a basket weave pattern of cornified cells. Alteration in these configurations is abnormal. For example, chronic persistent rubbing (such as in lichen planus and lichen simplex chronicus) and epidermolytic hyperkeratosis exhibit compact orthokeratosis on nonplantar-palmar skin, while laminated orthokeratosis is found in seborrheic keratosis.

"Dyskeratosis" refers to premature or abnormal keratinization of individual keratinocytes. These cells will not be uniformly placed or spaced in the epidermis. The condition appears to be associated with rapid transit of cells through the epidermis. Dyskeratosis has been categorized as benign (in Darier's disease) and malignant (as in Bowen's disease).

"Parakeratosis" refers to retention of elongated nuclei in the cells of the stratum corneum. This is the result of incomplete cornification and is usually the result of increased epidermal turnover (epidermopoesis), although not every case of increased epidermopoiesis results in parakeratosis (6). Parakeratosis is seen in many inflammatory dermatoses and is an indication of a recent pathologic process within the epidermis. It must be noted that areas of parakeratosis occur normally in some areas of the buccal mucosa (physiologic parakeratosis).

Disorders of keratinization may produce quantitative and qualitative changes in the stratum spinosum. Increased thickness constitutes acanthosis, while acantholysis refers to a lack of cohesion of prickle cells (see Chapter 3).

Hyperkeratosis, an increase in thickness of the stratum corneum, is a feature of many chronic skin diseases, including the genetic disorders of keratinization, as well as being the result of repeated trauma (corn, callus). The condition will result from increased production of the stratum corneum due to increased mitotic rate of the basal cells, or decreased shedding of cells of the stratum corneum. Both of these processes alter the normal balance between production and loss of stratum corneum. Although granular layer hypertrophy usually accompanies hyperkeratosis, reduction or absence of this layer occurs in autosomal dominant ichthyosis (see below), and epidermal atrophy may be found in chronic discoid lupus erythematosus, chronic actinic skin, and Kyrle's disease.

ICHTHYOSES

The ichthyoses are a group of disorders characterized by varying degrees of dry, scaling skin. The name is derived from the Greek word for fish. This group of disorders is easily recognized and has been known throughout history (Fig. 7.1). However, much confusion about these disorders exists. Many names have been used for the same condition, several variants for each may exist, and the condition may be associated with other minor abnormalities. Although three major categories of ichthyoses have been described (hereditary, acquired, and as part of a syndrome), discussion will be limited to the most common of the ichthyoses—the hereditary forms.

Hereditary Ichthyosis

Ichthyosis vulgaris (xeroderma, ichthyosis simplex, ichthyosis nitida, hyperkeratosis cognita) is the most common of the genodermatoses, estimated to affect 1% of the population (7). It is transmitted as an autosomal dominant disorder with onset in early childhood, usually between 1 and 4 years of age. The condition tends to improve with age. This is the mildest and least debilitating of the ichthyoses. It often ap-

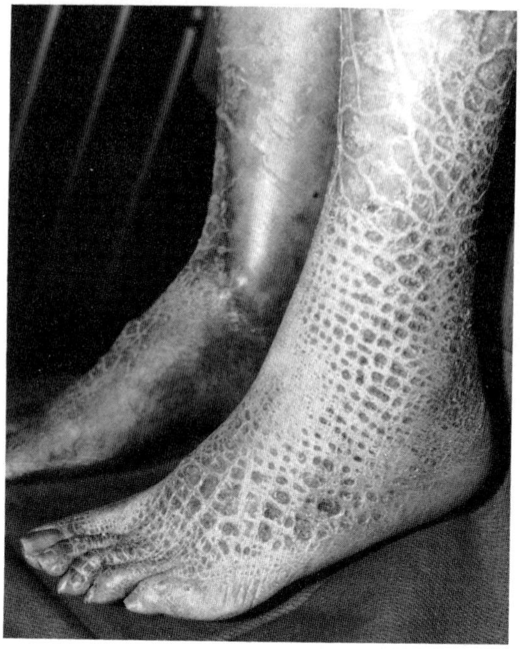

Figure 7.1. Typical "fish scale" appearance affecting the feet and legs of an elderly Caucasian female patient.

pears as mild xeroderma or fine, small, continuously shed white scales. Occasionally, fissures may develop and become infected. Severe forms in which large scales are present, giving the skin the appearance of that of a snake or alligator, have been reported.

The dryness and scaling are worse in the winter because of decreased sebaceous and sweat gland activity. Although usually asymptomatic, patients may complain of mild itching. Affected skin tends to be more sensitive to irritants than otherwise uninvolved skin. Nearly half of affected individuals demonstrate atopy, and many also are affected with keratosis pilaris. Ichthyosis vulgaris characteristically spares the axillae and antecubital and popliteal fossae. The areas most frequently affected are the elbows, knees, forehead, sides of the arms and thighs, and the palms and soles. The affected palms and soles demonstrate increased skin markings.

Transit time of the keratinocytes implicated in ichthyosis vulgaris is normal. This indicates that this form involves a disorder of cell retention. Synthesis of keratohyaline is likely abnormal, as few small abnormal keratohyaline granules are noted. Microscopic examination reveals mild hyperkeratosis which may show areas of parakeratosis. The granular layer is diminished or absent, and the stratum spinosum is thinned. Sweat and sebaceous glands show degenerative changes, and there is hypoplasia of hair follicles. Follicular plugging may be seen.

Sex-linked ichthyosis (ichthyosis serpentine, ichthyosis sauroderma, ichthyosis vulgaris, ichthyosis simplex) is characterized by large, infrequently shed dark scales. It is an x-linked disorder, having full expression only in males, with mild forms reported in female carriers. The disorder initially presents as mild scaling at or shortly after birth. Some infants are born with a membrane-like covering which is shed and replaced with scales. The scaling may increase in extent and severity with age, sparing only the palms and soles. In children, the most frequently affected areas are the scalp, neck, and sides of the face. Adults have the abdomen and legs involved. Corneal opacities have been reported to develop in some patients.

Increased synthesis of normal keratohyaline has been described and, recently, deficiency of steroid sulfatase has been reported (8). Histologic studies reveal marked hyperkeratosis, acanthosis, and hypertrophy of the stratum granulosum. More follicular plugging than in ichthyosis vulgaris is noted. The rete ridges are elongated and occasionally branched. Sweat and sebaceous glands are found in normal numbers, and perivascular lymphocytic and histiocytic infiltration is seen.

Lamellar ichthyosis (nonbullous congenital ichthyosiform erythroderma) is transmitted as an autosomal recessive disorder. It is more severe than ichthyosis vulgaris or x-linked ichthyosis. Affected individuals are usually born with a membrane-like covering (collodion baby) which produces eversion of the lips (eclabion) and eyelids (ectropion). Shedding of this jacket occurs shortly after birth, leaving a generalized erythroderma. Large yellow or yellow-brown plate-like scales loosened at their margins and attached at their centers then develop. These scales, generally affecting the flexor surfaces, are periodically shed (usually in spring and fall), which may result in partial remission, most often in summer (9). The palms and soles may be hyperkeratotic. The condition tends to increase in severity with age.

There is an increase in epidermopoiesis, with transit time being reduced to fewer days. All cell layers are thick, and sweat and sebaceous glands are normal. Mild perivascular infiltration of histiocytes and lymphocytes is present.

Epidermolytic hyperkeratosis (bullous ichthyosiform erythroderma) is an autosomal dominant disease which initially appears at or shortly after birth as widespread bullae. These open, leaving raw, oozing tender areas which subsequently develop large, thick, dark scales. This early feature of blistering occurs less frequently later in life, at which time the disease is characterized by keratotic or verrucous lesions affecting especially the flexural areas and the palms and soles.

It is believed that a defect in tonofibril formation, with loss of their normal arrangement in the stratum spinosum and a loss of desmosomes in spinosal cells, plays a role in the disease. Marked hyperkeratosis is noted, and the cells of the upper epidermis are vacuolated. Coarse keratohyaline granules are found in cells of the granular layer. Perivascular infiltration may be seen.

Differential Diagnosis

These several hereditary forms of ichthyosis can be distinguished from one another by virtue of their clinical features (onset, scale type, and location) and histopathology. Among other disorders to be considered in the differential diagnosis are psoriasis (which can be differentiated by family history, nail changes, onset, and response to sunlight), exfoliative dermatitis (which tends to be of "recent" onset and rapidly worsens), and other conditions such as contact dermatitis, atopic dermatitis, and seborrheic keratosis, all of which have "recent" onset histories. Epidermolysis bullosa and Ritter's disease may be confused with lamellar ichthyosis in infants. However, epidermolysis bullosa does not show scaling or erythroderma, and Ritter's disease will have cultures of *Staphylococcus aureus* (9).

Treatment

Treatment of the ichthyoses is generally directed towards hydration of the skin. This can be accomplished through the application of a variety of topical agents. Among suggested treatments are bathing with oil and application of mineral oil or other lubricants following bathing. The use of 20 to 40% urea in ointment, and 50% aqueous propylene glycol under plastic film occlusion, has been suggested. Retinoic acid applied under occlusion has been reported to be effective in lamellar ichthyosis and epidermolytic hyperkeratosis. Caution must be used especially on sun exposed areas because of the possible carcinogenic effect of the medication. Systemic treatment with methotrexate has been attempted in lamellar ichthyosis and epidermolytic hyperkeratosis. Isotretinoin (13 *cis*-retinoic acid, 2.0 mg/kg/day) has been used in lamellar ichthyosis and etretinate (Ro-10-9359, Tigosin, 1.0 mg/kg/day) has been used in ichthyosis vulgaris. Systemic corticosteroids may be necessary, even lifesaving, in cases of epidermolytic hyperkeratosis.

KERATINIZING DISORDERS OF THE ADNEXA

Among the keratinization disorders are a group of conditions involving the pilosebaceous apparatus.

Darier's disease (dyskeratosis follicularis, keratosis follicularis, Darier-White's disease) in an autosomal dominant disorder affecting males and females in equal distribution. It is a progressive disorder starting in late adolescence or the early 20s as skin-colored papules. These enlarge and coalesce to produce the characteristic dirty brown, waxy-greasy keratotic papules. The lesions in intertriginous areas tend to be verrucous, hyperkeratotic, and malodorous (as a result of maceration and bacterial growth). Lesions on the palms and soles appear as punctate keratosis or pits, and the nails may develop subungual hyperkeratosis and hypertrophied ridges.

Other major sites of predilection are the face, postauricular areas, neck, chest, upper back, axillae, inguinal area, nails, and oral and genital mucous membranes. Exposure to ultraviolet light results in exacerbation of the disease, which may explain why the disorder tends to be worse in summer and improve in winter. Individuals with Darier's disease have been reported to be susceptible to bacterial and viral infection of the skin, particularly vaccinia and herpes simplex (10).

Defects in synthesis, organization, or maturation of the tonofilament-desmosome complex are believed to play a role in the pathogenesis of the disease (11). The disease is characterized histologically by the presence of "corps ronds" cells and "grains." Corps ronds cells are large keratinocytes, found high in the epidermis, which show an eosinophilic cytoplasm with large circular nuclei. These go on to produce the grains which are dyskeratotic eosinophilic, parakeratotic cells. Follicular hyperkeratosis and epidermal clefts are also seen.

Among the differential diagnosis, in addition to the other follicular keratoses, is seborrheic dermatitis, which must be considered when a mild form of Darier's disease is suspected. In this case the warty papules characteristic of Darier's disease must be carefully looked for. Warty nevi should be considered when a localized linear form exists. Another consideration is acanthosis nigricans, which occurs in flexural areas and is pigmented.

Histologically, solitary warty dyskeratoma (transient acantholytic dermatosis, Darier variant of Grover's disease) (12, 13) is reported as indistinguishable from Darier's disease. Other disorders which appear in the histologic differential diagnosis are benign familial pemphigus (Hailey-Hailey disease), the pemphigus group of disorders, superficial hidradenoma, and nevus syringacystadenomatosus papilliferas (13).

Treatment, which is generally unsatisfactory, has included use of oil baths with emollients, antiseptic and hexachlorophene soap, 2% salicylic acid in petrolatum, 1% vitamin A acid in equal parts of alcohol and propylene glycol applied for 48 hr under occlusion, etretinate (50 mg/day for 3 to 4 weeks with reduction to 35 mg/day and then 25 mg/day), and a short course of 200,000 IU of vitamin A (50,000 IU 4 times per day).

Keratosis pilaris is a common autosomal dominant disorder affecting the upper posterior arms, upper lateral thighs, and buttocks that produces a characteristic "gooseflesh" appearance. It affects both sexes and can occur at all ages, although it is more commonly seen in women and adolescents. An association with ichthyosis vulgaris has been reported as having associations with hypothyroidism, Cushing's syndrome, and vitamin A intoxication (14). Keratosis pilaris is characterized by asymptomatic, symmetric, multiple, discrete hyperkeratotic papules occurring at the openings of hair follicles. Mild erythema may be present about the follicle. The condition tends to be worse in cold weather.

Microscopic examination reveals hyperkeratosis of the follicular opening with dilation and plugging. A hair may be found in the center of the papule.

Among the clinical differential diagnoses to be considered are lichen spinulosis, which is rare. It occurs in children and undergoes spontaneous remission. Pityriasis rubra pilaris affects the face and neck with scaling and erythema and produces horny papules on the dorsa of the fingers. Darier's disease affects the back, neck, and scalp with characteristic greasy, brown isolated hyperkeratotic lesions. Ichthyosis starts at or shortly after birth and tends to produce dry and scaling skin. Secondary syphilis mimics several skin diseases and can be detected through appropriate blood studies.

Treatment for keratosis pilaris is generally not required. The patient should be warned that the condition will be aggravated by hot baths, soap, wool, and rough clothing. Two percent salicylic acid in hydrophilic ointment has been used as has 20% urea cream, solution or cream of tretinoin, and a short course of vitamin A (100,000 IU).

Pityriasis rubra pilaris is a rare, chronic, exfoliating condition characterized by circumscribed follicular keratosis, palmoplantar keratoderma, and eythroderma. No systemic manifestations have been reported, the only complaints being occasional itching. The disease can arise at any age from childhood through the 80s. Two peaks of onset have been reported, giving rise to two "classical" forms—juvenile and adult. An atypical form has also been reported.

The juvenile form appears before age 10, tends to be mild, and is lifelong in duration. The adult form appears between ages 40 and 60 with a sudden onset which often follows systemic illness. Myasthenia gravis and neuromuscular disease have been implicated (10). This form follows a course of generalized involvement and exfoliation with spontaneous remission after 1 to 3 years.

Pityriasis rubra pilaris begins as multiple, reddish, hyperkeratotic perifollicular papules, usually on the scalp, face, posterior neck, trunk, and extremities. These papules coalesce to form red scaling plaques. The condition may become generalized and erythrodermic, with sparing of small salmon-colored islands. White streaks may be found on the oral mucosa (15). The presence of papules with horny follicular plugs on the dorsal surface of the fingers is an important feature. The palms and soles are thickened and may fissure.

Biopsy reveals follicular hyperkeratosis with basal cell layer degeneration and perivascular inflammation. A more significant finding is a horizontal and vertical alternation of orthokeratotic and parakeratotic cells (12). An increased turnover of epidermal cells and increased rate of nail growth has also been reported.

Disorders within the differential diagnosis of pityriasis rubra pilaris are follicular psoriasis in children, seborrheic dermatitis, keratosis pilaris, phrynoderma, and lamellar ichthyosis.

Among the numerous reported treatments of this condition are the topical use of emollients, bath oils, keratolytics, vitamin A under occlusion, and the avoidance of soap. Systemic therapy consists of vitamin A (100,000 to 500,000 units/day), oral methotrexate (5 mg/day), and azathioprine (100 mg/day) (10).

Kyrle's disease (hyperkeratosis follicularis and hyperkeratosis parafolliculosis) starts as small, horny plugs which may increase in size to as much as 1.5 cm in diameter. The lesions spare the palms and soles, are most common on the legs and forearms, and may be surrounded by a zone of erythema. Onset is between 30 and 60 years of age, with males and females equally affected. There is some indication that the disorder may be associated with abnormal glucose metabolism or hepatic disease.

Early histologic changes include a laminated adherent hyperkeratosis, thinning of the stratum malphigii, and flattening of the rete ridges. Later, parakeratotic plugs may produce a foreign body giant cell reaction in the dermis.

Treatment

Accepted therapeutic plans involve the use of keratolytics, localized cautery, and cryotherapy.

Keratosis pilaris atrophicus occurs in childhood and is characterized by follicular papules affecting the eyebrows, cheeks, and scalp. These subsequently become inflamed and atrophy with destruction of the follicle and hair loss. The condition often accompanies keratosis pilaris.

Lichen spinulosis (keratosis spinulosa) is a rare disorder consisting of patches of symmetrical, flesh-colored papules 1 to 2 inches in diameter. Horny spines extend from the follicles. Children, especially boys, are affected. The neck, lateral arms, abdomen, buttocks, thighs, and popliteal fossae are the common sites of involvement. The lesions slowly involute and disappear after several months. Treatment, if necessary, consists of use of 2% salicylic acid in hydrophilic ointment or 1% hydrocortisone in hydrophilic petrolatum.

Phrynoderma is an acquired follicular keratosis, associated with nutritional deficiency. Lack of vitamin A, the B group, C and fatty acids have been implicated. It is characterized by the formation of horny follicular plugs on the elbows, thighs, and buttocks. It can occur at any age.

Plantar-palmar keratoderma, the condition of thickening of the stratum corneum of the palms and soles may be either inherited or acquired. Attempts have been made to classify the former as to mode of inheritance, precise extent of involvement of the palms and soles, and presence of associated features. No one method has yet been found to be totally acceptable from a taxonomic point of view.

Unna-Thost disease (tylosis, diffuse palmoplantar keratoderma, keratosis palmaris et plantaris hereditarium) is an autosomal dominant disorder developing during the first 3 months of postnatal life. It first appears as areas of erythema and tenderness on the palms and soles which progress to become well demarcated diffuse hyperkeratoses which persist throughout life. The nails may also be affected, and the condition may be accompanied by hyperhidrosis. Increased thickness of the stratum corneum and hypergranulosis are the prominent histologic findings.

Greither's syndrome, believed to be a variant of Unna-Thost disease, begins in infancy but progresses in extent and severity over many years and affects the dorsum of the hands and feet and elbows and knees, in addition to the palms and soles.

Keratoma hereditarium mutilans (Vohwinkel's disease) is an autosomal dominant condition presenting in infancy with diffuse palmar-plantar keratoses demarcated by erythematous borders. Additional striate, honeycomb, or starfish-shaped keratoses develop on the elbows, knees, and dorsal aspects of the hands and feet. Associated features are scalp alopecia, hearing loss in the high frequency range, bullous lesions of the sole, and ainhum-like constricting bands developing around the lesser digits progressing to autoamputation (15). Such bands have also been reported in Mal de Meleda, pityriasis rubra pilaris, pachyonychia congenita, leprosy, and scleroderma (11).

Howel-Evans syndrome, palmoplantar keratoderma associated with squamous cell carcinoma of the esophagus, is an autosomal dominant condition which thus far has been limited to two families. The keratosis is of late onset, occurring between the ages of 5 and 14, with the malignancy developing at 40 to 50 years. Cases of acquired palmoplantar keratoderma associated with internal malignancy, especially of the esophagus and bronchi, have been reported.

Pachyonychia congenita, another autosomal dominant disorder, appears to be a trauma-related keratoderma. The nails are the first areas affected, becoming thick during infancy as a result of scratching.

Disseminated palmoplantar keratoderma has a postpuberty onset, is autosomal dominant in nature, and is associated with corneal dystrophy. The keratoses arise as fine punctate areas on the palms and soles with some extension to adjacent areas. The lesions enlarge to produce hyperkeratotic papules with deep-seated nuclei.

Punctate keratoderma most commonly develops between the ages of 15 and 30 and is characterized by many well-demarcated plugs or papules over the palms and soles. They range in size from 2 to 10 mm but may become larger when subjected to trauma. The keratotic plugs often slough spontaneously and fall out, leaving a depression with a keratotic wall. These lesions must be differentiated from arsenical keratoses. Excisional biopsy reveals hypertrophied stratum corneum with cone-shaped keratotic plugs. The stratum granulosum remains normal.

Many variants of punctate keratoderma apparently exist, and the literature seems to indicate controversy as to frequency of occurrence. Acquired forms have also been reported.

Porokeratosis mibelli (hyperkeratosis excentrica, hyperkeratosis figurato centrifuga atrophica) is an autosomal dominant disorder which has been reported to affect individuals of Italian descent, with males outnumbering females by 3 to 1 (16). Many variants have been reported. These include disseminated superficial actinic porokeratosis, hyperkeratotic porokeratosis, multiple palmar and plantar porokeratosis, both disseminated eruptive as well as linear (17, 18).

The lesions, which begin in patients between the ages of 5 and 10, may exist in solitary fashion or may number several hundred. Regardless of distribution the lesions characteristically appear as slowly expanding hyperkeratotic rings with a shining, atrophic center. These well-defined keratotic borders are the most important clinical feature of this condition.

This hyperkeratotic skin condition follows a slowly progressive course with new lesions occasionally appearing. There have been some reports of such lesions differentiating as skin cancers such as squamous cell carcinoma and Bowen's disease (19, 20).

Porokeratosis mibelli tends to affect the

fingers, dorsa of the hands and feet, ankles, face, neck, and mucous membranes. When sectioned through an advancing edge, a feather-like plug of parakeratosis (cornoid lamella) is identifiable. The stratum granulosum is absent in the area, and the epidermal cells are vacuolated. A moderate chronic inflammatory infiltrate of lymphocytes and histiocytes is found in the upper dermis, especially under the cornoid lamella. Dermal atrophy and skin appendage loss may also be found. Treatment of such localized lesions consists of electrocoagulation, surgical excision, or the topical application of 5-fluorouracil.

Among the clinical differential diagnoses for the various forms of porokeratosis mibelli are verrucae, linear verrucous nevus, chronic discoid lupus erythematosus, and secondary syphilis.

Mal de Meleda, an autosomal recessive keratoderma is a hyperkeratotic skin disorder which arises between 2 and 6 months of age. The initial presentation is that of a diffuse erythema which progresses to become a callosity with an erythematous border. Such keratoses may also develop on the dorsal aspects of the hands and feet as well as on the elbows and knees. Additionally, the nails may become dystrophic, and the condition is often associated with hyperhidrosis and bromhidrosis.

Severity of this rare condition peaks after 10 years of the disease with spontaneous, and sometimes permanent, remission developing during pregnancy. Marked thickening of the stratum corneum, along with a thick stratum granulosum and lucidum and marked acanthosis, are found on microscopic examination.

Papillon-Lefèvre, an autosomal recessive disorder, exhibits gingival dysplasia and intracranial calcification of the falx cerebri, tentorium, and choroid plexus, in addition to the symmetrical well-demarcated keratoses of the palms, soles, elbows, knees, and the skin overlying the Achilles tendon (15). Gingivitis, alveolar bone changes, and erythema of the palms and soles are early changes noted at the postpartum age of approximately 6 months. Hyperkeratosis replaces the original erythema at about the time the "baby" teeth appear: Remission occurs when these teeth are lost with the reactivation of the disease when permanent teeth develop. The histology is one of hyperkeratosis, acanthosis, focal porokeratosis, and some perivascular infiltration.

Richner-Hanhart syndrome (keratosis palmoplantar circumscripta) is characterized by corneal dystrophies, bradyphalangia, oligophrenia, and mental retardation in addition to the palm and sole keratoses. These patients have been reported to have tyrosinemia, with low tyrosine diets resulting in some improvement in the eye and skin conditions.

Treatment of the palmoplantar keratodermas is directed toward reduction of the thickening, prevention of fissures and subsequent infection, and the elimination of odor. Treatment plans currently employ modifications of footgear designed to reduce friction such as insole modifications and shoe therapy.

Additionally, reduction of the hyperkeratoses, surgical excision of the stratum corneum, application of keratolytics, application of 0.05 to 0.3% retinoic acid, use of topical or intralesional costerosteriods, and administration of oral retinoids are employed.

Acquired palmoplantar keratoderma reportedly has been associated with many conditions ranging from trauma as in the mechanically induced corn and callus to ingestion of toxic agents. Plantar-palmar keratoses have been reported to be associated with internal malignancy in Howel-Evans syndrome (esophageal carcinoma), pachydermoperiostosis (carcinoma of the lung), malignant acanthosis nigricans, Seizary syndrome, and acrokeratosis paraneoplastica (Bazex' syndrome, malignancy of the upper respiratory-digestive tract, or metastatic disease to the neck lymph nodes) (21–24). The presence of these keratoses is, however, not a sign of internal malignancy (20, 25).

Ingestion of arsenic as well as chlornaphthalenes, oils, greases, and wood preservatives has been reported to be associated with keratoses of the palms and soles (10). The lesions of chronic arsenic intoxication appear as yellow-brown punctate keratoses or velvety hyperkeratoses on the palms and soles (26). Histologic examination reveals hyperkeratosis with parakeratosis, acanthosis, and papillomatosis. Treatment involves electrodesiccation, cryotherapy, or application of 5-fluorouracil.

References

1. Elias PM: Stratum corneum lipids in health and disease. In Fleischmajer R (ed): *Progress in Diseases of the Skin*, chap 1. New York, Grune & Stratton, 1982, vol 2.
2. Steinert PM, Peck GL, Idler WW: Structural changes of human epidermal-keratin in disorders of keratin. *Curr Probl Dermatol* 10:391, 1980.
3. Baden, HP: Keratinization in the epidermis. *Pharmacol Ther* 7(2):393, 1979.
4. Bowden PE, Wood, EJ, Cunliffe WJ: Comparison of prekeratin and keratin polypeptides in normal and psoriatic epidermis. *Biochem Biophisica Acta* 783:172, 1983.
5. Yoshiike T, Negi M, Manabe M, Hattori M, Ogaua H: Fractionation and characterization of the human epidermal stratum corneum in keratinization disorders. *J Dermatol* 9(3):243, 1982.
6. Ackerman, AB: Sherlock Holmesian dermatopathology. Parakeratosis as a diagnostic clue. *Am. J Surg Path* 2(1):71, 1978.
7. Watson W: *Selected genodermatoses. Pediatr Clin North Am* 25(2):263, 1978.
8. Gonzalez E, Baden, HP: Ichthyosiform Dermatoses. In Madden S (ed): *Current Dermatologic Therapy.* Philadelphia, W.B. Saunders, 1982.
9. Esterly NB: The ichthyosiform dermatoses. *Pediatrics* 42(6):990, 1968.
10. Shelly WB: *Consultations in Dermatology II, with Walter B. Shelly.* Philadelphia, W.B. Saunders, 1974.
11. Ebling FJ, Rook A: Disorders of keratinization. In Rook A, Wilkinson DS, Ebling FJG (eds): *Textbook of Dermatology*, ed 3, chap 37. Oxford, Blackwell, 1979.
12. Ackerman AB: Subtle clues to diagnosis by conventional microscopy. Marked compact hyperkeratosis as a sign of persistent rubbing. *Am J Dermatopathol* 2(2):149, 1980.
13. Milne JA: *An Introduction to the Diagnostic Histopathology of the Skin.* Baltimore, Williams & Wilkins, 1972.
14. Garwood JD: Keratosis pilaris. *Am Fam Physician* 17(2):151, 1978.
15. Hilton L, Simpson RR, Simpson RR: Differential diagnosis of plantar palmar keratoderma. *J Am Podiatry Assoc* 68(8):578, 1978.
16. Butterworth T, Strean LP: *Clinical Genodermatology.* Baltimore, Williams & Wilkins, 1962.
17. Mehregan AH, Khalili H, Fazel Z: Mibelli's porokeratosis of the face. *J Am Acad Dermatol* 3:394, 1980.
18. Witkowski JA, Wood MG: Porokeratosis of Mibelli: a perforating disease of the epidermis. *Cutis* 29:171, 1982.
19. Razach EMA, Natarajan M: Ulcerative systematized porokeratosis (Mibelli). *Arch Dermatol* 113:1583, 1977.
20. Gilbertsen VA, Bean SF, Fusaro RM: Palmar keratoses and visceral cancer. A spurious relationship. *Arch Dermatol* 105:222, 1972.
21. Gibbs RC: Alterations of palms and soles. Indicators of internal disease. *NY State J Med* 65(107):1220, 1965.
22. Millard LG, Gould DJ: Hyperkeratosis of the palms and soles associated with internal malignancy and elevated levels of immunoreactive human growth hormone. *Clin Exp Dermatol* 1:363, 1976.
23. Kerdel FA, MacDonald DM: Palmo-plantar keratoderma associated with carcinoma of the bronchus. *Acta Derm Venereol (Stockh)* 62:178, 1981.
24. Highet AS, Rook A, Anderson JR.: Acrokeratoelastoidosis. *Br J Dermatol* 106:337, 1982.
25. Stolman LP, Kopf AW, Garfinkel L: Are palmar keratoses a sign of internal malignancy? *Arch Dermatol,* 101:52, 1970.
26. Hamada T, Horiguchi S, Nakano H: Cutaneous manifestations of occupational chronic arsenical poisoning. *Osaka City Med J* 23(1):9, 1977.

Suggested Readings

Baden HP: Treatment of hyperkeratotic dermatitis of the palms. *Arch Dermatol,* 110:737, 1974.

Bowden PE, Cunliffe WJ: Modification of human prekeratin during epidermal differentiation. *Biochem J* 199:145, 1981.

Domonkos AN: *Andrews' Diseases of the Skin.* Philadelphia, W.B. Saunders, 1982.

Fitzpatrick TB, Arndt KA, Clark WH Jr, Eisen AZ, Van Scott EJ, Vaughan JH (eds): *Dermatology in General Medicine.* New York, McGraw-Hill, 1979.

Haneke E: The Papillon-Lefèvre syndrome: keratosis palmoplantaris with periodontopathy. *Hum Genet* 51:1, 1979.

Holevich Y: Surgical treatment of palmar and plantar keratosis. *Acta Chir Plast (Prague)* 9(1):34, 1967.

Kisner WH, Hendrix, JH Jr: Keratosis palmaris et plantaris. *Plast Reconstr Surg* 51(4):424, 1973.

Lemont H: Comments on the histologic differentiation of genetic and mechanically induced

keratoses of the soles. *J Am Podiatry Assoc* 66(4):259, 1976.
Madden S (ed): *Current Dermatologic Therapy.* Philadelphia, W.B. Saunders, 1982.
Maltosy AG: Keratinization. *J Invest Dermatol* 67:20, 1976.
Marks R, Finlay AY, Holt PJA: *Br J Dermatol* 104:667, 1981.
Montagna W, Lobitz WC Jr (eds): *The Epidermis.* New York, Academic Press, 1964.
Moschella, SL, Pillsburg DM, Hurley HJ Jr: *Dermatology.* Philadelphia, W.B. Saunders, 1975.
Potter GK: Histopathology of clavi. *J Am Podiatry Assoc* 63(2):57, 1973.

CHAPTER 8

Psoriasiform Disorders

LEE J. SANDERS

Identification of papulosquamous disorders on the lower extremities can be extremely challenging for the student, resident, and physician. Several inflammatory disorders of the skin may present with a similar erythematous, papular scaling appearance. Investigative curiosity, clinical and familial history, physical examination, and laboratory studies will help to establish the diagnosis.

The disorders which will be discussed in this chapter include psoriasis, lichen planus, pityriasis rubra pilaris, and secondary syphilis. In addition to these entities, dermatophytosis and dyshidrosis should be included in the differential diagnosis for psoriasiform disorders. In order to establish a diagnosis, consider obtaining: a skin biopsy, a KOH prep to rule out fungous infection, and a serology to rule out syphilis.

PSORIASIS

Psoriasis is a common, papulosquamous skin disease which is chronic, recurrent, and inflammatory. The degree of skin involvement may vary from a lesion which measures just a few millimeters to generalized involvement of the whole skin. It affects 0.25 to 1.5% of the population (1) and can occur at any age. There is an undisputed genetic role, with a familial pattern seen in 30% of the cases (2–4). It occurs uncommonly in blacks, and rarely, if at all, in American Indians. It is seen with equal frequency in men and women.

The etiology of psoriasis is as yet unknown, and there is no reliable cure. Treatment will often be needed over an individual's entire lifetime, with clearing of the skin from time to time, followed by the development of new lesions. Lower extremity skin and nail involvement is quite common. Interphalangeal and metatarsophalangeal joint involvement (psoriatic arthropathy) are at times encountered in a small percentage of patients with psoriasis (5), requiring the practitioner's careful evaluation.

Etiology and Pathogenesis

The cause of psoriasis is still unknown, but genetic predisposition and immunological and environmental factors clearly play important roles. The mode of inheritance appears to be a dominant trait. It is not yet clear whether several genes or a single major gene is responsible for the disease. Some of the genetic factors predisposing to psoriasis are known to be closely linked to the major histocompatibility (HLA) antigens. The major histocompatibility complex (MHC) is a closely linked group of genes that provides the code for the structure of cell surface antigens and several plasma proteins, as well as for factors that regulate immune responses to a variety of antigens (6).

The following HLA antigens have shown associations with psoriasis: HLA-B13, HLA-Bw17, HLA-Bw16, HLA-Bw37, HLA-B8, HLA-B27, and HLA-Cw6 (7–10). Cw6 has recently been demonstrated to be the most frequent HLA antigen to be detected in psoriasis patients (4). HLA-B8 is associated with persistent palmar-plantar pustulosis (9, 11). There appears to be a fivefold greater susceptibility to psoriasis in individuals with B17, and their disease appears to have an earlier age of onset (4). There is a significantly greater frequency of HLA-B27 in patients with psoriatic arthritis and with pustular psoriasis (7, 11).

The pathogenesis of psoriasis still remains unclear. There are alterations in epidermal replication and maturation, manifested by abnormal keratinization with a high number of mitoses. This is characterized histologically by hyperkeratosis, parakeratosis, and regular acanthosis. It takes 3 to 4 days for a psoriatic keratinocyte to travel from the basal cell layer to the stratum corneum and to be cast off, in contrast to the 26 to 28 days for normal keratinocytes (12). This is reflected clinically by the abnormal profuse scaling which one sees in these patients.

Research has provided us a greater understanding of the pathogenesis of this disease; however, experimental data have been limited in some ways by the lack of a good animal model. Voorhees *et al.* (13) have studied the cyclic nucleotides, cyclic adenosine monophosphate (cAMP), and cyclic guanosine monophosphate (cGMP) and their relationship to the regulation of epidermal cell growth. It is now postulated that the increased epidermal proliferation in psoriasis may be induced by an increase in cGMP and by an increase in the cGMP/cAMP ratio. Closely related to the function of the cyclic nucleotides are the prostaglandins, which also play a role in the regulation of epidermal cell proliferation and the possible mediation of the cellular and vascular response (14). Prostaglandins dilate cutaneous blood vessels and participate in inflammatory reactions.

Other studies have shown the polyamines (low molecular weight amines) to be involved in the regulation of cellular proliferation (4, 15, 16). In a study of involved and uninvolved epidermis of patients with psoriasis, as well as of normal epidermis, polyamines were found to be in higher concentrations in involved epidermis, higher in uninvolved epidermis of psoriasis patients than in normal epidermis, and higher in urine from patients with psoriasis than in urine from control subjects (4, 16, 17).

Clinical Features

The cutaneous lesions of psoriasis have a predilection for the scalp, nails, extensor surfaces of the extremities (especially the knees, elbows, and shins), and lumbosacral and gluteal cleft areas. Eruptions are usually symmetrical and may vary in presentation from a solitary pink or dull red macule to numerous plaques. These lesions are characterized by well-defined, rounded, erythematous, dry, scaling plaques of various sizes, covered by grayish-white or silvery-white scales (Fig. 8.1).

The scales are the result of parakeratosis. They are micaceous, and although attached centrally, they are loose toward the periphery of the plaque. Upon removal of the scales, bleeding points appear (Auspitz's sign). Another characteristic clinical feature of the disease is the appearance of new psoriatic lesions at the sites of injuries to the skin. This response is known as the Köebner or isomorphic phenomenon. This may also be seen in lichen planus, in vitiligo, with flat warts, and in active eczematous dermatitis. The Köebner phenomenon has medicolegal importance and should be carefully considered when prescribing therapeutic or elective surgical treatment for psoriatic patients. As a point of interest to the surgeon, psoriatic plaques harbor bacteria, and cutting through them should be avoided.

On the palms and soles psoriasis may present as typically scaly patches, thick fissured plaques, small erythematous papules, or pustules (Fig. 8.2). Initial presentation may be a sudden shower of small

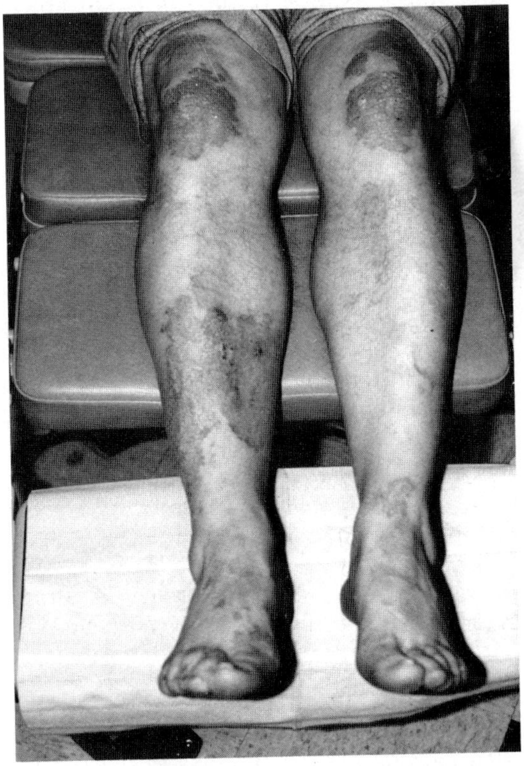

Figure 8.1. Psoriasis of both lower extremities.

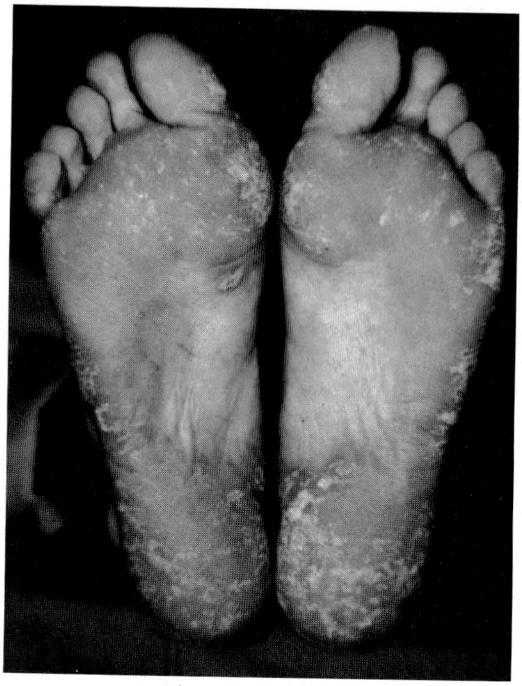

Figure 8.2. Psoriasis of the soles.

drop-like (guttate) lesions on the trunk and lower extremities, especially in children and young adults. This often follows a "strep throat" (streptococcal pharyngitis).

Psoriasis may be divided into psoriasis vulgaris (ordinary psoriasis), which occurs in various forms and in which pustules are usually absent; generalized pustular psoriasis (von Zumbusch), considered to be the most severe type; and localized pustular psoriasis (18, 19).

There are two types of localized pustular psoriasis which specifically affect the hands and feet: (*a*) localized acrodermatitis continua of Hallopeau (also known as acrodermatitis perstans and dermatitis repens). This usually begins on a single digit as a localized, unilateral, infected ulcer or paronychia which is posttraumatic. The lesion begins on the skin around the distal phalanx adjacent to the nail. Small blisters or pustules appear, which burst and eventually become crusted. New lesions appear by extension or confluence (Fig. 8.3).

Pustular psoriasis of the palms and soles (pustulosis palmaris et plantaris) usually occurs without any other manifestation of psoriasis but may be seen in association with psoriasis vulgaris. This entity, which

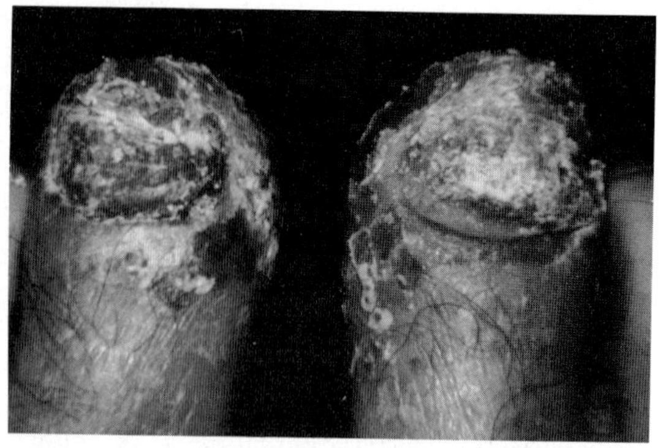

Figure 8.3. Acrodermatitis continua involving both great toes. Courtesy of Dr. Kenneth Canter.

was initially described by Barber in 1930 (20), is bilateral and symmetrical. Patches develop on the midportion of the soles with recurring crops of small pustules. These sometimes fuse to form "lakes of pus." As a rule the pustules do not rupture but tend to dry up, leaving behind brown crusts. This condition is characterized by periods of quiescence and exacerbation and is extremely resistant to treatment.

One should consider vesicular tinea pedis and pustular secondary syphilis in the differential diagnosis for pedal pustular eruptions.

Histopathology

The histologic picture of psoriasis vulgaris is characterized by:

1. Marked hyperkeratosis and parakeratosis.
2. Regular elongation of the rete ridges with thickening in their lower portion.
3. Elongation and edema of the dermal papillae.
4. Atrophy over the dermal papillae (thus explaining Auspitz's sign. Auspitz's sign is due to bleeding of ectatic vessels in the papillae under the thin epidermis.
5. Absence of granular cells.
6. Small collections of neutrophils (Munro microabscesses) may be present in the stratum corneum (Fig. 8.4). Biopsy in localized pustular psoriasis of the palms and soles is characterized by the presence of large rounded intraepidermal unilocular pustules which contain many polymorphonuclear leukocytes and which may extend into the underlying dermis (Fig. 8.5).

Nail Involvement

There are several characteristic nail changes and clinical signs which may be seen in the nails of patients with psoriasis.

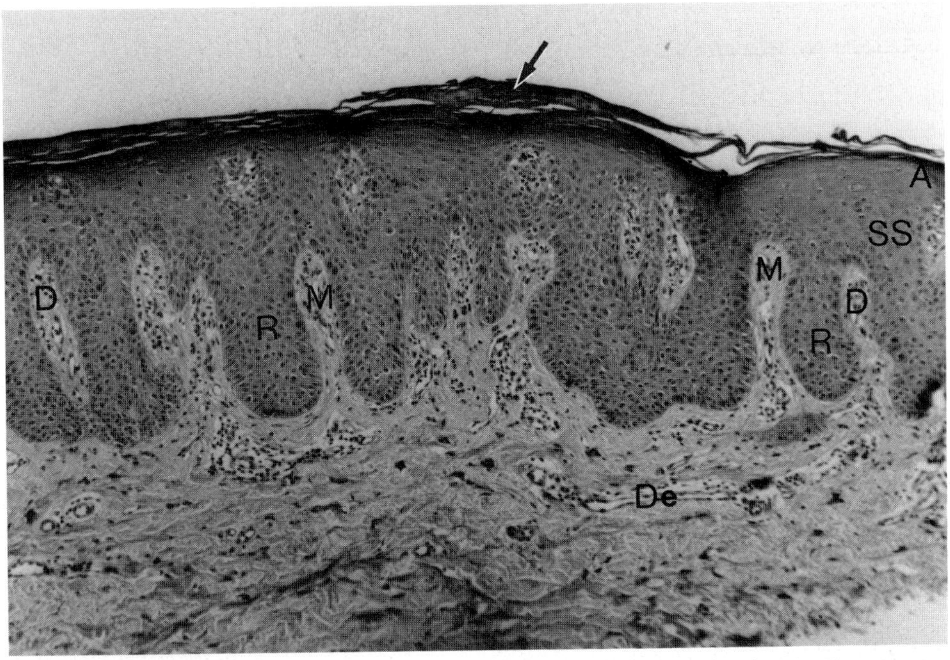

Figure 8.4. Photomicrograph of psoriasis. Retention of nuclei in the horny layer (*arrow*), regular elongation of the rete ridges (*R*), and elongation and clubbing of dermal papillae (*D*). *M*, Munro microabscess; *SS*, stratum spinosum; *De*, dermis. Original magnification, × 63.

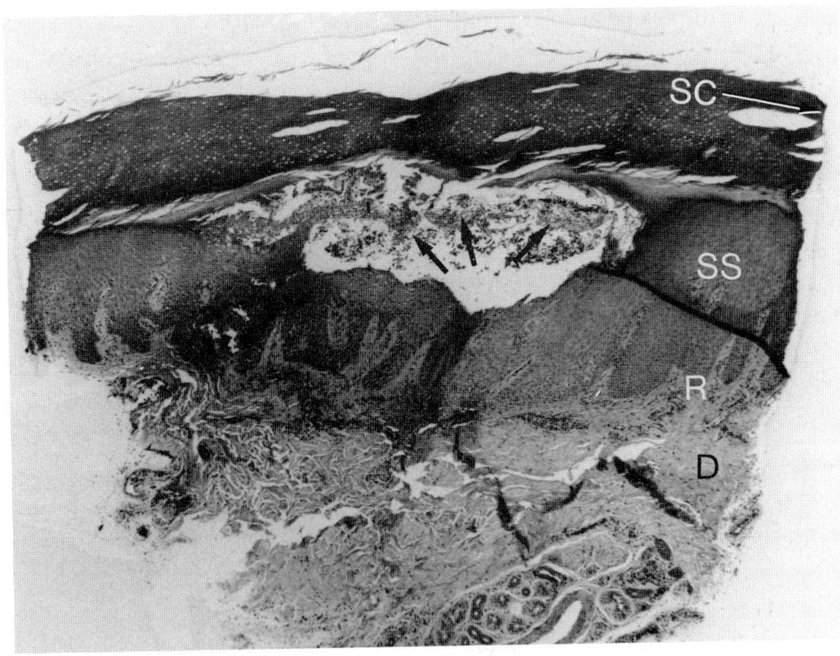

Figure 8.5. Photomicrograph of localized pustular psoriasis. Hyperkeratosis with a large intraepidermal unilocular pustule (*arrow*). Many polymorphonuclear leukocytes are present within the cavity of the pustule. *SC*, stratum corneum; *SS*, stratum spinosum; *R*, rete pegs; *D*, dermis. Original magnification ×25.

These are:

1. Pits in the surface of the nail plate, like dents made with a needle
2. Leukonychia with a smooth or rough surface
3. Tan spots under the nail plate (oil spot sign)
4. Onycholysis
5. Crumbling of the nail plate
6. Subungual hyperkeratosis
7. Splinter hemorrhages

It should be made clear that although these nail changes strongly suggest psoriasis, they are not pathognomonic. Careful examination of the skin should be done to seek out confirmatory evidence of psoriasis. In addition, onychomycosis, lichen planus, and traumatic dystrophic nail changes should be ruled out.

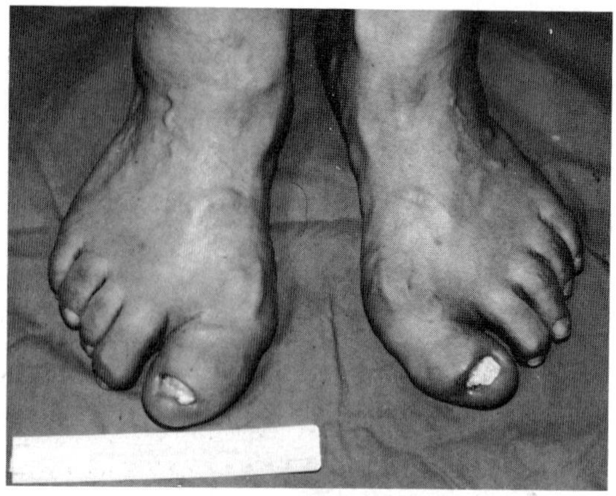

Figure 8.6. Psoriatic arthritis. Sausage deformity of both great toes with nail dystrophy.

Psoriatic Arthritis

Psoriatic arthritis is defined as psoriasis associated with inflammatory peripheral arthritis, spondylitis, or both. The association between psoriasis and arthritis was first mentioned in 1818 by Jean Louis Alibert (23). Since that time, psoriatic arthritis has gained acceptance as a distinct clinical entity seen in as many as 5 to 7% of patients with psoriasis (23, 24). It is an asymmetrical inflammatory condition of the joints which tends to cause less pain and disability than rheumatoid arthritis. There is almost equal distribution between males and females. Patients usually have a negative serologic test for rheumatoid factor. Most authors have found HLA-B27 to be positive in over 90% of patients with psoriatic arthritis and spondylitis (5, 25).

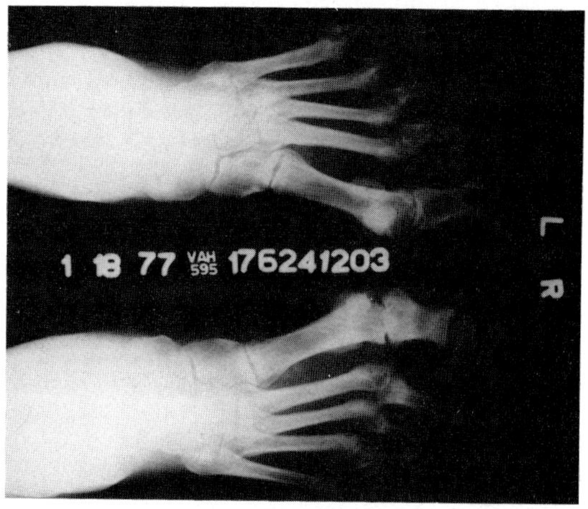

Figure 8.7. Anteroposterior (AP) radiograph of patient in Figure 8.6, showing destruction of the interphalangeal joint of both great toes, with subluxation of the metatarsophalangeal joints.

Classicially the term psoriatic arthritis has been used to describe an arthritis affecting the distal interphalangeal joints; however, in Moll's view this may account for only 5% of the cases. More frequently involved are the metatarsophalangeal and proximal interphalangeal joints (Fig. 8.6 and 8.7). Involved digits may develop a "sausage" appearance (25). In addition a destructive polyarthritis, arthritis mutilans, may be seen in a small percentage of cases. This is characterized by osteolysis of the phalanges, metatarsals, and metacarpals, resulting in deformity and subluxation of joints.

Nail involvement has been noted in approximately 80% of patients with psoriatic arthritis, in contrast to 30% of psoriatic individuals without arthritis. There is thought to be a close temporal relationship between nail and joint changes (23–25).

In a group of patients with psoriatic arthritis studied by Baker et al. (26), psoriasis preceded the onset of arthritis in 64% of the cases, while both skin and joint involvement occurred simultaneously in 23% of the cases. Arthritis preceded skin manifestations in 13% of the cases. Canter and Reese (5) provided a concise review of the pathologic and clinical aspects of this entity.

Treatment

Treatment for psoriasis has typically involved the use of a variety of bathing routines (tar baths and oils) and topical preparations applied alone and in combination. Ultraviolet light (UVA and UVB) has been incorporated to enhance the effectiveness of the treatment. Oral retinoids (retinol, tretinoin, isotretinoin, and etretinate), cytotoxic agents [topical 5-fluorouracil (5-FU) and systemic methotrexate], and photochemotherapy (PUVA) are the most recent additions to the therapeutic approach (4, 27).

The physician's choices for treatment are influenced by many factors, including: extent of involvement, severity, duration, patient's age, compliance, previous treatment, ease and convenience of therapy, cost, rate of improvement, and possible side effects. Clearly, benefit-risk judgments for new therapies must be defined and carefully considered before initiating treatment.

A common approach is to begin treatment with one of the following topical agents: glucocorticosteroids, keratolytics, anthralin, or crude coal tar plus UVB (Goekerman regimen).

The corticosteroid ointments and gels are often effective. The efficacy can be enhanced when used under occlusion with plastic wrap. Topical steroids lose their effectiveness over time, and psoriasis tends to rebound promptly when they are withdrawn. The clinician should recognize that both local and systemic side effects may develop. The local side effects of striae, atrophy (thinning of the skin), purpura, and telangiectasies are well recognized. These effects are seen with prolonged topical steroid therapy and especially with the use of more potent fluorinated compounds, particularly when used with occlusion. Systemic absorption of these more potent corticosteroids increases the risk of pituitary-adrenal suppression.

Intralesional steroids (triamcinolone, 2.5 mg/ml to 5 mg/ml) injected into the posterior nail fold in a quantity of 0.2 to 0.3 ml have been used for treatment of psoriatic nail disease (21, 28–30).

It is generally agreed upon by most dermatologists that systemic steroids should be avoided, as they can lead to severe flares of the disease and may precipitate life-threatening pustular psoriasis.

Keratolytics are used to aid in the removal of hyperkeratotic plaques. Of these preparations, salicyclic acid seems to be the most effective and least toxic. It is frequently used in a strength of 6% and is commercially available as a gel. The skin is hydrated by soaking for approximately 5 minutes before application of the gel. The benefit is enhanced by the use of plastic wrap for occlusion at bedtime. Prolonged use over large areas could result in salicylic acid toxicity, manifested by nausea, vomiting, hearing changes, lethargy, or mental confusion.

The use of crude coal tar and ultraviolet light (UVB), first reported by Goekerman, is one of the safest and most effective treatments available (31). This treatment is best carried out in a psoriasis day care center or hospital, due to the prolonged nature of the treatment (2 to 4 weeks) and the staining properties of the tar.

Anthralin is an antipsoriatic drug with local irritant effect which is effective in the treatment of psoriasis, when used according to the Ingram technique (32). This combines the use of a coal tar bath, ultraviolet light exposure, and application of an anthralin paste. Because anthralin causes irritation of the skin, and discolors the skin, nails, and clothing, it may result in poor patient compliance. A simplified treatment program alternating topical corticosteroids with low strength anthralin pastes eliminates the irritant reactions and has a higher degree of patient acceptance (33).

Photochemotherapy (PUVA) combines the use of oral psoralens and long wave ultraviolet light (UVA). This treatment has been used since 1974 when it was reported by Parrish et al (34). Treatment consists of giving oral methoxsalen in a measured dose, followed 2 hours later by a measured dose of UVA, repeated 2 to 3 times per week until the psoriasis clears. Patients are then put on a maintenance schedule. Side effects include erythema, nausea, increased pigmentation, development of skin cancers, and the possible development of cataracts. This treatment has been reported to be only about 50% successful for the treatment of pustular psoriasis of the palms and soles (4, 35). However, Menné (36) found clearing or improvement in 23 of 24 patients maintained for 1 month on oral PUVA therapy. Morison et al reported that 18 of 20 cases of recalcitrant plantar pustulosis were resolved with at least 2 months of therapy.

In severe recalcitrant cases of psoriasis,

where all other attempts at treatment were unsuccessful, methotrexate may be the drug of choice. This drug is a potent folic acid antagonist which appears to function by inhibiting DNA synthesis and thereby reducing epidermal cell turnover time. Caution is required when using this drug, as it is reported to be hepatotoxic. A 3 to 5% incidence of cirrhosis has been reported in patients treated with methotrexate (4).

Topical fluorouracil has been used by Fredrikson to treat psoriatic nail dystrophy. He applied 1% FU under occlusive wrap and reported achieving a 75% reduction in pitting and hypertrophy of the nail in 17 of 20 patients after 4 to 6 months of treatment (38, 39). Tsuji and Sugai observed prompt resolution of plaque-type psoriasis in 7 to 9 days in 13 patients who were treated with occlusive 5% FU (38, 40). It should be noted that this topical treatment could be very irritating to the skin, with erythema, soreness, swelling, and pain.

Clinical trials with etretinate have shown impressive improvements in severe psoriasis in patients unresponsive to other therapy, with particularly good results in palmoplantar, pustular, and erythrodermic psoriasis. The incidence of side effects with this treatment is relatively high. Cheilitis occurs in 80% of patients, dry oral and nasal mucous membranes and skin desquamation in about 35% each, and thinning of the skin in 25%. Hair loss occurs with an incidence of 22% and is one of the major reasons for discontinuing therapy (41). At this time etretinate is not yet FDA-approved.

LICHEN PLANUS

Lichen planus (LP) is a relatively common papulosquamous disease of the skin and mucous membranes. It is a pruritic inflammatory dermatosis which is bilaterally symmetrical and is characterized by distinctive clinical and histologic features. It affects men and women equally, usually during young adulthood and middle age.

Etiology and Pathogenesis

The etiology of lichen planus is unknown, but several causes have been proposed, including (*a*) viral infection; (*b*) emotional upset (psychogenic factors); (*c*) exposure to certain drugs and chemicals (42), and (*d*) an immune-mediated injury. Indirect evidence for the role of the immune system is supported by the presence of lymphocyte infiltration at the dermoepidermal junction, with a predominance of T cells in the dermis, in addition to which LP patients have shown decreased serum IgA and IgM, and deposits of immunoglobulin in their skin (43). Olsen et al (44) have demonstrated a lichen planus-specific antigen (LPSA) in granular and deep prickle epithelial cells from the LP lesion. Sera from seven out of eight patients tested contained an antibody to LPSA.

Association of HLA-A3 has been reported in patients with LP, and this may represent a susceptibility factor in lichen planus (43, 45).

Fellner believes that LP is an allergic reaction pattern, particularly following exposure to different chemicals including dyes, color film developers, and gold (42). He has compiled the following list of drugs capable of producing lichen planus:

1. Gold
2. Demeclocycline HCL
3. Streptomycin
4. Tetracycline HCL
5. Arsenic
6. Mercury
7. Iodides
8. Chloroquine
9. Quinacrine
10. Quinine
11. Quinidine
12. Paraphenylenediamine
13. CD2 color film developer
14. Antimony
15. Phenothiazine
16. Paraaminosalicylic acid
17. Chlorothiazide
18. Hydrochlorothiazide
19. Amiphenazole

The morphology and histology of LP induced by drugs and chemicals may look exactly like other types of lichen planus.

Clinical Features

Lesions are small, polygonal, flat-topped, violaceous, papules. The surface of the lesion may demonstrate a delicate scaling or grayish-white cross hatching known as Wickham's striae. These can be seen better using a drop of mineral oil, and a magnifying lens. Common sites of involvement are the flexor surfaces of the arms (especially the wrists), extensor surfaces of the lower extremities (especially the ankles), sides of the feet, buccal mucosa, and glans penis (Fig. 8).

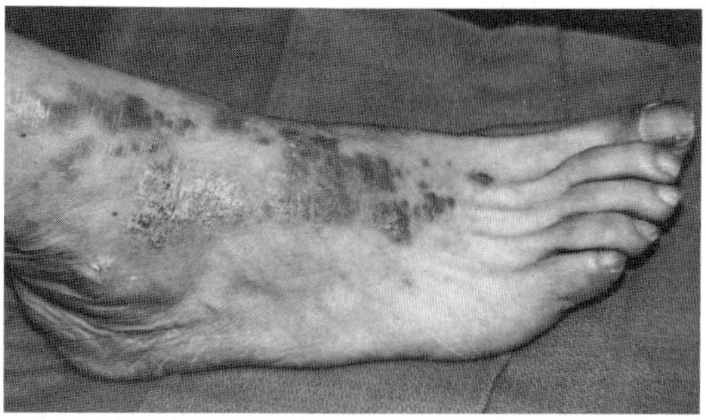

Figure 8.8. Lichen planus.

Of podiatric interest are the characteristic nail changes seen in 1 to 10% of the patients with LP (46–48). Oral mucosa lesions characterized by small whitish hyperkeratotic papules, in a lace-like pattern on the inner cheek, are seen in 30 to 70% of patients (42). The disease may manifest itself in a variety of other clinical forms, such as hypertrophic, ulcerative, bullous, linear, and atrophic LP.

An interesting finding in LP, as well as in psoriasis, is skin lesions produced in scratch marks, the Köebner phenomena. Deep pigmentation of healed lesions is characteristic and may persist for months.

Variations of lichen planus which affect the lower extremities include the following.

(*a*) Ulcerative LP of the Feet—A rare variant of lichen planus characterized by crippling ulcers of the feet and toes, permanent loss of toenails, and cicatricial alopecia of the scalp (49–51).

(*b*) Hypertrophic LP—Characterized by verrucous, heavily scaling lesions, which occur most often on the lower limbs, especially around the ankles (Figs. 8.9 and 8.10). The development of hypertrophic lesions greatly lengthens the course of the disease. This variant of LP can be extremely pruritic and may persist for years. Hypertrophic lichen planus must be distinguished from lichen simplex chronicus.

(*c*) Linear LP—Characterized by long narrow linear lesions, which may extend the whole length of a limb. These may resemble a linear nevus. The histology is characteristic and distinguishes this lesion from other linear dermatoses, including linear psoriasis.

(*d*) Guttate LP—Characterized by discrete, widely scattered lesions which may resemble psoriasis.

Secondary syphilis may masquerade as LP and should be considered in the differential diagnosis of any lichenoid dermatosis.

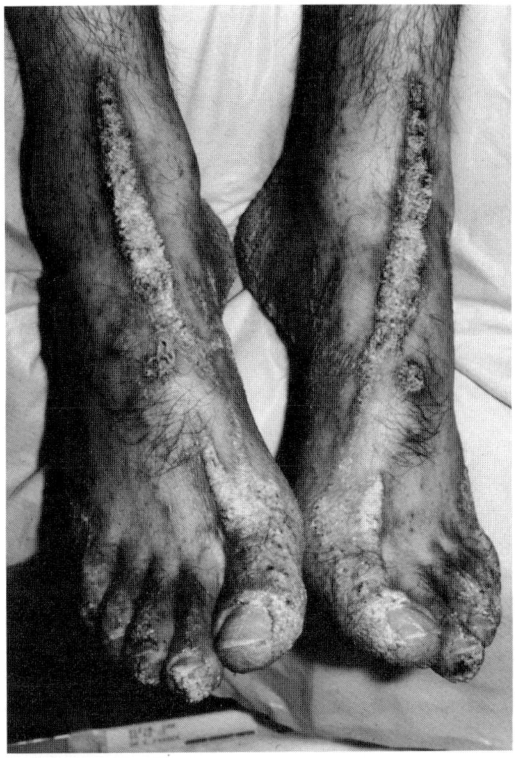

Figure 8.9. Hypertrophic lichen planus. Courtesy of Dr. Walter Koerber.

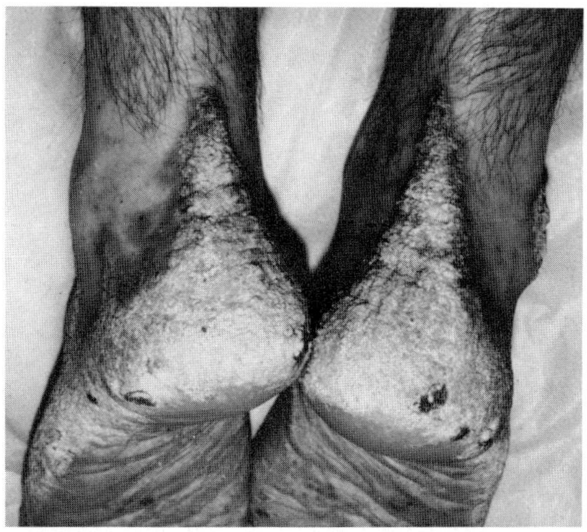

Figure 8.10. Hypertrophic lichen planus. Courtesy of Dr. Walter Koerber.

NAIL CHANGES

Lichen planus produces nail changes which can be traced to disease activity in one or more parts of the nail unit. These changes are nonspecific and not pathognomonic, as they are sometimes associated with other disorders. Nail changes in LP must be differentiated from those seen with onychomycosis, psoriasis, peripheral vascular disease, and traumatic nail dystrophies. The most frequent types of nail alteration are:

1. Irregular longitudinal grooving, ridging, and splitting of the nail plate.
2. Thinning of the nail plate,
3. Focal destruction of the proximal nail plate with fusion of the proximal nail fold to the nail bed (pterygium),
4. complete loss of nail plate, and
5. Subungual keratosis.

The predominant feature of this nail disease process is destruction and atrophy following inflammation. Thinning of the nail plate results from a marked reduction in size and function of the matrix. Another condition which may mimic these nail changes is severe erythema multiforme.

Histology

Histologically, typical lesions of LP are characterized by the following cardinal features (Fig. 8.11):

1. Hyperkeratosis.
2. Hypergranulosis, with a thickened granular cell layer.
3. Irregular acanthosis.
4. "Saw-toothed" appearance of the rete ridges.
5. Liquefactive degeneration of the basal layer.
6. Colloid bodies are seen in the lower epidermal layer.
7. A band-like upper dermal infiltrate of lymphocytes and histiocytes.

Epidermal changes seen in LP consist of continuous destruction of the keratinocytes followed by replacement with normal epidermal cells. These destroyed keratinocytes then form colloid bodies.

Treatment

The prospect for permanent remission in LP is better than in psoriasis. Two-thirds of all patients may clear spontaneously. Treatment is generally geared toward symptomatic relief. Administration of steroids is the basic treatment for lichen planus, with topical fluorinated steroids in-

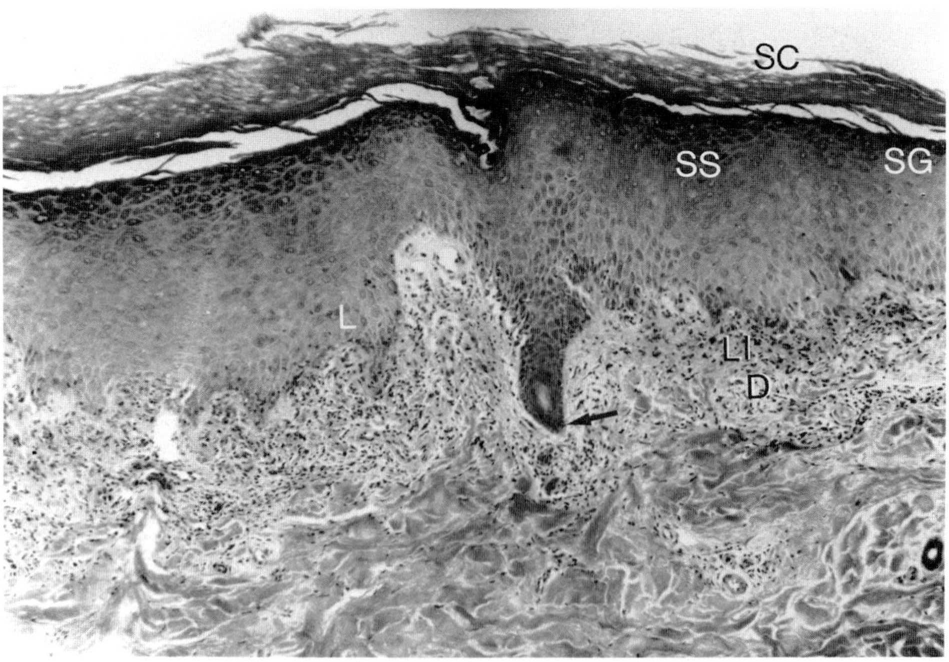

Figure 8.11. Photomicrograph of lichen planus, illustrating irregular acanthosis with "saw-toothed" appearance of the rete ridges (*arrow*). There is a band-like lymphocytic infiltrate in the upper dermis. *SC*, stratum corneum; *SS*, stratum spinosum; *LI*, inflammatory infiltrate; *L*, areas of liquefaction. Original magnification, × 63.

dicated for mild to moderate disease and systemic steroids (prednisone) indicated for severe reactions.

Antihistamines are helpful in relieving pruritis, especially at bedtime. Photochemotherapy (PUVA) may also be a consideration for the treatment of moderate to severe disease which has not been responsive to other treatments.

PITYRIASIS RUBRA PILARIS

Pityriasis rubra pilaris (PRP) is a rare, idiopathic papulosquamous disorder which is characterized by follicular plugging, perifollicular erythema, and palmoplantar hyperkeratosis. Although its incidence has been reported to be not more than 1 in 5000 new patients (52, 53), it bears mentioning because of its very striking podiatric presentation. The impressive, yellow-orange hued keratoderma of the soles associated with this disease has been referred to as the "keratodermic sandal" of pityriasis rubra pilaris.

Gross *et al.* (54) analyzed data on 173 case reports of PRP from the English language literature. Griffiths (52) reported on a personal series of over 100 patients. Their findings revealed no significant age or sex predilection, with onset of PRP at any age from birth to 70 years. Other investigators have found a bimodal distribution, with peaks in the first and fifth decades (55).

Etiology and Pathogenesis

The etiology of PRP is unknown. It has been reported to be both acquired and familial, with an autosomal dominant mode of inheritance. Gross et al. (54) reviewed four family groups in his analysis and found that in three groups a father or mother and one or more sons or daughters had PRP. In a follow-up study of 57 patients reported by Davidson et al (55) heredity was a factor in two children. Both children were the first of three generations in which PRP was noted. In five children the disease was preceded by infection or trauma.

Several authors have reported on physical factors which may have precipitated PRP. These include sunburn, chemical and electrical burns, infections, and parturition. PRP has also been observed in isolated instances in association with many diseases. These include syphilis, tuberculosis, hypertension, rheumatic fever, asthma, syringomyelia, diabetes, myasthenia gravis, Legg-Calvé-Perthe disease, and Downs syndrome. The significance of these associations is not known and may be fortuitous.

Porter and Shuster (56) have shown that the epidermal renewal rate is greatly increased in the lesions of PRP and psoriasis. Cell kinetic parameters are increased above normal but are less than in psoriasis. In a study by Niemi et al (57), HLA typing in 11 patients with PRP showed no difference from that of controls.

Clinical Features

Initially it may be difficult to distinguish PRP from psoriasis, and final discrimination may depend upon evolution of the disease.

Diffuse thickening of the soles and palms may be the first sign of this disease, or will be seen during the course of the disease. In the analysis of Gross et al (54) analysis, 67% of the patients had involvement of the soles, and 50% had involvement of the legs and dorsum of the feet during the course of their disease. The skin on the soles may appear smooth, shiny, yellow-orange hued, and hyperkeratotic. Plantar fissures may develop (Fig. 8.12).

The basic lesion of PRP is follicular hyperkeratosis. A small acuminate cone of compact keratin forms at the mouth of a follicle and is pierced by a hair at its summit. These pointed, plugged follicles may appear as black dots on the dorsum of the proximal phalanges of the toes and fingers.

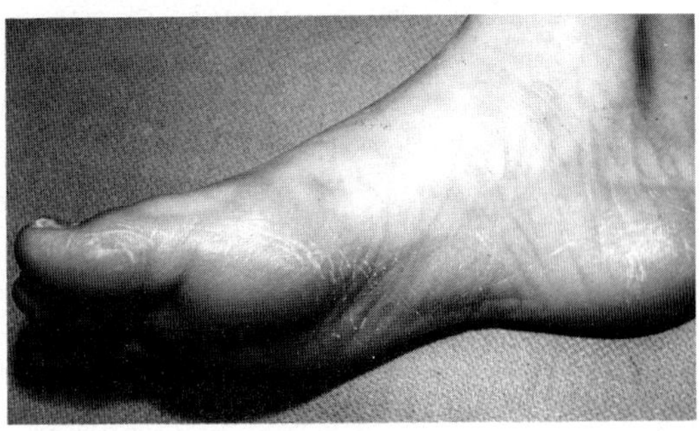

Figure 8.12. Pityriasis rubra pilaris. Courtesy of Dr. Walter Koerber.

Initially, follicular lesions may be prominent on the knees and elbows, but later these lesions become flat, thick, and psoriasiform at these sites. Perifollicular erythema and scaling may extend to involve the whole skin surface with islands of normal looking skin scattered over the erythema. As the erythema extends, the follicular component is often lost.

NAIL INVOLVEMENT

When the soles and palms are involved in PRP, the nails may show well marked changes. These include longitudinal ridging of the nails, subungual hyperkeratosis, splinter hemorrhages and, occasionally, psoriasiform pits. Gross et al reported in their analysis that 19% of patients showed toenail involvement, and 21% had fingernail involvement.

The differential diagnosis for PRP should include the following: psoriasis, seborrheic dermatitis, vitamin A deficiency (phrynoderma), follicular eczema, drug eruption, follicular ichthyosis, and lichen planopilaris.

Pityriasis rubra pilaris may have a duration of from 3 months to more than 7 years. About half of the patients remit completely within three years.

Histopathology

Histological examination of a skin biopsy specimen is necessary in order to establish the diagnosis of PRP. The essential pathologic process is follicular hyperkeratosis. In addition, there are diffuse hyperkeratosis, focal parakeratosis, and moderate acanthosis (Fig. 8.13).

Treatment

PRP has been described as having a capricious course, characterized by exacerbations and remissions. As a result it is difficult to assess the effectiveness of various treatments. Oral vitamin A, topical and systemic steroids, methotrexate, penicillin V, and antituberculous drugs have all been tried, without consistent results. In Davidson's study (55), many patients commented that therapy made little differences in the evolution or resolution of their disease. Schmidt stated that lesions clear no matter what therapy is given (55, 58).

Griffiths recommends symptomatic care with simple emollients. Goldsmith et al.

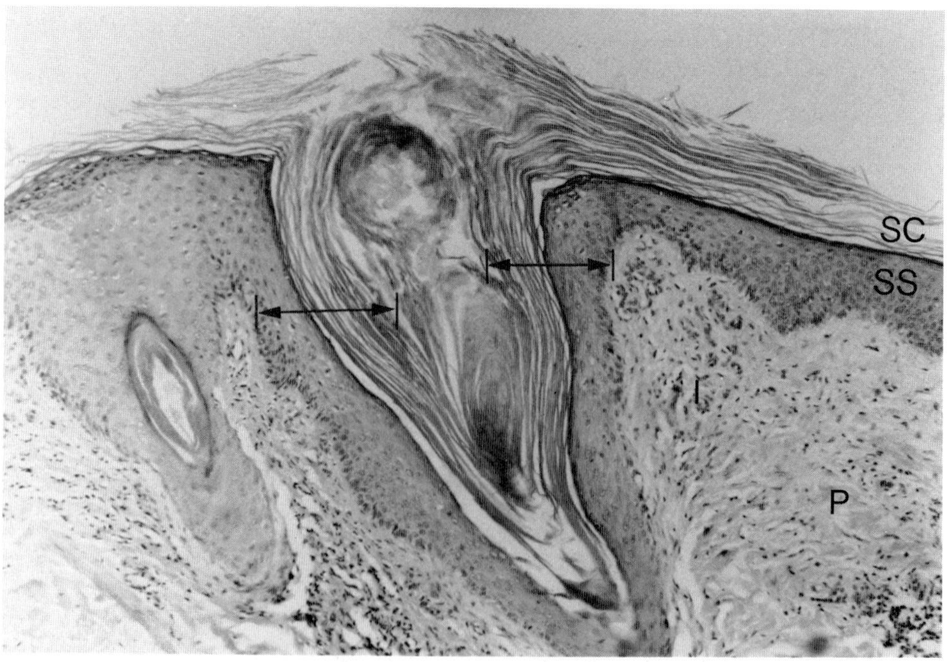

Figure 8.13. Photomicrograph of pityriasis rubra pilaris, illustrating follicular hyperkeratosis and a slight degree of acanthosis (*arrows*). *SC*, stratum corneum; *SG*, serratum granulosum; *Li*, lymphocytic infiltrate; *D*, dermis; *L*, area of liquefaction.

(59) reported on 45 patients treated with 13-*cis*-retinoic acid (isotretinoin). They reported marked improvement in the degree of erythema, induration, and scaling noted within 4 weeks. Remission or maintained improvement persisted after stopping therapy in many of the patients. Randle et al (60) reported using toxic doses of vitamin A (500,000 to 1 million IU/day) for 5 to 14 days in seven patients who were disabled by PRP. Within 72 hours, the patients began to exfoliate the hyperkeratotic and keratodermatous lesions. The skin of six of the seven patients was virtually cleared by the treatment, and none suffered a relapse.

Podiatric care should be directed to symptomatic treatment of the keratoderma. Keratolytic ointments or gels, as well as emollients, may be of some benefit. Samitz (61) reports seeing a dramatic response with vitamin A acid (0.1 to 0.5%) under occlusion.

SECONDARY SYPHILIS

Secondary syphilis is a disease entity which needs to be considered in the differential diagnosis for maculopapular, papulosquamous, and psoriasiform lesions on the soles and palms. Admittedly this entity is rarely seen today, with a decline in the number of patients with syphilis. However, it is still important for the physician to be familiar with the essential signs and symptoms of the disease and to recognize that the soles and palms may be the most frequent sites of involvement.

Secondary syphilis is that stage of syphilis which affects the skin and mucous membranes. There is generally an interval of 6 to 8 weeks between the appearance of the primary lesion (chancre) and the secondary eruption. The serum Venereal Disease Research Laboratory (VDRL) test is reactive in all patients with secondary syphilis, and a fourfold rise in the titer is indicative of acute disease. These patients are infectious and present a hazard to the clinician and surgeon. Dark-field microscopic examination and the Warthin-Starry silver stain may be used to demonstrate spirochetes in these skin lesions.

Clinical Features

Early cutaneous syphilis is very often inconspicuous, with subtle signs and symptoms which can easily be missed. The hallmark of secondary syphilis is its ability to mimic a variety of other skin diseases. These include psoriasis, lichen planus, pityriasis rosea, erythema multiforme, drug eruptions, and tinea pedis. Identification requires a high index of suspicion and reliance on confirmatory serologic tests to establish the diagnosis. Podiatrists should be aware that interdigital condyloma latum is a clinical sign of lues.

The cutaneous lesions of secondary syphilis are macular, papular, papulosquamous, or pustular. The majority of the patients in a prospective study by Chapel (62) had maculopapular and papulosquamous lesions. The distribution of lesions is generally bilateral and symmetrical, with color that varies from that of raw ham to red to brown (63). Lesions may have a coppery hue. Involvement of the palms and soles has been reported to occur in from 60 to 80% of patients (62, 63).

Discrete hyperkeratotic papular lesions are encountered usually on the nonweight-bearing surface of the soles. They may appear as deep-seated, flat-topped papules or scaly papulosquamous lesions (Fig. 8.14). Infrequently these papules may ulcerate and become crusted and pustular. These lesions are teeming with *Treponema pallidum.*

Patients may present with one or more of the following constitutional symptoms: sore throat, malaise, headache (characteristically worse at night), muscle aches, fever, and hair loss. A generalized lymphadenopathy has been observed in 50 to 85% of patients with secondary syphilis (62).

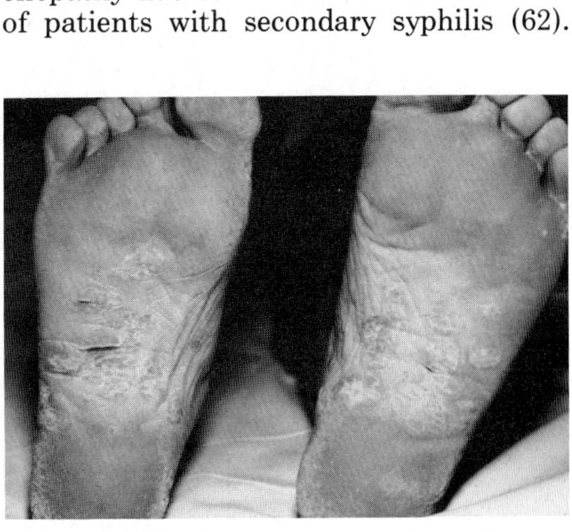

Figure 8.14. Secondary syphilis of the soles.

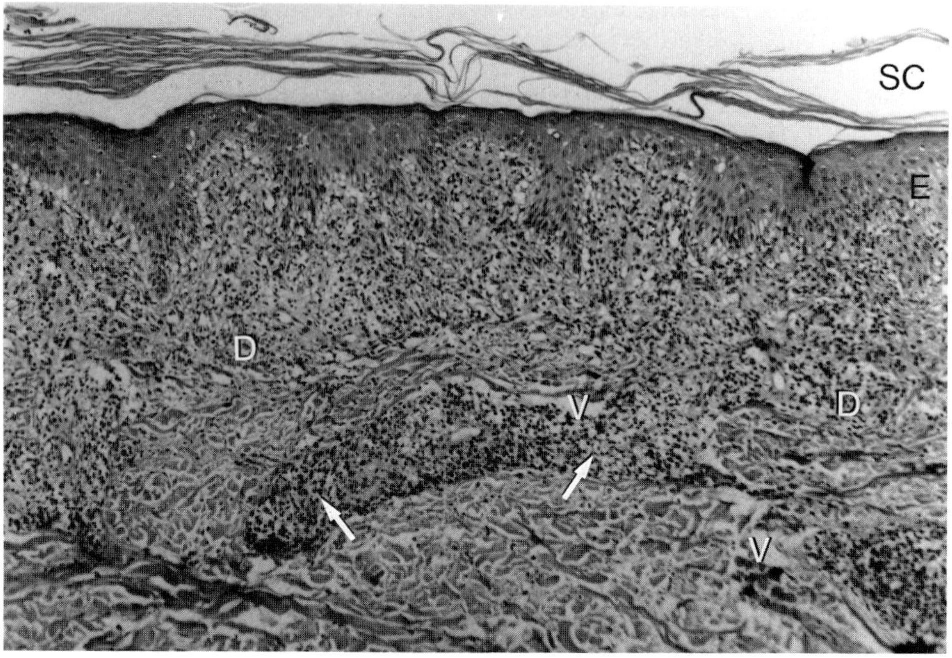

Figure 8.15. Photomicrograph of cutaneous syphilis, illustrating perivascular infiltrate (*arrows*). *SC*, stratum corneum; *E*, epidermis; *D*, dermis; *V*, blood vessels. Original magnification, × 63.

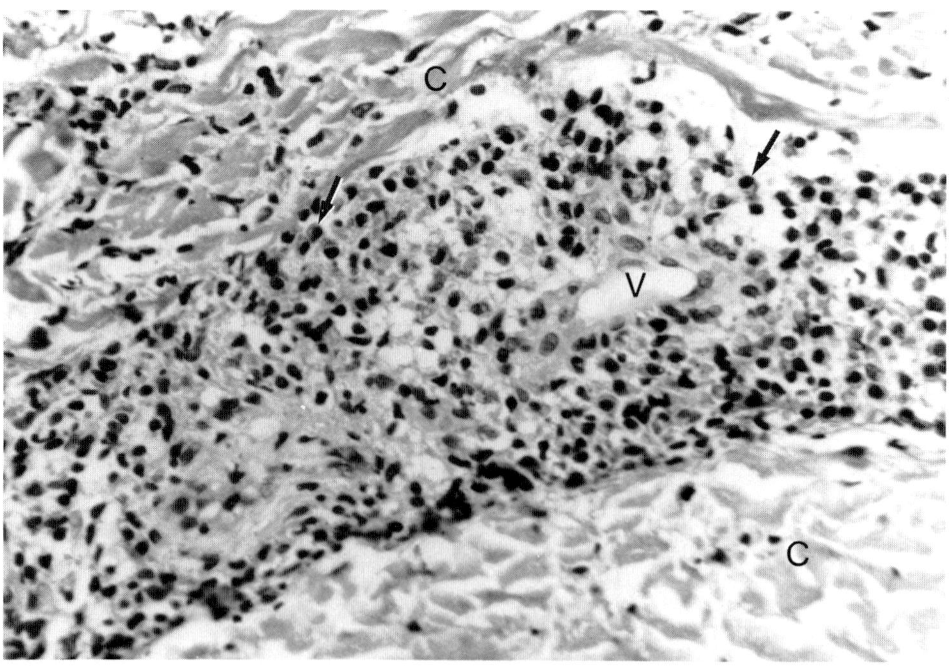

Figure 8.16. Higher magnification of Figure 8.15. Perivascular infiltrate contains plasma cells (with eccentrically placed nuclei) (*arrows*). Original magnification, × 250. *C*, collagenic fibers; *V*, blood vessels.

The lymph nodes are enlarged but not painful and have a hard, rubbery feel.

Histology

The superficial and deep vessels of the dermis show marked endothelial swelling and proliferation and are surrounded by a pronounced infiltrate containing many plasma cells. This perivascular coatsleeve-like arrangement stands out very clearly in the lower dermis (64) (Figs. 8.15 and 8.16).

Treatment

The physician must be alert to the physical signs and serological evidence of infectious syphilis. Once the diagnosis has been established, the recommended treatment is 2.4 million units of benzathine penicillin G, given as an intramuscular injection at two sites weekly for 2 weeks (total, 4.8 million units) (65). Two to six hours after the first treatment with penicillin, the patient may develop chills, fever, headache, and joint pain. This is a Jarisch-Herxheimer reaction and should not be confused with an allergic reaction to penicillin.

Patients who have a history of penicillin allergy are given tetracycline hydrochloride orally (500 mg four times daily for 15 days).

ACKNOWLEDGMENTS

I wish to express my sincere thanks to Mrs. Barbara E. Deaven, medical librarian, and Mr. David E. Falger, Chief of Library Service, VA Medical Center, Lebanon, PA, for their assistance. In addition, I would like to thank Dr. P. Michael Olmstead for his help in preparing the photomicrographs used in this chapter.

References

1. Domonkos AN, Arnold HL, Odom RB: Andrew's diseases of the skin. In *Clinical Dermatology*, ed 7. Philadelphia, W.B. Saunders, 1982, p 226.
2. Abele DC, Dobson RL, Graham JB: Heredity and psoriasis: study of a large family. *Arch Dermatol* 88:90–99, 1963.
3. Watson W, Cann HM, Farber EM, Nall ML: Genetics of psoriasis. *Arch Dermatol* 105:197–207, 1972.
4. Cram DL: Psoriasis: current advances in etiology and treatment. *J Am Acad Dermatol* 4:1–14, 1981.
5. Canter KG, Reese DL: Psoriatic arthritis relative to the foot. *J Am Podiatry Assoc* 70:437–441, 1980.
6. Goldman JN, Goldman MB: What the clinician should know about the major histocompatibility complex. *JAMA* 246:873–876, 1981.
7. Ritzmann SE: HLA patterns and disease associations. *JAMA* 236:2305–2309, 1976.
8. Krulig L, Farber EM, Grumet FC et al: Histocompatiblity (HL-A) antigens in psoriasis. *Arch Dermatol* 111:857–860, 1975.
9. Ward JM, Barnes RMR: HLA antigens in persistent palmoplantar pustulosis and its relationship to psoriasis. *Br J Dermatol* 99:477–483, 1978.
10. McMichael AJ, Morhenn V, Payne R et al: HLA C and D antigens associated with psoriasis. *Br J Dermatol* 98:287–292, 1978.
11. Svejgaard A, Staub-Nielson L, Svejgaard E et al: HLA in psoriasis vulgaris and pustular psoriasis. Population and family studies. *Br J Dermatol* 91:145–153, 1974.
12. Van Scott EJ, Ekel TM: Kinetics of hyperplasia in psoriasis. *Arch Dermatol* 88:373–380, 1963.
13. Voorhees JJ, Chambers DA, Duell EA et al: Molecular mechanisms in proliferative skin disease. J Invest Dermatol 67:442–450, 1976.
14. Adachi K, Yoshikawa K, Halprin KM et al: Prostaglandins and cyclic AMP in epidermis. *Br J Dermatol* 92:381–388, 1975.
15. Voorhees JJ: Polyamines and psoriasis. *Arch Dermatol* 115:943–944, 1979.
16. Proctor MS, Wilkinson DI, Orenberg EK: Lowered cutaneous and urinary levels of polyamines with clinical improvement in treated psoriasis. *Arch Dermatol* 115:945–949, 1979.
17. Russell DH, Combest WL, Duell EA et al: Glucocorticoid inhibits elevated polyamine biosynthesis in psoriasis. *J Invest Dermatol* 71:177–181, 1978.
18. Pitlosh JP, Taubman MR, Tench W: Pedal pustular psoriasis: a review of the literature and case report. *J Am Podiatry Assoc* 72:429–435, 1982.
19. Benedetto AV, Bergfield WF: Papulosquamous disorders of the feet. *J Am Podiatry Assoc* 66:526–530, 1978.
20. Barber HW: Acrodermatitis continua vel pertans (dermatitis repens) and psoriasis pustulosa. *Br J Dermatol* 42:500, 1930.
21. Norton LA: Nail disorders: a review. *J Am Acad Dermatol* 2:451–467, 1980.
22. Zaias N: Psoriasis of the nail: a clinical-pathologic study. *Arch Dermatol* 99:567–579, 1969.
23. Rodnan GP, Schumacher HR: Psoriatic ar-

thritis. In *Primer on the Rheumatic Diseases*, ed 8. Atlanta, Arthritis Foundation, 1983, pp 91–92.
24. Anderson TF, Voorhees JJ: Psoriasis and arthritis. *Cutis* 21:790–800, 1978.
25. Moll JMH: The clinical spectrum of psoriatic arthritis. *Clin Orthop* 143:66–75, 1979.
26. Baker H, Golding DN, Thompson M: Psoriasis and arthritis. *Ann Intern Med* 58:909–925, 1963.
27. Bryant BG: Treatment of psoriasis. *Am J Hosp Pharm* 37:814–820, 1980.
28. Abell E, Samman PD: Intradermal triamcinolone treatment of nail dystrophies. *Br J Dermatol* 89:191–197, 1973.
29. Abell E: Treatment of psoriatic nail dystrophy. *Br J Dermatol* 86:79–82, 1972.
30. Bedi TR: Intradermal triamcinolone treatment of psoriatic onychodystrophy. *Dermatologica* 155:24–27, 1977.
31. Goeckerman WH: The treatment of psoriasis. *Northwest Med* 24:229–231, 1925.
32. Ashton RE, Andre P, Lowe NJ et al: Anthralin: historical and current perspectives. *J Am Acad Dermatol* 2:173–192, 1983.
33. Farber EM, Harris DR: Hospital treatment of psoriasis. A modified anthralin program. *Arch Dermatol* 101:381–389, 1970.
34. Parrish JA, Fitzpatrick TB, Tannenbaum C et al: Photochemotherapy of psoriasis with oral methoxsalen and long wave ultraviolet light. *N Engl J Med* 291:1207–1212, 1974.
35. Murray D, Warin AP: Photochemotherapy for persistent palmoplantar pustulosis (PPP). *Br J Dermatol* 101(Suppl 17):13–14, 1979.
36. Menné AT: Treatment of psoriasis of the palms and soles and pustulosis palmaris et plantaris with 8-methoxypsoralen and long-wave ultra-violet light. *Ugeskr Laeger* 138:3119–3122, 1976.
37. Morison WL, Parrish JA, Fitzpatrick TB: Oral methoxsalen photochemotherapy of recalcitrant dermatoses of the palms and soles. *Br J Dermatol* 99:297–302, 1978.
38. Goette DK: Topical chemotherapy with 5-fluorouracil. *J Am Acad Dermatol* 4:633–649, 1981.
39. Tsuji T, Sugai T: Topically administered fluorouracil in psoriasis. *Arch Dermatol* 105:208–212, 1972.
40. Fredriksson T: Topically applied fluorouracil in the treatment of psoriatic nails. *Arch Dermatol* 110:735–736, 1974.
41. Ward A, Brogden RN, Heel RC, et al: Etretinate a review of its pharmacological properties and therapeutic efficacy in psoriasis and other skin disorders. *Drugs* 26:9–43, 1983.
42. Fellner MJ: Lichen planus. *Int J Dermatol* 19:71–75, 1980.
43. Flamenbaum HS, Safai B, Siegal FP: Lichen planus in two immunodeficient hosts. *J Am Acad Dermatol* 6:918–920, 1982.
44. Olsen RG, Duplessis D, Barron C et al: Lichen planus dermopathy: demonstration of a lichen planus specific epidermal antigen in affected patients. *J Clin Lab Immunol* 10:103–106, 1983.
45. Lowe NJ, Cudworth AG, Woodrow JC: HLA antigens in lichen planus. *Br J Dermatol* 95:169–171, 1976.
46. Ronchese R: Nail in lichen planus. *Arch Dermatol* 91:347–349, 1965.
47. Norton LA: Nail disorders: a review. *J Am Acad Dermatol* 2:451–467, 1980.
48. Samman PD: The nails in lichen planus. *Br J Dermatol* 73:288–292, 1961.
49. Rook A, Wilkinson DS, Ebling FJG: Lichen planus and lichenoid eruptions. In Rook A et al (eds): *Textbook of Dermatology*. Philadelphia, F.A. Davis, 1969, vol 2, pp 1203–1204.
50. Cram DL, Kierland RR, Winkelmann RK: Ulcerative lichen planus of the feet. Bullous variant with hair and nail lesions. *Arch Dermatol* 93:692–701, 1966.
51. Thorman J: Ulcerative lichen planus of the feet. *Arch Dermatol* 110:753–755, 1974.
52. Griffiths WAD: Pityriasis rubra pilaris. *Clin Exp Dermatol* 5:105–112, 1980.
53. Griffiths WAD: Pityriasis rubra pilaris—an historical approach. *Clin Exp Dermatol* 1:37–50, 1976.
54. Gross DA, Landau JW, Newcomer VD: Pityriasis rubra pilaris. *Arch Dermatol* 99:710–716, 1969.
55. Davidson CL, Winkelman RK, Kierland RR: Pityriasis rubra pilaris. *Arch Dermatol* 100:175–178, 1969.
56. Porter D, Shuster S: Epidermal renewal and amino acids in Psoriasis and pityriasis rubra pilaris. *Arch Dermatol* 98:339–343, 1968.
57. Niemi KM, Kousa M, Storgårds K, Karvonen J: Pityriasis rubra pilaris—a clinicopathological study with a special reference to autoradiography and histocompatibility antigens. *Dermatologica* 152:109–118, 1976.
58. Schmidt FR: Discussion. *Arch Dermatol* 40:832–833, 1939.
59. Goldsmith LA, Weinrich AE, Shupack J: Pityriasis rubra pilaris response to 13-*cis*-retinoic acid (isotretinoin). *J Am Acad Dermatol* 6:710–715, 1982.
60. Randle HW, Diez-Perez JL, Winkelman RK: Toxic doses of vitamin A for pityriasis rubra pilaris. *Arch Dermatol* 116:888–892, 1980.
61. Samitz MH: *Cutaneous Disorders of the Lower Extremities*, ed 2. Philadelphia, J.B. Lippincott, 1981, p 173.
62. Chapel TA: The signs and symptoms of

secondary syphilis. *Sex Transm Dis* 7:161–164, 1980.

63. Costello MJ, Gibbs RC: *The Palms and Soles in Medicine.* Springfield, IL, Charles C Thomas, 1967, p 454.
64. Lever WF, Schaumburg G: *Histopathology of the Skin*, ed 5. Philadelphia, J.B. Lippincott, 1975, pp 300–301.
65. Fiumara NJ: Infectious syphilis. In Felman YM (ed): *Symposium on Sexually Transmitted Diseases: Dermatologic Clinics.* Philadelphia, W.B. Saunders, 1983, pp 3–21.

CHAPTER 9

Pyodermas

MARC A. BRENNER

The term pyoderm is a general one referring to any condition involving some purulent (pyo) affection of the skin (derma, dermia). It may occur in a relatively benign fashion, or it may fulminate to an acute life-threatening medical problem. Normally, the intact skin provides an effective barrier between the delicate internal environment of the body and a sometimes hostile external environment. The organ known as the skin, however, is not inviolate and can be injured.

The human integument reflects much concerning the general health of individuals; at the same time it provides a resilient but tough tissue covering which is host to many microorganisms. Under normal circumstances, this microbial flora exists in an equilibrium which is not harmful to the body. The delicate balance of the host-parasite relationship can be disturbed by conditions which favor invasion of microbes whenever their numbers increase greatly. This phenomenon is usually accompanied by micro- or macrotrauma which devitalizes the skin. Additionally, the relative virulence of involving organisms can increase as more delicate deep skin tissues are encountered. Trauma, together with increased numbers and virulence of organisms, can result in an inflammatory response of the integument; phagocytic cells of the body attempt to arrest the progression of the invading microbes, and pus is formed. These are the prevailing conditions for that broad spectrum of skin diseases identified as pyoderma.

Staphylococcal species to a greater extent and streptococcal species to a lesser extent can be cultured at any given time from normal intact skin. However, under adverse conditions these organisms are quick to colonize and multiply rapidly so as to establish a primary pyoderm. Common expressions of these pyogenic infestations include impetigo, paronychia, and erysipelas. Staphylococcal species are common Gram positive organisms which typically are seen in grape-like clusters. They are especially prone to involve deep tissues, resulting in infections causing abscesses, cellulitis, and lymphangitis. Resulting toxic reactions may potentially desquamate and otherwise disrupt large areas of the involved skin. Staphylococcal species may become resistant to antibiotic control, with serious sequelae such as staphylococcal scalded skin syndrome, toxic shock syndrome, and bacteremia.

It has been said that "*Staphylococcus aureus* is the microbe that gives the word 'germ" a bad reputation" (1). Because the organism is so common and is usually medically manageable, it is easy to underestimate its potential. Resistant strains of *Staphylococcus* involving surgical wounds are potentially fatal hospital nosocomial infections.

Medical researchers of the late 19th century involved themselves in heroic self-experimentation in an effort to understand the pathogenicity of *Staphylococcus*.

Garré applied an inoculum of an active staphylococcal culture from a recently fatal case of osteomyelitis to his own forearm. As a consequence of this act, multiple pustules and a carbuncle formed with great rapidity (2). Somewhat later Bockhart repeated this type of self-inoculation and developed cutaneous pustules and furuncles (3).

These rather crude types of experimentation were not always reproducible, and controversy continued as to the cause and effect relationships of pyoderm. However, with the dawn of the 20th century, such conditions as impetigo were clearly established as being associated with staphylococci and streptococci.

Basic human dermatological experimentation was activated during the decade beginning in 1935 by Epstein (4) and Sheehan and Fergusson (5). Elek and Conen (6) gave special emphasis to precisely what qualities of human skin predisposed to skin infection (1956–1957).

The effect of numbers of bacteria necessary to induce infection was experimentally determined to be between 2 and 3 million per ml of inoculum. An attempt to modulate these minimal infective doses by various means was then attempted: The presence of human plasma and mucin and even staphylococcal toxin did not appear to reduce this critical number.

However, greater susceptibility to infection in the presence of a significant decrease in microbe number was demonstrated when foreign bodies were introduced locally. Suture materials are good examples of this, and pedal tumors such as verrucae and porokeratosis plantaris discreta (of Steinberg) predispose to local skin infections.

Viruses, parasites, and bacteria in association with mechanical trauma so derange the skin of the foot as to make the extremity especially prone to pyoderm. The injury to the pilary complexes in shaving or plucking of hairs has been implicated in pyoderma such as impetigo.

Significant variation relative to susceptibility and resistance to staphylococci between different individuals and differing environment was demonstrated by Kligman and Maibach (7) in 1959. In general, however, it can safely be stated that staphylococcal species meet the requirements of Koch's postulates relative to pyoderm. Organisms are always associated with lesions; they can be cultured; and under suitable circumstances, their reinoculation can reproduce a like infectious lesion.

The variation in treatment plans for the pyodermas speaks to the art component in the practice of medical science. What was successful in the treatment of one case is not necessarily going to be efficacious in another.

Complex interactions between the host and microbial flora vary, and the homeostasis that may favor the host at one point in time can be shifted to favor the pyogenic bacterium. Underlying medical problems may also contribute to pyoderma, but most patients with recurrent pyoderma have no demonstrable predisposing disease.

Two decades have passed since Biro, Gibbs, and Leider implicated antibiotics and adrenal glucocorticoids with a statistical increase in the incidence of staphylococcal skin infections. Tetracycline appeared to sometimes increase the transmissibility of infections due to staphylococcal skin infection (8). Additional data demonstrated that antibiotics suppress some organisms and alter the indigenous microbial flora. Such changes can favor an overgrowth of staphylococcal and other species.

There is presently little doubt that the ingestion of corticosteroids can aggravate infections of the skin and other organs. The mechanism for this phenomenon is not fully understood. There is evidence that corticosteroids can delay mobilization of polymorphonuclear leucocytes necessary for the phagocytosis of microorganisms (8). All podiatrists have been challenged at one time or another by patients afflicted with rheumatoid arthritis treated with corticosteroids. As useful as these drugs may be, such patients usually have atrophic skin which is prone to ulceration. Infections of these lesions, particularly when the extremities are involved, are extremely resistant to conventional therapies.

The quality and integrity of the skin reflects the patient's general condition. Protein depletion, starvation, and poor habits of hygiene are frequently associated with pyodermas. Physiologic or psychological shock, emotional upset, and a crowded environment are often overlooked as being partially etiologic in dermatological disease. Blood vessels and nerves supplying the skin are controlled by the autonomic nervous system, and inflammatory conditions of the foot may be reflecting this generalized state.

The evaluation of a primary pyoderma, therefore, needs to include the patient's total state of health, both mental and physical. This truism would seem to be self-evident, but experience has shown that the obvious is easily overlooked.

Secondary pyodermas are often sequelae

of a primary pruritic dermatitis. Skin conditions which itch invite scratching: Scratching with fingernails provides an ideal situation for inoculating the already devitalized skin with *Staphylococcus* or one of many other potential pathogens. Iatrogenic introductions of skin pathogens by means of intravenous infusions is yet another source for establishing a pyoderma.

Traumatic means of disrupting skin so as to permit the introduction of pyogenic pathogens are too many to enumerate. Surgical incisions are of particular interest to podiatrists in this regard, however. The foot is the most distal of body parts. It is subject to circulatory deficiency as well as to trauma. Surgical incisions disrupt normal tissue planes. Moreover, excessive instrumentation with clamps, retractors, and suturing can devitalize these tissues. Alterations of homeostasis, hemorrhage, and hematoma formation can also adversely affect the skin and favor colonization by skin pathogens. These contingencies are mentioned elsewhere in this text for additional emphasis.

SYSTEMIC DISEASE

Pyogenic involvements of the skin may be influenced by underlying systemic disease. Chief among these concerns is diabetes mellitus. While some may argue as to whether or not pyodermas are predisposed to by diabetic states, it is universally accepted that once a cutaneous infection is established, its management is much more complicated in diabetic patients. There is presently substantial evidence of linkage between diabetes mellitus, mucormycosis, and candidiasis. Circulatory changes of the skin secondary to microangiopathy and functionally defective polymorphonuclear leukocytes have been cited as contributory to cutaneous diabetic complications. Recurrent and persistent plantar foot ulcerations and bullae are common diabetic skin manifestations which can easily become complicated so as to develop as a secondary pyoderma (9). A complete discussion of the pedal manifestations of diabetes mellitus is an encyclopedic matter and is beyond the scope of this chapter.

Substance Abuse

Toxic substances, bacteria, talc, and the like may be introduced into the skin by the injection of drugs by addicted individuals. Such activities may lead to pyodermas, dermopathy, ulcerating nodules, and typical atrophic scars (10).

Alcoholic intoxication may predispose to certain pyodermas. The precise linkage for this, however, remains obscure.

Nutritional habits and poor hygiene have obvious deleterious effects on the skin which can predispose to pyoderma. The fact that alcoholics have a high incidence of pulmonary infection has led some investigators to believe that there is a direct link to pyodermas, but this is by no means certain.

Skin infections occur with much greater frequency among patients suffering from myelogenous leukemia and hypogammaglobinemia than in the general population. Perillie and Finch have demonstrated a sharp reduction in the mobilization of phagocytic cells in traumatized skin in leukemia (11).

These patients doubtless have some degree of immunologic deficiency which permits the more aggressive establishment of pyoderma (Fig. 9.1). Staphylococcal skin infections may become more readily established if degenerative localized skin and subcutaneous conditions develop. These factors are not well understood, and addi-

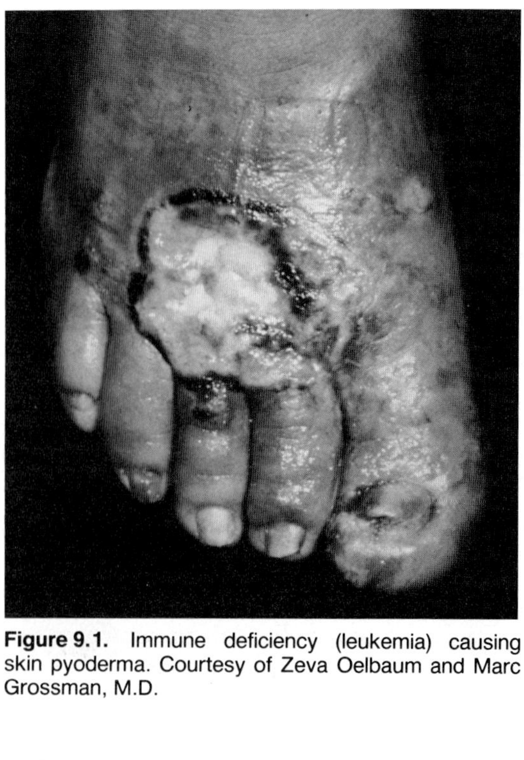

Figure 9.1. Immune deficiency (leukemia) causing skin pyoderma. Courtesy of Zeva Oelbaum and Marc Grossman, M.D.

tional study is needed relative to immune competency and structural integrity in local skin infections.

COMMON PEDAL PYODERMAS

Primary pedal pyodermas are the result of direct bacterial invasion into the otherwise normal skin of the foot. Secondary pyogenic infections develop in already devitalized denuded or damaged integument. Chronic pruritic dermatosis, trauma, insect bites, and the like are commonly implicated.

Pyodermas are rarely reported by physicians for statistical purposes. Some cases respond to self-treatment while others resolve spontaneously. Consequently, it is not possible to statistically evaluate the incidence of the condition.

This group of pyogenic skin conditions are primarily staphylococcal and streptococcal infections. Variations of their clinical expressions can be categorized as follows.

Impetigo Contagiosum

Impetigo contagiosum is presently the most commonly encountered pyogenic infection of the skin. Infants and children are most commonly affected. Half of all such infections are mixed, involving streptococcal and staphylococcal species. Group A β-hemolytic streptococci are also common offenders. Impetigo occurs most commonly in summer and fall as a superficial pyogenic skin infection. It is a highly contagious condition usually transmittable through direct contact between individuals. Factors favoring the developing of impetigo contagiosum include crowded living conditions and poor personal hygiene, hot and humid weather, and hyperhidrosis.

Streptoccocal Impetigo

Impetigo due to streptococci is typically nonbullous and encrusted. This is in contrast to that caused by *Staphylococcus*, which tends to be bullous (Figs. 9.2–9.3).

The nonbullous forms of impetigo begin as a small vesicle which soon becomes pustular and then crusts over. The lesions multiply as the condition progresses, and the encrustation is thick and of a golden coloration. These yellowish-brown clusters tend to favor the exposed areas of skin. It

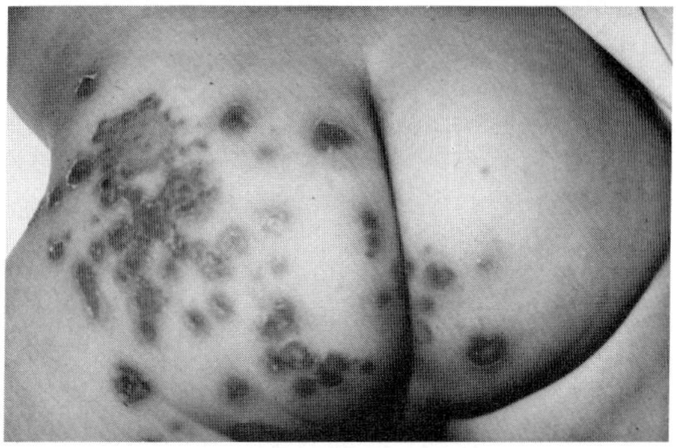

Figure 9.2. Impetigo contagiosa. Courtesy of Zeva Oelbaum and Marc Grossman, M.D., Columbia Presbyterian Medical Center.

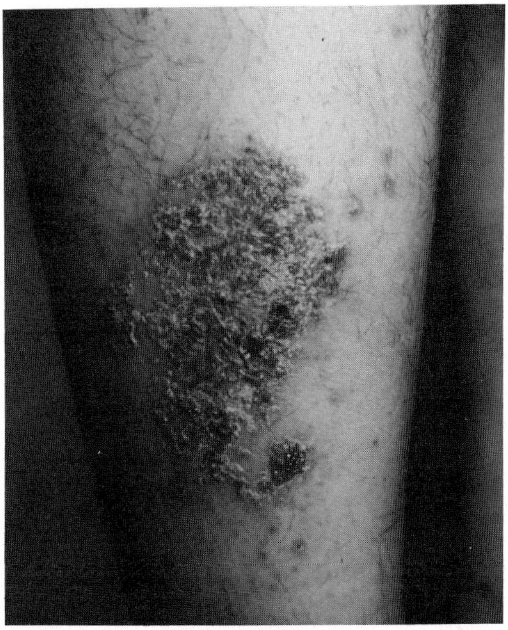

Figure 9.3. Impetigo contagiosa. Courtesy of Richard Gibbs, M.D., New York City.

is important, however, to examine the patient completely for other lesions: Impetigo is most common on the face, but it may occur on the buttocks, legs and arms, hands, and feet.

If crusts are removed, a red weeping border is exposed, and another crust is rapidly formed.

Streptococcal pyodermas commonly present a spreading erythema and is commonly associated with the lower extremities (Figs. 9.4 and 9.5). Tissue necrosis, lymphangitis, and regional lymphadenopathy are reasonably typical to this condition.

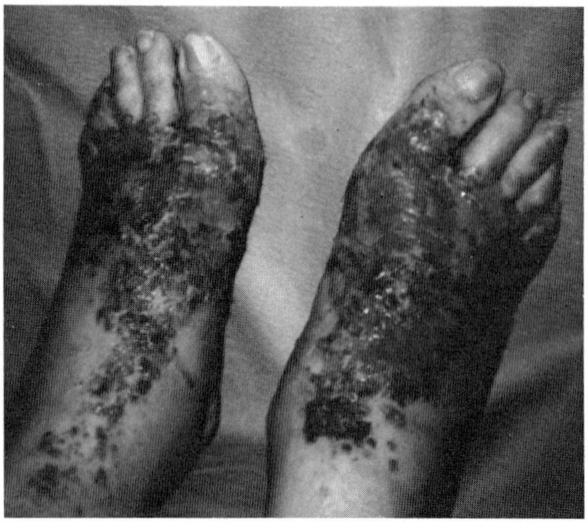

Figure 9.4. *Streptococcus pyoderma* before treatment. Courtesy of Marc A. Brenner, D.P.M., Queens, NY.

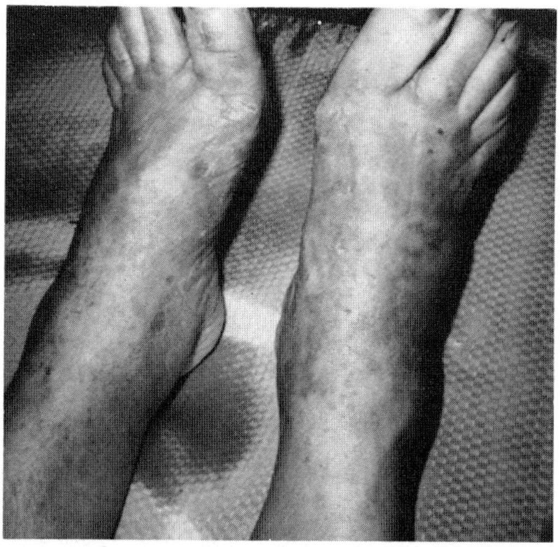

Figure 9.5. *Streptococcus pyoderma* after 2 weeks of therapy. Courtesy of Marc A. Brenner, D.P.M.

Individual lesions heal without scarring in 7 to 10 days. Untreated lesions may become widespread and are more difficult to control. Such lesions can become chronic. Old lesions resolve only to have new ones form. Rapidly spreading lesions often mimic superficial tinea involvements. Pruritis and burning are common concomitant complaints.

Systemic antibiotics reduce the contagion of the disease; however, this condition remains communicable until all lesions have dried completely.

The local organism may spread to the respiratory tract, and systemic involvement results (12). Streptococcal impetigo may progress to initiate nephritis in children under 6 years of age. Nephritis follows the acute pyoderma which follows a latent period of about 3 weeks. Hematuria can be determined microscopically on occasion, even during acute skin infection. Routine urinalysis should be performed whenever streptococcal infection is active. Such testing should be repeated in 2 weeks for signs of glomerulonephritis.

Rheumatic fever has no known association with streptococcal pyoderma.

ECTHYMA

Ecthyma is a severe variant expression of impetigo characterized by multiple crushed lesions which extend more deeply into the dermis. It frequently involves the lower limb with punched-out ulcerations appearing as the infection becomes progressive. Group A β-hemolytic *Streptococcus pyogenes* is usually implicated, although *Staphylococcus* species can be involved. Lesions are characterized by large encrustations which demonstrate a purulent ulcerous base when debrided (Fig. 9.6). Scar

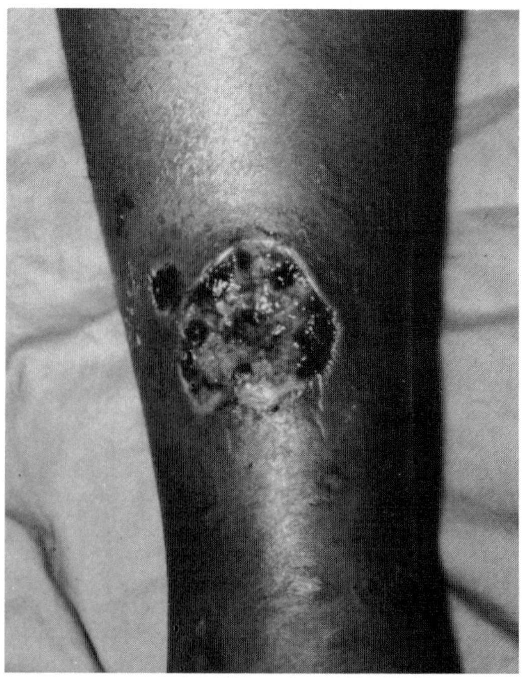

Figure 9.6. Ecthyma. Courtesy of Richard Gibbs, M.D., New York City.

formation and, at times, gangrene are commonly associated with this condition. Individuals in poor health, debilitated alcoholics, and even children may be affected by ecthyma.

PARONYCHIA

Whitlow or acute paronychia is a localized infection involving the posterior, medial, and/or lateral nail fold. *S. pyogenes* is most often the causal organism. This condition is the pyoderma most frequently encountered by specialists treating the feet. The nail of the involved digit acts as a foreign body which penetrates the contiguous nail fold. Predisposing causes include the hereditary malformations of the nail, direct trauma, shoe pressure, and improper care of the nail. Such factors can wedge a spicule of nail into the soft tissues which inoculates and infects the region. While Gram positive organisms are usually involved, Gram negative organisms such as *Pseudomonas* can be identified on occasion.

Treatment plans vary according to the severity of the infection. Adequate drainage should be established by removing the offending nail spicule, but total nail avulsion may be required if the condition is extensive. Antiseptic astringent wet dressings or soaks are helpful, and a topical antiseptic or antibiotic medication can be employed.

CELLULITIS

Cellulitis is an extensive pyogenic infection involving both dermis and subcutaneous tissues. Group A β-hemolytic streptococcal organisms are usually implicated, but *S. aureus* and *Haemophilus influenzae* among others can be involved.

The involved area is warm to the touch, erythematous, edematous, and painful. It may or may not be possible to identify the lesion whereby the infecting organism gained entry. Patients may appear ill and febrile. Lymphangiitis and/or lymphadenopathy is often present.

Hemolytic streptococcal species produce a particular superficial type of cellulitis or erysipelas known as "St. Anthony's fire." It is associated with young debilitated patients having a recent history of acute upper respiratory infection (AURI). Erysipelas can occur on the extremities, but it is most often seen on the face. Lesions are characterized by warm, tender, indurated bright red raised plaques. They are sharply demarcated and grow rapidly for several days (Fig. 9.7). Children are especially susceptible to high body temperatures and delirium when cellulitis is active.

LYMPHANGIITIS

Lymphangiitis involves infection and inflammation of the lymphatic system which is so extensive in the lower extremities. Group A β-hemolytic streptococci is commonly involved. Red, painful linear streaks can be seen extending from usually minor parts of entry such as paronychias, intertrigo, or tinea. Multiple systemic manifestations, including malaise, fever, and chills, can be present, and regional lymph nodes are usually palpable as the condition progresses toward bacteremia or septicemia. The white blood cell count is now elevated, and the differential blood smear demonstrates the left shift. Additional complications include bacterial endocarditis and recurrences of the original inflammation.

CARBUNCLES AND FOLLICULITIS

Folliculitis is a bacterial infection of a hair follicle. Carbuncles are deeper pyogenic infections involving several hair fol-

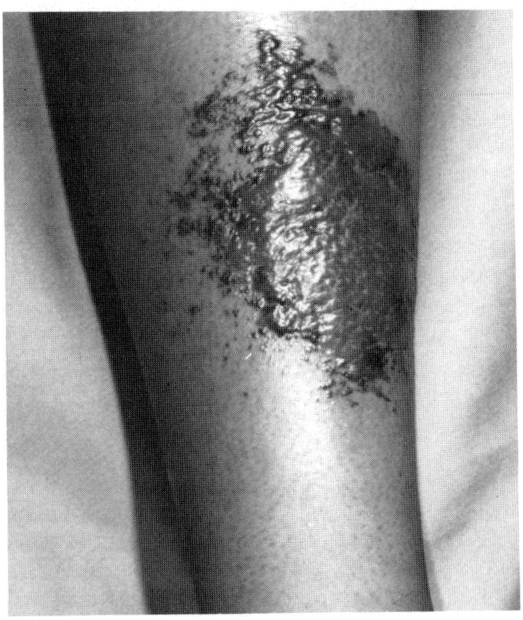

Figure 9.7. Erysipelas. Courtesy of Richard Gibbs, M.D., New York City.

licles. Such lesions are extremely painful. They are erythematous, indurated, pustular, and may develop multiple drainage points. Deeply seated abscesses may demonstrate interconnected channels. It is not uncommon to see a hair piercing one or more lesions. Mechanical factors such as rubbing, picking, or plucking the hair are often instrumental in introducing staphylococcal species into the deeper tissues. Blacks are especially prone to carbuncle formation. Their use of hydrating substances such as vegetable shortening and white petrolatum for hydration of the skin produces an occlusive situation favorable to the development of bacteria.

Boils or furuncles are pyodermas involving staphylococcal abscess formation of the perifollicular regions. The posterior aspect of the neck, axillae, gluteal region, and inner thighs are common areas of involvement. The lower limb may also be affected by the pain and erythema of furuncles. Bacteremia is a potential complication of boils and fever, and malaise can occur.

ERYTHRASMA

Erythrasma is a Gram negative bacterial infection caused by the rod-shaped bacillus, *Corynebacterium minutissemum.* Prior to 1960, such bacterial infections were thought to be a form of scaling intertriginous tinea. Diagnosis is confirmed by its characteristic coral red fluorescence under Wood's light examination.

A common site for erythrasma involves the interspaces between the lateral digits of the feet. Special care needs to be taken in diagnosing intertrigo in these regions. This is especially necessary for differentiating fungus or monilial involvements from gram negative rod infections. This emphasis has been made elsewhere in this book. The treatment of erythrasma varies widely.

Erythrasma responds well to erythromycin in dosages of 250 mg four times daily. Such a treatment plan, however, would not be at all helpful for fungus or monilial involvements.

The differential diagnosis of the primary and secondary pyodermas can be aided by considering the topography of lesions (13). For example, bilateral eruptions on the thin-skinned dorsal aspects of the feet might well suggest a contact dermatitis. Unilateral inflammatory lesions might indicate trauma, foreign body reactions, insect bites, neuropathic tissue necrosis, and secondarily infected tinea involvements.

Some pyogenic skin infections are extremely rare but can be potentially devastating diseases. For example, massive disruption of the skin of the foot has been described in gram negative pyodermas involving meningococcemia (Fig. 9.8). Certain extensive tumorigenic conditions of the feet such as epithelioma cuniculatum and tuberculosis cutis verrucosa may be so disfiguring as to require amputation. The last-named condition is presened here as a pyoderma because of superinfestation by *Moraxella phenylpyruvica* (Fig. 9.9). Other uncommon conditions include:

1. Scalded skin syndrome (by *staphylococcus*)
2. Toxic shock syndrome
3. Scabies
4. Tularemia
5. Arthrax
6. Maduromycosis
7. Sporotrichosis
8. Blastomycosis
9. Orf
10. Cat scratch disease
11. Drug abuse dermopathy

THERAPEUTIC PRINCIPLES FOR THE PYODERMAS

Precise dermatological diagnosis may be elusive, particularly when secondary and tertiary lesions exist as a result of neglect

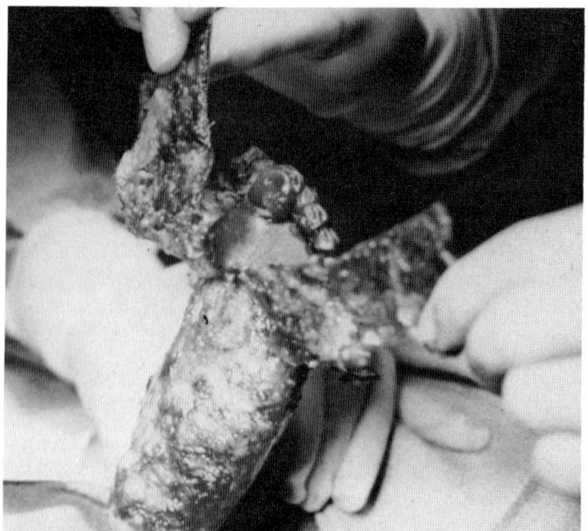

Figure 9.8. Meningococcemia, gram negative pyoderma, massive skin disruption. Courtesy of A. Kaynan, M.D., Queens, NY.

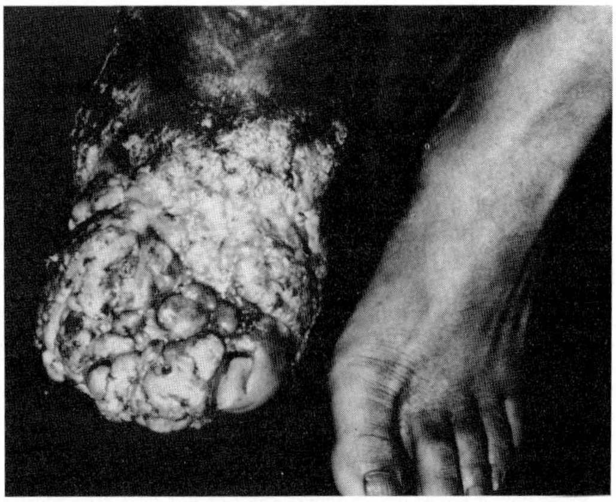

Figure 9.9. Chronic pyoderma, possible tuberculosis cutis verrucosa superinfected with *Moraxella phenylpyrouvica.* Courtesy of Dr. Ichiro Kikuchi, Miyazaki Medical College, Kiyotake, Japan, and Marc A. Brenner, D.P.M., Queens, NY.

or self-treatment by the patient. Success in treatment for the pedal pyodermas is especially dependent on accurate diagnosis. The effects of inflammatory responses resulting from overzealous improper treatment must be neutralized.

Dahl has implicated professionals such as physicians and pharmacists in treating skin diseases symptomatically on the basis of their appearance at that moment in time without a proper diagnosis in hand (1). The application of a steroid cream to arrest the inflammation of a pyoderma may temporarily mask its symptoms, but it inevitably exacerbates the infection.

Podiatrists should be especially aware of the complexities of dermatological conditions of the foot and have special responsibilities in this regard. Where pyodermas are concerned, the shoe is an incubator where warm, moist, dark conditions exist. Moreover, many exogenous factors associated with hosiery and shoes can adversely effect skin infections of the foot.

Oversimplification of skin conditions by the categorization of the similarity of the appearance of the lesions for purposes of treatment is to be avoided. Occasionally even when the correct dermatological diagnosis is in hand, good therapeutic results can be elusive. Modern medicine has provided many specialty and subspecialty resource persons who are eager to render assistance. The best interests of the patient demand that first consideration be given their needs and appropriate consultation be quickly sought whenever difficulty is encountered in dealing with a pyoderma.

Medical photography is an important adjunct in developing and accumulating dermatological experience and judgment. Study and review of all skin conditions, including the pyodermas over time, will instill an ever-increasing confidence in treating these conditions. The podiatric dermatological index of suspicion needs to be kept constantly sharp. Laboratory assistance in assessing pyodermas may need to involve gram stains, KOH preparations, urinalysis, and biopsies, together with appropriate blood chemistries and counts. This emphasis has been repeated many times in this book and cannot be overemphasized.

Once a pyoderma has been established, the equilibrium between intact skin and its normal microbial flora has been radically shifted to favor the bacteria. This alteration results in a devitalizing inflammatory response characterized by infection and purulence. These adverse changes need to be quickly and effectively reversed. In destroying the infecting organism(s) associated with a skin lesion, it is important to encourage the vitality and integrity of the integumentary system.

The use of topical antibiotics for the treatment of pyodermas came under serious challenge in the 1970s (14). Recent literature, however, supports the clinical use of topical antibiotics and antimicrobials when appropriately prescribed. Obviously, the involved organism needs to be susceptible to the antibiotic, or it may have adverse effects.

It is necessary to maintain strict cleanliness of the skin throughout the course of treatment for the pyodermas: This will decrease the numbers of surface organisms present on the skin. Cleansing also stimulates regeneration of the devitalized skin so as to restore the protective barrier of the involved integument.

There are numerous antibacterial agents commercially available which lend themselves to topical use in the home, office, and hospital. Gram positive organisms are especially susceptible to solutions of chlortiexidine gluconate (Hibiclens), hexachlorophene (Phisohex), and povidone-iodine (Betadine).

Prophylactic daily scrubbing with these

materials is beneficial not only during the active course of a pyoderma but also as a preventive measure against recurrence of the condition (15, 16).

Topical use of such antibiotics as bacitracin, neomycin, and polymycin B, in combination or separately, can be very useful. Neomycin, however, has demonstrated some problems with sensitization. Gentamycin may be effective and is available for both topical and systemic administration.

Antibiotics in topical form should be restricted to short-term use because of the possibility for yeast overgrowth. In addition, it is important that they be applied two or three times daily over clean surfaces.

Antiseptics which are not antibiotic in nature should not be overlooked when treating pyodermas. Gentian violet in 2% concentrations and 0.5% silver nitrate are medications which are both antibacterial and antifungal. Some practitioners, however, disapprove of their use because of their uncontrollable discoloring properties. Patients are interested in results, however, and are not always as concerned with cosmetic appearances as some practitioners may think. A very real problem exists, however, whenever an involved part is so deeply stained by medications that monitoring the progress of the skin disease is obscured.

Many pyodermas, such as impetigo and ecthyma, are characterized by the formation of scabs and crusts: Gentle debridement by means of sterile gauze wipes or by a cutting instrument under aseptic conditions is indicated. Astringent and antiseptic effects of warm solutions made up of aluminum subacetate (Burow's solution) soaks or wet to dry dressings are invaluable in pyodermas. They need to be applied frequently for 10 minutes, four to six times daily. Patient compliance is clearly imperative in dealing with pyodermas. Potassium permanganate solutions are also useful but tend to be messy and stain the foot and footwear.

Astringent antiseptic applications of solutions appear to dehydrate purulent lesions of pyoderma so as to make the integumentary environment inhospitable to the bacterial invaders associated with the infection. Dehydrated tissues formed as a result of wet dressings or soaks afford a more stable mechanical external barrier to infection. Such surfaces are also less able to support large numbers of microbes necessary to establish a pyoderma.

MAINTENANCE THERAPY

A localized pedal pyoderma represents a potential source of infection to the skin of other body parts. Moreover, such local infections can become septemic problems with life-threatening consequences. Spread of these infections to other individuals is an additional consequence of skin infection. Consequently, good general hygiene needs to be emphasized for patients demonstrating skin infection. This is equally true for all persons coming into contact with purulent skin infections.

All individuals involved with pyoderma should wash their hands frequently. This principle, enunciated many years ago by Lister, needs to be reinforced constantly. One needs only to view the many admonitions to professional staff along hospital corridors designed to reduce nosocomial infections to be convinced of this.

Patients need to be assisted in order to prevent progression of their localized skin infection. Their fingernails should be kept short and clean, and gloves can be employed in cases where pruritis is so extreme as to demand the almost irresistible scratching of pruritic lesions. Whenever possible, a cool dry climate should be provided. Home care should emphasize the use of separate wash basins, disposable towels and linens etc., to contain the infection.

Moist conditions favor the progression of local skin infections. Therefore, it is mandatory that patient compliance to the treatment plan prescribed be adhered to. Aeration of the part is critical; avoidance of occlusive foot wear such as is common with man-made synthetic materials employed in hosiery and shoes is important. Aeration of shoes or special disinfecting processes applicable to footgear may need to be employed.

ACUTE SEQUELAE OF PEDAL PYOGENIC MANIFESTATIONS

Most podiatric pyodermas respond to local therapeutic regimens; treatment plans may be topical, systemic, or combinations of both modalities. However, whenever life-threatening sequelae of a localized pyoderma is involved, more heroic treatment plans must be instituted, and appropriate consultation is required.

The administration of antibiotics by oral, intramuscular, or intravenous routes is based on indications determined by culturing the organisms involved and determining their sensitivities. Gram stain preparations are of value in the initial phases of treatment. Penicillin G is an effective antibiotic which covers a wide spectrum of organisms. It has a rather high incidence of sensitivity among patients, however. Individuals who show signs of allergic responses usually do well on erythromycin. Oral administration in doses of 250–500 mg every 4 to 6 hr PO is therapeutic for both drugs.

Patients who tolerate the penicillins well may also be given cephalexin (Keflex) in essentially the same dosage as for penicillin. β-hemolytic streptococcal species respond to a wide variety of first and second generation cephalosporin antibiotics (Table 9.1). Most physicians adopt several antibiotics with which they become comfortable for general usage.

When fever, malaise, and lymphadenopathy are present, bed rest, elevation of the involved part, and antipyretic medications are employed. At times, it becomes necessary to hospitalize patients when pyodermas are especially acute. Some organisms, such as methicillin-resistant *Staphylococcus*, require carefully selected intravenous antibiotics over considerable periods of time, and expert care and monitoring of patients are required (infection control specialists).

There are times when 5 million or more units of penicillin G administered by continuous intravenous infusion is necessary. Cefoxitin is an excellent alternative antibiotic if patients do not exhibit sensitivity or allergy to it. Serious pyodermas may require the administration of oral antibiotics over time in order to prevent reoccurrences in addition to appropriate local skin care.

It is important to consult the appropriate product information sources in order to become familiar with indications, contraindications, side effects, etc., of all drugs employed.

In general, streptococcal pyodermas affect the lower extremities more seriously than is the case with staphylococcal species. The difficult pyogenic skin infections need to be treated with high antibiotic dosages until a good response is observed. Dosages can than be reduced by one-half for the following week. An additional 14-day period devoted to appropriate topical care is wise.

Minor pyodermas usually respond to topical therapy. When the proper response is achieved, an additional 4 days of prophylactic care should be imposed.

Children usually respond well to orally administered antibiotics in cases of pyoderma. Smaller doses are indicated, and the amount prescribed is determined on the basis of age and weight.

SUMMARY

Pyodermas of the lower extremities are no respectors of age, sex, or race. Such afflictions most commonly are associated with young, poor, and unkempt individuals. In general, these conditions are relatively minor to moderate illnesses: They may, however, lead to major complications, and they can become so severe as to require hospitalization.

Group A β-hemolytic streptococci- and penicillinase-resistant *Staphylococcus* account for most variant forms of pyoderma. Treatment plans require strict hygiene, frequent cleansing with antimicrobials, removal of crusts and other skin debris, and warm antiseptic and astringent soaks.

Systemic therapy is usually preferable to topical antibiotic administration in cases involving streptococcal species.

Adequate local management is always indicated as part of the treatment plan and may be all that is required.

The total patient, together with his or her psyche, needs to be considered in dealing with all dermatological conditions of the lower extremity. Pyodermas can be especially vexing problems and should not be viewed too simplistically.

References

1. Dahl M: *Editorial: Current Concepts in Skin Disorders*, no. 3, 1983, p 4.
2. Garré, C. *Fortschr Med* 3:165–173, 1885.
3. Bockhart M: *Monatschr Prakt Dermatol* 6:450–471, 1887.

4. Epstein S: Beitrag zur staphlogenen impetigo contagiosa. *Dermatol Z* 70:328–340, 1935.
5. Sheehan HL, Fergusson AG: Impetigo aetiology and treatment. *Lancet* 1:547–550, 1943.
6. Elek SD, Conen PE: The virulences of *Staphylococcus pyogenes* for man. A study of the problems of wound infection. *Br J Exp Pathol* 38:573–586, 1957.
7. Maibach H, Kligman A: The biology of experimental human cutaneous moniliasis (*Candida albicans*) *AMA Arch Dermatol* 85:233–257, 1962.
8. Biro L, Gibbs RC, Leider M: Staphylococcal infections. A study of incidence on a dermatologic ward. *AMA Arch Dermatol* 82:205–211, 1960
9. Brenner MA: An ambulatory approach to the neuropathic ulceration. *J Am Podiatr Assoc* 64 (11):862–868, 1974.
10. Kallick C: Diagnosis of Infected Lesions Associated with Abscesses and Ulcerations. Indianapolis, IN, Eli-Lilly Series 2, 1978.
11. Perillie PE, Finch SC: Quantitative studies of the local exudative cellular reaction in acute leukemia. *J Clin Invest* 43:425–430, 1964.
12. Moschella SL, Hurley HJ: *Dermatology*, ed 2. Philadelphia, W.B. Saunders, 1985.
13. Sarkany I, Tapin D, Blank H: Erythrasma—Common bacterial infection of the skin. *JAMA* 177:130–132, 1961.
14. Marples RR, Kligman AM: Limitations of paired comparisons of topical drugs. *Br J Dermatol* 88:61–67, 1973.
15. Rinaldi R, Sabia ML: A double controlled study: Betadine solution treatment of athlete's foot. *Arch Podiatr Med Foot Surg* 3 (1):1–10, 1976.
16. American Medical Association: Dermatological preparations. In *AMA Drug Evaluations*, ed 5, Chicago, American Medical Association, 1983, chap 62, pp 1385–1386.

CHAPTER **10**

A New Look at Dermatophytosis and Atopy

CARL ABRAMSON

INTRODUCTION

Dermatophytoses are probably the most common, prevalent, and insidious of all human infectious diseases. Although they are not generally fatal except, rarely, in immunosuppressed patients, they tend to become chronic and, many times, severely debilitating. Tinea pedis has been reported to affect nearly every human being who wears shoes throughout the world at one time or another. Dermatophytes occur ubiquitously in our daily environment on fomites such as towels, clothing, furniture, walls, floors, etc., as well as hairs and squames from infected persons. These all contribute to the continuous availability of the dermatophytes for transmission through indirect contact. Although almost everyone comes in contact with dermatophytes at one time or another during his or her daily life, and a large percentage of this populace becomes colonized with the fungus, clinical dermatophytoses occur in moderation. Most of the population coming in direct or indirect contact with dermatophytes develops an occult or symptomless tinea pedis infection as the result of colonization. Predisposing factors such as trauma combined with temperature and/or stress and moisture seem to be necessary prerequisites to convert a subclinical infection into a symptomatic clinical disease process (1). Many have indicated that tinea pedis is a highly contagious disease and that direct contact with infectious squames and/or tissue is the sole requisite for successful transmission (2–5). Genetic predisposition such as has been reported to occur with the atopic-chronic dermatophytosis syndrome has been alluded to involve persons who have a family history of hay fever, asthma, or atopic dermatitis (5, 6). They report that certain genetically predisposed patients with chronic dermatophytosis produce different types and amounts of amino acids in their sweat, which act as contributing factors to the maintenance of chronic dermatophytosis by stimulating the growth of a variety of dermatophytes. There are many clinical responses to dermatophytes, such as increased or decreased susceptibility, infection, reinfection, recrudescence, subclinical infection, and chronic infection. Each of these are based on the individual's host response to the dermatophytic invader, as well as the specific dermatophytic species. The clinicoanatomic site of infection, regardless of the involved dermatophyte, is the basis for the classification of dermatophytosis (Table 10.1). In the following sections of this chapter, we will discuss the many aspects of dermatophytoses that will reflect the complex nature of this disease process. Areas covered will include historical background, clinical disease, pathogenesis, immunology, genetic predisposition, diagnosis, differential diagnosis, and treatment. Dermatophytes causing tinea pedis will be emphasized.

HISTORICAL BACKGROUND

One of the first reports of a dermatophyte infection was recorded by the Roman Aulus Cornelius Celsus in 30 A.D., who described a suppurative infection of the scalp in a publication of the times named "*De Re*

Table 10.1
Classification of Dermatophytosis by Clinicoanatomic Site of Infection

Name	Site
Tinea capitis	Head
Tinea corporis	Body
Tinea imbricata	Body
Tinea barbae	Beard
Tinea cruris	Groin
Tinea manum	Hands
Tinea unguium	Nails
Tinea pedis	Feet

Medicina." The lesion became known as "kerion of Celsus." The Romans were also responsible for naming the clinical disease of dermatophytosis as "tinea" after associating the lesions with insect larvae that made holes in wool and destroyed keratin. The Greeks recognized that the clinical lesions formed a circular or ring form and called the disease "herpes." It was not until the 16th century that the English combined the Roman and Greek description into the term "ringworm." Both terms, tinea and ringworm, are still retained as the descriptive clinical terminology for dermatophytic disease (7).

In 1837, Robert Remak, a Polish physician at the Berlin University Medical School, was the first to report that hyphae were found in the lesion of a man with the disease known as "favus" (8). In 1839, Schoenlein confirmed this observation by identifying the filaments seen by Robert Remak as filaments belonging to molds (9). In 1841, David Gruby, A Hungarian physician working in Paris, was the first scientist to establish that a fungus was responsible for causing a human disease (10). He isolated the fungus from the favus lesion, grew it on potato slices, and reproduced the disease in man by inoculation of the cultured fungus into human skin. This method for identifying an etiologic agent associated with a specific disease was to become known 40 years later as "Koch's postulates." Other contributions of David Gruby included naming of the genus *Microsporum* in 1843, discovery of the dermatophyte *Microsporum audouinii*, description and definition of ectothrix and endothrix infections due to tinea capitis, as well as identifying and naming the etiologic factor of thrush, the yeast *Candida albicans* (11). The Swedish scientist Per Hendrick Malmsten described the second important genus *Trichophyton* in 1845, as well as *Trichophyton tonsurans* (12). *Trichophyton mentagrophytes* was described and named in 1847 by Charles Robin, who was also the first to recommend topical therapy for dermatophytoses. The third and last major genus, *Epidermophyton* sp., was discovered and named by Raymond Sabouraud. His total scientific work and discoveries were published in 1910 in the volume *Les Teignes* (13). Included in this historic publication was his classification system for the identification and differentiation of the three genera of dermatophytes, which is basically still in use today. Although dermatophytic infections have been reported in Greek and Roman literature, it wasn't until 1888 that tinea pedis, per se, was noted as a specific dermatophytic disease by Pellizari (14). In the late 19th and early 20th centuries, Sabouraud in France and Whitfield in England described clinical, diagnostic, and laboratory methods for identification of tinea pedis, all of which were published by Kaufman-Wolf in 1914 (15). It became the most common worldwide disease to infect the shoe-wearing population of the world. For the next 50 years a variety of minor changes in taxonomy occurred in the 1920s, 1930s, and 1950s. It wasn't until 1959 that the discovery of the perfect stage of the ascomycetous form (sexual stage) of many dermatophytes occurred (7). The ascigerous genus for *Trichophyton* is *Arthroderma* and for *Microsporum* is *Nannizia.* These sexual stages are important in the scientific determination and taxonomic classification of the dermatophytes along with the classic methods of antigenic analysis, as well as study of cultural, physiologic, and morphologic characteristics. In 1958, James C. Gentles, a Scottish mycologist, reported that oral administration of griseofulvin cured experimental dermatophytosis in a guinea pig (16). Later that year, the first patient was treated with griseofulvin and cured of tinea capitis, soon to be followed by treatment and cure of tinea pedis. This was the beginning of the antifungal chemotherapeutic revolution for the treatment of dermatophytosis. This author had the good fortune of having Dr. C. James Gentles visit the microbiology laboratory at the Pennsylvania College of Podiatric Medicine (Fig. 10.1). Soon to follow were other specific antidermatophytic agents such as tolnaftate, haloprogin, clotrimazole, miconazole, cyclopirox, and ketoconazole. These will be discussed in the section on therapy.

IMMUNOLOGIC ASPECTS

Infection by dermatophytes may result in a variety of clinical responses based on factors related to the invading fungus, the environment, the host, and the interaction between the fungus and the host. The host-parasite relationship and/or response will vary from an acute, short-lived, easy to treat infection to a chronic, long-term, therapeutically resistant infection. Other contributing factors that must be considered are the species or strain of dermatophyte, its source [geophilic (soil); zoophilic (animal); anthropophilic (human)], and the site of the infection (hair, nails, and glabrous or intertriginous skin) (Table 10.2). Zoophilic and geophilic species of dermatophytes more than often cause inflammatory infections which may heal spontaneously and confer resistance to reinfection, whereas anthropophilic species usually do not confer resistance to reinfection and may result in chronic infections.

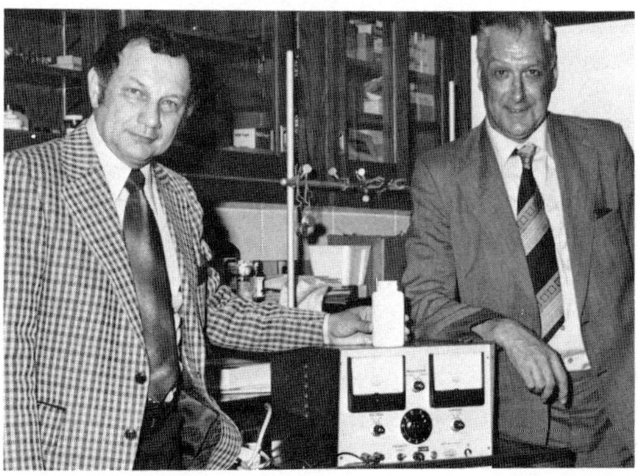

Figure 10.1. Dr. James C. Gentles (RT) visiting the Pennsylvania College of Podiatric Medicine, Department of Microbiology, to discuss a collaborative research effort with Dr. Carl Abramson, Professor of Microbiology, Immunology, and Pathology.

Other contributing factors regarding the host are age, sex, genetic predisposition, as in atopic-chronic dermatophytosis, infectious history, and therapeutic modalities which affect the immune response, such as x-rays, corticosteroids, and immunosuppressive therapy.

Trichophytin as an Indicator of the Immune Response

Cutaneous hypersensitivity to dermatophytes was first introduced in 1902 by Neisser and Plato, who studied the preparation and use of the "trichophytin" intradermal test (17). Both delayed (tuberculin type) and immediate (wheal and erythema) type reactions were elicited following infection. It has been reported that the delayed reaction is caused by the protein or peptide fraction of the dermatophyte and the immediate reaction by the carbohydrate fraction (18, 19). The procedure has been extensively used as a screening test for dermatophytic infection, although there is reported low specificity and cross reactivity with other fungi such as *Alternaria* sp., *Aspergillus* sp., *Cladosporium* sp., and *Penicillium* sp (20). This cross reactivity should diminish as trichophytin preparations from dermatophytes are further purified using newer technologies (21).

Early experiments showed that patients became hypersensitive to trichophytin 7 to

Table 10.2
Classification of Dermatophytes by Source

Geophilic (soil)	Anthropophilic (man)	Zoophilic (animal)
Microsporum gypseum	*Epidermophyton floccosum*	*Microsporum persicolor*
Microsporum fulvum	*Microsporum ferrugineum*	*Microsporum nanum*
Trichophyton ajelloi	*Microsporum audouinii*	*Microsporum canis*
	Trichophyton concentricum	*Microsporum distortum*
	Trichophyton mentagrophytes var. *interdigitale*	*Microsporum gallinae*
	Trichophyton megninii	*Trichophyton equinum*
	Trichophyton schoenleinii	*Trichophyton simii*
	Trichophyton soudanense	*Trichophyton verrucosum*
	Trichophyton rubrum	*Trichophyton mentagrophytes* var. *mentagrophytes*

10 days after infection and remained positive up to 3 years following therapeutic or immunologic cure. They also showed that repeated dermatophyte infections and trichophytin injections produced decreased inflammatory reactions, suggesting an acquired immunity.

Patients with acute inflammatory disease infected with geophilic or zoophilic species of dermatophytes, such as *T. mentagrophytes* elicit a delayed-type hypersensitivity reaction to trichophytin, as shown by induration and erythema in 24 to 48 hr. In contrast, patients infected with chronic anthropophilic *Trichophyton rubrum* present with an immediate-type hypersensitivity reaction within 15 minutes (wheal and flare). It has been suggested that delayed hypersensitivity be correlated with immunity, but its absence, replaced by the presence of immediate type hypersensitivity, correlates with chronic or recurrent dermatophyte infections (22–24).

Patients with atopy have also been reported to fall into this category and will be discussed in the next section.

Atopic-Chronic Dermatophytosis Syndrome

Since the 1950s, a number of diseases have been found to be related to the HLA (human leucocyte antigen) genetic system. The best known is the association between ankylosing spondylitis and HLA-B27. The HLA system is also known as the human major histocompatibility complex (MHC) system. The predominant host immune response to a donor's MHC antigen when exposed to foreign cells results in graft rejection. The HLA system, therefore, plays a major role in effecting transplant rejection, as well as in predicting patients at risk or increased susceptibility to chronic rheumatic, inflammatory, and immunologic diseases (25). The first report of human disease related to HLA typing was in 1967 with Hodgkin's disease. Since then, HLA has been related to over 50 skin diseases, as well as numerous arthritic and immunologic diseases (26). The relationship between HLA antigens and atopic diseases, genetic predisposition, the immune response system, and serum IgE levels predispose certain patients to atopic-chronic dermatophytosis syndrome (6). It has been shown that specific IgE immune responses are associated with certain HLA haplotypes. Human IgE antibody response is also related to the IgE serum level, which itself is controlled by a single gene independent of the major histocompatibility locus; therefore, the genetic control of the reaginic antibody formation is found to involve many separate genes (27).

Normal human immunoregulatory network exists and maintains a delicate balance between helper and suppressor subsets of T lymphocytes. It is well documented that T and B cell function is normally modulated by a complex interaction between helper and suppressor T cells. Overactive suppressor cells have been demonstrated in patients with hypogammaglobulinemia and other acute infectious diseases. Deficiencies in suppressor T cell function have been associated with autoimmune and collagen diseases. Therefore, the regulation of excessive IgE production may be due to an absence or deficiency of suppressor cells. These suppressor cells are T lymphocytes. Patients with atopic diseases are identified by abnormalities of IgE synthesis. T lymphocytes are found to be depressed; therefore, depression of cell-mediated immunity is found as a clinical manifestation of atopy. These patients demonstrate decreased delayed hypersensitivity reactions to a panel of antigens, specifically, trichophytin. Studies of atopics have shown a lack of delayed hypersensitivity reactivity but an increased immediate hypersensitivity reaction to trichophytin. Patients with chronic tinea pedis infections showed 66% immediate and 33% delayed response to trichophytin. Delayed reactivity to trichophytin in such atopic patients is similar when tested with airborne and dermatophytic antigens other than *T. rubrum*. Delayed reactivity to trichophytin is related to resistance to dermatophytic infections, and immediate reactivity is related to susceptibility. Patients with chronic tinea pedis or chronic onychomycosis show a lack of delayed hypersensitivity but frequent occurrence of immediate hypersensitivity to trichophytin challenge (23, 24). Persons with longlasting tinea infections showed a higher immediate reactivity and diminished delayed reactivity. One can assume that imparied T cell function must be considered to be a primary cause of the immunologic reactions in certain kinds of atopy that are followed by a decreased resistance to dermatophyte infection. These are usually followed by a clinical dermatophyte infection with a chronic course, especially in patients infected with *T. rubrum.* Another mechanism occurs whereby the activation of B cells produce IgE antibodies against any allergen. This may occur during an infection and may precipitate allergic disease. Allergic "breakthrough" may result from a temporary disturbance of the normal regulatory T suppressor cell-dependent damping mechanisms on IgE synthesis controlled at the genetic level. Thus, allergic sensitization may occur in individuals with genetically determined T cell deficiency upon allergenic stimulation during certain periods when T cell suppressor activity is usually low, or the production of IgE by B cells is increased because of mitogenic stimulation (27, 28).

It has repeatedly been observed that patients suffering with hyperimmunoglobulin E syndrome usually have recurrent microbial infections, chronic dermatitis, or hyperimmunoglobulin E-associated disease. Patients with this syndrome show associated defects of T cell functions, neutrophil chemotaxis, and/or neutrophil phagocytosis. Serum inhibitors against lymphocytes or neutrophils inhibiting their function also have been found in patients with this syndrome. These patients present with severe abscesses of the scalp, forehead, groin, and extremities caused by *S. aureus*, as well as purulent rhinitis, severe dental caries, onychomycosis, and chronic dermatophytosis (29). In recent years, a relationship has been noted between atopy and chronic, extensive dermatophyte infection. Severe atopic dermatitis has been associated constantly with generalized *T. rubrum* infection. Dermatophytosis studied in prison inmates found that 40% of the inmates harbored chronic extensive dermatophyte infections and were found to be atopic. Their atopic manifestations were almost exclusively hay fever and/or asthma. Chronic dermatophytosis was three times more frequent in those inmates having atopic disease. Approximately 50% of patients examined with chronic *T. rubrum* infection had a history of atopy. There are specific predisposing factors associated with chronic extensive dermatophytosis. These conditions include atopy, hay fever, asthma, diabetes, lymphoma, thymoma, Cushing's syndrome, and primary immunodeficiency disease, as well as patients receiving immunosuppressant medication. The immunosuppression from systemic medications and topical steroids may be observed to heighten susceptibility to fungal infections, including dermatophytosis. These medications suppress the immune response (30–32). As alluded to earlier, an impairment in the function of T suppressor cells, as well as B cells and macrophages leading to an imbalance between suppressor and helper T cells, may be responsible for the hyperproduction of IgE. Since the T cells are involved in delayed reactivity and since we indicated earlier that delayed reactivity to trichophytin was reduced in patients with atopic disease, then one finds a relationship which may be identified as the atopic-chronic dermatophytosis syndrome (6). This is evident in patients with a genetic predisposition for hyperproduction of immunoglobulin E, as in atopic disease, which is controlled by HLA antigens which in turn are genetically controlled from the sixth chromosome. Clinically, the atopic-chronic dermatophytosis patient is a male with infection beginning during the second decade of life (33). History of the patient presents with clinical dermatophytosis commonly caused by *T. rubrum.* The chronic lesion is characterized by pruritis, erythema, scaling, and hyperkeratosis. The initial inflammation is usually intense but diminishes with time. The patient develops a "moccasin"-type, erythrodermic, hyperkeratotic foot lesion. Palmar and plantar skin surfaces develop painful fissures, as well as tinea cruris and onychomycosis. The general description may be that of an exfoliative erythroderma. Immunologic findings in patients with chronic-atopic dermatophytosis syndrome have increased serum IgE and immediate hypersensitivity reaction to trichophytin with the delayed reaction weak or absent. Trichophytin-specific IgE may be identified by the *R*adio-*A*llergo*S*orben*T* (RAST) test. The immune responsiveness of the patient shows enhanced synthesis of IgE to trichophytin but failure to express cell-mediated immunity to trichophytin, both in vivo and in vitro. There is a positive correlation between cellular immunity to dermatophytes and intact host defense. When the cellular immunity to trichophytin is compromised, there is an associated susceptibility to infection. As the dermatophyte proliferates rapidly through susceptible tissues, the host has little capacity to incite intense inflammation. However, an immunized host expresses cell-mediated immunity to dermatophyte antigen at the site of infection, and the skin becomes acutely and intensely inflamed. Development of intense inflammation results in the disappearance of the dermatophyte and subsequent resolution of the infection. This suggests that host defense against dermatophytes requires intact cell-mediate immunity and an intense cutaneous inflammatory response of the delayed type. The intense inflammation impedes fungal invasion by damaging the epidermis and permitting inhibitory plasma factors access to the pathogen. In atopic patients with chronic dermatophyte infection, one finds that the infection is intensely inflamed for only a short period of time. This aborted inflammatory response suggests an altered host immunity reflected by a diminished degree of inflammation. At this point, there is usually a dramatic emergence of immediate hypersensitivity to trichophytin with a disappearance of delayed hypersensitivity to the same allergen. The host-parasite interaction of delayed type hypersensitivity to trichophytin decreases, resulting in the infected lesions becoming less inflammatory. IgE, measured at this point, shows an increase in synthesis to the dermatophyte antigen and is found to be central to the defect in host resistance. It is believed that this mechanism predisposes the patient to the atopic-chronic dermatophytosis syndrome. The basic mechanism includes the role of IgE in immune modulation of T-effector cells. IgE is critically involved through the mast cells and its complement of pharmacoactive mediators in the modulation of T-effector cell function in chronic dermatophytosis. During the infective stage of *T. rubrum*, water-soluble trichophytin diffuses into the dermis from the fungus. Trichophytin in the dermis binds specifically to sensitized T-cells or specific antibody. Thereby mast cell-fixed antitrichophytin IgE becomes a trigger that activates mast cell secretion of pharmacologic mediators. Histamine released locally would then act on antigen activated T-effector cells, prohibiting further activation and release of lymphokines or other mediators of inflammation. Histamine would, therefore, inhibit T-effector cell function and suppress delayed-type hypersensitivity-mediated inflammatory response. IgE mast cell mediator system is an important mechanism for in situ immunomodulation. The IgE mast cell mediator modulation mechanism explains the basis of atopic susceptibility to dermatophyte infection, as well as the decrease in inflammation concomitant with the appearance of trichophytin-specific IgE and the antigen-specific nature of the cell-mediated immune defect. It has been suggested that podiatrists who burr down fungal-infected hyperkeratotic onychomycotic nails and inadvertently inhale large amounts of nail dust aerosols exposé themselves to this sequelae. These podiatrists would be immunizing themselves through the respiratory passages with fungi that are antigenic and may induce the sequence of events previously described. This would result in an IgE response that later in life would thwart cell-mediated immune responses to antigen from pathogenic dermatophyte fungi penetrating their skin. It has been shown that the nonpathogenic molds contain cross-reacting antigens. Many individuals with asthma and hay fever synthesize IgE early in life in response to inhalation of airborne molds and fungi. Many of these individuals examined for cell-mediated immunity to trichophytin or other antigens of airborne molds do not express cell-mediated responses. They are found to exhibit strong immediate-type hypersensitivity to airborne molds, as well as to trichophytin antigens, but exhibit no delayed response. Therefore, although never infected with dermatophytes, these individuals exhibit the immune profile of the atopic-chronic dermatophytosis syndrome patient. In a recent study of 230 podiatrists who were selected to submit sera for a study to determine their immunologic response following inhalation of nail dust allergens, it was found that 30% produced high IgE values.

Thus, although recalling only a negative history of dermatophyte infection, these podiatrists exhibited an immune profile of the atopic-chronic dermatophytosis syndrome patient (34, 35). Should the skin of such an individual become infected with a dermatophyte, it would then seem that the cell-mediated immune mechanism would be diminished to trichophytin challenge. Therefore, in the presence of cross reactive IgE and by the modulation mechanism inhibiting T-effector cells the delayed reaction would be diminished or inhibited, resulting in a highly susceptible at-risk patient, that is at risk with regard to fungal infection. It is, therefore, necessary for the podiatrist to acquire a more comprehensive awareness of the relationship among genetic predisposition, altered immune mechanisms, and chronic-resistant-atopic dermatophytosis syndrome before embarking on a series of unsuccessful therapeutic modalities when treating or retreating chronic "athlete's foot."

Dermatophytids

"Id" reactions, also known as dermatophytids, epidermatophytids, favids, microsporids, and trichophytids, are believed to occur as a result of hematogenous spread of allergenic fungal elements or products from the initial focus of infection. The dermatophytid occurs as an eruption secondary to a primary lesion in a sensitized patient. This is usually the result of the reaction between circulating antigens and skin-sensitizing antibodies. Jadassohn, in 1918, was the first to recognize these lesions as an allergic process related to dermatophytosis (36). Some relate them immunologically to tuberculids, syphilids, and candidids, since they also have been reported to resemble these other "id" reactions histopathologically (37). In tinea pedis, lesions are usually found on the hands as well as the feet, suggesting a contact dermatitis type IV hypersensitivity which is T-cell-mediated rather than B-cell-mediated hypersensitivity as suggested above. In tinea pedis, the vesicles are usually grouped and tense (pompholyx type), but they may also be diffuse and bullous. In either case, they are sterile, containing a clear, viscous fluid which has been shown in our laboratories to contain immunoglobulins (C. Abramson, unpublished data). The following fungi have been reported to cause dermatophytids in children and adults: *M. audouinii*, *Microsporum canis*, *T. mentagrophytes* (zoophilic strain), *T. mentagrophytes* var. *interdigitale* (anthropophilic strain), *T. rubrum* and *Epidermophyton floccosum*. The most common site of dermatophytids other than the feet is the hands of patients with infections on the feet (23).

Treatment begins by elimination of the primary focus of infection, avoidance of hand to foot contact, as well as contact with shoes and socks worn during the infectious period. Also indicated is the use of topical steroids to involute the hypersensitivity response.

CLINICAL ASPECTS

Tinea Pedis

Most, if not all, dermatophyte infections begin with colonization of the horny layer of the epidermis, the stratum corneum. The ensuring clinical and pathologic process that follows is generally dependent on factors contributed by the host response, the environment, the anatomic site, the strain, the species, and the source of the dermatophyte. The resultant pathology varies from mild, chronic, noninflammatory, scaly lesions to an acute, inflammatory, vesicular, pustular to bullous syndrome. It may occur intertriginously and/or on the dorsal, lateral, or plantar surface and may spread by contiguous autoinoculation to any and all keratinous tissue, i.e., hair, skin, and nails of the patient. The dermatophytes most often associated with infections are *T. rubrum*, *T. mentagrophytes*, and *E. floccosum*, but characteristic tinea pedis may also be caused by *Trichophyton violaceum*, *Trichophyton megnini*, *M. canis*, and *Microsporum persicolor* or any other dermatophyte. *C. albicans,* many saprophytes, as well as a large number of bacteria, can mimic the clinical symptoms of "athlete's foot." It is therefore necessary that a microscopic KOH preparation, as well as a culture and sensitivity, be performed prior to specific therapy, so that the etiologic agent is identified. Repeated exposure to the fungus through contact with fomites carrying infected squames from community showers, pools, rugs, or other public facilities; poorly fitted shoes resulting in trauma followed by maceration; and increased moisture and/or humidity resulting in the "sweaty sock" syndrome all contribute environmentally as predisposing factors. In some cases, nonenvironmental genetic factors may be the primary predisposing underlying cause for clinical tinea pedis. It is also interesting to note that the natural resistance barrier of the skin, specifically, production of fungistatic lipids, is not part of the anatomical structure of the foot. Eccrine sweat glands do not provide this function. Tinea pedis has been classified into four clinical types: (*a*) chronic intertriginous; (*b*) chronic papulosquamous hyperkeratotic; (*c*) vesicular or subacute; and (*d*) acute ulcerative vesiculopustular (38). The first type presents with white, dead, macerated, peeling, fissured skin, usually between the third and fourth or fourth and fifth toes (Fig. 10.2). Hyperhidrosis and bromhidrosis are usually present. Removal of the debris reveals an erythematous, weeping epidermis teeming with viable fungus. The second type is chronic and presents with papulosquamous hyperkeratotic lesions that may be localized or cover the entire surface of the foot, i.e., "moccasin foot" (Fig. 10.3). Scaling may be rough and pronounced or subtle and fine, sloughing off like dandruff, as seen in infections with *T. rubrum*. The third type, caused primarily by *T. mentagrophytes*, presents with vesicles, vesiculopustules, and/or bullae and may occur as a patch-like network of lesions intertriginously, dorsally, and on plantar surfaces (Fig. 10.4).

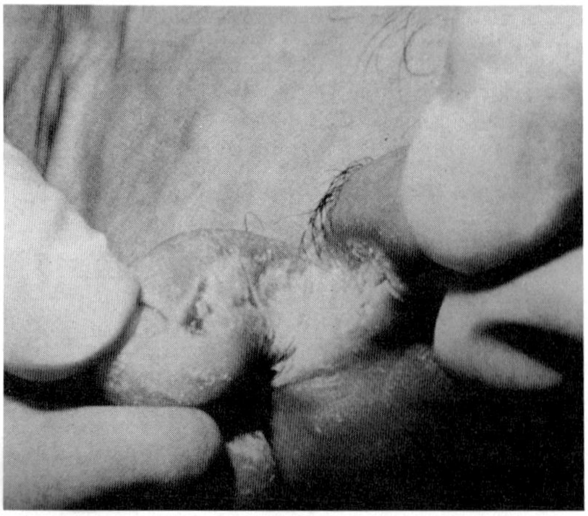

Figure 10.2. Intertriginous tinea pedis.

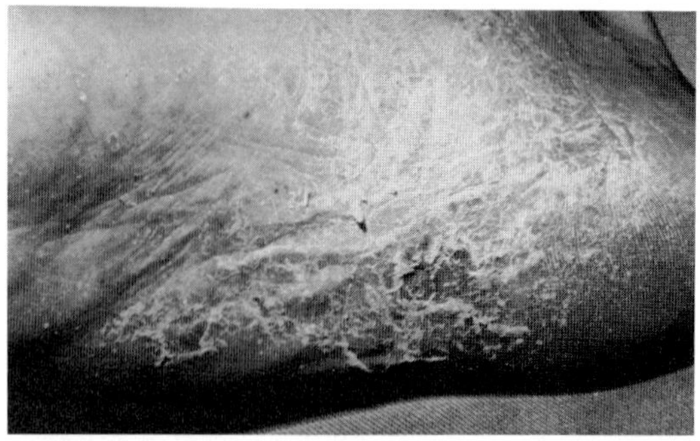

Figure 10.3. Chronic papulosquamous hyperkeratotic tinea pedis.

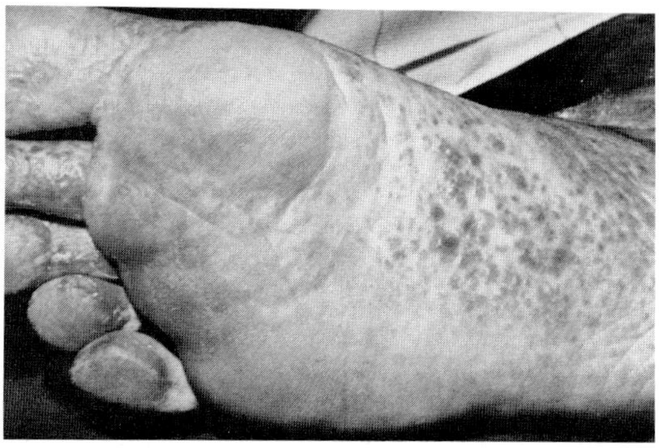

Figure 10.4. Vesicular tinea pedis.

Viable fungi are found on the inner surface of the roof of the vesicle, which can be demonstrated by cutting off the top of lesion and observing by the KOH procedure. The last clinical type in this classification presents as an eczematoid acute ulcerative vesiculopustular process, usually secondarily infected with bacteria. Cellulitis, pyrexia, lymphadenitis, lymphangitis, and overwhelming "id" reactions complicate the clinical picture and contribute to the worsening of the pathologic process. Observing the two extremes, namely, the first and last types of this classification, Leyden and Kligman introduced the term "dermatophytosis simplex" to describe the intertriginous type and the term "dermatophytosis complex" to describe the secondarily bacterial infected acute ulcerative vesiculopustular form. Attention to the differences with regard to infection by a single microbial type and species vs a mixed microbial flora (multiple types and species) determines therapeutic management and choice of antifungal and/or antibacterial agents (39).

As indicated elsewhere in this chapter, one should always be aware that tinea pedis may be mimicked by a large number of yeasts, saprophytic fungi, gram-negative and gram-positive bacteria and, therefore, it is essential to isolate and identify the etiologic agent prior to antimicrobial therapy.

Tinea Unguium (Dermatophytic Onychomycosis)

Although tinea unguium of the toenails is primarily caused by *T. rubrum*, *T. mentagrophytes*, and *E. floccosum*, any dermatophyte may cause this disease. Zaias has reported that about 25% of onychomycosis is caused by dermatophytes, 25% by bacteria and 50% by saprophytic fungi (40). Three clinical types are generally attributed to dermatophytic infection: (*a*) distal subungual; (*b*) proximal subungual; and (*c*) white superficial tinea unquium. The distal subungual is the most common type resulting from invasion of the fungus through the lateral or distal edge of the nail plate. Symptoms include minimal paronychia with involvement of the nail, resulting in a pitted or grooved, yellowish surface. The classic infected toenail is brittle, friable, discolored, thickened, and elevated distally at an angle of 45° due to the collection of subungual debris. Invasion of the nail plate usually occurs from the nailbed. A single nail or many nails may be involved. KOH preparations are difficult to visualize, and it may take 24 hours to digest and clear nail specimens. Cheesy subungual debris should be used for culture, and in vitro antimicrobial measures must be taken to inhibit bacterial and/or saprophytic fungal flora. The proximal subungual type of infection may begin following trauma and subsequent invasion of the lateral or proximal aspects of the nail folds. White superficial onychomycosis or leuconychia mycotica, also known as superficial white spot tinea unguium, infects the surface of the nail plate. This type presents with punctate, circumscribed, opaque, whitish lesions which may remain in a confined area or spread and cover the entire nail surface. Specimens from the surface of the infected nail by KOH preps show large, broad, mycelial filaments which have been called "eroding fronds" (40). Culture is an absolute necessity prior to therapy because of the large number of bacteria and saprophytic fungi that can mimic dermatophytic tinea unguium.

Gram-Negative Athlete's Foot

Classic tinea pedis, or athlete's foot, presents as a mild scaling to severe, soggy, whitish, hyperkeratotic, pruritic, intertriginous malodorous infection.

The initial phase of interdigital athlete's foot has recently been named "dermatophytosis simplex" (39). Eighty-seven percent of the total microbial flora found or recovered in dermatophytosis simplex include aerobic gram-positive bacilli, yeasts, and dermatophytes. Although the dermatophytes are a small percentage of the total flora, they have been recovered in 85% of infected interspaces. The primary invasion of the horny layer by dermatophytes compromises the integrity of the host tissue, thereby increasing the susceptibility of the patient to severe infection. With the advent of predisposing fators, such as trauma, hot weather, sweating, exercise, tight shoes, and constant shear, this hydrated, wet-environmental milieu contributes to a doubling of the bacterial population with the subsequent replacement of the fungal flora. Gram-positive cocci and bacilli are predominant, but *Proteus* sp. and *Pseudomonas* sp. begin to appear in significant numbers. Dermatophytes begin to decrease and are recoverable only in about 50% of cases. This form of tinea pedis is currently described as "dermatophytosis complex."

Progression of dermatophytosis complex to a more severe form presents with whitish, soggy maceration, extreme pruritus, bad odor, redness, edema, tenderness, and fissuring. The mean bacterial count triples from that of dermatophytosis simplex but still includes gram-positive cocci and bacilli. Gram-negative organisms, primarily *Proteus* sp. and *Pseudomonas* sp., are found in 65% of intertriginous areas. Dermatophytes under these conditions are only recoverable in 36% of the infected interspaces.

A fourth form of tinea pedis described as "gram-negative athlete's foot" has been described as the most severe form of intertriginous infection. Patients present with foul-smelling, whitish, painful, strongly macerated, hyperkeratotic interspaces with erosions, exudation, and intense inflammation. The hyperkeratotic, plaque-like lesion has a characteristic greenish tinge consistent with pigmented *Pseudomonas aeruginosa* infection (Fig. 10.5). The lesions are painful and disabling. The recovery of fungi in "gram-negative athlete's foot" is fruitless. It has been postulated that the disappearance of fungal flora may be due to the production of an inhibitory substance caused by the *Pseudomonas* population. A partially purified, extracellular, diffusible product from *P. aeruginosa* was shown to selectively inhibit dermatophytes, specifically *T. rubrum*, resulting in "gram-negative athlete's foot" (41).

LABORATORY IDENTIFICATION AND DIFFERENTIAL DIAGNOSIS

Examination of skin and/or nail scrapings or specimens is paramount in making a preliminary diagnosis, but it is essential that whether such results are positive or negative, a culture must be done. In preparation for a classic KOH mount, one must prepare the patient prior to removal of the specimen. Outer debris and macerated tissue from the plantar or intertriginous spaces should be removed, and the infected site should be cleansed with an alcohol sponge. Specimens should be removed from the periphery of the tinea pedis lesions using a sterile scalpel. Some of the epidermal scales should be placed on a clean slide, and 20% DMSO-KOH should be added, heated over a small flame, allowed to digest, and observed for classic long, refractile, tortuous, branching septate hyphae, arthrospores, and/or mycelia threading their way through the epidermal scales. They are differentiated from fibers, artifacts, and debris by the presence of internal structures such as nuclei, organelles, septations, and droplets in the hyphae. The addition of Parker Superchrome Blueback ink to the KOH solution is helpful in the differentiation and identification of true mycelia. Vesicles and bullae may be examined by clipping the tops of the lesions and observing microscopically following KOH digestion. Dry scales may be sent in a sterile envelope to a clinical lab for KOH and culture if they cannot be performed in your office laboratory. Scrapings or specimens for culture should be removed from suspected infected sites, followed by inoculation into appropriate media. The media should be inoculated by cutting into the surface with the scraping instrument using parallel streaks. Dermatophyte test media (DTM) of Sabouraud's dextrose agar containing cycloheximide and chloramphenicol support the growth of dermatophytes and selectively inhibit normal flora species of bacteria and saprophytic fungi. Growth of dermatophytes occurs in 10 days to 3 weeks at 25°C. There are exceptions for some rare strains.

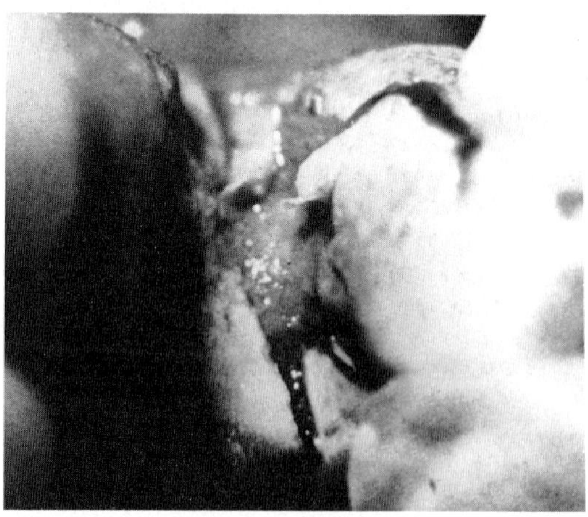

Figure 10.5. Gram-negative athlete's foot caused by *P. aeruginosa*.

Identification requires recognition of cultural characteristics (color, topography, and consistency of colony) (Fig. 10.6). Lactophenol cotton blue (LPCB) slide mount allows for an immediate determination of microscopic morphology. Based upon conidial formation and structure (macro- and microconidia), as well as ancillary mycelial morphology, one can identify the usual strain of dermatophytes in the genera *Microsporum*, *Trichophyton*, and *Epidermophyton*. The clinician must be aware of a spontaneous mutation that occurs in many dermatophyte species when clinical specimens are cultured. This phenomenon is called "pleomorphism." There is a loss of pigmentation and spore formation, making it impossible to identify the genus and species. All one sees microscopically are "sterile hyphae" with no sign of macro- or mi-

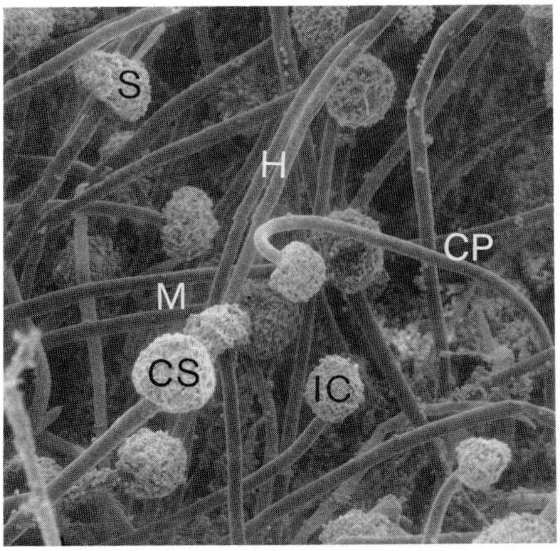

Figure 10.6. The morphology of *Aspergillus* is somewhat similar regardless of the species. This scanning electron micrograph is representative of *Aspergillus niger*, which is rare on the human foot. *CS*, conidiospores; *CP*, conidiophore; *H*, hyphae, *M*, mycelial mat; *IC*, individual conidiospores. Not seen are the foot cells which attach the fungal stalk to the mycelial mat, and the sterigmata and vesicle which extend from the end of the conidiophore.

croconidia. Under normal laboratory conditions, this mutation is irreversible (42).

Culture and microscopic analysis are essential prior to therapy because infections clinically similar to tinea pedis may be mimicked by saprophytic fungi and bacteria and will, therefore, not respond to classic antidermatophytic therapy. One example is gram-negative athlete's foot (41). As a result of predisposing factors, such as hyperhidrosis, occlusion by tight shoes, minute abrasions due to friction, and fungus-infected skin surfaces, dynamic overgrowth of opportunistic gram-negative bacilli prevails. As the gram-negative population increases, the recovery of dermatophytes dramatically diminishes, until a point is reached when no dermatophytes can be recovered from clinically symptomatic tinea pedis. *P. aeruginosa* is inhibiting its fungal competitor *T. rubrum* by producing a diffusible antifungal agent into the infectious environment of the intertriginous foot lesion. Clinically, the patient is diagnosed as having tinea pedis; laboratory culture for fungus and KOH are negative, and what was a paradox just a few years ago can currently be identified and treated appropriately as gram-negative athlete's foot by classical bacterial methods (43).

Intertriginous erythrasma caused by *C. minutissimum* will mimic dermatophytic tinea pedis but will not respond to antidermatophytic therapy (44). It is a chronic, superficial bacterial infection found most commonly in the more lateral interdigital areas. It presents with scaling, maceration, and fissuring between the fourth and fifth or third and fourth toewebs. Wood's lamp examination of infected toewebs or dorsal foot lesions show a classic coral red fluorescence. Bacterial culture should reveal the etiologic agent as *C. minutissimum* which also fluoresces in vitro.

THERAPEUTIC PRINCIPLES

Tinea pedis caused by members of the genera *Trichophyton*, *Microsporum*, and *Epidermophyton* infect the foot in a variety of clinical forms. As previously described, they include: (*a*) intertriginous; (*b*) papulosquamous hyperkeratotic; (*c*) vesicular; and (*d*) acute ulcerative vesiculopustular. The degree of skin damage, the intensity of inflammation, and the extent of skin and/or nail surface affected dictate the course and type of therapeutic management. Host-parasite interactions resulting from the immune response of the host, as well as the type and source of the dermatophyte, are important factors in your therapeutic approach. Zoophilic and geophilic-derived dermatophytes more than likely result in a vigorous, intense inflammatory response, followed by an early cessation of the infection. The intact cellular immune response in this series of events contributes to the clinical profile. Anthropophilic dermatophytes, on the other hand, meeting a diminished cellular immune response, result in an infection that may become chronic, more extensive, and less inflammatory. Other contributing factors, which dictate the course of infectious events, include: sex, genetic background, age, occupation, general health, and the environment.

If a lesion is severely inflamed, denuded, and weeping, symptomatic therapy in the form of soaks and/or compresses may be indicated. Topical therapy should be avoided, and oral antifungals should be considered. If the lesions are chronic, hyperkeratotic, thickened, and scaly, keratolytic agents which peel the area should be used in conjunction with topical antifungals. Drying antifungal powder, such as undecylenic acid, should be considered for maintenance therapy (45). In severe infections, elevation of the foot and/or bed rest is indicated. Corticosteroids may be used in the event of hyperergic "id" reactions.

For chronic infections requiring long-term therapy, culture and antifungal sensitivity testing is important because of resistance patterns which have developed among the dermatophytes, resulting in treatment failures (46).

Identification of the etiologic agent is essential prior to therapy. Most important is awareness of the toxic and/or adverse effects of long-term oral or intravenous antifungal therapy, interaction of drugs, and the profile of your patient's medical history. To detect onset of physiologic and/or anatomic abnormalities caused by the antifungal agent, the patient should be periodically monitored by classic clinical laboratory surveillance. Topical antifungals may be used for chronic, minimally inflamed intertriginous or hyperkeratotic infections. These include: tolnaftate, haloprogin, miconozale, ciclopirox, and clotrimazole. As previously suggested, a keratolytic may also be indicated with hyperkeratotic infections prior to or in between the application of the antifungal agent. In acute ulcerative or vesiculopustular tinea pedis, topical agents will only irritate or aggravate the inflammatory, weeping, vesicular area; therefore, the oral antifungals ketoconazole or griseofulvin, in conjunction with soaks or compresses, are indicated. It is reported that therapeutic effects of ketoconazole occur earlier and have a significantly higher cure rate than griseofulvin and that ketoconazole resistant strains of dermatophytes have not occurred as with griseofulvin (46). It has been suggested that griseofulvin may be delivered to the epidermal cells producing keratin, which cornifies forming the stratum corneum. The griseofulvin concentrates in the stratum corneum. More importantly, sweat carries the drug to the stratum corneum within a matter of hours. The griseofulvin is thought to interfere with nuclear mitosis by binding with the microtubular protein of the dermatophyte (38).

Delivery of ketoconazole is similar to that which occurs with griseofulvin. There is incorporation into basal cells that eventually becomes the stratum corneum and/or there is delivery carried by sweat traveling to the surface of the skin. The mechanism of action of ketoconazole acts through interference of the ergosterol synthesis in the dermatophyte, resulting in defects in the cell membrane (46). Some of the adverse reactions of oral griseofulvin include hematologic dyscrasias, peripheral neuropathy, gastrointestinal upset, proteinuria, porphyria, photosensitivity, and cross reactivity with penicillin hypersensitivity. Some of the adverse reactions of oral ketoconazole include gynecomastia, drug-associated hepatitis, pruritis, photophobia, gastrointestinal upset, and jaundice. Where applicable, one should use topical therapy first before considering the use of systemic therapy.

Chronic infections may take from 6 weeks to 1 year before complete recovery, with recurrences almost 100%. Acute inflammatory infections may be self-limiting or may be cured within weeks using topical therapy assisted by competent host-parasite reactivity. For specific therapeutic dosages, contraindications, etc., please consult your most recent edition of *Physician's Desk Reference*.

References

1. Baer RL, Rosenthal S: The biology of fungus infections of the feet. *JAMA* 197:1017–1020, 1966.
2. English MD: Tinea pedis as a public health problem. *Br J Dermatol* 81:705–707, 1969.
3. Georg LK: Epidemiology of dermatophytes. *Ann NY Acad Sci* 89:69–77, 1960.
4. Binazzi M, Simonetti S: Skin mycoses-geographic distribution and present day pathomorphosis. *Int J Dermatol* 22:92–97, 1983.
5. Svejgaard E, Albrectsen B, Baastrup N: The occurrence of tinea of the feet in 15 year old school children. *Mykosen* 26 (9):450–454, 1983.
6. Jones HE: The atopic-chronic dermatophytosis syndrome. *Acta Derm Venereol* (*Suppl*) (Stockh) 92:81–85, 1980.
7. Ajello L: Natural history of dermatophytes and related fungi. *Mycopathol Mycol Appl* 53:93–110, 1974.
8. Remak R: Zur Kenntnis von der planzlichen natur der parrigo lupinasa. *Med Zeitung*

9:73–74, 1840.
9. Schoenlein JL: Zur pathologie der impetigenes. *Arch Anat Phys Wiss Med* p. 82, 1839.
10. Gruby D: Surles mycodermes que constituent la teigne faveuse. *CR Acad Sci* 13:309–312, 1841.
11. Gruby D: Recherches sur la natur, le siege et le developpement du porrigo de calvans ou phytoalopecie. *CR Acad Sci* 17:301–303, 1843.
12. Malmsten PH: *Trichophyton tonsurans* der haarscheerende Schimmel. *Arch Anat Physiol Wiss Med* 1:1–19, 1845.
13. Sabouraud R.: *Les Teignes.* Paris, *Masson et Cie,* 1910.
14. Pellizzari C.: Recherche sur *Trichophyton tonsurans. G Italiano mal veneree* 29:8–40, 1888.
15. Kaufman-Wolf M.: Uber Pilzerkrankungen der Hande und Fusse. *Dermatologica* 21:385–396, 1914.
16. Gentles JC: Experimental ringworm in guinea pigs: Oral treatment with griseofulvin. *Nature* 182:476–477, 1958.
17. Neisser A: Plato's Versuche uber die Herstellung und Verwundung von Trichophytin. *Arch Dermatol Syphilol* 60:63–76, 1902.
18. Grappel SF, Bishop CT, Blank F: Immunology of dermatophytes and dermatophytosis. *Bacteriol Rev* 38:222–250, 1974.
19. Abramson C, Orlando J, Glickman H: *Trichophyton rubrum* fractions related to immediate and delayed hypersensitivity (abstr). *Bacteriol Proc:* 123, 1970.
20. Ahmed AR: Immunology of human dermatophyte infections. *Arch Dermatol* 118:521–525, 1982.
21. Kaaman T: The clinical significance of cutaneous reactions to trichophytin in dermatophytosis. *Acta Derm Venereol (Stockh)* 58:139–143, 1978.
22. Sorensen GW, Jones HE: Immediate and delayed hypersensitivity in chronic dermatophytosis. *Arch Dermatol* 112:40–43, 1976.
23. Jillson OF: Immunology of dermatophytosis. *Cutis* 301:27–35, 1982.
24. Hay RJ: Chronic dermatophyte infections. *Br J Dermatol* 106:1–7, 1982.
25. Tait BD, Finlay RI, Simons MJ: Serum HLA typing. *Tissue Antigens* 17:129–135, 1981.
26. Schaller JG, Hansen JA: HLA relationships to disease. *Hosp Pract:* 41–49, 1981.
27. Katz DH: The allergic phenotype: manifestations of "allergic breakthrough" of IgE antibody production. *Immunol Rev* 41:77–108, 1978.
28. Perlmutter L, Potvin L: Studies on T-lymphocytes of atopics and non-atopics. *J Allergy Clin Immunol* 65:2223–228, 1980.
29. Katona JM, Tata G, Scanlon RT, Bellanti JA: Hyper IgE syndrome: a disease with suppressor T cell deficiency. *Ann Allergy* 45:295–300, 1980.
30. Jones HE, Reinhardt JH, Rinaldi MG: Logical and immunological survey for dermatophytosis. *Arch Dermatol* 108:61–65, 1973.
31. Hanifin JM, Lobitz WC Jr: Newer concepts of atopic dermatitis. *Arch Dermatol* 113:663–670, 1977.
32. Rajka G, Barlinn C: On the significance of trichophytin reactivity in atopic dermatitis. *Acta Derm Venereol (Stockh)* 59:45–47, 1979.
33. Bazin H, Platteau B, Pavwels R: Genetic control of the IgE reaginic immune response. *Int Arch Allergy Appl Immunol* 66:19–24, 1981.
34. Abramson C, Wilton J, McGeady S, Shapero PA, McCarthy DJ: Serologic profiles following prolonged inhalation of onychomycotic aerosols. *Bacteriol Proc:* 399, 1983.
35. Davis RP, Ganderton MA, Savage MA: Human nail dust and precipitating antibodies to *Trichophyton rubrum* in chiropodists. *Clin Allergy* 13:309–315, 1983.
36. Jadassohn J: Uber die Trichophytien. *Berl Klin Wochenschr* 231:489–494, 1918.
37. Williams CM: Dermatophytid complicating dermatophytosis of the glabrous skin. *Arch Dermatol Syphilol* 13:661–669, 1926.
38. Rippon JW: Cutaneous infections. In Rippon JW (ed): *Medical Mycology,* ed 2. Philadelphia, W.B. Saunders, 1982, pp 154–248.
39. Leyden JJ, Kligman AM: Interdigital athlete's foot: The interaction of dermatophytes and resident bacteria. *Arch Dermatol* 114:1466–1472, 1978.
40. Zaias N: Onychomycosis. *Arch Dermatol* 105:263–274, 1972.
41. Abramson C: Athlete's foot caused by *Pseudomonas aeruginosa. Clin Dermatol* 1:14–24, 1983.
42. Koshy TK: The formation of macroconidia in dermatophytes following UV. Irradiation and temperature treatment. *Can J Microbiol* 23:1298–1301, 1977.
43. Hugh R, Gilardi GL: Pseudomonas. In Lennette EH, Ballows A, Hausler WJR Jr, Truant JP: *Manual of Clinical Microbiology,* ed 3. Washington, DC, American Society for Microbiology, 1980, p 288.
44. Maglietta T, Detwiler DE, Capogna L: Tinea pedis and erythrasma. *J Am Podiatry Assoc* 73:315–318, 1983.
45. Jones EJ: Therapy of superficial fungal infections. *Med Clin North Am* 66:873–893, 1982.
46. Robertson MH, Hanifin JM, Parker F: Oral therapy with ketoconazole for dermatophyte infections unresponsive to griseofulvin. *Rev Infect Dis* 2:578–581, 1980.

CHAPTER 11

Cutaneous Manifestations of Viral Diseases

FREDERICK J. BARTOLOMEI and DANIEL J. McCARTHY

HISTORICAL PERSPECTIVE

Clinical virology is an interdisciplinary field which has evolved and expanded at an accelerating rate, coinciding with the development of additionally sophisticated research methodologies. Nasemann reviewed the development of viral research beginning at the turn of the century (1). Löffler and Frosch, in 1897, determined that the etiologic agent of bovine foot-and-mouth disease is transmissible via cell-free filtrate. In 1904, Borrel employed a staining technique to demonstrate the fowl poxvirus. Three years later, Paschen observed the smallpox virus with the light microscope. Also in 1907, Lipschütz used light microscopy to visualize the molluscum contagiosum virus. The electron microscope was developed prior to 1938 when Ruska first began utilizing it for viral research. The basis for the study of viral morphology was established in 1941 when special staining techniques were used to demonstrate some 20 distinct viruses. In 1950, Enders improved contemporary tissue culture techniques and applied them to the beginnings of research in in vitro viral replication. Lwoff, in 1957, set forth the "virus concept" for categorizing viruses.

Viruses are distinguishable from other microorganisms by the application of specific criteria. The single most important differentiating feature is that viruses possess only one nucleic acid, either deoxyribonucleic acid (DNA) or ribonucleic acid (RNA). The present chapter considers only the DNA viruses with dermatologic relevance to the lower extremity of man. Specifically, it addresses the virus-induced diseases of molluscum contagiosum, herpes simplex and herpes zoster, and verruca, with verruca plantaris discussed as the prototype of the pedal verrucae. These disorders encompass the poxvirus, herpesvirus, and papovavirus groups of viruses containing deoxyribonucleic acid. Because cutaneous viral disorders may present a puzzling array of symptoms and may occasionally mimic nonviral diseases, the podiatric physician should be thoroughly versed in their etiology, clinical manifestations, and therapeutic alternatives.

PEDAL VERRUCAE

Pathogenesis and Pathology

The human papilloma virus invades the host through uncovered regions of the integument. The virus appears to directly penetrate the skin in areas especially susceptible to trauma, such as the periunguis, hands, and weight-bearing portions of the plantar surface of the foot. The virus produces a benign, infectious acanthoma (Figs. 11.1 and 11.2). Epidermal changes characteristic of the disease develop after inoculation.

Diagnosis

The accurate diagnosis of a verruca generally rests heavily upon clinical findings. The history, morphology, and distribution of the lesion(s) may support the initial impression. Additional diagnostic considerations include pinpoint hemorrhaging with debridement (2) and elicitation of a painful response with lateral pressure. Despite its characteristic clinical features, other disorders must be considered when atypical lesions or patients at low risk present with a suspected papillomavirus infection. The extensive differential diagnosis of

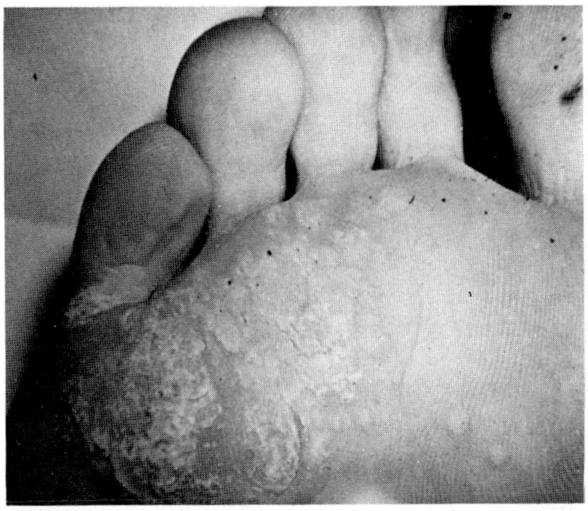

Figure 11.1. Clinical appearance of verrucae, mosaic type plantar to the head of the first metatarsal. Courtesy of Dr. J. Yale, *Podiatric Medicine*: 150, 1980.

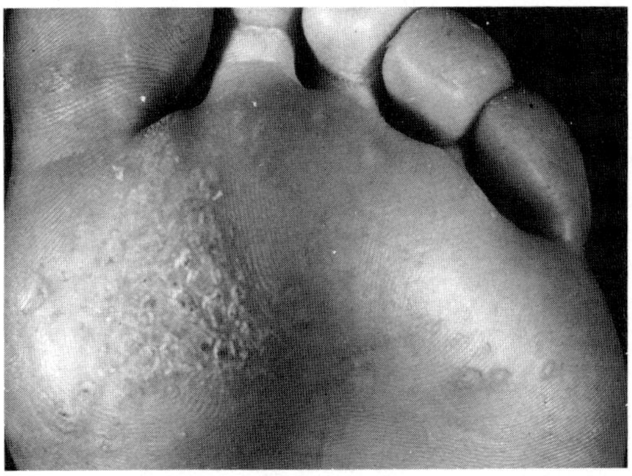

Figure 11.2. Clinical appearance of mosaic verrucae. Courtesy of Dr. Royal Montgomery.

pedal verrucae includes other benign neoplasms (3), malignant neoplasms, dermatoses (4), and miscellaneous lesions.

Among the benign tumors, the pigmented nevus, fibroma, xanthoma, glomus tumor, epidermoid cyst, and pyogenic granuloma must be excluded. Among the malignant tumors, the basal cell epithelioma, squamous cell carcinoma, and malignant melanoma must be excluded. Among the dermatoses, the arsenical keratosis, keratosis punctata, molluscum contagiosum, and radiation dermatosis must be excluded. Finally, the lesions of hyperkeratosis, eccrine poroma, porokeratosis plantaris discretum, heloma durum, and heloma milliare must be excluded. The last-named lesions are of the utmost importance to the podiatrist in terms of differential diagnosis since they are most commonly encountered.

Light Microscopy

The general morphologic characteristics of human skin involved in the wart response demonstrate essential similarities whether one speaks of verruca plana juvenilis, verruca vulgaris, verruca plana, verruca filiformis, or verruca digitata. The lesion has radial symmetry, and the much-elongated rete ridges always converge about a central moderately deep point within the dermis (Fig. 11.3). The elongate and centripetal direction of retia, together with an elevation of the circumscribed epidermis of the lesion, have given rise to the descriptive term "papillomatous." An exceedingly diagnostic feature of verrucae are the many basophilic inclusion bodies literally streaming up through the tissues toward the free surface of the skin (5). These have been shown to be viral DNA by immunofluorescent techniques and may be differentiated from pyknotic nuclei common to heloma durum by their rigidly spherical shape.

The cells of the most "papillomatous"

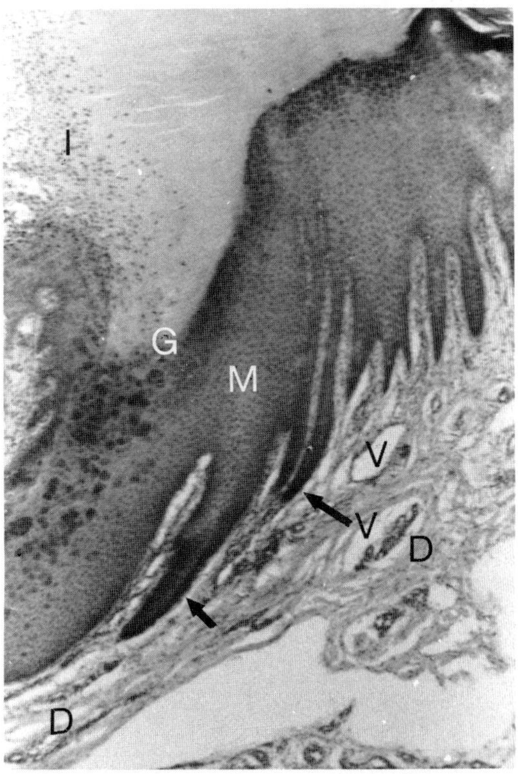

Figure 11.3. Light microscopic appearance of typical verrucae biopsy. Rete ridges are directed centripetally (*arrows*). *I*, inclusion bodies; *G*, stratum granulosum; *M*, stratum Malpighii; *D*, dermis; *V*, blood vessel.

portion of the lesion lack distinct definition and are said to be "vesicular." They are irregularly basophilic and often appear as coalescent masses.

It is characteristic for verrucae to demonstrate a well-delineated stratum granulosum, with well-formed deeply basophilic cells about the periphery of the lesion. This normal condition is lacking about those regions where cell kinetics seem most accelerated. Spherical DNA inclusion bodies appear to be pushing rapidly towards the free surface of the skin in great numbers, and it becomes difficult to estimate just where the stratum spinosum ends and the stratum corneum begins.

Still another feature of the verrucae is the apparent vascularity observed within the epidermis proper (Fig. 11.4). Vessels can be observed in cross, longitudinal, and tangential sections, although they are often poorly structured and appear to be sinusoid-like.

Scanning Electron Microscopy

Separation of epidermis from dermis in verrucae demonstrates some distinctive features when viewed by scanning electron microscopy. A flat section of normal epidermis which was free of verrucous changes was maintained at the periphery of the lesion. Rete ridging and concavities for reception of dermal papillae were shallow and comparatively regular in arrangement. The verruca itself, however, sat much like an inverted dome and represented a sharp departure from as the norm as it extended inward within the dermis (6). The apex of the lesion, which is the top surface of the dome, was a relatively structureless region, formed by a confluence of many rete ridges from all sides (Fig. 11.5). The central region, however, was deeply cavitated by penetration of the central arteriole or precapillary nourishing the lesion, and peripheral to this were several concavities representing perforations for the venous return from the epidermal portion of the verruca. Surrounding the relatively less structured apical area of the dome-shaped lesion, the wall of the epidural interface demonstrates relatively larger concavities for the reception of the dermal papillae, which at this peripheral margin were centripetally arranged and broadest at their bases, which were also the points of entry of the tapered dermal papillae into the epidermal interface. Nerves approach the lesion from below and

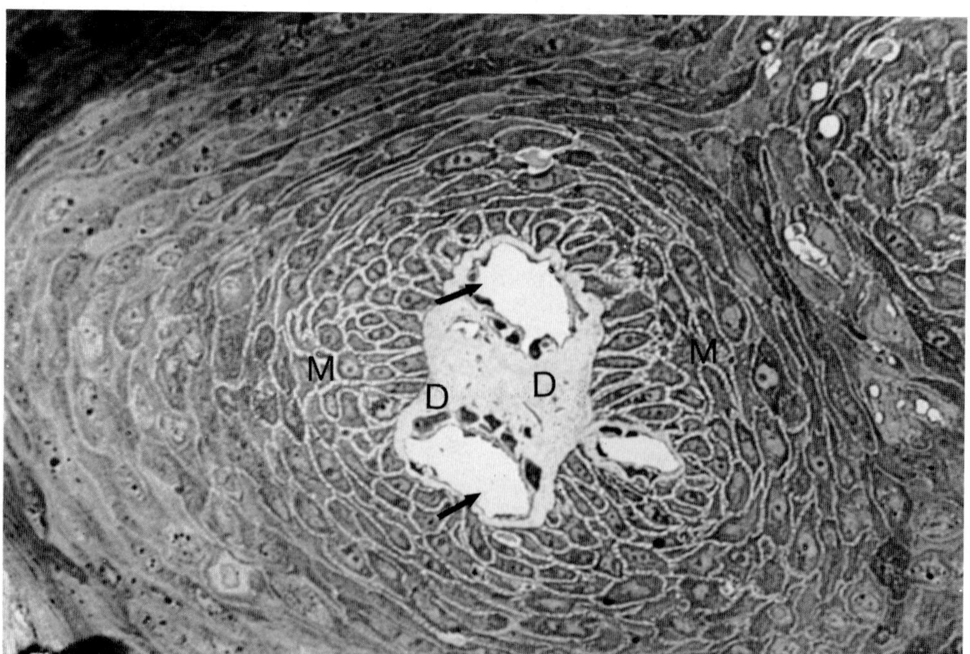

Figure 11.4. Apparent localization of blood vessels within the epidermis (*arrows*) is more apparent than real. Light microscopy in tangential section of tissue. *D*, dermal stroma; *M*, stratum Malpighii.

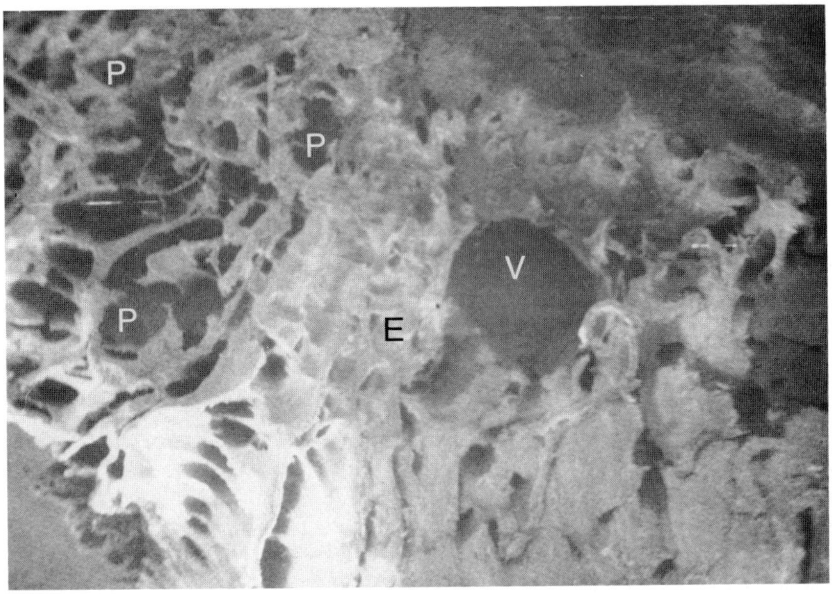

Figure 11.5. Scanning electron microscopic appearance of the epidermodermal interface in verrucae. Epidermal retia (*E*) converge about central blood vessel orifices (*V*). *P*, site of dermal papillae interdigitations.

converge upon the verruca. One quadrant, the upper right portion of the radially symmetrical lesion, is illustrated in the scanning electron micrograph.

Transmission Electron Microscopy

High magnification of verrucae demonstrates distinctive ultrastructural features. The upper wart-infected spinosal cells demonstrated that the inner and outer nuclear membranes of the nucleus underwent separation in some cells. The nucleolus appeared to be more electron-dense. Mitochondrial damage is apparent, and tonofibrils occurred as shorter, thicker fascicles in random arrangement (Fig. 11.6). Membrane-bound cytoplasmic vacuoles could be observed with some frequency, and the plasma membranes continued to be widened and somewhat tortuous (7). Endoplasmic reticulum and Golgi apparatus occurred sparsely in the attenuated cytoplasm. Some keratinocytes appear totally devoid of evidence of the presence of the papillomavirus, while some cells of the stratum spinosum demonstrated large numbers of virions in aggregation.

Signs of nuclear toxicity were evident in some cells from biopsies of verrucae plantaris. This took the form of cerebriform infoldings of the nuclear membrane. These were not deep enough to produce the so-called intranuclear pseudoinclusions (Fig. 11.7). Tonofilaments maintained essentially normal perinuclear orientation relative to cerebriform nuclei. However, in the cytoplasm of infected wart cells, the tonofilament-desmosome complex (TDC) was severely disrupted, and intercellular spaces were greatly expanded (Fig. 11.8).

Transmission electron microscopy revealed some detail of the nature of the infecting polyoma-papillomavirus implicated in the wart response. Portions of the endothelial cells lining the blood vessels are preserved, with matrix distributed about the vessels associated with collagen nearby within warty epidermis (Fig. 11.9). The virus particle is of icosahedral symmetry with a diameter of 52 nm with 72 individual capsomers, several of which have been identified with circles on the high resolution negatively stained insert (8). The confusion in the literature as to size and number of capsomers arises from artifact in preparation and failure of the early investigators to recognize that the virion was arranged in a skew fashion. As a result, some investigators derived too low a count, and others computed too great a number, depending upon the position of the virus investigated.

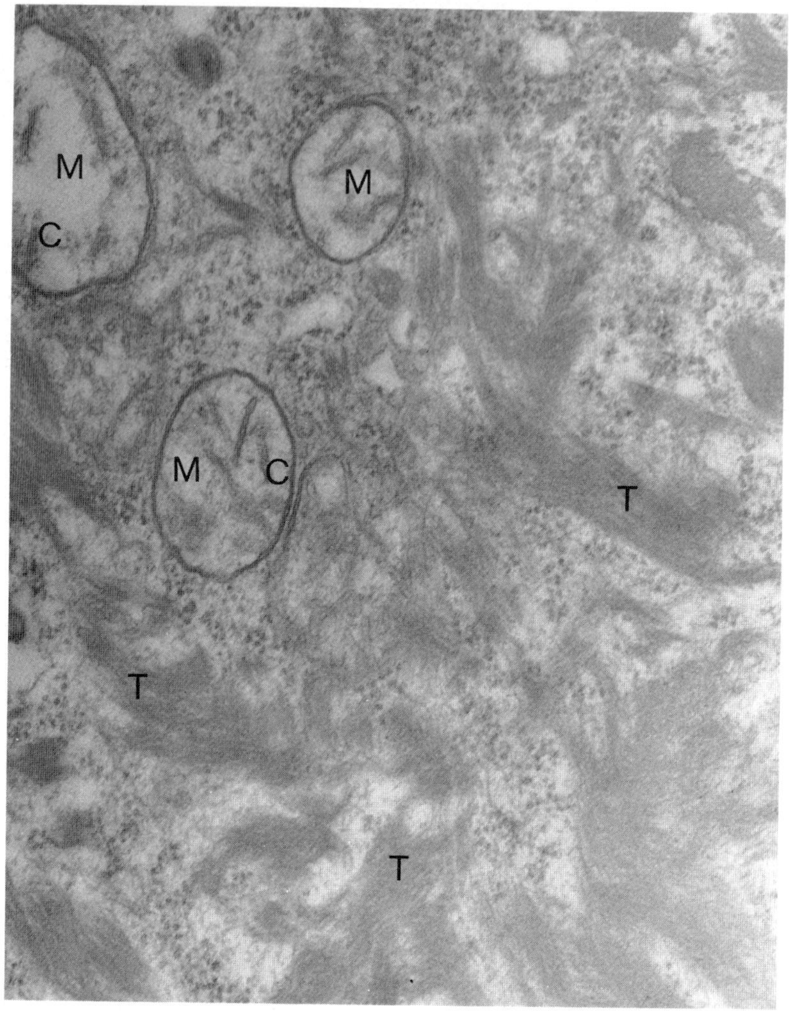

Figure 11.6. Mitochondrial damage in pedal verrucae (*M*). *C*, cristae; *T*, tonofilaments.

Treatment

The untreated lesion of verruca plantaris may assume a variable course and duration. Spontaneous disappearance is well documented (9, 10), and lesions may resolve during periods of emotional stress. The lesion may remain solitary or produce additional neoplastic lesions. Distant satellite lesions tend to remain independent, while nearby lesions may coalesce into a mosaic pattern. Treatment may reduce the duration and dimensions of the lesion and thereby lessen the likelihood of transmission or autoinoculation. However, because verruca plantaris is both benign and frequently self-limiting, ideal therapeutic modalities should be relatively innocuous. Reasons for treatment include discomfort, interference with asymptomatic ambulation, concern for transmission or autoinoculation, irritation of the involved skin, cosmetic considerations, age, and distribution of the lesions. The great number of treatment alternatives for verrucae suggests that no modality is universally effective in returning the hypertrophied prickle cell layer of the epidermis to the normal state. Various forms of treatment include posthypnotic suggestion therapy, electrodesiccation, ultrasound, irradiation, vitamins, steroids, enzymes, vaccines, antimetabolites, initiators of inflammation, cryoagents, and surgical intervention. Verrucae sometimes persist despite treatment, and alternative or adjunctive modalities may be necessary for resolution.

Posthypnotic suggestion therapy or psy-

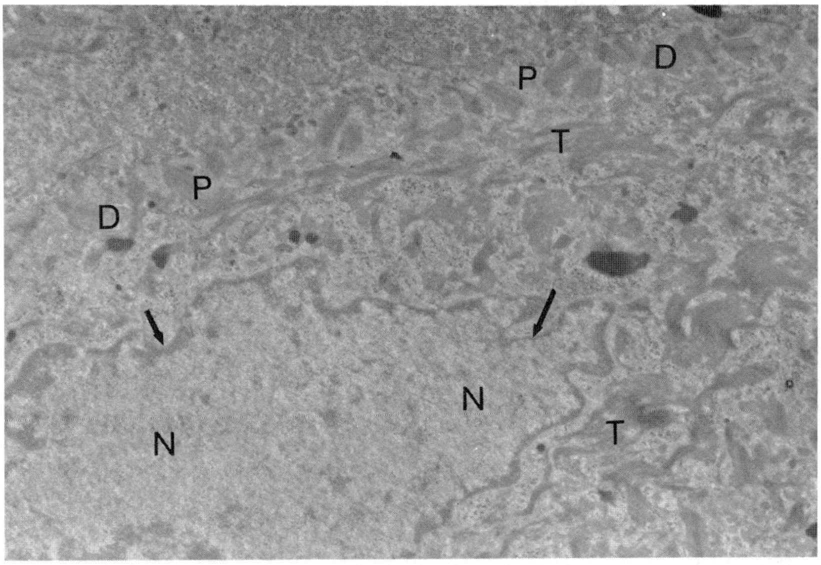

Figure 11.7. Cerebriform nucleus (*N*) in verrucae as demonstrated by transmission electron microscopy. *Arrows* indicate infoldings of the nuclear membrane. *P*, plasma membrane; *D*, desmosomes; *T*, tonofilaments.

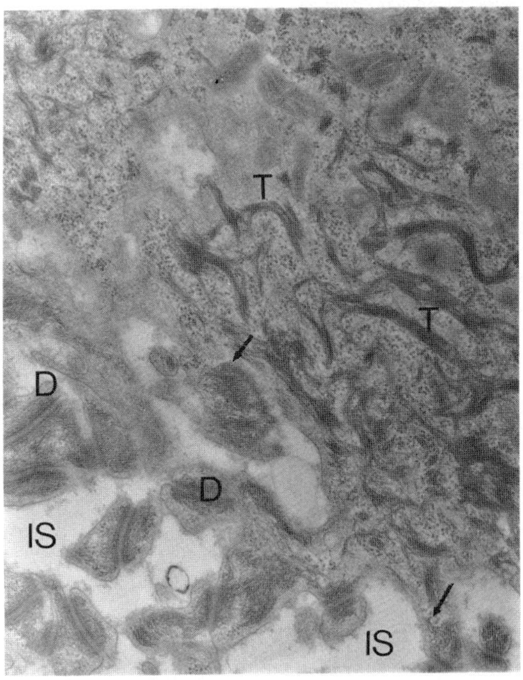

Figure 11.8. Greatly widened intercellular spaces and severe disruption of tonofilament-desmosome complex (TDC) as demonstrated by transmission electron microscopy (*arrows*). *IS*, intercellular spaces; *T*, tonofilaments; *D*, desmosomes.

chotherapy predate all other forms of treatment. They are still advocated by some practitioners (11). Whether suggestion therapy (or coincidental spontaneous regression) is responsible for resolution of the lesion remains the subject of considerable controversy.

Electrosurgery may be employed alone (12, 13) or adjunctively in the treatment of pedal verrucae. Both direct current (DC) in the negative galvanic technique and alternating current (AC) in the monoterminal or biterminal modalities are suitable (14). Tissue dehydration precedes charring, and cell death ensues with thrombosis of the small underlying blood vessels (15).

Ultrasonic energy provides still another therapeutic alternative. The protein molecules in the verrucous tissue selectively absorb the sound waves. A marked increase in temperature within the verruca may be responsible for its destruction (16). Ultrasound is typically applied at 1.5 W/cm^2 for 15 min at weekly intervals. It is ineffective in the eradication of widely separated plantar lesions (17).

X-radiation therapy involves the application of a tightly columnated roentgen beam to the verruca. The popularity of radiotherapy has declined steadily since the late 1960s, primarily over concern for potential ulceration or malignant transformation about the treatment site. Nonetheless, the proper administration of radiation therapy to verruca plantaris is still recommended by some physicians (18). In fact, a recent reexamination of 3675 verrucae pre-

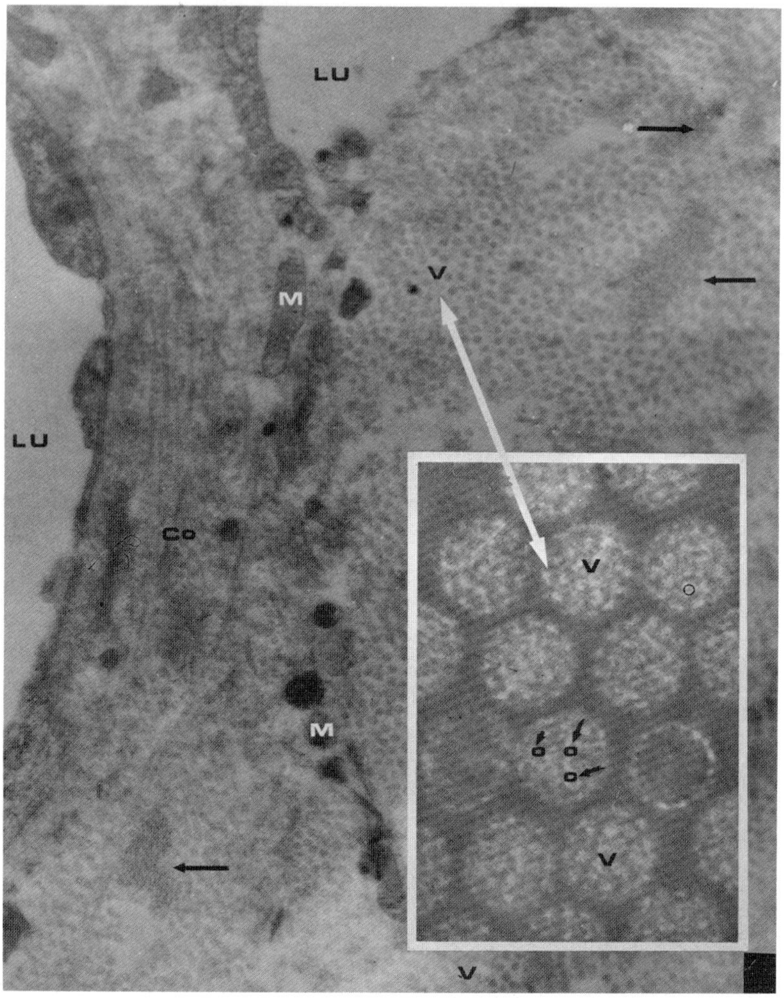

Figure 11.9. Papilloma virions (*V*) in verrucae have 72 unit capsomeres (*arrows*). *Lu*, blood vessel lumen: *Co*, collagenic fibers; *M*, mitochondria. *Inset* at *lower right* demonstrates capsomere morphology. The blank image at the right center is termed a "ghost."

viously treated with radiotherapy failed to uncover significant sequelae, except for changes in pigmentation, hyperkeratoses on weight-bearing surfaces, and subcutaneous atrophy in regions with a thin cutis (19). Side effects arose in 5 to 12% of the patients and were dependent upon the number of x-ray doses to the site (20).

Vitamin A compounds have been utilized orally and topically in the treatment of pedal verrucae, especially as an adjunctive agent (21). Although the usual oral dose is 50,000 IU (22), the dosing frequency is highly variable. In general, the use of vitamin A remains controversial (23, 24).

The topical application of corticosteroids have markedly reduced the size of some verrucae (25) and has initiated the total disappearance of others (26, 27). Apparently the verrucae respond to the anti-inflammatory property of the steroid.

Enzymes have been employed orally, topically, intralesionally, and subcutaneously in the management of plantar verrucae (28). The orally administered enzymes trypsin and chymotrypsin are most desirable as adjunctive agents (29). Fibrinolysin with deoxyribonuclease, in an ointment preparation, is topically administered (30). Direct application causes the fewest untoward effects and must be considered the preferred route.

Immunologic aspects of the papilloma virus are well known. Consequently, various vaccines have attempted to effect a cure. Both intralesional injections of the smallpox vaccine and subcutaneous injections of extracts from human verrucae have, in the past, received favorable reports (31, 32). Such substances attempt to block viral replication through the interferon system. The vaccines have numerous potential local and systemic side effects, and indications for their use no longer exist (33).

Antimetabolites and their derivatives inhibit the synthesis of viral and keratinocyte protein enzymes (7). The agents block cell division by substituting a competitive inhibitor in the production of nucleic acids. In essence, the antineoplastic antimetabolites deprive the papilloma virus (which is an obligate intracellular parasite) from the epidermal cell components which are necessary to sustain them. Intralesional (34) and topical (35) introduction of 5-fluorouracil to pedal verrucae has been evaluated by researchers worldwide. The intradermal injections consistently produced favorable results (34). However, results from the topical administration of the ointment are influenced by the frequency of application and the use of occlusive dressings (7, 35).

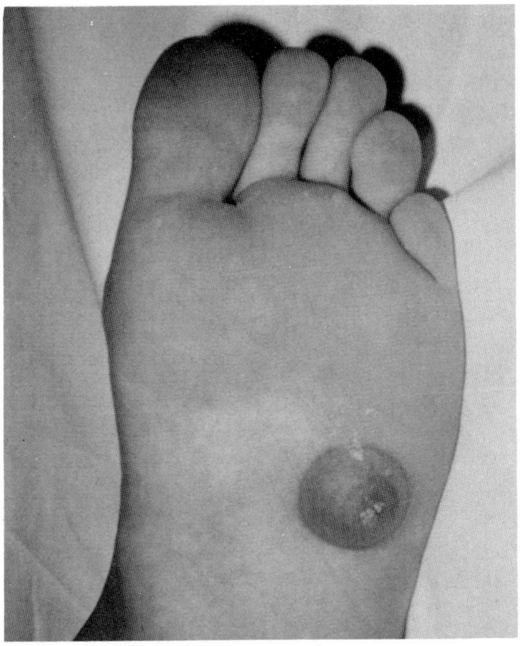

Figure 11.11. Appearance of plantar verrucae following cryocautery treatment. Courtesy of Dr. J. Yale, *Podiatric Medicine*: 151, 1980.

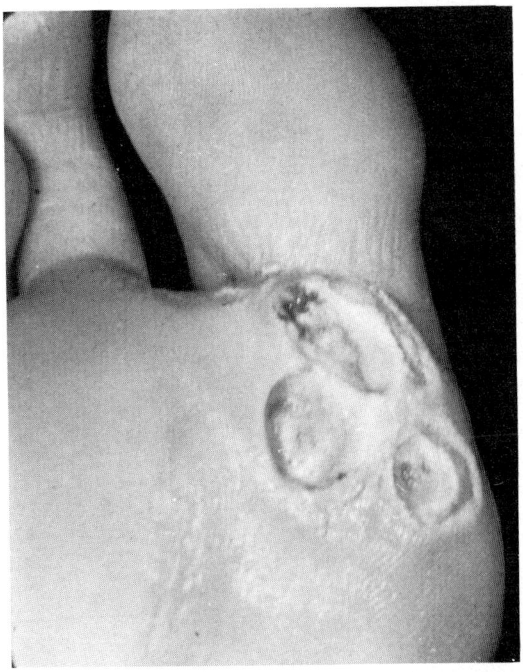

Figure 11.10. Appearance of plantar verrucae following treatment with 60% salicylic acid. Courtesy of Dr. J. Yale, *Podiatric Medicine*: 151, 1980.

Certain chemical agents irritate tissue and induce inflammatory processes with eventual necrosis of the verruca. Two general classes of chemical initiators of inflammation are the sclerotics and the escharotics. The sclerotics are seldom used. Among the escharotics, the acidic compounds act to oxidize tissue and the alkaline compounds act to dehydrate tissue (Fig. 11.10). The list of escharotic agents includes salicylic acid, salicylic-lactic acid, nitric acid, phenol, benzalkonium chloride dibromide (36), formalin (37), chloroacetic acids (38), cantharidin (39), and podophyllum resin (40).

The cryonecrotic activity of an agent is inversely related to its boiling temperature. Liquid nitrogen, liquid air, liquid oxygen, and carbon dioxide snow are cryotherapeutics capable of destroying verrucous tissue (Fig. 11.11). Necrosis occurs through ice formation, cellular dehydration and toxicity, thermal shock, denaturation of the lipoproteins, and vascular stasis (41). Immediately following the application, the verruca blanches; within hours an inflammatory reaction develops; and in 1 to 2 weeks the lesion hopefully sloughs. Rapid freezing followed by slow thawing produces optimal results (42). Cryotherapy may be utilized alone (43) or adjunctively (44) in the management of pedal verrucae.

The definitive treatment of pedal verrucae involves surgical intervention with excision of the lesion. A superficial incision is made to demarcate the boundaries of the verruca and to facilitate penetration of the dissecting instrument (45, 46) (Fig. 11.12). The blunt dissector separates verrucous from normal tissue. The lesion is "shelled-out" in toto, hopefully without violating the epidermal-dermal interface (47) (Fig. 11.13). The wound edges are saucerized via scalpel or scissors, and the cavity is curetted vigorously; fulguration (48), electrodesiccation (49), or caustics (50) may be adjunctively applied to the base. An absorbable gelatin hemostatic sponge is incorporated into a slightly compressive dry sterile dressing (51).

Utilization of the carbon dioxide laser in podiatric surgery remains in its formative stages. The intense beam of monochromatic light vaporizes precise amounts of tissue within a zone of hemocoagulation. The favorable results of a pilot study were recently reported (52).

Other miscellaneous treatment modalities reported in the literature include the antiviral agents idoxuridine (53) and acyclovir (54), the antibiotic bleomycin sulfate (55), and even the application of the inner side of a banana skin (56).

MOSAIC VERRUCAE

It is not uncommon for the normally well-circumscribed plantar wart to develop small satellite lesions which have a vesicular appearance. Such lesions tend to demonstrate a lesser degree of superficial keratinization. The parent lesion may have peripheral capillaries which radiate outward; satellite growths have central capillary tips oriented perpendicularly to the free surface of the skin (56).

When multiple verrucae with satellite lesions are left untreated in the presence of a compromised immunologic host response to the human papovavirus, mosaic verrucae may occur. The patchy irregularly outlined regions of this type of warty tissue have multiple cores which coalesce (Fig. 11.2). As a result of this phenomenon, mosaic warts demonstrate irregularity of depth: When shaved, they exhibit a propensity to bleed from the many capillaries which loop into the papillomatous superficial tissues.

Because of the immunologic problem, mosaic warts stubbornly resist most conventional means of therapy: Surgery, electrosurgery, psychotherapy, and treatment

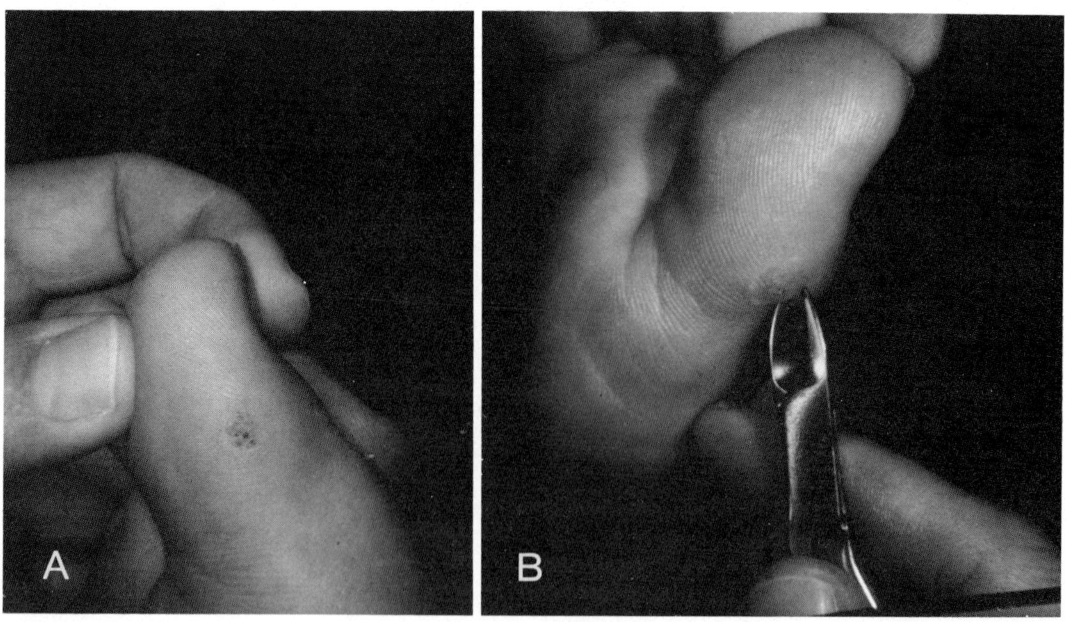

Figure 11.12. (*A*) Preoperative appearance. (*B*) Definitive excisional procedure for verrucae plantaris. The periphery of the lesion is sharply defined, and the incision is made.

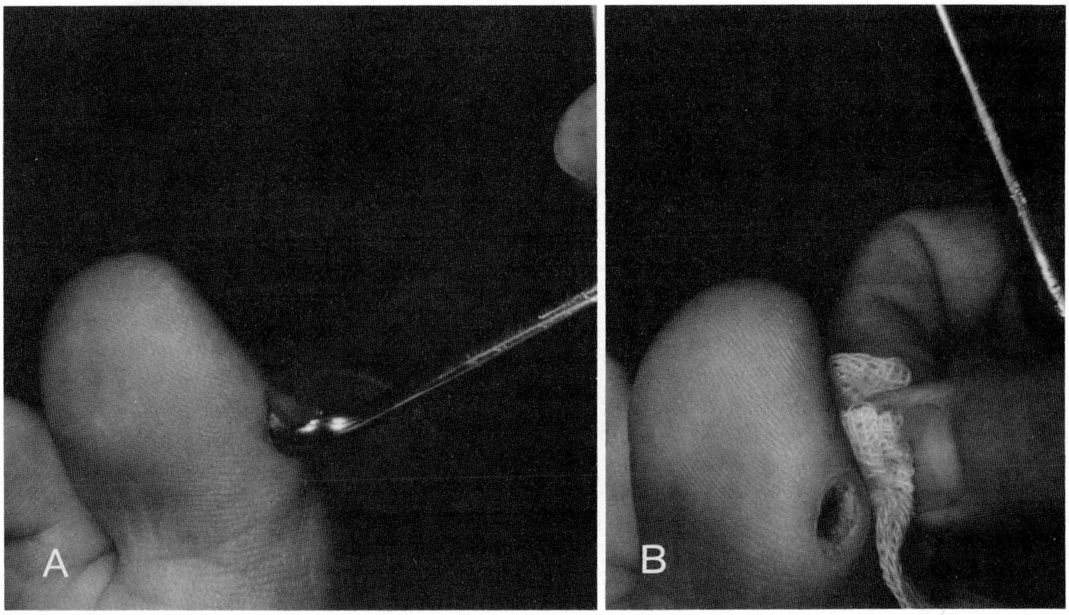

Figure 11.13. (*A*) Curettage of verrucae plantaris in toto following its initial delineation. (*B*) Postoperative appearance. Courtesy of Steven Berlin, D.P.M.

by means of topically applied acid compounds are usually doomed to failure. Radiotherapies and vaccinotherapy are absolutely contraindicated in this condition. Both patient and physician need to be prepared for a prolonged course of treatment. In general, the gentle regular application of combinations of acids over time is preferable to a heroic assault on these typically extensive lesions. Dr. Montgomery has found local applications of bichloroacetic acid and trichloroacetic acid covered with a 40% salicylic acid plaster to be especially helpful in the treatment of mosaic verrucae.

It is important not to overtreat this condition. Devitalization, tissue inflammation, and secondary infection are not likely to help the patient to develop resistance against the presence of the infecting virus. They must ultimately develop an immune response capable of dealing with this agent before the condition can be resolved. Above all, a positive favorable outlook must be maintained by both the patient and the physician.

MOLLUSCUM CONTAGIOSUM

Etiology

The molluscum contagiosum virus—an unassigned member of the mammalian poxvirus family or one of Nakano's group 2 poxviruses—is the largest true virus to cause human illness. It possesses structural characteristics midway between the variola group and the paravaccinia group of the poxviruses. The virus resembles other members of the poxvirus family in size, ultrastructure, genome, and chemical composition (58). The brick-shaped virus measures approximately 300 × 200 × 100 nm (59). A figure-8 shaped nucleoid lies within the inner membrane, which is separated from the outer membrane by two lateral bodies. The genome of the molluscum contagiosum virus is a linear, duplex DNA with terminal or near-terminal cross-links and a molecular weight of about 185×10^6 daltons (60). Like other poxviruses, the molluscum contagiosum virus replicates within the cytoplasm of the host cell and produces distinctive cytoplasmic inclusion bodies. Unlike other poxviruses, the virus can not reactivate heat-inactivated vaccinia virus (61), nor can it be cultured by methods suitable for the growth of other poxviruses (62).

Diagnosis

Because of its distinctive morphology, accurate diagnosis of molluscum contagiosum generally occurs "prima vista." The distribution of the lesions may support the initial impression based solely on morphology. Nonetheless, other disorders must be considered when atypical lesions or classic lesions in atypical locations or patients at low risk present with a suspected molluscum contagiosum infection. The extensive differential diagnosis of molluscum contagiosum includes inflammatory papules along with perforating lesions of granuloma annulare; histiocytoma, solitary Darier's disease, basal cell epithelioma (63), pyogenic granuloma, keratoacanthoma, leukoplakia (64), pyogenic molluscum pendulum, hidradenoma, intradermal nevus, lichen urticatus, neurofibromatosis, idiopathic keloid (63), dermatitis herpetiformis, atopic dermatitis, botryomycoma, and lichen planus. On the foot, molluscum contagiosum may resemble tylomas, helomas, and verrucae (65). Physical examination of the affected patient typically reveals between 5 and 20 growths, although much larger numbers have been documented. The individual lesion is an undisturbed state, possesses a smooth, spherical or dome-shape with a slight umbilication, pitting, or dell of the vertex (Fig. 11.14). The papular lesion usually measures 2 to 5 mm in diameter; however, nodules approaching 1 cm in diameter have developed. Initially the lesion appears firm and flesh-colored, changing to a softer texture and pearly white hue upon maturation (66). An easily expressible central core of caseous material, consisting of virus-packed clusters of epidermal cells, exists. Some lesions may be secondarily infected.

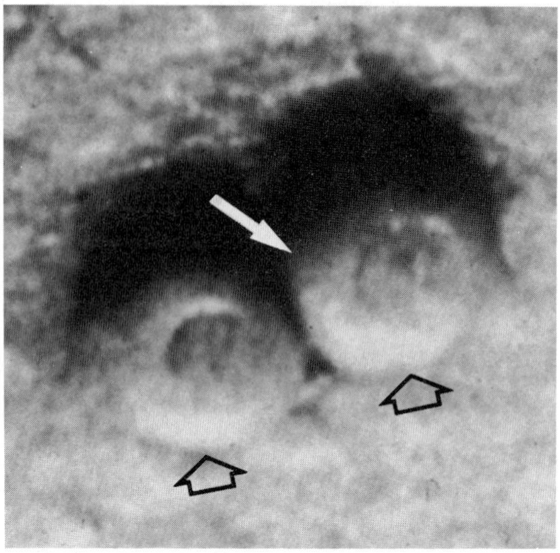

Figure 11.14. Clinical appearance of molluscum contagiosum. Courtesy of Ashur Rabinowitz, M.D.

Light Microscopy

Molluscum contagiosum appears clinically as an umbilicated papule with a caseating center. Microscopic examination at low power reveals the lesion to be an orderly lobulated mass with septations (Fig. 11.15). The lesion is a result of epidermal response to a large intracytoplasmic virus of the pox group. However, in any given lesion, most keratinocytes are normal. Diseased cells are dyskeratotic, many of which aggregate about a central chamber into which products of keratinization are discharged.

The stratum basale appears to be essentially normal at the light microscopic level, and the basement membrane is intact. The stratum spinosum is markedly acanthotic, and evidence of viral involvement can be detected in the lower levels of prickle cell aggregates. Intercellular spaces are widened, and desmosomes are conspicuous. Keratinocytes in the lower spinosum demonstrate a vesicular or hazy appearance, but as cells pass upward the nucleus becomes compressed and sickle shaped by these bodies.

Such cells assume a more oval appearance in the stratum granulosum. Transformation occurs in the keratohyaline layer so that hyalinized ellipsoid basophilic bodies pass upward through the hyperplastic epithelium. Such masses constitute the diagnostic molluscum bodies.

Their presence is pathognomonic and of considerable importance to the dermatohistopathologist. No evidence of virus formation can be identified in stratum basale cells, and the basement membrane is intact. Subcellular organelles may be reduced in numbers, although tonofilaments are plentiful.

Transmission Electron Microscopy

The stratum spinosum at high magnification reveals molluscum contagiosum virus as large brick-shaped virions measuring about 100 × 200 × 300 nm. Its DNA core is disc-like and biconcave. It is surrounded by an outer envelope which encapsulates a

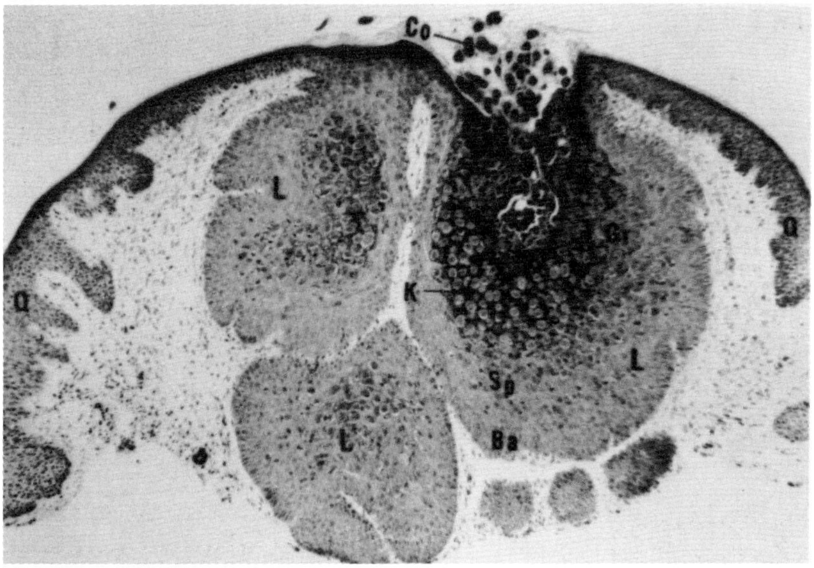

Figure 11.15. Light microscopic appearance of molluscum contagiosum at low power. *Q*, normal epidermis at either side of the centrally situated lesion: *L*, lobulations of acanthotic epidermis; *Ba*, normal-appearing basal cells associated with the lesion proper. *Co*, exfoliating virus infected cells; *K*, keratin surrounding abnormal cells of the stratum spinosum (*Sp*); *Gr*, stratum granulosum. From *Ultrastructure of Normal and Abnormal Skin*, Philadelphia, Lea & Febiger, 1967.

proteinaceous coat. This virus is a member of the poxvirus group which always replicates in the cytoplasm of host cells: In this case, it shows a tissue preference for keratinocytes of the skin.

Not all virions demonstrate the normal brick-shaped contours with typical centrally oriented dumbbell-shaped nucleoids. Certain viroplasmic regions of the cytoplasm of infected cells have areas of finely granular viroplasm in which viral membranes are delineated by alternately electron-dense and electron-lucid structures. Maturing virions appear spherical and more electron lucid than their mature counterparts; they are also bound by trilamellar membranes within which electron dense particles, presumably ribosomal particles can be identified (Fig. 11.16).

Treatment

Molluscum contagiosum is a self-limited cutaneous disease. Without therapy, the duration ranges from 6 months to 3 years with a particular lesion present for about 2 months. Spontaneous disappearance of the lesions is well documented (67, 68), and lesions may clear following posttraumatic inflammation (69) or secondary bacterial infection (70). Treatment may reduce the duration of the disease and, thereby, reduce the likelihood of transmission or autoinoculation. However, because the condition is both benign and self-limited, ideal therapeutic modalities should be relatively innocuous. Reasons for treatment include concern for transmission or autoinoculation, irritation or inflammation of the involved skin, cosmetic considerations, age of the patient, and distribution of the lesions. The great number of treatment alternatives for molluscum contagiosum suggests that no single modality is universally effective. Various forms of treatment include surgery, cryosurgery, and chemical initiators of inflammation. Despite the different mechanisms of action, each of the therapeutic agents attempts to mechanically eradicate the molluscum contagiosum virus from the infected epidermis. Classic surgical treatment involves incising the surface of the lesion and expressing the caseous core. Curettage, sometimes followed by light electrodesiccation, provides another surgical modality. Contemporary therapy includes cryotherapy with solid carbon dioxide or liquid nitrogen. Topical caustics or irritants, which desquamate the affected skin, include podophyllin (71), cantharidin (72),

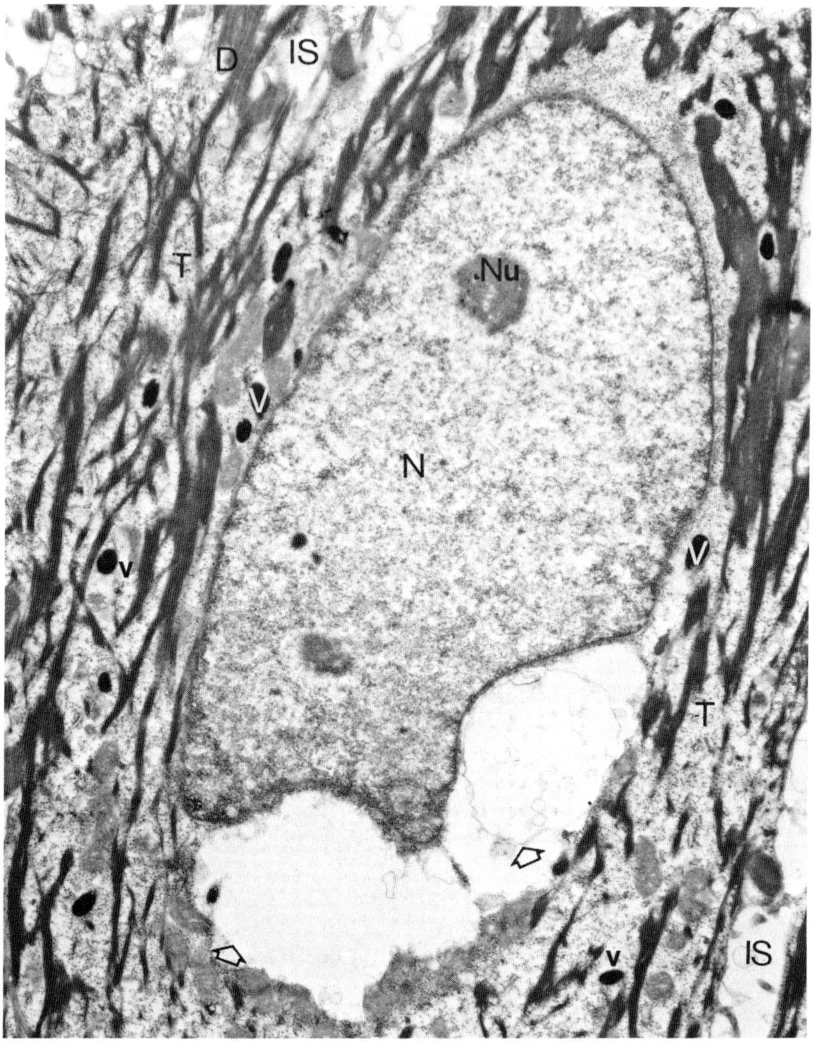

Figure 11.16. Molluscum contagiosum-infected keratinocyte as revealed by transmission electron microscopy. *Arrows* indicate a perinuclear vacuole. *N*, nucleus; *Nu*, nucleolus; *T*, tonofilaments; *D*, desmosomes; *IS*, intercellular spaces; *V*, virion of molluscum contagiosum.

silver nitrate (69), carbolic acid (73), tretinoin (74), phenol, mono-, di-, or trichloroacetic acid (63), tincture of iodine (70), and benzoyl peroxide. Salicylic acid and lactic acid produce inflammation of the skin. Alternative measures to local treatment encompass systemic medications such as griseofulvin (75), tetracycline, and the sulfonamides (57). The patient should be evaluated every week for 8 weeks to ascertain whether the lesions, including those clinically inconspicuous lesions, have resolved. The efficacy of the different treatment options has not been examined in controlled or blinded studies.

HERPES SIMPLEX AND HERPES ZOSTER

Etiology

The varicella-zoster virus—the common etiologic agent of chickenpox and herpes zoster—belongs to the herpesvirus family of deoxyribonucleic acid (DNA) tumorigenic viruses. Herpes zoster occurs by the reactivation of the varicella-zoster virus present in the body of a partially immune host (76). The virus resembles other members of the herpesvirus family in size, ultrastructure, genome, and chemical composition. The ovoid to brick-shaped virus measures approximately 130 to 200 nm in diameter (1). The varicella-zoster virus falls midway between the human papillomavirus and molluscum contagiosum virus in size and morphology. Like other herpesviruses, the virus replicates within the nucleus of the host cell and produces distinctive intranuclear inclusion bodies (77). The viral particles possess a 162-unit capsomere in an icosahedral arrangement (78).

The varicella-zoster virus is epidermotropic and grows well on human epidermis. The virus can not be cultured in eggs on the chorioallantoic membrane and can not be transmitted to laboratory animals. The virus can be cultured in vitro from specimens of infected cerebrospinal fluid. The etiologic agent will propagate on certain tissues such as human embryonic tissue and monkey kidney epithelium (1). The varicella-zoster virus is among the more readily cultured and propagated DNA viruses known to cause human disease (79). This characteristic of the virus has facilitated research on the replicative cells.

Pathogenesis and Pathology

The varicella-zoster virus initially invades the host through the mucous membrane of the respiratory tract. After the initial viremia the microorganism replicates within the reticuloendothelial system (79). The result of this primary infection is chickenpox. The disease is characterized by vesicular eruptions of the skin and mucous membranes (80). After the primary infection clears, the virus lies dormant in a latent form in the dorsal root ganglion or extramedullary cranial nerve root ganglion (1). Herpes zoster represents a reactivation of the virus and a resultant secondary viremia (81). It is believed that some type of provocation (for example, trauma and malignant processes) permits or stimulates the reactivation. Unlike chickenpox, which produces a disseminated eruption, herpes zoster typically remains confined to the dermatome supplied by the affected ganglion (32). However, the specific factors limiting the eruptive pattern remain unknown. Epidermal changes characteristic of herpes zoster develop after reactivation. Essentially, zoster is an inflammatory process with arteritis, arteriolitis, and capillaritis (1).

Massive ballooning and reticular degeneration within the infected epidermis produce tense intraepidermal vesicles (83). The inflammation of the blood vessels causes a markedly erythematous margin. The prickle cells initially demonstrate edema and loss of intracellular bridges with resultant acantholysis. Early lesions show unilocular vesicle evolving to multiloculations as the septae undergo lysis.

Clinical Features

The postulated clinical incubation period varies from 1 to 3 weeks (1). This estimate is based upon the observation of children with a negative history of chickenpox developing characteristic lesions of varicella 1 to 3 weeks after exposure to the contents of a herpes zoster vesicle. Prodromal symptoms of anorexia, malaise, and low grade fever precede the development of viral exanthems (80). Intense segmental pain in the dermatome(s) of the affected nerve(s) lasts for 3 to 5 days and typifies the preeruptive stage. Clusters of maculopapules appear and evolve into vesicles. Physical examination of the affected patient with a herpes zoster eruption typically reveals unilateral groups of small vesicles restricted to the nerve segment(s) of the involved posterior ganglia (82). The individual mature lesion, in an undisturbed state, possesses a translucent vesicle on an erythematous base (Fig. 11.17). The papulovesicular lesion usually measures 2 to 5 mm in diameter. The easily expressible central contents of serous material contain multinucleated giant cells with eosinophilic nuclear inclusions. Secondary infection of these lesions is a distinct possibility. Herpes zoster is frequently a self-limiting disease with a favorable prognosis. The duration of the uncomplicated attack varies from 2 weeks to 1 month and is somewhat dependent upon the age of the patient (82).

The primary sites of involvement for herpes zoster are those dermatomes supplied by nerve segments in the thorax, neck, face, sacral, and lumbar regions (66). Although uncommon, the cutaneous disorder has been described on various locations of the lower extremity, including the foot (82). Typically, the lesions are confined to a single, unilateral dermatome corresponding

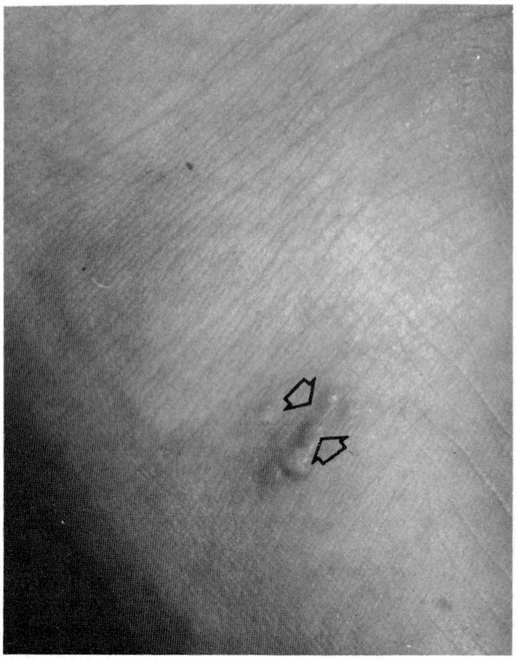

Figure 11.17. Clinical appearance in herpes simplex involving the arch area of the foot. Courtesy of Royal Montgomery, M.D.

to the nerve segment of the involved posterior ganglia.

Diagnosis

The accurate diagnosis of herpes zoster generally occurs solely upon clinical findings. The history, morphology, and distribution of the lesions may support the initial impression. The pathognomonic triad of clusters of vesicles, unilateral segmental distribution, and intense pain facilitates the diagnosis (1). Despite its characteristic clinical features, other disorders, such as unilateral vesiculation in poison ivy, must be considered in the preeruptive phase with neuralgic pain or when patients at low risk present with a suspected herpes zoster infection.

Light Microscopy

Herpes zoster or varicella demonstrates the presence of multinucleated giant cells with distinctive intranuclear inclusions. Such cytological features are best obtained at the light microscopic level, using scrapings from the bases of vesicular lesions and using Giemsa histologic staining techniques. Rapidly processed biopsies of the lesion may provide equally efficacious results.

Transmission Electron Microscopy

The best evidence for the analysis of zoster varicella virus is obtained by transmission electron microscopy. Such studies indicate that the stratum basale is the location at which the virus can be identified. The nuclei of such cells indicate a centripetal dispersion of chromatin in a manner which is typical for other viral conditions of the human skin.

Zoster virions are somewhat unique with respect to their ability to situate themselves at a variety of locations within the keratinocyte. Pleomorphism also characterizes the virions themselves in the intranuclear situation. In some instances, they possess a single-layered capsule which surrounds nucleoids of circular or elliptical shapes. Alternately, they may have a double-layered capsule which surrounds a central core of low electron density (Fig. 11.18).

The varicella-zoster virus, in addition to its outer envelope, has a capsid of 162 capsomeres (84). It is a DNA virus of the herpesvirus group which has a dimension of 160 nm when all replicative processes are complete. Their exit from basal cell nuclei can be accomplished in several ways (85): nuclear membrane disruption, reduplication of nuclear membrane, or nuclear pores may provide egress (Fig. 11.19).

Once in the host cell cytoplasm, virions may lie free and uncoated. Others are enclosed by smooth membrane bound vesicles; actually, the capsular membrane of virions seen in the cytoplasm may have been added by the host cell nuclear membrane during passage. Other virions appear to have been encapsulated by dilated rough endoplasmic reticulum.

Pleomorphism characterizes herpesvirus in the host basal cell keratinocytes: They may demonstrate one, two, or three capsular layers. An outer envelope is added to the virions by the host plasma membrane as it continues its passage out of the basal cell (85).

Once in the stratum spinosum, acantholysis occurs as the prickle cells lose their desmosomal attachments, round up, demonstrate degradation of subcellular organelles and, finally, lyse.

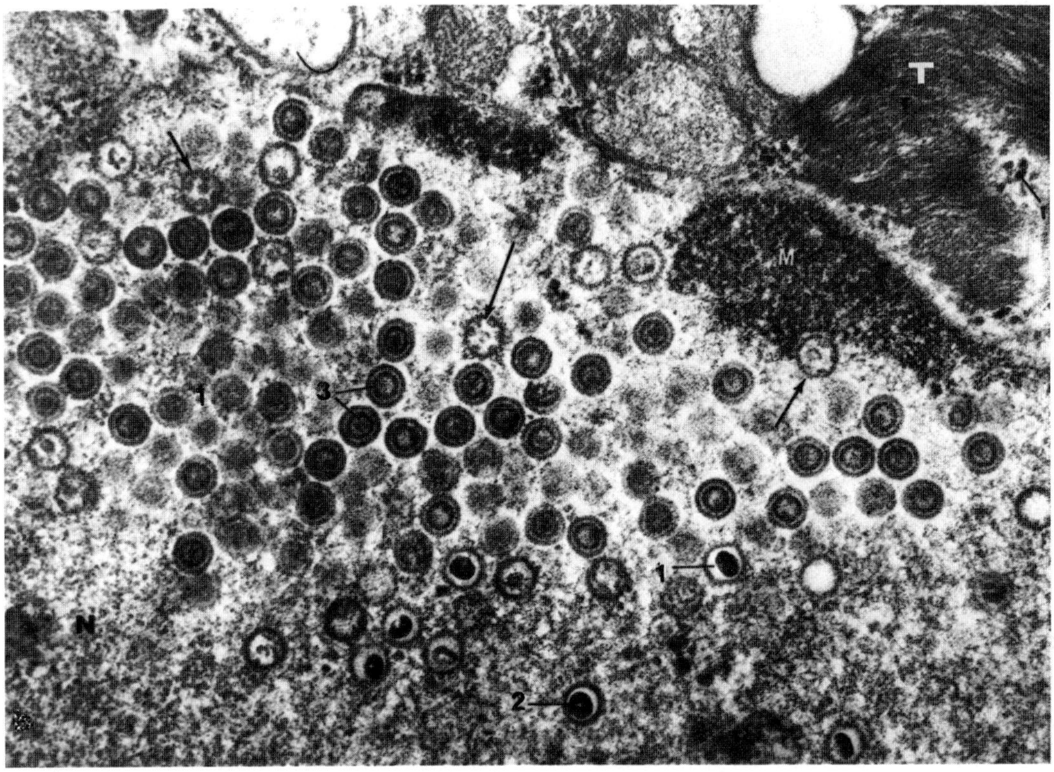

Figure 11.18. Four types of virions identified within the nucleus of keratinocyte herpes zoster infection. Types 1, 2, 3 are numbered for identification: the *arrows* mark a special type with an outer capsule with six circular structures symmetrically arranged on its inner surface and one circular structure in the center. *N*, nucleus; *M*, marginated chromatin within the nucleus; *T*, tonofibrils; *r*, ribosomes.

Treatment

Herpes zoster is usually a self-limiting cutaneous disease, although postherpetic complications sometimes arise. The duration of the uncomplicated attack ranges from 2 weeks to nearly 1 month (86). Treatment may reduce the duration of the disease and, thereby, reduce the likelihood of transmission to children who have not contracted chickenpox. Reasons for treatment include concern for transmission, symptomatic relief of pruritis, fever, and pain, reduction of the likelihood of protracted neuralgia, and avoidance of secondary bacterial infections (81). Various forms of treatment include local and systemic procedures. Topical application of astringent compresses are soothing and promote drying of the lesions. Typically, gauze bandages saturated with calamine lotion, zinc oxide, or iodochlorhydroxyquin are used. A flexible colloidin painted over the eruption diminishes hyperesthesia to contact with clothing. Later, a topical steroid cream and/or an antibiotic ointment may be employed. Systemic medications include analgesics, corticosteroids, gamma globulin, interferon and, in potentially fatal cases, lysozyme. The need for strong analgesics exists in most cases of herpes zoster. A frequent therapeutic regimen involves aspirin or acetaminophen with 15 to 60 mg of codeine by mouth every 4 hr (80). Large initial oral doses of steroids, equivalent to 40 to 60 of prednisone in single or divided daily doses, are tapered weekly over a 3- to 6-week period (87). Gamma globulin (approximately 0.5 ml/kg), has been advocated in both the treatment of chickenpox and herpes zoster (88). Some investigators claim success with interferon and interferon inducers. Severe cases of herpes zoster might warrant the use of lysozyme (500 mg/day intravenously for 1 week, then orally for 2 weeks (1)).

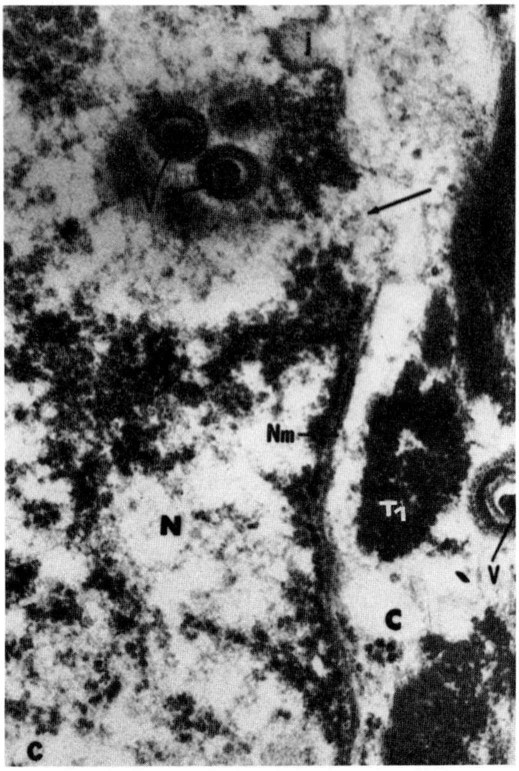

Figure 11.19. Virions exiting through the nuclear membrane results in separation of its trilamellar structure. *V*, represents virions lying near the location of a disruption (*arrow*) of the nuclear membrane (*Nm*). *J*, site of evagination of the nuclear membrane; *V*, virion, *C*, cytoplasm; T_1, tonofilaments in cross section; *T*, tonofilaments in longitudinal section.
From *Ultrastructure of Normal and Abnormal Skin*, Philadelphia, Lea & Febiger, 1967.

References

1. Nasemann T: *Viral Diseases of the Skin, Mucous Membranes and Genitals.* Philadelphia, W.B. Saunders, 1977.
2. Scranton PE: The management of superficial disorders of the forefoot. *Foot Ankle* 2:238, 1982.
3. Gibbs R: Calluses, corns, and warts. *Am Fam Phys* 3:92, 1971.
4. Montgomery RM: Diagnosis of plantar warts. *Cutis* 3:1233, 1967.
5. McCarthy DJ: A morphogenic and histochemical analysis of pressure prone verrucae of the human foot. *J Am Podiatry Assoc* 67:377, 1977.
6. McCarthy DJ: Alterations in the morphology of dermo-epidermal interface of pedal verrucae as revealed by scanning electron microscopy. *J Am Podiatry Assoc* 66:505, 1976.
7. McCarthy DJ, Berlin SJ: The ultrastructural effects of 5-fluorouracil in the management of pedal verrucae. *J Am Podiatry Assoc* 72:302, 1982.
8. McCarthy DJ, Rusin V: The implications of ultrastructural modifications induced by cryocautery in pedal verrucae. *J Am Podiatry Assoc* 67:312–322, 1977.
9. Bauer, MB: Treatment of plantar warts with acyclovir. *Am J Med* 73:313, 1982.
10. Gibbs, RC, Costello MJ: *Palms and Soles.* Chicago, Charles C Thomas, 1967.
11. Wygant L: Hypnosis in a case of multiple verrucae. *J Am Podiatry Assoc* 51:660, 1961.
12. Isreal RM: How I treat plantar warts. *Postgrad Med* 46:215, 1969.
13. Weisfeld M: Understanding porokeratosis plantaris discreta. *J Am Podiatry Assoc* 63:138, 1973.
14. Kligman I: Irradication of verrucae with negative galvanic. *J Foot Surg* 6:84, 1967.
15. Maddin S: *Current Dermatologic Management.* St. Louis, C.V. Mosby, 1970.
16. Bartolomei FJ, Biggs EW: Ultrasonic energy in the treatment of verruca plantaris. *Curr Podiatry* 31: (2):16, 1982.
17. Tropp BE: Ultrasound in verruca plantaris: report of a study. *J Am Podiatry Assoc* 57:326, 1967.
18. Shair HM: On radiotherapy for plantar warts. *J Dermatol Surg Oncol* 5:257, 1979.
19. Veien NK, Norholm A, Hattel T, et al: Late effects of x-ray treatment of warts. *J Dermatol Surg Oncol* 8:275, 1982.
20. Shair HM, Hanshaw WJ, Drayson LD: Radiation therapy for plantar warts. *J Dermatol Surg Oncol* 4:635, 1978.
21. Harris L: Combined electro-desiccation and chemo-surgery for plantar verruca. *J Am Podiatry Assoc* 56:100, 1966.
22. Lieberman H: An empirical treatment for mosaic verrucae. *J Am Podiatry Assoc* 50:737, 1960.
23. McLaughlin RR: Treatment of plantar warts. *Arch Dermatol* 106:129, 1972.
24. Gunther SH: Retinoic acid vs. placebo in linear verrucose nevi, scaly, lichenified eczema, and verruca plantaris. *Br J Dermatol* 89:317, 1973.
25. Harry TV: Treatment of warts with dexamethasone. *Practitioner* 203:356, 1969.
26. Babu TN: Treatment of warts with dexamethasone. *Practitioner* 210:478, 1968.
27. Yeretsian KH: The vanishing warts. *Practitioner* 194: 824, 1965.
28. Cramer L: Parenzyme injection for plantar warts. *J Am Podiatry Assoc* 48:526, 1958.
29. Bornstein B: Effects of oral chymotrypsin on surgical sequellae. *J Am Podiatry Assoc* 53:349, 1963.
30. Owens RE: More and more verrucae. *J Foot Surg* 6:200, 1967.

31. Biberstein H: Immunization therapy of warts. *Arch Dermatol Syphilol* 50:12, 1944.
32. Hutchinson R: The treatment of warts by viral interference. *Practitioner* 204:700, 1970.
33. Memorandum on Vaccination Against Smallpox, 1967. London, Ministry of Health Stationary Office.
34. McCarthy DJ, Tate R, Rusin J: Intradermal use of 5-fluorouracil in human pedal verrucae. *J Am Podiatry Assoc* 69:587, 1979.
35. Bunney MH: The treatment of plantar warts with 5-fluorouracil. *Br J Dermatol* 89:96, 1973.
36. Hellier FF, Roberts S, Whitefield M: The treatment of warts. *Practitioner* 202:67, 1969.
37. Anderson I: The treatment of plantar warts. *Br J Dermatol* 75:725, 1972.
38. Gibbs RC: Conservative management of plantar warts by gentle chemocautery. *J Dermatol Surg Oncol* 4:915, 1978.
39. Ormond CS: Cantharone, a cantharidin tincture as a useful agent in treating intractable plantar lesions. *J Am Podiatry Assoc* 52:427, 1962.
40. Beckman H: *Dilemmas in Drug Therapy.* Philadelphia, W.B. Saunders, 1967.
41. Zacarian SA: *Cryosurgery of Skin Cancer and Cryogenic Techniques in Dermatology.* Chicago, Charles C Thomas, 1969.
42. Purdey EJ: Liquid air in the treatment of warts *J Am Coll Health Assoc* 18:225, 1970.
43. Kingland HD: Cryotherapy in the treatment of verrucae. *J Am Podiatry Assoc* 52:435, 1962.
44. Oliver WW: Conservative treatment of verruca plantaris for children. *J Am Podiatry Assoc* 49:413, 1959.
45. Lerner L: Management of plantar verruca via excision and curettage. *J Am Podiatry Assoc* 49:11, 1959.
46. Overcase VC: Curetting verrucae with minimum hemorrhage. *J Natl Assoc Chirop* 47:187, 1957.
47. McGregor RR, Wehr GV: Blunt dissection of plantar verrucae using a new instrument. *J Am Podiatry Assoc* 64:92, 1974.
48. McLaughlin CR: Plantar warts—a plea for rationale treatment. *Lancet* 1:168, 1948.
49. Lapidus PW: Orthopedic skin lesions of the soles and toes. *Clin Orthop* 45:87, 1966.
50. Schenkman SP: Curettage and cautery of verrucae. *J Am Podiatry Assoc* 51:659, 1961.
51. Silver CM, Simon SD, Litchman HM: The use of orahesive in the surgical treatment of plantar verruca. *Rhode Island Med J* 52:680, 1969.
52. Borovoy M, Fuller TA, Holtz P et al: Laser surgery in podiatric medicine—present and future. *J Foot Surg* 22:353, 1983.
53. Manilla GT, Hood TK, Eakin NR: Treatment of plantar warts. *Rocky Mountain Med J* 63:42, 1965.
54. Bauer DJ: Treatment of plantar warts with acyclovir. *Am J Med* 73:313, 1982.
55. Koenig RD, Horowitz LR: Verruca plantaris—effective treatment with bleomycin: review of the literature and case presentations. *J Foot Surg* 21:109, 1982.
56. Warszawer-Schvarcz L: Treatment of plantar warts with banana skin. *Plast Reconstruct Surg* 68:975, 1981.
57. Montgomery RM: Painful cutaneous lesions of the foot. *South Med J* 63:615–619, 1970.
58. Nakano JH: Comparative diagnosis of poxvirus disease. In Kurstak E, Kurstak C: *Comparative Diagnosis of Viral Diseases.* New York, Academic Press, 1977.
59. Kwittken J: Molluscum contagiosum: some new histological observations. *Mt Sinai J Med* 47:583, 1980.
60. Postlethwaite R: Molluscum contagiosum: a review. *Arch Environ Health* 21:432, 1970.
61. Brown T, Butler P, Postlethwaite R: Nogenetic reactivation studies with the virus of molluscum contagiosum. *J Gen Virol* 19:417, 1973.
62. McFadden G, Pace W, Purres J et al: Biogenesis of poxviruses: transitory expression of molluscum contagiosum early functions. *Virology* 94:297, 1979.
63. Olansky S, Clair A: How we treat molluscum contagiosum. *Postgrad Med* 47:259, 1970.
64. Hartzell MB: The epidemic of epithelioma (molluscum) contagiosum, with some new observations concerning the "molluscum bodies." *Med Rec* 81:1171, 1912.
65. Campanelli M, DiCenso F: Molluscum contagiosum: a case report. *J Am Podiatry Assoc* 68:566, 1978.
66. Fitzpatrick T, Polano M, Suurmond D: *Color Atlas and Synopsis of Clinical Dermatology.* New York, McGraw-Hill, 1983.
67. Reed RJ, Parkinson RP: The histiogenesis of molluscum contagiosum. *Am J Surg Pathol* 1:161, 1977.
68. Kipping HF: Molluscum dermatitis. *Arch Dermatol* 103:106, 1971.
69. Jacobs PH: Molluscum contagiosum. *Aerospace Med* 41:1196, 1970.
70. Kaye JW: Problems in therapy of molluscum contagiosum. *Arch Dermatol* 94:454, 1966.
71. Curtin BJ, Theodore FH: Ocular molluscum contagiosum. *Am J Ophthalmol* 39:302, 1959.
72. Funt TR: Cantharidin treatment of molluscum contagiosum. *Arch Dermatol* 83:504, 1961.
73. Paton EP: Seven cases in which operation wounds were infected with molluscum con-

tagiosum. *Westminster Hosp Gazette* 16:11, 1909.
74. Papa CM, Berger RS: Venereal herpes-like molluscum contagiosum: treatment with tretinoin. *Cutis* 18:537, 1976.
75. Kapur TR: Griseofulvin therapy in molluscum contagiosum: a case report. *Ind J Dermatol Venereol Leprol* 42:90, 1976.
76. Hata S: Cell-mediated immunity to varicella-zoster virus demonstrated by lymphocyte transformation in herpes zoster. *J Dermatol* 10:13, 1983.
77. Kurtis B: Laboratory diagnosis of cutaneous herpes simplex and varicella-zoster infections. *Trans St John's Hosp Dermatol Soc* 61:35, 1975.
78. Benn RA: Laoratory of diagnosis of microbiological skin disease. *Intern J Dermatol* 16:476, 1977.
79. Domonkos AN, Arnold HL Jr, Odom RB: *Andrews' Diseases of the Skin Clinical Dermatology*, ed 7. Philadelphia, W.B. Saunders, 1982.
80. Berkow R (ed): *The Merck Manual of Diagnosis and Therapy*. Rahway, NJ, Merck, 1977.
81. Fitzpatrick TB, Arndt KA, Clark WH: *Dermatology in General Medicine*. New York, McGraw-Hill, 1971.
82. Samitz MH: *Cutaneous Disorders of the Lower Extremities*. Philadelphia, J.B. Lippincott, 1981.
83. Hope-Simpson RE: The nature of herpes zoster: a long-term study and a new hypothesis. *Proc R Soc Med* 58:1, 1965.
84. Holmes LH, Watson DH: Electron microscopic study of the attachment and penetration of herpes virus in BHRU cells. *Virology* 21:112, 1963.
85. Morgan C, Ross HM, Holden M et al: Electron microscopic observations on the development of herpes simplex virus. *Exp Med* 110:643, 1959.
86. Moschella SL, Pillsbury DM, Hurley HJ Jr: *Dermatology*. Philadelphia, W.B. Saunders, 1975.
87. Eaglestein WH, Katz R, Brown JA: The effects of early coticosteroid therapy on the skin eruption and pain of herpes zoster. *JAMA* 211:1681, 1970.
88. Krugman S, Ward R: *Infectious Diseases of Children*, ed 3. St. Louis, C.V. Mosby, 1964.

CHAPTER 12

Cutaneous Infestations

JAMES R. BLACK and NEIL A. FENSKE

This discussion of podiatric cutaneous infestations is limited to six common clinical entities: larva migrans, mites, ticks, fleas, spiders, and ants. This is not a definitive discussion of all cutaneous infestations but represents the authors' clinical experience.

LARVA MIGRANS

Larva migrans, commonly referred to as "creeping eruption," is a cutaneous disorder named for its clinical description. The condition is caused by a variety of different nematodes, the larvae of which migrate or burrow under the skin.

Although man is not a natural host for the larvae, infestations occur through contact with warm, damp sand or dirt where the larvae are hatching. Gardeners, children, people who go barefoot, and workers who are required to crawl under houses are the most likely victims. The condition is more prevalent in the Southeastern region of the United States and in South America; however, documented cases have been reported in the Eastern coastal states as far north as New Jersey (1).

Clinical Manifestation

The initial contact with the larvae may present a nonspecific dermatitis at the point of entry. Generally, the infected sight is characterized by itching and the formation of small reddish papules. The larvae may hibernate for hours or even months before migrating through the epidermis. The larvae then migrate aimlessly throughout the skin until they are rejected or die.

Once the larvae begin to burrow, small thread-like tunnels, characteristic of the infestation, start to form. These lesions form on the superficial surface of the skin, often interrupted by the small red papules that appear when the larvae are at rest. There may be singular or multiple linear eruptions, depending on the extent of the infestation (Fig. 12.1).

The pinkish lesions are approximately 2 to 4 mm in width and slightly elevated. The burrows may be straight, looped, curved, or the shape of whatever course the larvae venture to take (Fig. 12.2). These larvae tracks can continue to lengthen up to an inch or more daily.

It is relevant for the podiatric physician to consider that the clinical presentation on weight bearing surfaces may not resemble the classical description. Specifically, the urticarial tracts may be less discreet and less elevated than on nonweight-bearing areas (Fig. 12.3). Additionally, the thickness of the stratum corneum on the plantar aspect of the foot may be a causal factor in contributing to an altered appearance of the lesion. For these reasons, cutaneous larva migrans on the sole of the foot have been inappropriately diagnosed and treated as bacterial cellulitis and lymphangitis (12).

The eruptions are extremely pruritic and may be so severe as to inhibit sleep. The intense scratching resulting from the pruritus often leads to eczema followed by secondary infection. In severe cases, systemic involvement may occur as the larvae migrate to the lungs and other organs.

Etiology

The usual source of larva migrans in the United States and South America is due to intestinal hookworms in dogs and cats. The most common is *Ankylostoma braziliense*; however, *Ankylostoma canium* is also present in these domestic animals. In Europe, the dog hookworms commonly seen is *Uncinaria stenoceophala.* Other forms of larva

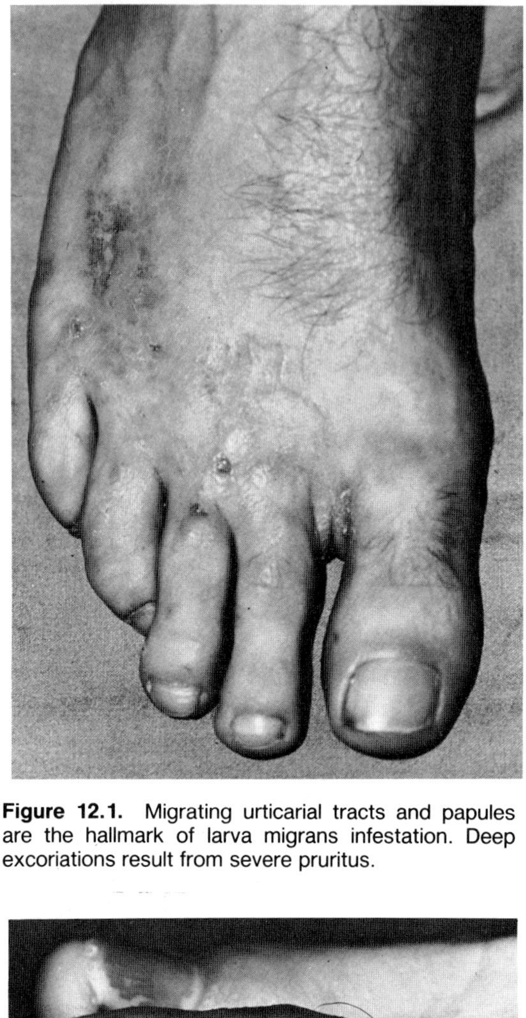

Figure 12.1. Migrating urticarial tracts and papules are the hallmark of larva migrans infestation. Deep excoriations result from severe pruritus.

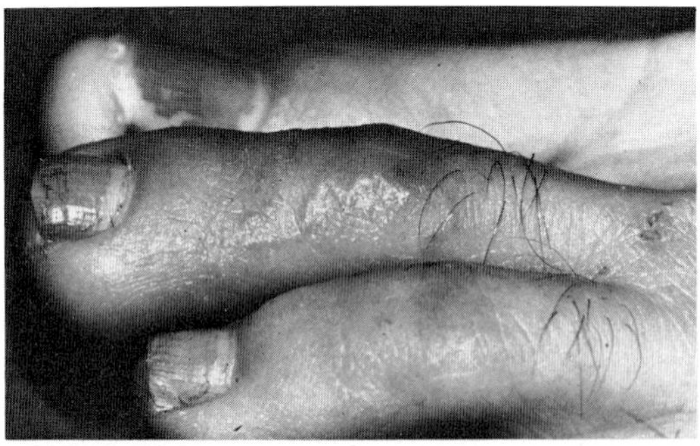

Figure 12.2. Close-up tract showing characteristic serpiginous configuration of the eruption.

migrans which may present are *Ankylostoma ceylonicum*, *Gnathostoma spinigerum*, *Bunostomum phlebotomum*, *Dirofilaria conjunctivae*, and *Capillaria* sp.

The *A. braziliense* passes from the intestines of its natural hosts (dogs and cats) when its ova is deposited in the animal's excrement. When the feces is dropped in an environment where the soil is warm and

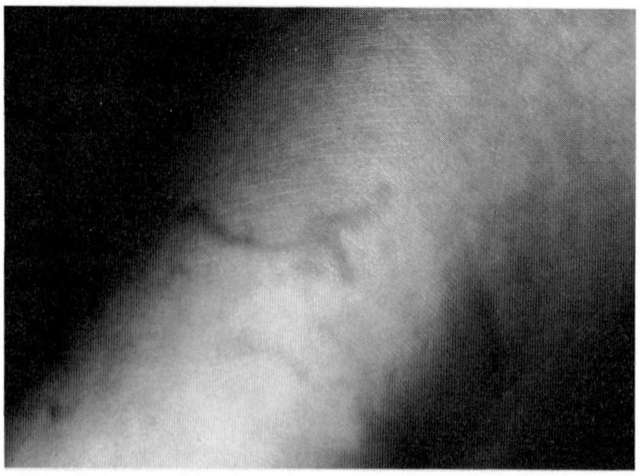

Figure 12.3. Infestation of the palmar-plantar surface may mimic lymphangiitis due to the thickened stratum corneum occurring in these anatomic sites.

damp, the larvae hatch and flourish. This infected larvae can penetrate the human skin upon contact.

Eruptions may also be caused by certain types of fly larvae such as the *Gastrophilus* (horse bot fly) and the *Hypoderma* (cattle warble fly) (3).

Human intestinal infections caused by *Strongyloides stercoralis* can mimic larva migrans in the perianal area. This is referred to as larva currens (4).

Differential Diagnosis

The serpiginous lesions are atypical and easily recognized. However, the diagnosis is often confused by eczema and secondary infections resulting from intense scratching by the patient.

Definitive Diagnosis

As stated earlier, the irregular, migrating burrows are characteristic of larva migrans. As the larva advances, the early tunnels crust, thus contributing to the intense pruritus.

It is important to determine if the patient has been exposed to the environmental conditions associated with larva migrans. If a dog or cat stool sample is available from the environmental area of infestation, it may reveal the hookworm ova (5).

It is generally impossible and unnecessary to extract the larva specimen from the patient because of its microscopic size. Lab tests, however, may show the presence of eosinophilia.

Treatment

When bacterial infections and eczema inhibit the definitive diagnosis, it may be advisable to prescribe antibiotics or topical steroids to control the itching.

The primary course of treatment is aimed at destroying the larva and separating it from the host. Small, localized infestations can be destroyed by cryosurgery (6). Carbon dioxide snow, ethyl chloride spray, or liquid nitrogen can be used. The freezing must be aimed just ahead of the burrow, where the larva is located.

The treatment of choice is thiabendazole (Mintezol), taken internally or used as a topical suspension. For topical application, the suspension is applied twice per day for 1 to 3 weeks with little or no resulting side effects. Internal treatment with thiabendazole is very effective when given in dosages of 25 mg per kg of body weight, twice daily for 2 days. However, side effects have been reported, and it should be used with caution in patients with liver disease (7). Dizziness, nausea, vomiting, abdominal pain, and headaches are possible side effects associated with oral thiabendazole.

MITES

Although mite infestation is a highly contagious condition, the incidence of this entity has been grossly underestimated. For simplification, we will focus this discussion on "human itch mites" or scabies. We will also discuss the other types of mites seen in a podiatric practice, which have other natural hosts but occasionally infest humans.

Sarcoptes scabiei var. *hominis*, causes an extremely pruritic skin condition, more commonly known as scabies. Ancient historical references to scabies go as far back as the Babylonian and later Roman eras (8). Scabies have always plagued soldiers because the highly contagious infestation flourishes when war conditions force people to live in close, filthy surroundings.

Scabies is acquired through physical contact with an infested person. It is commonly spread to other family members, bed partners, close acquaintances, and among schoolchildren. It is not limited to any one sector of society.

Clinical Manifestation

The initial contact is generally followed by an incubation period of 3 weeks to 1 month before the patient exhibits any symptoms. The skin is then apparently sensitized to the mite and reacts with extreme pruritus. At this point there are very few organisms present. The itching worsens in the nocturnal hours and often prevents sleep.

The primary site is a tiny, greyish burrow. A papular rash with vesicles soon develops. Unlike the larva migrans, these initial burrows are much narrower, noninflammatory, and limited to a few millimeters in length. They are often indistinguishable (Fig. 12.4). Both the male and female mites inhabit the area. The females are twice as large as the males and are continually depositing eggs. These eggs hatch within days, and the larvae continue to spread over the skin.

The common areas of infestation are on the nipple region in females, on the genital area in males (Fig. 12.5), and on the abdomen, wrists, elbows, axillae, hands, and feet. Usually, more than one area is affected. The primary lesions and burrows are most apparent in the interdigital spaces of the hands and feet (Fig. 12.6). The extent of the infestation between the toes relates directly to hygiene.

It is uncommon for scabies to primarily infest the feet. However, in the April 1980 edition of the *Journal of the American Podiatry Association* (*JAPA*), a case study outlines a scabies outbreak on the feet of a

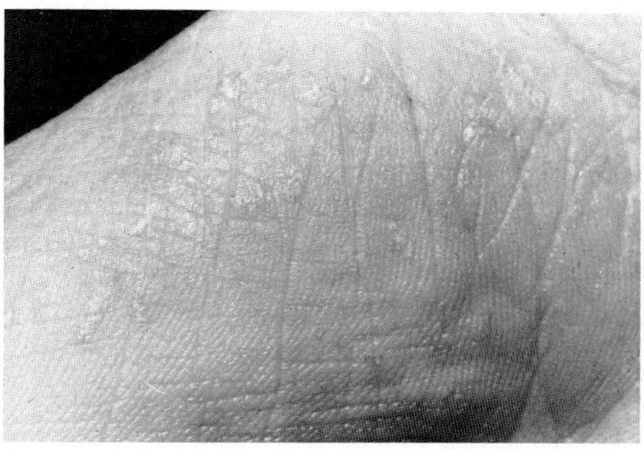

Figure 12.4. Subtle, superficial, noninflammatory burrows on this patient's foot are the hallmark of scabies infestation.

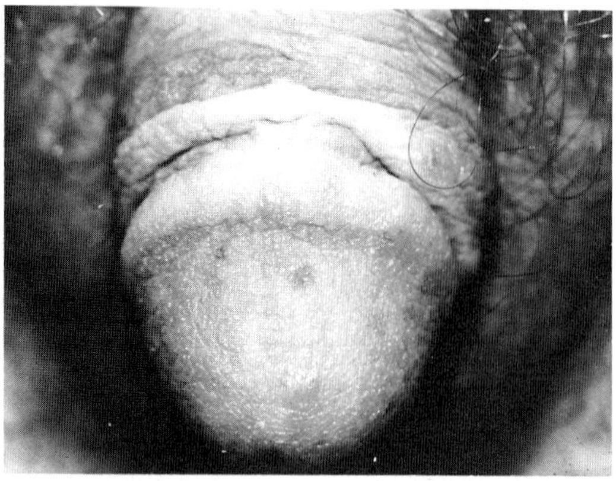

Figure 12.5. The genitals are frequently affected in scabies. Here the condition is often manifest as scabietic nodules. These represent an allergic phenomenon, thus they do not respond to antiscabietics but, instead, to topical corticosteroids.

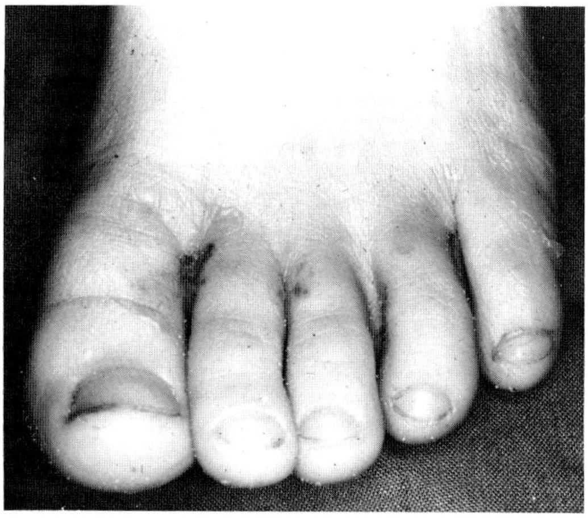

Figure 12.6. The interdigital spaces of the hands are commonly affected by scabies. The feet may be similarly involved. Lesions consisting of noninflammatory burrows, inflammatory papules filled with larvae, and excoriations.

25-year-old man who was treating the infestation as a fungal infection for weeks prior to seeking help (9).

In extremely severe cases, such as in Norwegian scabies, crusting occurs (Fig. 12.7) as millions of mites inhabit the infested areas. The toenails and fingernails are common sites of invasion (Fig. 12.8).

Etiology

Although the primary source of scabies is through physical contact with an infested person, the disease can also be spread through infected linen and clothes. These

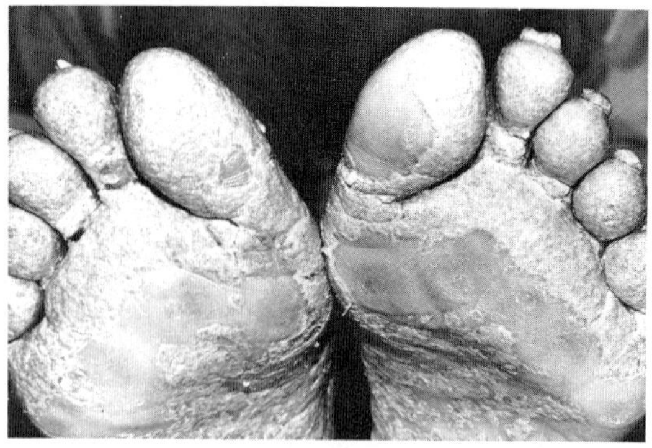

Figure 12.7. Severe scabies infestation occurring in immunocompromised patients is known as Norwegian scabies. Hyperkeratotic areas are loaded with organisms.

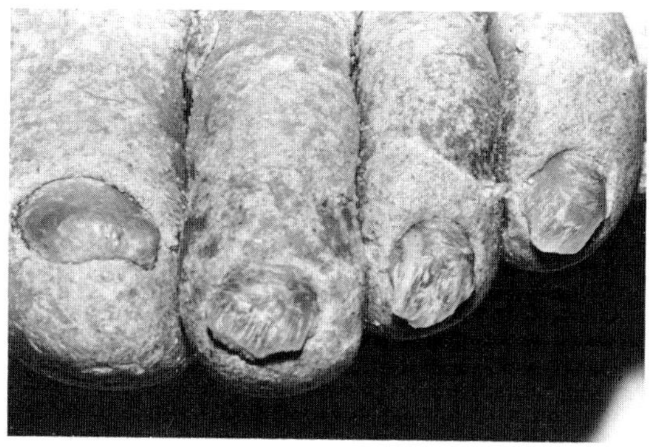

Figure 12.8. Invasions of toenails and fingernails is common in Norwegian scabies.

mites, however, cannot live away from the skin for more than a few hours.

As stated earlier, other types of mites can accidentally be transmitted to man from its natural host. Among those are the food mites *Glyciphagus* (grocery mite), *Tryophasgus* (copra mite), and *Acarus siro* (cheese mite). When one is carrying infested sacks of food, these mites can crawl into cracks in the epidermis. It is generally seen around the shoulder and neck areas. The disease is self-limiting, but treatment may be necessary for the associated pruritus.

Animal mites are another source of infestation. However, this presentation is atypical and is generally limited to the site of immediate contact, such as the hands, arms, or chest. *Sarcoptes scabiei* is found in many mammals, including dogs, cows, horses, pigs, sheep, and goats. *Notoedres cati* is seen in the cat population, as is *Cheyletiella yasguri*. The rabbit is the natural host of *Cheyletiella parasitovorax*. Many of these infestations are self-limiting because of the inability of the mite to thrive on the foreign host. The outbreak usually ceases with removal of the infected animal.

Rats, mice, and birds can also be mite carriers. *Ornithonyssus bacoti* and *Allodermanyssus sanguineus* are the species seen in rats and mice. People who work in stockyards or warehouses are the most susceptible. *Dermanyssus gallinae* are the mites that infest fowl. The mites can fall from the nests of infested chickens and pigeons and temporarily cause skin lesions on humans. People who work with poultry or around offices plagued by pigeons may be exposed.

Grain mites, *Pyemotes ventricosus*, feed on the larvae of insects that are generally found in grain, straw, hay, and stored plants (10). People who work with these products or sleep on straw mattresses are likely candidates. Contact produces urticarial papules and vesicles. The treatment is the same as in scabies.

Finally, *Trombicula alfreddugesi* and *Trombicula splendens* are rampant throughout the United States and are more commonly known as harvest mites or "chiggers." This mite attaches itself to the skin, rather than burrowing in, and injects the saliva which produces extreme pruritus. The lesions are usually apparent around the sites of clothing restriction, such as an elastic sock band or belt line. The mite is usually disengaged upon scratching or falls off within hours. The itching continues, however, for several days. Clear fingernail polish applied to the site is reported to give relief.

Differential Diagnosis

The clinical symptoms mimic a number of skin diseases. Eczema, superficial pyococcal infection, papular urticaria, pruritus hiemalis, and pediculosis capitis must also be considered (11).

Diagnosis

Diagnosis can be made by scraping the lesions thoroughly with a scalpel, applying the scraping to a glass slide in mineral oil, and viewing the material under a microscope. The mite, ova, or fecal material may be viewed, thus confirming the diagnosis (Fig. 12.9). To help isolate the mite, saline or mineral oil can be used to induce activity. Avoid the use of potassium hydroxide (KOH) as used for fungal examination, since it will kill the organism.

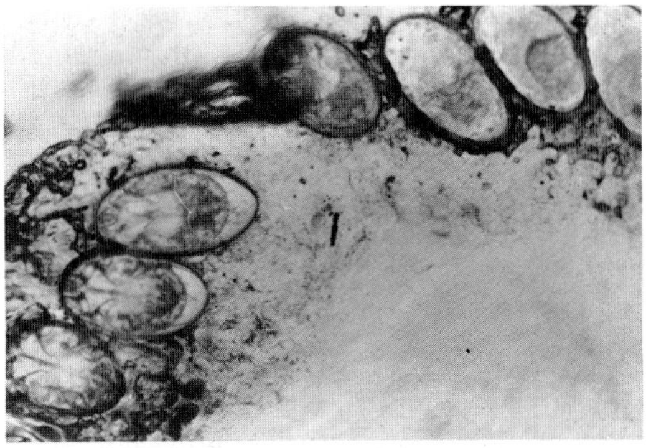

Figure 12.9. Microscopic examination of scraping from affected area reveals eggs, some ready to hatch, and small dark pieces of fecal material.

Treatment

A very rigid course of treatment must be followed to eradicate the infestation. Anyone who is regularly in close contact with the patient should be treated simultaneously.

First, the patient must soak in a hot, soapy bath and thoroughly scrub off any crusty or scaly areas. Antiscabietics must then be applied to the entire body surface below the neck. Kwell cream or lotion has proven effective when left on overnight and washed off in the morning. This procedure must be repeated again in 24 hr. After two applications, the bed linens should be changed and washed thoroughly to decrease the risk of reinfestation.

Although the organisms are dead, the remnants are still present in the epidermis. Thus, the patient will continue to itch due to the allergic reaction for several days after treatment. It is imperative that the patient understand this phenomenon of postscabietic pruritus and not continue to overtreat with the drying antiscabietic.

Consequently, the physician should restrict the amount of antiscabietic prescribed. Topical corticosteroid therapy is initiated after completion of the antiscabietic. Scabietic nodules, in particular, are pruritic and, if recalcitrant, may even require the intralesional injection of corticosteroids. The postscabietic phenomenon may last for 4 weeks.

In children, dilute the Kwell by half and only apply for 2 hours. Avoid having the children lick their fingers. There is reference to the possibility of the drug crossing the blood-brain barrier and developing central nervous system sequala.

TICKS

Ticks are large, bloodsucking parasites that are scientifically classified with mites as members of the order *Acarina.* Most dermatological reference books separate the two entities because of the clinical dissimilarities. For that same reason, we will continue to treat ticks as an entity apart from mites.

Ticks live on the grass and brush in wooded areas, waiting for a host. They prey on animals, birds, reptiles, and man. Adults are generally attacked on the feet and legs when walking through wooded areas. Children, because of their smaller size, are more likely to be attacked on the scalp and other areas.

Ticks are dark, greyish brown with a leather-like exterior. They are distinguishable from other types of insects because they have eight legs, two body sections, and no wings. Insects generally have six legs, three body sections, and wings. There are two type of ticks. The *Argasidae* is a soft-bodied tick, and the *Ixodidae* is a hard-bodied tick.

Ticks expand in size as they fill with blood from the host. Often the tick will grow to many times its normal size while feeding.

Tick bites produce some dermatological symptoms, but the significance of the parasite lies in its ability to transmit disease to and from its hosts.

Clinical Manifestation

There is generally little or no pain when the tick initially attacks its host. The tick anchors itself firmly to the epidermis, head first. It is generally detected when it increases in size as it fills with blood. In a 1967 article in the *Journal of the American Podiatry Association*, Dr. Zebrack reported a case where a woman was rushed to his office complaining of a tumor that was growing so fast it "hung down over the top of her foot." In this case, the soft-bodied tick was described as "completely pliable and skin-like, even to color" (12).

In some cases the tick bite may produce a severe localized skin reaction. These bites have an erythematous halo which may be followed by small pruritic nodules. These itchy nodules may persist long after the offending tick is removed.

More serious systemic complications may arise from the pathogenic bacteria, viruses, and rickettsiae that may be transmitted through tick bites. Diseases such as Rocky Mountain spotted fever, tick-borne relapsing fever, Colorado tick fever, tularemia, erythema chronicum migrans, and Western equine encephalitis (10) have been associated with tick bites.

In select species, the tick injects a salivary neurotoxin into its host. This toxin slows the motor nerve conduction and can cause a progressive but reversible paralysis. The patient may first show signs of irritation and diarrhea. When the toxic tick has been feeding upon its host for a few days, weakness and poor leg control of the patient may be the first active signs of motor involvement. If the tick is removed at this stage, the paralysis should subside and completely reverse within days. In very severe cases, however, the paralysis can extend to the respiratory system, resulting in death (13).

Etiology

The soft-bodied ticks (*Argasidae*) feed quickly at night and are primarily bird parasites. Because these ticks prefer several hosts, the chances of disease transmission is increased. In this group of ticks, you will find *Argus persicus* (the poultry tick), and *Argus reflexus* (the pigeon tick). Another soft-bodied species responsible for disease transmission is *Otobius megnini*, the tick found on many domestic animals.

The hard-bodied ticks (*Ixodidae*) include a number of species with no particular host preference. These ticks may feed for several days before dropping off. *Ixodidae* ticks include the following genre: *Dermacentor, Ixodes, Rhipicephalus, Haemaphysalis, Hyalomma, Boophilus,* and *Amblyomma.*

The tick responsible for paralysis in Canada and the Northwestern United States is the *Dermacentor andersoni* or wood tick. In the Southeastern states, *Dermacentor variabilis* or the dog tick has been implicated. Other species such as *Ambylomma americanum* (the Lone Star tick), *Amblyomma maculatum* (the Gulf Coast tick), and *Ixodes scapularis* (the black-legged deer tick) have also been reported as sources of tick paralysis. In Australia the offending species is *Ixodes holocyclus* and in Europe and South Africa it is *Ixodes pilosus* (4).

Differential Diagnosis

Deeply imbedded soft-bodied ticks may resemble warts or tumors. Tick bite marks may resemble papular urticaria, dermal fibrosis, fibroxanthoma or histiocytoma.

Definitive Diagnosis

When the tick is still attached, location of the tick will provide a definitive diagnosis. If the tick has already dropped off, the presence of a single nodule with a necrotic center may aid in the diagnosis.

Treatment

Prompt removal of the tick is highly recommended. Care must be taken to encourage the tick to loosen its grip; otherwise, the head of the parasite may remain in the epidermis when the body is plucked off. A heated nail, match, or a few drops of chloroform applied directly to the tick's body should loosen its grip and enable you to pull it out intact. If a portion of the tick is retained in the skin, a punch biopsy will remove it.

Prevention is the best cure for tick bites. Patients should be encouraged to spray their clothes and shoes with commercial repellents such as Deet, Indalone, or benzyl benzoate before entering wooded areas.

FLEAS

The flea is similar to the tick because it is also a bloodsucking parasite that infests both animals and humans. This characteristic encourages the transmission of bacteria, rickettsia, and other parasitic diseases from host to host.

Fleas are more prevalent in the summer and tend to breed in dust or dirt, carpets, floorboard crevices, birds' nests, garbage, and animal kennels. The tiny, wingless parasites are very resilient: Fleas can survive for months without feeding.

The flea can jump incredible distances relative to its size, several feet at a time. It is attracted to and will attack moving subjects. The most common site of infestation in man is around the feet and ankles migrating upward (14).

There are two families of fleas. The *Sarcopsyllidae* family contains species found in the South American and African tropics which feed by burrowing under the skin of its host. The more common fleas belong to the *Pulicidae* family. These fleas are found worldwide and simply bite its host, extracting blood.

Clinical Manifestation

The degree of individual sensitivity determines the extent of the dermatitis. Sensitivity is highest during initial exposure, especially in children or adults who are moving into an infested area for the first time. Repeated bites increase sensitization until the bites become completely innocuous.

In extremely sensitive people, the bite may present as a wheel or papule with a hemorrhagic punctum. The bites, which usually occur in the lower extremities, are generally grouped in irregular clusters and are intensely pruritic (Fig. 12.10). In severe cases large urticarial lesions, bullae (Fig. 12.11) and even small necrotic ulcers may develop.

Scratching may lead to bacterial infections and impetigo (Fig. 12.12). Plague and rickettsial murine typhus may be transmitted through contact with rodent fleas.

The burrowing flea, *Tunga penetrans*, has more severe dermatological effects. Although it is generally found in tropical countries such as South America, Africa, and the West Indies, a few cases have appeared in North America. It is also referred to as the chigoe or jigger flea (13). This is not to be confused with the chigger mite.

Unlike other types of fleas, the chigoe flea is a poor jumper. The female usually attaches herself to the skin and slowly digs deeper and deeper until only the posterior segment protrudes. As the flea feeds on the host's blood, it will increase in proportion, often reaching the size of a small pea.

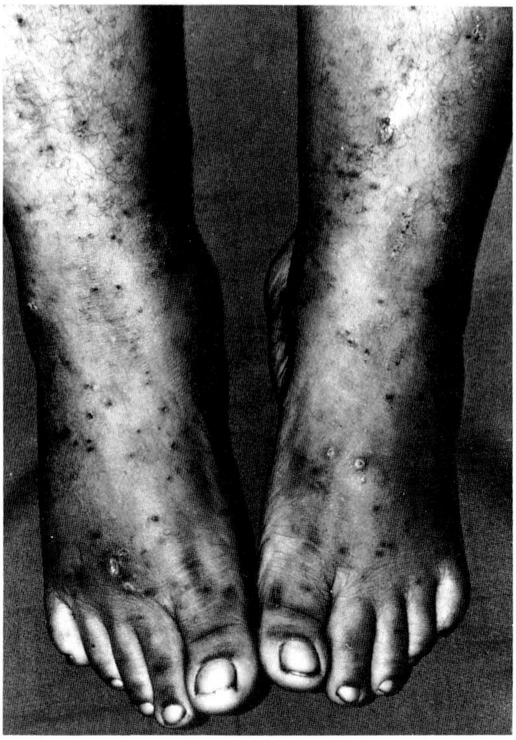

Figure 12.10. Flea bites characteristically manifest as discrete and grouped inflammatory papules or papulovesicles. Often the lesions are excoriated and secondarily infected, as seen in this patient.

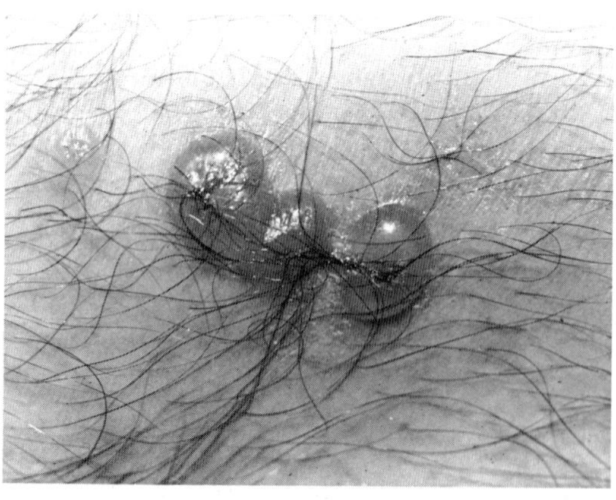

Figure 12.11. In patients highly sensitive to flea bites, blisters may occur. Note the clustering of lesions, a pattern typical of insect bites.

The resulting lesions are usually situated between the toes, on the soles of the feet, and under the toenails. If the lesions are neglected and the flea is not removed, deep ulceration, secondary infections, and even gangrene could result.

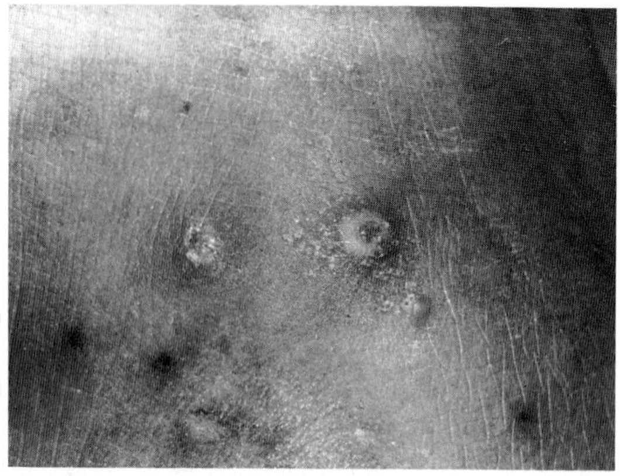

Figure 12.12. Secondary infection is common following insect bites. Purulent lesions should prompt appropriate antimicrobial therapy.

Etiology

The human flea *Pulex irritans* is the parasite responsible for most human infestation. However, fleas from dogs (*Ctenocephalides canis*) and cats (*Ctenocephalides felis*) also attack man.

The life cycle of a flea may be completed within weeks if the ideal environmental temperatures exist. Fleas thrive in warm, humid, sandy areas. Fleas can survive for long periods of time without feeding; hence the persistence of fleas in uninhabited apartments and basements.

The female flea will lay her eggs in crevices, in dust, or in the dirt. If eggs are deposited on the host, they will fall to the gound. The larvae form cocoons and go through three stages before reaching the adulthood. Under certain environmental conditions, the larvae may stay in the cocoon stage for up to a year (15).

Differential Diagnosis

Flea bites in sensitive individuals may be confused with various insect bites because the results resemble papular urticaria (Fig. 12.13), bullae, and necrotic ulcers. Secondary infections caused by intense scratching may also confuse the diagnosis.

Definitive Diagnosis

It is important to determine if the patient is exposed to a flea-infested environment. Brushings from domestic pets and house dust samples may be examined for signs of flea infestation.

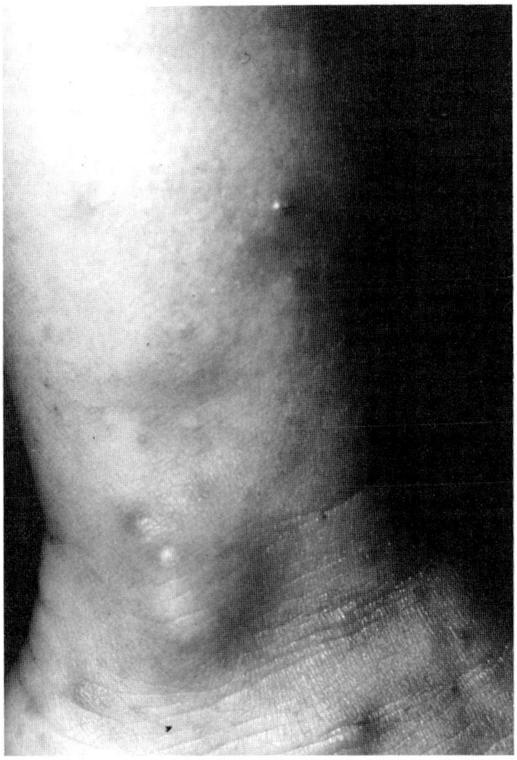

Figure 12.13. Papular urticaria is a descriptive term for inflammatory urticarial papules due to insect bites of any etiology. This child was bitten by several mosquitoes.

If *T. penetrans* is suspected, first determine if the patient has recently visited any tropical countries where the parasite may exist. In these cases, the flea may be extracted from the skin for a definitive diagnosis and treatment.

Treatment

Surgical removal of the burrowing chigoe flea is recommended by puncturing the site with a sterile needle and forcing the flea out. An ether-soaked gauze or cotton ball applied to the lesion will kill the flea prior to extraction. Antiseptic dressing or antibacterial cream should be applied once the flea is removed.

Desensitization has been suggested for successful elimination of flea bites; however, the patient will eventually become desensitized after repeated exposure. Hydrocortisone cream will help relieve the pruritus caused by the flea bites.

Elimination of the fleas from the environment is necessary to halt the infestation. This may be accomplished by using DDT sprays and powders on all suspected breeding grounds. Commercial flea sprays and powders should also be used on the domestic pets. Cats must be prevented from licking the toxic powder. This procedure must be repeated every 2 weeks to eliminate newly hatched fleas.

Commercial flea repellents such as Deet and Off should be used on the susceptible patient. This will help prevent future attacks until the environment is free from the flea infestation.

SPIDERS

Spiders are easily identified by their unique appearance. Members of the order *Araachnida*, spiders have no wings or antennae, and their bodies are divided into two segments (8). Spiders are characterized by their four pairs of long legs.

Although there are over 2000 species of spiders, only a few are of medical significance. In the United States, almost all of the spider bites are caused by two types of spiders: the black widow spider (*Latrodectus mactans*), and the brown recluse spider (*Loxosceles reclusa*). For this reason, we will limit our discussion on spiders to these two genera.

Clinical Manifestation

The feet, buttocks, and genitalia are the most common sites of spider bites. There may not be an immediate sensation of pain when the bite occurs, and often the patient is unaware of the spider's presence (16). A localized reaction generally appears shortly after the incident, followed by systemic complications hours or even days later.

A burning and stinging sensation may occur within minutes at the site of the black widow spider (*L. mactans*) bite. Two small red puncta may be seen as the area becomes swollen and erythematous.

Within an hour after the initial bite, severe muscle cramping and abdominal pain develop. This pain intensifies and peaks about 3 hours later. Nausea, weakness, vomiting, profuse sweating, and dizziness may accompany the pain. The pain will gradually subside, but the symptoms may recur for 2 or 3 days following the incident.

In extremely severe cases, paralysis and convulsions have been noted. Respiratory failure and cardiac arrest may cause death as a result of the bite in children and the elderly. The mortality rate from black widow spider bites is over 5% (4).

The brown recluse spider (*Loxosceles reclusa*) bite may cause a mild stinging and pruritus at the site within moments. The local pain intensifies as the puncture blisters, often followed by ischemic necrosis and deep ulceration (Fig. 12.14). The site may become gangrenous (Fig. 12.15).

Systemic complications resulting from the brown recluse spider bite may include nausea, vomiting, chills, weakness, and muscle pains. In severe cases, signs of hemolysis, hemoglobinuria, renal failure, and hemolytic anemia may develop within days. Death has been reported in severe cases, usually involving children.

Etiology

L. mactans is found throughout the United States. It has been named the black widow spider because the female immediately kills the male after copulation. The female black widow spider is distinguished by a red or orange hourglass marking on its underside.

The black widow spider is often found in dark, unused sheds, lumber stacks, and in outdoor privies. Many cases involving bites on the buttocks and genitalia are reported to be received when using outdoor privies. The female spider often lays her eggs under the seats of outdoor privies and bites the intruder in self-defense.

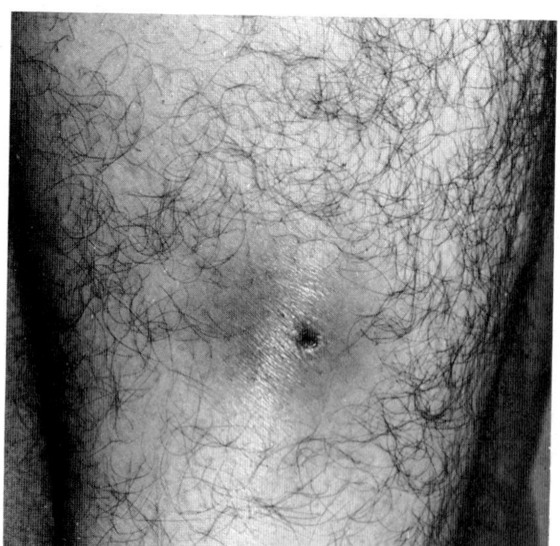

Figure 12.14. Tender induration, intense bluish-red discoloration, and central necrosis are typical changes following brown recluse spider bites.

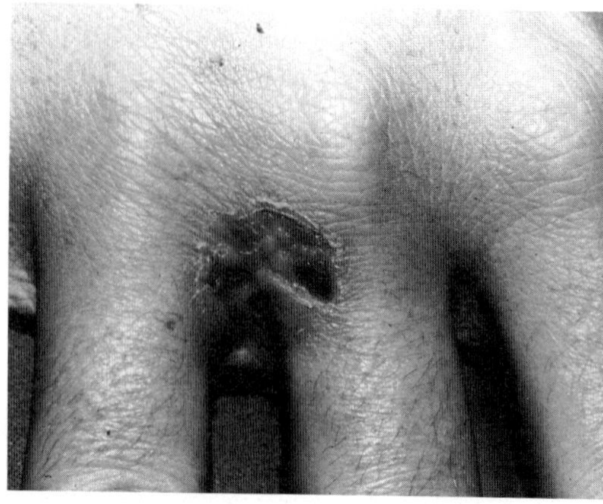

Figure 12.15. Extensive necrosis, followed by deep scar, can result from the bite of a brown recluse spider, as occurred in this patient.

The black widow spider injects venom into its victim through its fangs. The neurotropic venom is said to be 15 times more potent than the venom of a rattlesnake. However, because of the small size of the spider in relation to its victim, the dose is usually not lethal.

The red-legged widow spider (*Latrodectus bishopi*) is found in Florida. It injects a milder form of venom into its victim as a means of self-defense.

L. reclusa, or brown recluse spider, is also known as the violin spider because of its shape. It is a yellowish-brown spider, approximately 10 to 15 mm long. These spiders are commonly seen in the Southern and Midwestern states. *Loxosceles arizonica* and *Loxoscles unicolor* are other common, poisonous brown spiders.

These brown spiders are generally found in lumber, under rocks, and in homes. Most of its victims are bitten at home while sleeping or dressing.

Differential Diagnosis

The systemic complications resulting from the bites of these two species of spiders can mimic a number of conditions. Renal colic, coronary occlusion, tetanus, strychnine poisoning, tabetic crisis, lead colic, and porphyria (13) should all be ruled out first.

The abdominal pains seen in black widow spider bites are often confused with pancreatitis, volvulus, or perforated ulcers.

The differential diagnosis must also take conditions such as dermatitis venenata, epidermoid carcinoma, epidermolysis bullosa, diabetic neurocutaneodystrophy, and factitial ulceration into consideration (17).

Definitive Diagnosis

The abdomen should not be tender to the touch, despite the accompanying pains. The conditions listed in the differential diagnosis section seldom have additional pain in the extremities.

A good examination of the feet may produce signs of the two red puncta marks in cases of the black widow spider bites and blisters or ulcerations with the brown recluse spider bites.

Treatment

The treatment for black widow spider bites should be aimed at providing relief from the cramps and neutralizing the neurotoxin. If available, the specific antiserum should be obtained and administered as soon as possible, particularly in children and the elderly.

A hot bath will give immediate, temporary relief from the muscle spasms. Intravenous injection of 10 ml of 10% calcium gluconate is also therapeutic.

The treatment for the brown recluse spider bite primarily involves local wound management. The course of the wound will be less severe if corticosteroids, antihistamines, and antibiotics are administered as soon as possible. Skin grafting may be necessary in severe cases involving ulceration.

ANTS

Ants are members of the large *Hymenoptera* order of insects. Many adult insects in this group have poisonous glands and can inject the venom by stinging or biting. The venom may be used in self-defense or as an offensive measure for obtaining food. Bees and wasps are also members of the *Hymenoptera* order.

Allergic reactions to ant venom can cause death in extremely hypersensitive people. The incidence of death from *hymenoptera* insects in the United States is almost twice as high as deaths caused by snake venom.

Clinical Manifestation

An immediate burning pain is produced by the poisonous ant sting or bite. This burning sensation is generally followed by localized redness and swelling. Mass attacks are common in ant bites and may cause severe diffuse edema.

Fire ants, *Solenopsis saevissima*, are particularly toxic and can cause intense local and systemic reactions. Within a moment after experiencing the painful sting, a wheal appears which may increase up to 10 mm in diameter. After 24 hours, a small pustule may develop, surrounded by an intense erythematous ring (Fig. 12.16). In older or hypersensitive individuals, fire ants have been known to cause extensive vesiculation, skin necrosis, and even systemic toxicity (Fig. 12.17).

An estimated 2% of the population has a severe allergic reaction to hymenopteran venoms. Systemic reactions include urticaria, angioedema, asthma, and gastrointestinal distress. In extremely hypersensitive cases, the patient may go into anaphylactic shock with fever, rapid pulse, low blood pressure, and even coma. Women may also experience uterine contractions (8). The degree of hypersensitivity may increase with each exposure and could be potentially fatal.

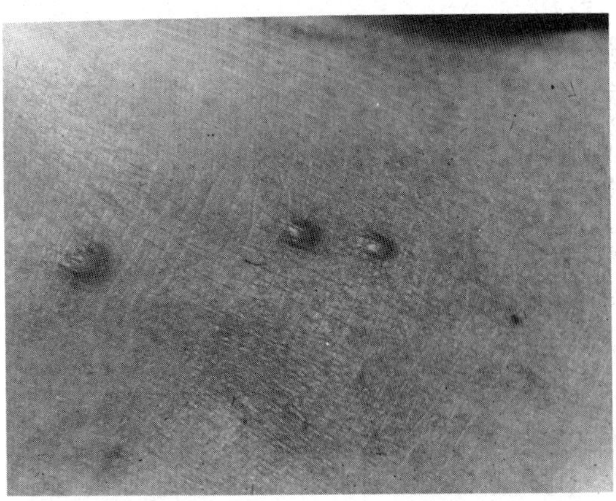

Figure 12.16. Discrete pustules surrounded by intense erythema are typical of fire ant bites. Like most insect bite reactions, the lesions are usually grouped together.

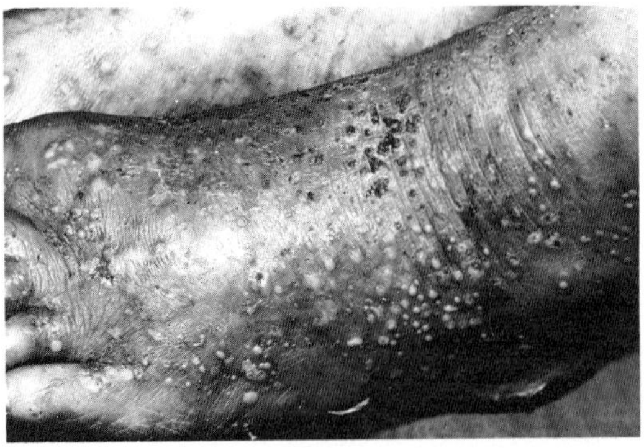

Figure 12.17. This alcoholic patient "passed out" on a fire ant hill, resulting in a myriad of bites and systemic toxicity.

Etiology

Ants belong to the super family *Formicidae*. The fire ant (*S. saevissima*) was imported from South American and is now commonly found in the Southern United States. The pharaoh ant (*Monomorium pharaonis*) is also commonly found in the warmer Southern states and has a mild bite. The tiny brown ant is a household pest. Multiple Harvester ant bites (*Pogonomyrmex*) are common because the ants attack when their earth mounds are disturbed (4).

Hymenoptera venoms are hemolytic and neurotoxic. They contain histamines, hyaluronidase, phospholipases, and various kinins (26).

Differential Diagnosis

The severe local reaction caused by fire ants may be confused with the bite of a brown recluse spider. The lesions are also very similar to those induced by other insect bites or stings, especially bees and wasps.

Definitive Diagnosis

A thorough examination of the affected area should help identify the lesions, accompanied with the history of onset. The discrete pustules with surrounding erythematous rings are pathognomonic. Ant bites generally occur in a grouped distribution and are therefore distinguishable from the single wheals produced by bees or wasps.

Treatment

Availability of treatment is essential for patients who have a known hypersensitivity to *Hymenoptera* venom. These patients should carry and learn to self-administer adrenaline. Sublingual sympathomimetic drugs, such as isoproterenol, should also be carried by the allergic patient. Sting kits are commercially available (13).

A cool compress, antipruritic lotions and oral antihistamines will alleviate local irritation caused by the sting or bite.

Desensitization is recommended for anyone who exhibits an allergic reaction to the *Hymenoptera* venom. Hypersensitive individuals should also avoid any contact with ants by always wearing shoes when outdoors. Bright color clothes and perfumes also attract the insects and should be avoided.

References

1. Kleger SJ, Feldman B: Larva migrans. *J Am Podiatry Assoc* 56:324, 1966.
2. Belsole R, Fenske N: Cutaneous larva migrans in the upper extremity. *J Hand Surg* 5:178, 1980.
3. Domonkos AN, Arnold HL, Odom RB: *Andrews' Diseases of the Skin—Clinical Dermatology*, ed 7. Philadelphia, W.B. Saunders, 1982, p 544.
4. Rook A, Wilkinson DS, Ebling FJG: *Textbook of Dermatology—Volume One*, ed 3. Oxford, Blackwell Scientific Publications, 1979, p 878.
5. Boland TW, Agger WA: Cutaneous larva migrans—recent experience in the La Crosse area. *Wis Med J* 79:32, 1980.
6. Zebrack SD: Creeping eruptions (larva migrans)—a case report. *J Am Podiatry Assoc* 64:105, 1974.
7. Stewart WD, Danto JL, Maddin S: *Dermatology—Diagnosis and Treatment of Cutaneous Disorders*, ed 4. St. Louis, C.V. Mosby, 1978, p 339.
8. Fitzpatrick TB, Arndt KA, Clark WH, Eisen AZ, Van Scott EJ, Vaughan JH: *Dermatology in General Medicine.* New York, McGraw-Hill, 1971, p 1944.
9. Dockery GL: Human scabies—a review of diagnosis and current therapy. *J Am Podiatry Assoc* 70:177, 1980.
10. Moschella SL, Pillsbury DM, Hurley HJ: *Dermatology.* Philadelphia, W.B. Saunders, 1975, vol 1, p 1514.
11. Hall-Smith P, Cairns RJ, Beare RLB: *Der-*

matology, ed 2. New York, Grune & Stratton, 1973, p 133.
12. Zebrack SD: Parasitic tick on the foot—a case report. *J Am Podiatry Assoc* 57:276, 1967.
13. Isselbacher KJ, Adams RD, Braunwald E, Petersdorf RG, Wilson JD: *Harrison's Principles of Internal Medicine*, ed 9. New York, McGraw-Hill, 1980, p 925.
14. Rasmussen JE: Parasites. In Roenigk HH: *Office Dermatology*. Baltimore, Williams & Wilkins, 1981, p 126.
15. Stewart WD, Danto JL, Maddin S: *Synopsis of Dermatology*, ed 2. St. Louis, C.V. Mosby, 1970, p 242.
16. Istell R, Bodmer EJ, Buchbinder E: Black widow spider (latrodectus mactans)—bite of the foot. *J Am Podiatry Assoc* 69:562, 1979.
17. Cangialosi CP, Schnall SJ: Pedal spider bite (arachnidism)—report of two similar cases. *J Am Podiatry Assoc* 71:385, 1981.

CHAPTER 13

Contact Dermatitis and Atopic Dermatitis

LEONARD A. LEVY

The first responsibility of a clinician is to follow principles that will minimize the risk of adverse reactions that may follow treatment. Obviously, physicians should avoid, to the degree possible, prescribing or exposing the patient to drugs or environmental agents which may have a relatively high risk of causing such reactions. Moreover, they must also be aware of the sensitizing potential of those drugs which may cause the patient to adversely react to a necessary medication administered later during the course of treatment. By understanding the way these problems may occur, it is frequently possible to protect patients, especially those with a high risk of developing such problems.

The subject of contact dermatitis, environmental irritants, and allergic and other adverse reactions to drugs could and does fill many articles, monographs, and texts. However, the emphasis of this discussion will be confined to the relationship of such reactions as they relate to practitioners having a special interest in problems affecting the foot and its contiguous structures.

This study will include summaries of problems resulting from primary irritants, mechanical injuries, and allergic and pharmacologic agents. The environment we provide for the foot in most of the industrialized world places it in contact with a number of potential allergens. The lower extremities are exposed to hundreds of chemical and physical agents used in various occupations, as well as in the home.

SKIN TESTING

In essence, the patch test provides a model of the disease being tested in a relatively safe manner. It is one of the most direct methods of medical testing. The results of properly performed and interpreted patch tests are accepted as scientific proof of the cause of dermatitis and have medicolegal significance (Figs. 13.1 to 13.3).

A test series or battery is the grouping together of allergens for patch testing. When the offending agent cannot at least be suspected from the history obtained from the patients, the use of a standard series of screening allergens is very helpful. If a positive result is demonstrated one must attempt to fit it into the history and physical examination. Sometimes after obtaining a positive result, one finds that the result is not due to the primary cause of the contact dermatitis but rather to a cross reacting chemical. However, this still may be useful in determining the true etiological agent. An example that can be cited is one in which there is a positive reaction to a mixture of "caine" anesthetics. The "caines" may not be the primary cause of the dermatitis. Instead, the dermatitis may be due to paraphenylenediamine, para-aminobenzoic acid, or other chemicals with a structural formula having an amino acid radical in the para position. A weak reaction from a cross reacting substance is a clue to look for the primary agent in one of the related derivatives.

As many as 40 to 50 substances can be tested simultaneously by the patch method. Mixtures allow these numbers to be increased substantially by having four to five related substances mixed together. The North American Contact Dermatitis Group (NACDG), a task force of the American Academy of Dermatology, recommends mixes of "caines," parabens, and fragrances, and that four sets of rubber chemi-

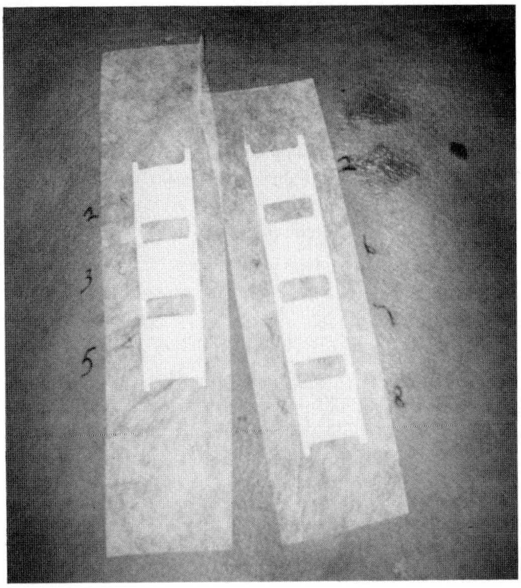

Figure 13.1. Strips used for patch testing. Each opening contains a different substance being tested.

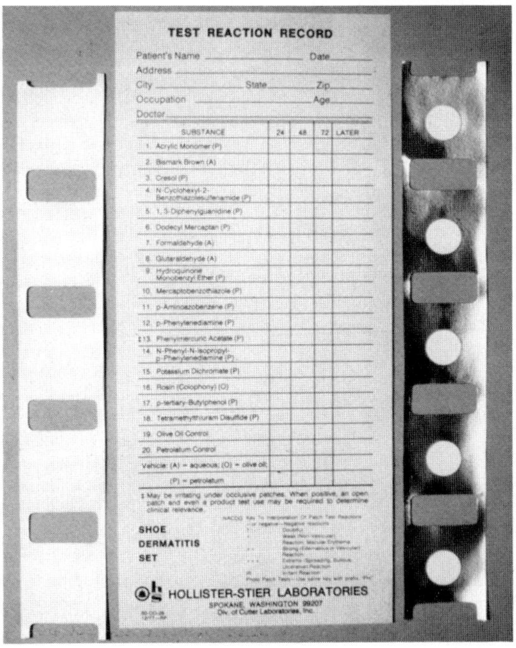

Figure 13.2. Test Reaction record for evaluating shoe dermatitis.

cals be employed. Caution must be taken, however, in using such mixtures since a patient sometimes may have a negative reaction to such a test but a positive response to one of the ingredients tested separately. This is probably because the concentration of the test substance in the mix may be lower than that in the individual test material. The concentration of each chemical in a mix, therefore, must be high enough to stimulate a reaction. In addition, the ingredients in the mix must not chemically react and cause an irritation which may be interpreted as a false-positive reaction or cause an opposite reaction resulting in deactivation of the ingredients in the mix and yielding a false-negative reaction.

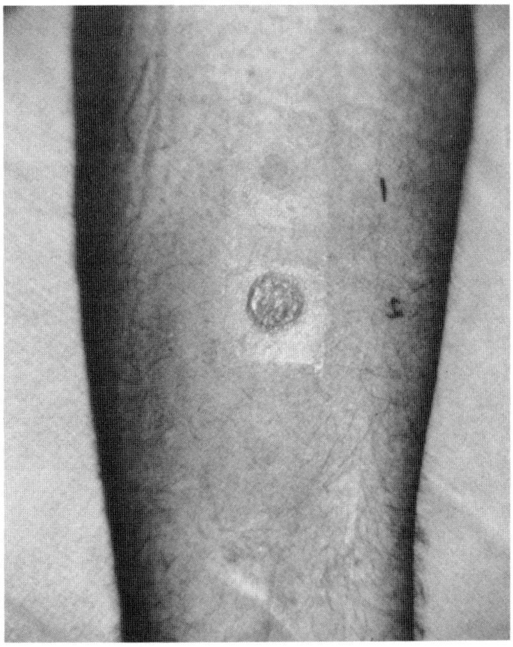

Figure 13.3. Positive patch test.

To avoid false-positive and false-negative results, one should use standard procedures that have been adopted for performing patch testing. Variation from the classic methods is to be avoided. Those test modifications as subtle as changing the backing material from filter paper to gauze or cotton to the changing of the vehicle from an aqueous solution to a petrolatum mix are to be avoided. Such methods have been adopted as standards for patch testing recognized all over the world. They are the results of tests on thousands of patients which determined the appropriate concentration of the chemical that was to be used.

There are a relatively few places where the materials for the standard series can be obtained. These include the following:

1. American Academy of Dermatology, 1576 Maple Avenue, Evanston, IL, 60201

2. Hollister-Stier Laboratories, Box 3145, T.A., Spokane, WA 99220, telephone: (509) 489-5656
3. TRO-LABS, Laboratory for Dermatologic Patch Tests, Hyorups Alle 1, 2900 Hellerup, Copenhagen, Denmark

The methods used worldwide most typically are the closed A1 patch test and the Finn Chamber. A1 patch testing uses a cellulose disc. Discs are attached to a polyethylene-coated aluminum backing which comes in rolls. A hypoallergenic tape is used to attach the patch to the skin, such as Scanpor.

Scanpor has a polyacrylate adhesive. The tape itself is a finely meshed paper with a large number of perforations per square centimeter. It is not occlusive and, therefore, after it is applied, a vehicle, commonly white petrolatum, is used. The polyethylene aluminum backing of the A1 patch makes for an impermeable covering.

The Finn Chamber is another recommended method. It consists of a round aluminum chamber 8 mm in diameter and provides a test area of 50 mm. These chambers are available individually or attached to a Scanpor tape and are provided with a removable paper covering. More patches can be applied using the Finn Chamber, and the reaction sites are smaller then the A1 test.

Patches remain in place for 48 hr. The back is the site recommended for testing. Areas normally covered by clothing should be selected because strongly positive reactions may last for many weeks. In addition, these areas may scar, and increased or decreased pigmentation may result. Patches should not be applied over hairy areas. If excessive burning or itching occurs over any site, that particular patch should be removed without disturbing the other ones. Patients must be advised to keep the patches dry and not to disturb them in any way. Activities that increase sweating should be avoided.

When the 48-hr period ends, patches are removed and encircled with a felt pen or gentian violet. The patient is advised that these stains will soil clothing. However, an almost colorless ultraviolet paint is now available which shines bright yellow-green when exposed to black light (Ultraviolet Products, Inc., San Gabriel, CA). It remains on the skin about 36 hrs if not washed off. When reading the patches, the "ultraviolet" paint should be reapplied so that any late reaction can be diagnosed.

One of the reasons patch testing produces fewer false negatives than some of the other methods is because it allows for deeper penetration as a result of the occlusive technique that is used.

The open test is yet another method that is used if liquids, gels, or creams are suspected to be the causes of a dermatitis. Substances which are being tested are applied full strength to normal skin without being covered. This is done twice daily for at least 2 days. Patients are advised to cease the regimen if an irritation results. Reading the sites is done in the same manner as with the patch tests, except that the areas are observed after the first 15 to 30 min to see if any contact urticaria occurred.

A third method is that used to help confirm the closed testing method (i.e., patch test) which had previously been found to be positive. It is called the "provocative" use test and is performed by rubbing the suspected substance onto normal skin of the antecubital fossa twice daily for a week. This is usually done over an area 3 cm in diameter. If no reaction is observed, it is considered to be a negative test.

Injury to the skin due to nonmechanical sources occurs when a person comes in contact with certain substances which release pharmacologically active substances and physical agents like those producing cold or heat. This category of dermatitis essentially affects all persons that come in contact with these substances as long as the concentration of material is high enough. These materials or agents are referred to as primary irritants and show a response in the skin within minutes or hours of exposure.

In contrast, it requires time to acquire hypersensitivity to an allergen in order to produce an allergic response resulting in an inflammatory reaction of the skin. Individuals must have previous exposure to the allergen to acquire the hypersensitivity.

People with skin that is macerated as a result of high humidity, exposure to water, heat, cold, pressure, or friction are more vulnerable to primary irritant contact dermatitis. Skin that is dry or thick is less likely to react to contactants. Thin skin is more reactive than thick to such irritants. In the case of repeated exposure to mild irritants, the skin sometimes builds up a resistance to the effects of such contactants.

CONTACT DERMATITIS

General Clinical Findings

The typical local skin reaction to contact dermatitis is erythema, edema, vesicles, papules, oozing, and scaling. Pruritis is the usual accompanying symptom. Longstanding conditions are generally characterized by scaling, fissuring, lichenification, and thickening of the skin. Changes in pigment and pigmentation of the integument are also common. Microscopically, the acute lesions show spongiosis, vesiculation, and infiltration of inflammatory cells. Vascular dilation is typically seen in the upper dermis. Chronic conditions present a modified histological picture of acanthosis, hyperkeratosis, parakeratosis, and an infiltrate in the upper dermis which is mainly lymphocytic.

Reactions to Primary Irritants

While most people are unlikely to accidentally receive exposure to pure alkalis, many activities of daily living, ranging from showering and bathing to house cleaning, may expose the skin to dilute amounts of such chemicals. The foot may receive such exposure through the use of soaps and detergents associated with normal washing habits. While it is less likely that the foot and ankle will be exposed to such alkali or alkali preparations as lye, drain pipe cleaners, bleaches, ammonia preparations, or toilet bowel cleaners, such events would certainly not be considered rare. Patients have been seen on occasion who have elected to soak their feet in bleach compounds. More often, exposure of the foot to these preparations is due to accidental occurrences associated with housecleaning or occupationally related activities. It would be far more likely, however, for such exposure to involve the hands or some other exposed part of the body.

Exposure to many of these noxious substances usually occurs through domestic or industrial accidents. However, such occurrences most frequently spare the feet, which are protected by shoes.

Primary irritant dermatitis due to strong acids causes corrosive damage. Nitric acid, for example, causes a deep burn with yellow staining. Hydrochloric acid produces more superficial damage, resulting in blistering burns. Charring of the skin and a brown coloration occurs with sulfuric acid exposure. Ulceration which heals slowly occurs under the charred area. Phenol (carbolic acid) causes protoplasmic poisoning with a white eschar on the surface of the skin. In addition, phenol causes a temporary local anesthesia.

Allergic Contact Dermatitis

Allergic contact dermatitis is due to a specific acquired hypersensitivity of the delayed type. It occurs when an allergenic substance comes into contact with skin that has been previously sensitized. Sometimes the dermatitis may occur on a sensitized area of skin when the allergen is taken internally.

The most useful of diagnostic procedures is that of patch testing. While quite simple to perform, the test requires experience and objectivity for accurate interpretation. It is used frequently to discover a specific chemical responsible for dermatitis. A positive patch test indicates prior sensitization. This could have taken place years before the dermatitis occurred or only a few days previously, if the test results and the dermatitis are related. Relevant positive patch test reactions that demonstrate the agent causing the contact dermatitis are not numerically large. However, test results usually range from 25 to 35% positive, which is more accurate than most other diagnostic procedures employed.

While the affect on the skin of certain caustics, acids, and physical agents is obvious, allergic dermatitis is not so easily distinguishable. Some drugs may produce reactions that only appear to be allergic. The Jarisch-Herxheimer phenomenon is an example of a condition in which fever, chills, skin rash, edema, and headache may occur during the course of penicillin treatment for syphilis. Even the syphilitic skin lesions may flare during such therapy. However, the reaction tends to disappear as the treatment continues, indicating that the response was not of allergic origin. The release of endotoxins or microbial antigens or both are thought to be the agents responsible for the Jarisch-Herxheimer phenomenon. Reports of similar reactions in treating fungal diseases have been reported.

Over 50% of patients with infectious mononucleosis or lymphatic leukemia, as well as those individuals taking allopurinol for gout and who are given ampicillin, develop rashes. It is interesting to note that urticaria and other skin eruptions can occur with placebo treatment during controlled clinical drug trials.

The choice of an allergic reaction occurring in patients who do not have a history of a previous drug reaction is less than 3% for most drugs and, for some, close to zero. It should be noted that the skin is the organ which is most frequently involved in the majority of allergic reactions. A Boston survey of more than 22,000 inpatients identified only 22 drugs that were the possible causes of five or more reactions. Reaction rates over 2% occurred among patients using such commonly prescribed drugs such as semisynthetic penicillins, corticotropin, and erythromycin. Fifty drugs were given to over 500 patients, including aspirin, tetracycline, and hydrochlorothiazide, and no adverse reactions were experienced.

The risk of developing allergic sensitivity to a drug is influenced by its route of administration. Topical medication is the most likely to sensitize while oral is the least likely. Ideally, attempts to identify the potentially allergic patient should be done before the allergic reaction occurs to the degree possible. Age, sex, and atopic background should be considered important enough to influence therapeutic decision. In addition to skin testing, a history of a previous reaction clearly increases the risk of an allergic response.

Among the skin reactions that may occur as a result of an allergic response to a drug or some other substance is urticaria. This symptom may be manifest, together with anaphylaxis, angioedema, serum sickness, or simply with the urticaria alone. The reaction may develop suddenly or several hours or days after exposure to the allergic material. It may be expressed as a small papule or as 20-cm lesions with clear centers.

Allergic contact dermatitis may occur when a drug is applied topically. This usually expresses itself initially with the appearance of pruritus and erythema (Table 13.1). This is followed by induration, which may be followed by vesiculobullous lesions whenever topical administration of the allergen is continued. Usually, cessation of the application of the substances results in remission of the lesions. The patch test simply is a miniature reproduction of the primary allergic lesion and provides proof implicating the agent causing the sensitivity.

Fixed Drug Eruptions

Eruptions appearing in the same place each time a drug is administered are called fixed erruptions. They, like allergic contact dermatitis, may be eczematous or sometimes bullous. The lesion may also simply express itself as a macule. The color of the lesion varies from pink to red or brown. Most often there is no pruritus, which is typical for allergic contact dermatitis. Hyperpigmentation of the skin may remain after resolution of the eruption. Drugs that are commonly the cause of these lesions are the penicillins, tetracyclines, gold salts, phenolphthalein, meprobamate, barbiturates, analgesics, and sulfonamides.

Prevention of Contact Dermatitis

The most important aspect of patient management in treating allergic and other types of contact dermatitis is to prevent exposure to the known or suspected causative substances. Drugs should not be prescribed haphazardly. Many of them may not cause any harm initially but may sensitize patients to react at some later date when a necessary course of treatment is indicated. By using drugs with a low sensitizing potential to the greatest degree possible, the possibility of sensitizing patients to a drug is reduced. Van Arsdel lists a number of drugs which rarely are responsible for allergic reactions. Many of these

Table 13.1
Natural History of Signs and Symptoms of Contact Dermatitis

Erythema
Pruritis
Induration
Vesiculation

are drugs which are part of the therapeutic armamentarium of practitioners involved in the care of foot disorders. These include antihistamines, aspirin, atropine, local anesthetics, nystatin, opiates, steroid hormones, and tetracyclines. Whenever it is therapeutically appropriate, these drugs should be considered for patient administration, instead of others which may present a greater risk of sensitizing a patient.

A careful history of allergies should be taken prior to administering a drug. If the patient reports what may be allergy symptoms to the drug being contemplated for use or to a chemically related drug (e.g., penicillins and cephalosporins), caution must be employed before proceeding with such a choice of therapy. Skin tests are reliable for determining sensitivity to foreign proteins found in drugs. If the drug being considered is the best for the patient's medical problem and is thought to be essential but the patient has a history of an allergic reaction to the drug or to one related to it, skin testing is indicated.

Patients with suspected penicillin or local anesthetic allergies require such testing. Penicillin testing is accomplished by using penicilloyl polylysine and a fresh saline solution of benzyl penicillin, (penicillin G) in a dilution of 10,000 U/ml. Initially, scratch tests or prick tests are performed with these solutions. If the tests are negative, a skin test is performed intracutaneously using 0.01 to 0.02 ml of solution. If after 15 to 20 minutes no wheal or erythema occurs, it is concluded that the risk for penicillin treatment is no greater than for patients with no history of an allergic reaction.

Patients having a history of allergy to a drug and a positive skin test can usually be given an alternative drug. In any event, they should not be given the drug to which they have demonstrated a sensitivity. If this can not be accomplished and the only one effective for the patient's problem is the one to which he or she is sensitive, then desensitization can be accomplished. This should be done by an allergist and can be achieved in 2 to 3 hr in most cases.

Patients who are treated with a drug who develop skin symptoms that include pruritus should be given antihistamines with sedative and tranquilizing properties. Those recommended include cyprohepta dine, diphenhydramine, and hydroxyzine. Topical corticosteroids are not appropriate for pruritus associated with urticaria but could be used in situations in which eczema is present with or without bullous skin reactions. Glucocorticoid therapy should be used promptly if a severe inflammatory reaction occurs, just as is the case for severe contact dermatitis. One should not be too concerned with the risks of such therapy, according to Van Arsdel. The duration of treatment is short, and one can expect quick resolution to the patients inflammatory problem in a great percentage of cases. Urticaria, on the other hand, if it develops rapidly after taking a drug, may progress to systemic anaphylaxis. Such conditions should be treated initially with 0.3 to 0.5 mg of epinephrine administered subcutaneously. Other signs of anaphylaxis should be watched for, and appropriate preparations should be made (e.g., oxygen availability, airway establishment if needed, maintenance of plasma volume, treatment of bronchospasm).

Shoe Dermatitis

Dermatitis due to shoe materials usually is a result of the rubber in the toe box, the cements used in shoe manufacturing, and the dichromate used in tanning leather. In some instances the cause is due to the presence of felt, cork liners, dyes with formaldehyde components, asphalt, and tar. Because of the location of shoe dermatitis, many patients are misdiagnosed as having fungal disease and are treated with antimycotic agents which not infrequently aggravate the dermatitis. While not conclusive, one finding observed in the examination of the contact dermatitis patient is the absence of any interdigital lesions, which often are involved in patients with fungal disease. Like patients with fungal disease, severe contact dermatitis of the feet may produce id reactions on the hands. Dermatitis due to shoe materials most often starts on the dorsum of the toes and the instep. It usually remains confined to these locations. Weeping, crusting, erythema, and lichenification may occur in complicated cases, in addition to secondary infection. This type of dermatitis occurs frequently enough to have resulted in the development of a special patch testing kit consisting of components of shoes (Hollister-Stier) (Figs. 13.4 to 13.7).

In the event rubber is proven to be the sensitizing substance, shoes should be worn either without a toe box or with a toe box constructed from Celastic. While it is not universally true, more expensive shoes tend not to have rubber toe boxes or rubber adhesives. Frequent sensitizing substances in shoes include monobenzylether of hydroquinone, which is a rubber antioxidant, and rubber accelerators such as mercaptobenzothiazole. Chromate sensitivity is the cause of 20% of shoe dermatitis. It is more common in people with hyperhidrosis. Chromates are included in the tanning process of leathers. Aldehydes such as formaldehyde may be used in tanning white leather and can be the responsible agent in some cases of contact dermatitis due to shoes.

Red dyed shoes should be avoided because of the frequently inadequate binding of the dye with the leather. While one may then resort to leather substitutes and corfam, the linings of such shoes may contain formaldehyde and dyes, and may have been tanned with chromates.

Shoe companies which manufacture or sell special shoes for people with a hypersensitivity to standard shoe materials are listed in Table 13.2.

Poison Ivy

The feet and ankles are frequently the sites of a contact dermatitis due to poison ivy, poison oak, and poison sumac. Such eruptions are referred to as Rhus dermatitis: It appears within about 48 hr after one has been exposed to these plants. Intense itching is the first symptom, followed by inflammation, vesicles, and even bullae. The most characteristic diagnostic feature is the typically linear pattern exhibited by

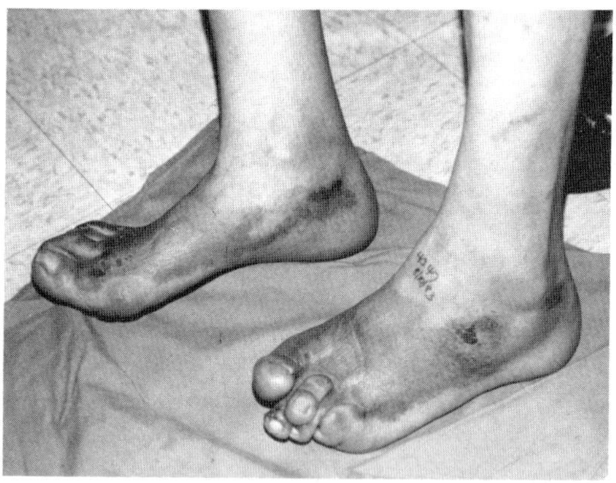

Figure 13.4. Shoe dermatitis.

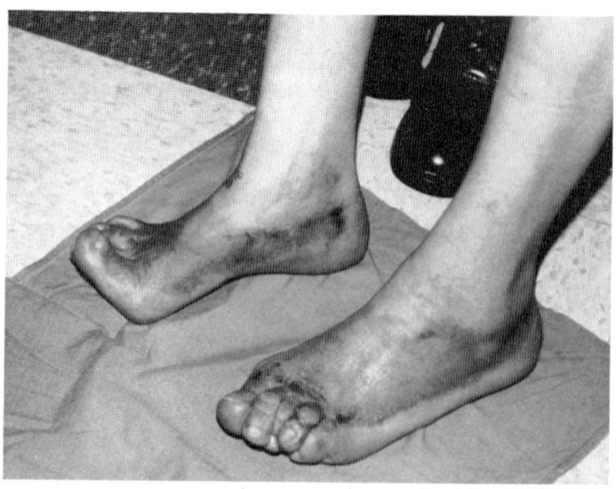

Figure 13.5. Shoe dermatitis.

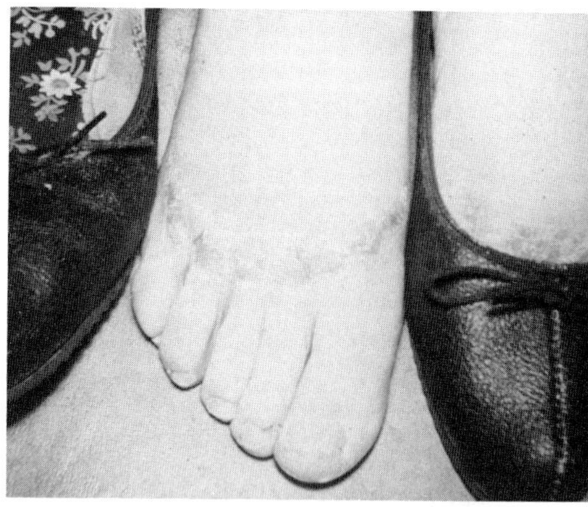

Figure 13.6. Shoe dermatitis.

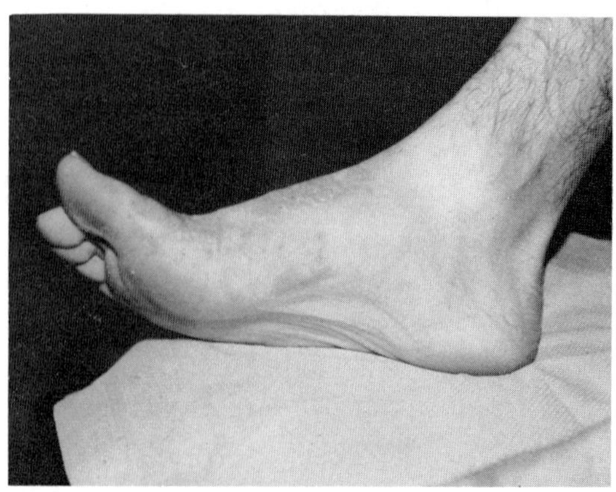

Figure 13.7. Shoe dermatitis.

Table 13.2
Sensitizing Material

Shoe company	Rubber cement	Dichromate	Other
Alden Shoe Company Taunton Street Middleborough, MA 02346 (Derma-Pedic shoes)	x	x	
Siboney Shoe Company Division of Suave Shoe Co. Miami, FL	x		
American Footwear Co. Altoona, PA (for women)	x		
Vo Gal Shoe Co. Appleton St. Lawrence, MA (for children)	x		
Foot-So-Port Shoe Co	x	x	x
or			
Musebeck Shoe Co., Inc. Oconomowoc, WI 53066	x	x	x

the groups of vesicles. Attacks last about 2 to 3 weeks, and then lesions dry and become crusted.

The dermatitis is caused by an oleoresin called urushiol. The active antigen is pentadecylcatechol. No difference exists in the lesion caused by poison ivy, as compared to that from poison oak and sumac. A 2% poison ivy oleoresin in acetone is used for patch testing.

Treatment must include avoiding exposure to the plant and articles that have come in contact with it, such as shoes, other articles of clothing, pets, and tools. Contaminated clothing should be laundered to get rid of the oleoresin, and the patient should bathe using regular bath soap.

Topical corticosteroids may be applied every 3 to 4 hr. Vesicles should be opened with a sterile sharp object such as a needle or scalpel, then touched with alcohol. During acute inflammatory states, when the lesions are producing fluid, compresses should be used with 1:5000 potassium permanganate solution or Burow's solution (1:20 every 4 hr for 20 to 30 min). This may be followed by applications of corticosteroid lotion, cream, or aerosol spray. Because topical antihistamines and local applications of "caine" derivatives are potentially sensitizing, their use should be discouraged. In severe cases oral or injectible corticosteroids are useful. A single dose of 40 to 60 mg of triamcinolone acetonide or 12 mg of betamethasone may be administered intramuscularly. This dosage is repeated in 3 or 4 days if necessary. Oral doses are given in decreasing amounts over 7 to 10 days. Oral antihistamines may also be helpful.

Dermatitis from Fabrics or Other Clothing Material

Contact dermatitis due to clothing appears to be more common in those people who have dry and or thin skin or who perspire considerably. Cotton is almost never the cause of a dermatitis. Only the sizing used in cotton may sensitize the skin and cause a dermatitis. Wool rarely acts as a sensitizing agent. However, it may act as a primary irritant in some people due to the barbs on the fibers. This is particularly a problem in people with atopic dermatitis. A positive patch test to wool generally is due to dyes added to the material. Silk and synthetic fibers are very rarely a sensitizers. Again, it is usually only the dyes that are the cause of a contact dermatitis rather than the fibers themselves. Spandex, the stretchable polyurethane fiber found in certain clothes, such as socks, does not produce allergic contact dermatitis if the material is produced in the United States. The spandex made outside of this country may contain mercaptobenzothiazole, which may cause contact dermatitis. Permapress cloth contains formaldehyde byproducts which may produce dermatitis in the lower extremities.

Atopic Eczema

Atopic eczema is a chronically relapsing inflammatory skin disease with altered immune and pharmacological responses. It is usually seen in patients with a personal or family history of asthma, allergic rhinitis, or atopic dermatitis. Wise and Sulzberger suggested "atopic dermatitis" as a term which could include lichenification and dry lesions as well as weeping eczematous lesions which are more typical in children. Because of the differences in the presentation occurring between infancy and adulthood, the evolutionary stages have been referred to as infantile eczema between birth and 2 years of age, childhood neurodermatitis for those aged 2 to 12, and then the adult form.

It has been shown that 85% of patients had their initial onset of atopic eczema before they were 5 years of age. Sixty percent of this group developed symptoms in their first year of life (Rajka). While adult disease does occur, it is very atypical and more often is due to another diagnosis. The estimated prevalence of atopic dermatitis appears to be between 7 to 24 per 1000.

No distinct diagnostic features are evident on histological examination. Parakeratosis, hyperkeratosis with irregular acanthosis, and spongiosis are seen. Vesicles are rare. Small vessels are noted on the upper dermis and mid-dermis, which are prominent. In addition, there is lymphatic dilation.

Langerhans cells are believed to be an abnormal finding in atopic dermatitis. However, in chronic lesions an increased number of Langerhans cells were noted in the epidermis, which is also thickened and acanthotic. This increase of Langerhans cells does not appear to be present in acute lesions or in uninvolved skin of the atopic patient. The familial nature of the disorder seems to be accepted but the method of inheritance still is not known. The likelihood of a child developing allergic symptoms with one parent having a history of allergies is 58%. If both parents are affected, the probability increases to 79%.

Vascular responses of the skin are seen typically in patients with atopic dermatitis. A subtle facial pallor is often present, but the reason for it is still not clear. The white line that appears after stroking the skin of patients with atopic dermatitis is a phenomenon referred to as white dermographism. Normal skin, when stroked with a blunt instrument, will leave a red line which is called the triple response of Lewis. The linear pallor on stroking atopic skin is probably a phenomenon due to vasoconstriction.

Response to cold and heat in atopic dermatitis is altered. Digits in atopics cool more rapidly in cold environments and rewarm more slowly in warm environments compared to those of normal persons.

Management of atopic eczema in infants and children begins with avoiding external irritation which may precipitate an attack. This includes avoiding sudden changes in temperature, too frequent bathing, friction, chafing, heavy tight clothing, and medicated oils. Avoiding soap and water and using mild soap substitutes such as Cetaphil lotion (Texas Pharmacal) is recommended. Eggs, cow's milk, and wheat products may aggravate the condition and should be avoided by substituting other foods for them. For example, goat's milk or soybean emulsion may be used in lieu of cow's milk. Rice products can substitute for those made from wheat (e.g., rice flakes, puffed rice, boiled rice, Ry-Krisp).

Adults with atopic dermatitis also should avoid stress and temperature extremes as well as exposure to soaps and greases. They should avoid wool since it often is physically irritating. The use of room humidifiers is helpful, especially in the winter, when the skin may become xerotic. Coffee, tea, cola, chocolate, and other stimulants should be limited.

Pruritus may be relieved with antihistamines and cyproheptadine (Periactin), trimeprazine (Temaril) or hydroxyzine (Atarax or Vistaril) also is helpful to suppress itching.

Severe cases of adult atopic eczema are treated with systemic corticosteroids while milder cases may be treated adequately with topical preparations of these drugs. Intramuscular triamcinolone acetonide suspension (30 to 60 mg every 4 to 6 weeks) is safer than an oral regimen. It decreases the possibility of the many side effects associated with oral corticosteroids since it permits recovery from any adrenal suppression before a subsequent dose is given. Acute weeping lesions should be treated with wet compresses of Burow's solution such as Domeboro packets (Dome) and Aluwets. Applications (20- to 30-minute) of a 1:5000 solution of potassium permanganate are also effective alternatives. After using the compresses a mild cream such as Acid Mantle (Dome) can be applied.

The most important topical medications include corticosteroids in spray, cream, lotion, or ointment form. If these preparations fail to result in improvement, one should suspect that the patient may have a sensitivity to one of the frequently used preservatives employed, such as paraben. If neomycin is one of the ingredients, sensitivity to that drug should also be considered.

Xerotic skin, which is often associated with atopic eczema, can be treated with hydrophilic creams or 1% hydrocortisone in 10% urea cream (Carmol HC cream-Ingram). Coal tar (1 to 5%) in white petrolatum or hydrophilic ointment (USP) is still used, and a soluble gel preparation of 5% tar (Estar Gel-Westwood) is an alternate topical medication.

Soap substitutes are recommended because of the irritating nature of washing. Alpha Keri, Dove, Basis, Neutragena, and Emulave are acceptable, less irritating soaps. Scholz advocates cleansing daily with a lipid-free lotion (Cetaphil lotion, Texas Pharmacal). All greases, soaps, ointments, internal steroids, and bathing are stopped. Erythromycin is taken in the event any secondary infection occurs since many strains of *S. aureus* implicated in these patients have been found to be resistant to penicillin. A corticosteroid cream is rubbed into the skin daily, and 50,000 units of vitamin A are taken by mouth daily for 6 months. Dessicated thyroid (30 to 60 mg) or Euthroid is taken daily, as long as the drug given is tolerated by the patient. When internal corticosteroids are stopped, it may be necessary to prescribe antihistamines, phenobarbital, and ataractic agents. The goals of the therapy used to treat atopic dermatitis is to reduce pruritus, hydrate the skin, and restore its integrity to thwart opportunistic organisms.

The role of allergy in atopic dermatitis has still not been resolved completely. However, patients with atopic dermatitis in some instances demonstrate excessive serum levels of IgE. There does not appear to be much of a correlation, however, between the severity of the dermatitis and the IgE serum level. In addition, there are patients without atopic conditions who have elevated IgE levels. T-cell function has been reported to be deficient in atopic individuals, possibly due to the elevated IgE levels.

Among the implications of these immunologic phenomena to the physician is the fact that depressed T-cell function makes the patient more susceptible to viral infection. This may include an increased risk of such conditions as verruca vulgaris and molluscum contagiosum, which may make their appearance on the foot.

CHAPTER 14

Pedal Vesiculobullous Diseases

THOMAS DeLAURO

Complex skin changes frequently produce a variety of integumentary lesions which make dermatologic diagnosis difficult and confusing.

A frequent diagnostic error is failure to distinguish which among many different lesions is primary. Such an exercise tends to reduce the complex to a more simplistic solution.

Blistering of the skin presents one such dilemma. Man is unique in possessing the only integument capable of blister formation.

It is necessary to differentiate between two fluid-filled skin lesions. A distinction is made simply on size differences. Vesicles are palpable fluid-filled skin lesions less than 1 cm in diameter. Bullae are similarly defined except that they demonstrate larger dimensions (Figs. 14.1 and 14.2).

Vesiculobullous lesions can be localized as to whether they are intraepidermal or subepidermal. Subepidermal lesions result, in the main, from hypersensitivity reactions. Erythema multiforme is one example of such a reaction. This condition is characterized by large bullae which dissect and extend along the epidermal-dermal interface.

Diseases of the skin demonstrating intraepidermal diseases, however, are composed of more minute vesicles. This classification may be further subdivided into two groups: the spongiotic type, which includes tinea pedis, contact dermatitis, dyshidrosis, pityriasis rosea, etc., and the acantholytic types, which are characterized by suprabasilar separations and include viral diseases, such as herpes simplex and herpes zoster. Acantholysis is the term given to epidermal cells which become edematous and lose their cohesiveness and separate from one another.

The induction of blisters for experimental study is often performed by means of a suction technique (1). The application of 50% ammonium hydroxide has produced similar results (2). Aging seems to have some interesting effects on blister induction. Older adults exhibit a more rapid initial response time to stimuli than that seen in younger patients, suggesting enhanced diffusion through appendiceal shunts or loss of the stratum corneum. The time to produce a full blister is greatly increased in the elderly. This is probably secondary to a reduced number of capillaries, which are needed to fill the blister. These findings have suggested that "full blister time" may be an indicator of chronologic age (2).

Investigators warn that clinical, histologic, and immunologic parameters must be used together to assess a blistering disease if the correct diagnosis is to be made and proper therapy instituted (3).

An adequate nerve supply seems to play some role in preventing blister formation; neuropathies may be associated with "trophoneurotic bullae" (4).

Psychosomatic induction of blisters has been known to occur, but continued experiments in hypnotic suggestion have resulted in limited reproducibility (5).

It is well-known that large burns may result in multiple immunologic disturbances. The recent discovery that blister fluid from such patients could suppress the lymphocyte blastogenic response may provide a partial explanation for this phenomenon (6).

Concentrations of antibiotics in skin blister fluid may be used as an indicator to

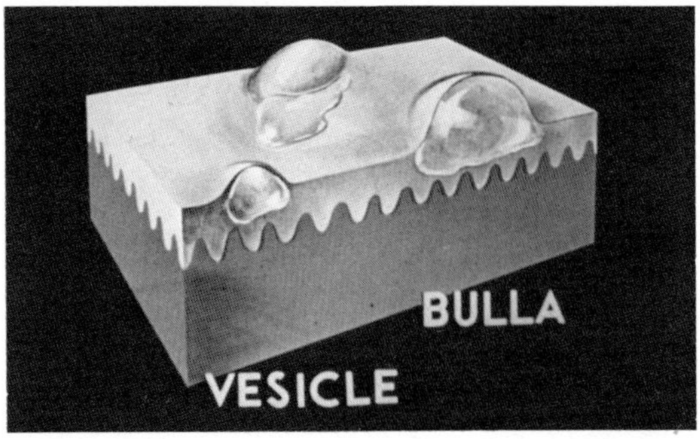

Figure 14.1. Graphic illustration of vesicle and bulla.

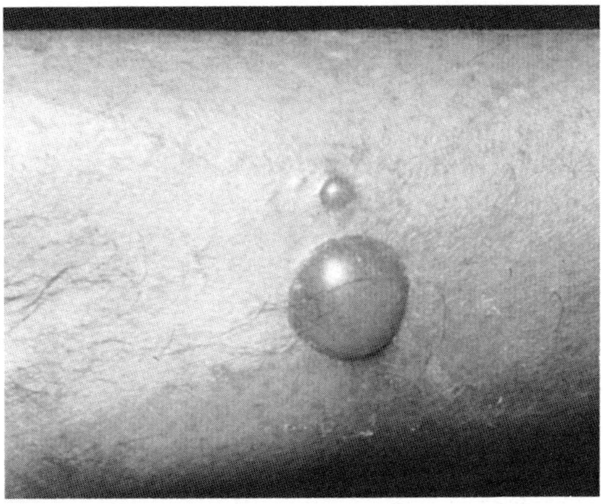

Figure 14.2. Vesicle superiorly and bulla inferiorly.

detect an antibiotic's ability to penetrate the extravascular space after oral administration (7).

A basic understanding of these findings will permit a continuity for brief descriptions of each vesiculobullous disease. Only those major details that facilitate diagnosis will be discussed.

To provide relatively accurate and rapid differential diagnosis, the following groupings is suggested:

a. Diseases limited to the feet and/or hands
b. Diseases limited to the extremities
c. Generalized diseases (affecting face and torso as well).

The first group, those confined to the feet and/or hands, consists of *common*, and *uncommon* subgroups. According to Gibbs, the most common pedal blistering diseases are dyshidrosis, tinea pedis, and contact dermatitis.

Dyshidrosis (8–10), also known as pompholyx, is a chronic disorder of unknown etiology. It is composed of deep-seated, pruritic vesicles which may become pustular. These recurrent vesicles are symmetrically located at the sides of the soles and/or palms (Fig. 14.3). Minimal inflammatory signs are present. Hyperhidrosis is a frequent concomitant finding, and this can predispose patients to contact dermatitis.

The lesions of *tinea pedis* (Fig. 14.4), with or without dermatophytid, are classically pruritic, with foot involvement preceding the appearance of hand lesions. While these "id" lesions share the same location and sterility of dyshidrotic lesions, vesicular tinea pedis is inflammatory and provides positive KOH preparations as well as dermatophyte growth on Sabouraud's agar cultures. Tinea pedis usually begins in the lateral interdigital spaces and spreads to

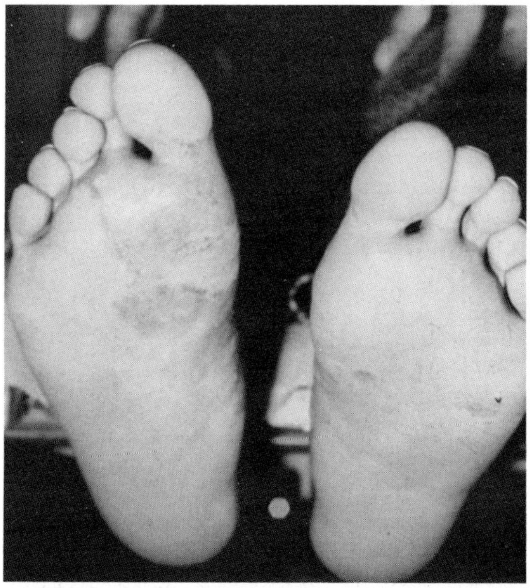

Figure 14.3. Dyshidrosis. Note the predilection for the borders of the feet and toes.

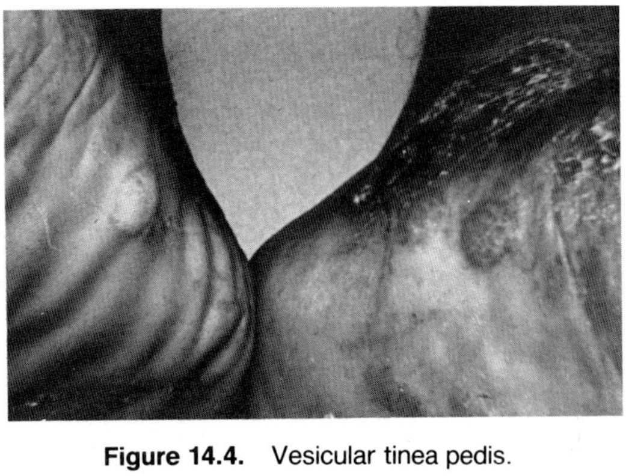

Figure 14.4. Vesicular tinea pedis.

the plantar surface of the foot (11). One should remember that vesicular tinea pedis is usually caused by *Trichophyton mentagrophytes*.

When medications are the cause of dermatologic disease, the term dermatitis medicamentosa is applied. Any of several reactions may occur, including vesiculobullous types. Drug toxicity or allergy is the usual cause for the eruption, rather than idiosyncrasy or intolerance. It has been correctly stated that "... almost any drug can produce any type of cutaneous eruption at any time."

On occasion, drug ingestion evokes a skin response in the same location each time the drug is taken. This phenomenon is known as a fixed drug eruption and has been reported with penicillin, heparin, and phenolphthalein, among others. On the plantar surface of the foot these fixed drug eruptions usually resemble erythema multiforme or, as in the case of gold dermatitis (rheumatoid arthritis (RA) patients), plantar bullae are common.

Aside from internal medications, external drug contact may result in a vesiculobullous dermatosis.

CONTACT DERMATITIS (8)

Contact dermatitis (also known as dermatitis venenata) is further categorized into primary irritant and allergic types. Only the acute forms are vesiculobullous and are usually diagnosed by the sharply demarcated nature of the dermatosis (Fig. 14.5), which often consists of numerous, closely set, intact blisters. Although irritant substances can potentially cause this dermatosis in any patients, allergic substances require individuals to be susceptible, and an incubation period is usual.

Podiatrists must be familiar with every component of the topical medications they use, since any one of them may cause such pruritic disorders. These include vehicles and therapeutic agents such as topical corticosteroids. This last consideration becomes more important in patients with chronically injured skin who have become sensitized by the use of topical medications over prolonged periods (12).

Shoe dermatitis is probably the most common form of contact dermatitis that a podiatrist treats, with rubber compounds being the usual offender. The dorsum of the foot, especially the hallux, is most often affected, since the thin dorsal skin allows for easier penetration of these chemicals. Less common shoe materials that cause this disease include dyes, tanning agents, and metals such as nickel which are used in buckles, eyelets, etc. Pedal hyperhidrosis serves to leach these chemicals out of shoe materials, and this condition must be treated concomitantly.

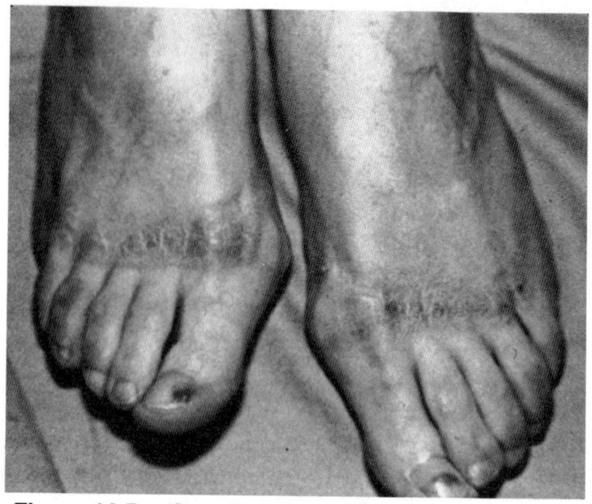

Figure 14.5. Chronic shoe dermatitis. Note the sharply demarcated nature of the dermatosis.

LESS FREQUENTLY ENCOUNTERED PEDAL BLISTERING DISEASES

Bacterial eczemas of the foot are usually secondary to *Staphylococcus aureus* and/or hemolytic *Streptococcus*. They often localize themselves to the medial interdigital spaces and spread to the dorsum of the foot. Some investigators feel that such eczemas result from preexisting sensitization rather than direct infection (11).

Hand, foot, and mouth disease (8), caused most often by infection with the Coxsackie A16 (and sometimes A5) virus, was originally found to be epidemic in girls' schools. Patients usually admit a history of gastrointestinal upset (e.g., diarrhea, "upset stomach"). The resulting dermatosis, which is composed of football-shaped vesicles with narrow red alveolae on the feet, buccal mucosa, tongue, and hands, follows the constitutional symptoms. On the soles, vesicles or just reddish papules may appear. These are especially common on the heels.

Often, several members of a family have

this condition, or it may spread between members of separate families. Mild oral and constitutional symptoms may precede this disease of normally abrupt onset, then subside as the exanthem appears. Hemorrhage can occur into these vesicles: The disease requires no specific therapy since it generally regresses spontaneously within several days.

"Tight-shoe" eczemas have been documented, which most often localize themselves to the back of the foot, the base of the toes, and about the ankles (11).

Herpes gestationis is an extremely pruritic inflammatory papulovesicular eruption that has a predilection for the extremities, palms, and soles of women. It usually begins in the 5th or 6th month of pregnancy or during the postpartum period. Immunologic studies reveal linear deposition of C3 along the basement membrane (13). Pustular herpes gestation is without any history of vesiculobullae is a rare occurrence, but it has been reported (14). Although some studies have indicated that miscarriages and maternal complications do not increase with this condition (13), herpes gestationis may herald the possibility of fetal death or premature delivery.

Second degree burns are an obvious cause of pedal vesiculobullous disease. Patients always admit a history of such trauma, except for those with peripheral neuropathy.

Bullous impetigo is representative of the staphylococcal toxin syndromes, all of which are characterized by intraepidermal cleavage secondary to a *S. aureus* exotoxin. Although most occurrences are generalized, bullous impetigo may exist in a localized form. It presents with flaccid bullae which undergo spontaneous rupture in 5 to 7 days, and heal without scarring. A Nikolsky sign is absent, as are constitutional symptoms. Leukocytes are found in blister fluid, but bacteria are noticeably absent. Cultures of denuded skin are characteristically positive for *S. aureus* (15).

The herpes virus is the causative agent in two closely related vesiculobullous diseases: herpes simplex and herpes zoster (Fig. 14.6). Although both conditions rarely affect the foot, herpes zoster is most frequently seen. Both appear as groups of vesicles on an erythematous base, and both

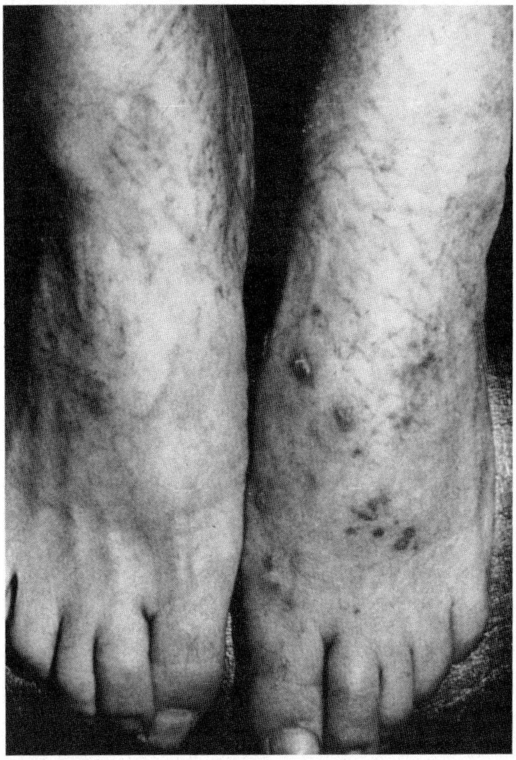

Figure 14.6. Herpes zoster. Note the dermatomal distribution that is a characteristic of this eruption.

are painful. Pain may even precede the development of herpes zoster vesicles by days. Herpes zoster is a unilateral disorder, occurring only once. The vesicles follow the course of a cutaneous nerve. In addition, a history of varicella can often be elicited in the zoster patient (varicella itself can affect the foot by contiguous spread). Such findings are absent in herpes simplex, where vesicles recur at the same location. Hemorrhage may occur in the zoster vesicles, which should alert the clinician to search for an underlying leukemia or lymphoma (8).

Diabetes bullosus (8), also called phlectenular dermatosis, is a rare asymptomatic disorder that presents with periungual vesicles and bullae (Fig. 14.7). No history of trauma can be elicited, and very often these patients have or are found to have diabetes mellitus. Recent studies have demonstrated an increased susceptibility to skin blistering in insulin-dependent diabetics relative to the normal population. Histologic differences have not been recorded in these two groups (16).

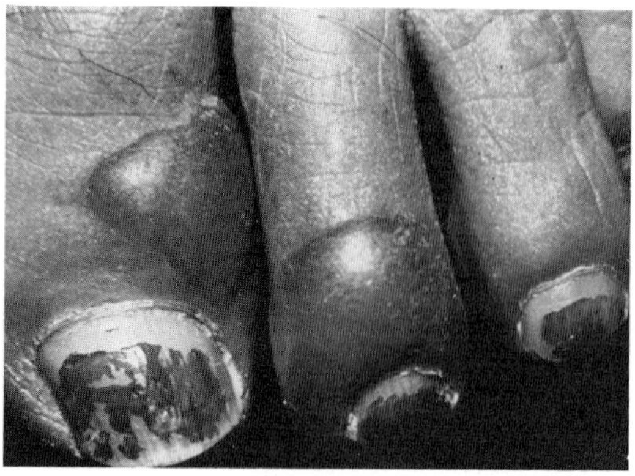

Figure 14.7. Diabetes bullosus.

Congenital syphilis (8, 9) exhibits a bullous eruption of the palms and soles, together with the characteristic finding of Hutchinson teeth and "sabre shins." It is interesting to note that syphilis is never vesicular in adults, due to the firm attachment between the epidermis and dermis that exists in patients of this age group.

Gonococcemia (9) may present as a vesicular disease, with patients admitting a history of urethral discharge, pelvic pain which worsens a day or so after the menstrual period, or other signs of pelvic inflammatory disease. Skin changes usually begin as tiny erythematous macules which soon transform into purpuric macules or vesicopustules, both affecting the palms and soles. It should be emphasized that gonorrhea may be an underlying cause of heel pain. Bouts of fever and arthralgia usually accompany the cutaneous eruption of gonococcemia.

Infantile acropustulosis is an uncommon dermatosis which seems to have a predilection for black male infants. Small, pruritic, vesiculopustules appear on the distal extremities before 1 year of age and resolve spontaneously between 2 and 3 years of age. Lesions are subcorneal, may contain eosinophils, and may be associated with eosinophilia. The only effective therapy seems to be sulfones (dapsone) (17–19).

Six separate diseases compose the *acropustuloses* (8), which are characterized by groups of sterile pustules (except for Streptococcal acrodermatitis) at the distal aspect of one or more extremities. They are included here because pustules (when small) are sometimes mistaken for vesicles, and also because these diseases may originate as vesicles.

Acral vesiculation coupled with digital gangrene, cyanosis, or ulceration is a sure indicator of *cryoglobulinemia*. These abnormal serum proteins precipitate within blood vessels upon exposure to cold, producing the vascular changes just mentioned.

The *bites and stings* of animals and insects (Fig. 14.8) may result in vesiculobullous eruptions. Skin lesions secondary to mites ordinarily occur within minutes to hours after the bite. The summit of each blister often exhibits a small but distinct punctum. Trombiculid ("chigger") mites attack the feet and ankles. Clinicians should search for red blood spots (crushed mites) on clothes and bedclothing. Skin lesions are secondary to toxins or the normal secretions of mites (20).

In India, linear or circular blistering eruptions on the lower legs or dorsa of the feet may indicate reaction to the acidic secretion of the "blister beetle" (*Mylabris* sp.). This "seasonal blistering dermatitis" gains its name from the predominance of cases during the months of June, July, and August (21).

The following are those pedal blistering diseases *limited to the extremities*, generally sparing the face and torso.

The *mechanobullous diseases* (22) are characterized by their hereditary nature, and all exhibit blistering eruptions at sites of trauma, thereby making the foot a major area of involvement. In the past, the rarely seen prototype for the group was epidermolysis bullosa; however, this designation

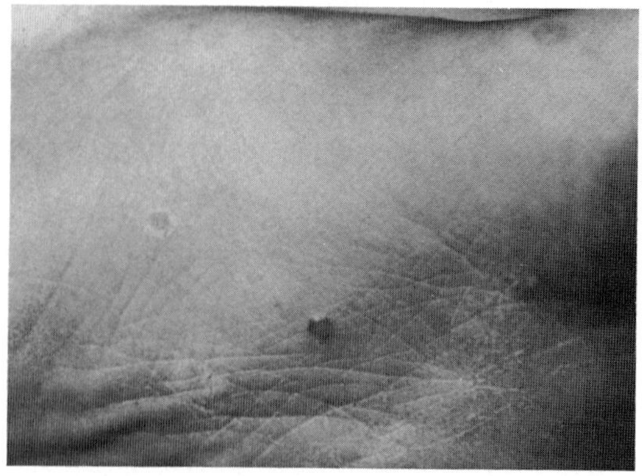

Figure 14.8. Scabies. The mite is frequently resting at the site of the vesicle.

has since been discarded because it does not truly represent the complete disease spectrum. Scarring and nonscarring forms of the mechanobullous diseases exist. The nonscarring variety as a group has been termed epidermolysis bullosa simplex, and all are worse in summer.

NONSCARRING MECHANOBULLOUS DISEASES

Several variants of nonscarring mechanobullous diseases can be categorized: (*a*) a generalized form, affecting the foot only fortuitously; (*b*) the Ogna type, which is coupled with easy bruisability and onset in infancy. Otherwise, the Ogna type is similar to the localized form; (*c*) a localized form, known as Weber-Cockayne disease, or recurrent bullous dermatosis of the feet (8, 9). This type is autosomal dominant, has its onset in childhood or later life, and is characterized by thick-walled blisters affecting the hands and feet while sparing the nails and mouth. Reported complications involve only the infection of blisters. Exacerbations of this illness are noted after prolonged walking and marching as well.

SCARRING MECHANOBULLOUS DISEASES

The scarring mechanobullous diseases uniformly exhibit milia formation and nail dystrophy. The autosomal dominant forms (dermolytic bullous dermatosis) are not life-threatening and exist in two subtypes.

A Cockayne-Touraine form, with onset in infancy or early childhood, is usually localized to the extremities. Scarring may be hypertrophic, with keratoses developing within the scars themselves. Nails may be lost completely but the teeth and mouth usually remain unaffected.

A Pasini, or "albopapuloid" type, also has onset during birth or infancy. Once again, blisters usually appear confined to the extremities. In contrast to the Cockayne-Touraine type, the Pasini form heals with atrophic scars, and mouth blisters are more common, although not severe. Trunk lesions described as albopapuloid (hypopigmented papules) are a part of the syndrome, as is increased urinary chondroitin sulfate excretion.

The recessive scarring form is indeed life-threatening. At the very least, mutilating syndactyly and contractures transform feet and hands to "mitten-like" structures secondary to repeated cycles of infection and healing with fibrosis (Fig. 14.9).

The final scarring type is a so-called "acquired" variety. Although the mechanobullous diseases are classically hereditary in nature, the acquired form lacks a genetic pattern. Blisters are again localized to the extremities: They heal with atrophic scars and/or milia. Oral lesions may or may not be present, and nails may be normal or dystrophic. Instead of appearing in infancy, the acquired form presents in adult life. Indeed, this type is difficult to classify, as it possesses elements of each of the mechanobullous diseases already described. It has been reported as occurring in association with dysglobulinemia (23), and in cases of systemic amyloidosis, with plasma cell dyscrasia (24, 25).

Erythema multiforme is the other blistering skin disease that limits itself to the extremities (8). It represents an allergic response (i.e., to drugs), and exists in both major and minor forms. Any variety of skin lesions may occur, including vesicles and bullae. The initial lesions, however, have an acute onset and usually have symmetric, vivid, erythematous macules on the dorsum of the hands and feet, the palms and soles, and the elbows and knees. The trunk is usually spared unless the limbs are markedly affected. The macules soon become annular or target-shaped. In the major or most severe form, bullae that are usually nonpustular arise within the center of these

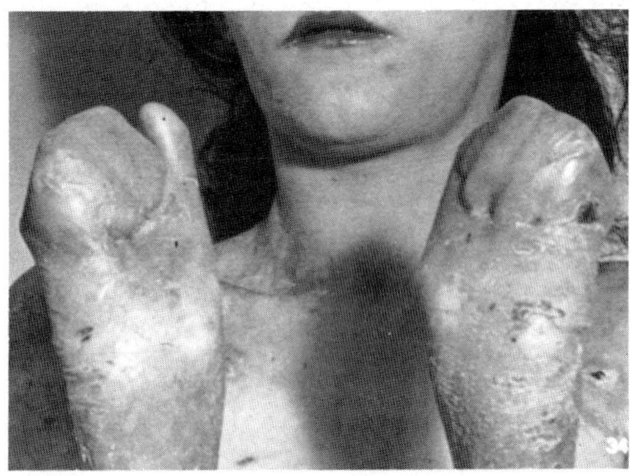

Figure 14.9. Autosomal recessive form of scarring mechanobullous disease.

annular lesions, and these may become hemorrhagic. All in all, the rash itself is more startling than the symptoms it evokes (i.e., pruritus). Fever, toxemia, a prodromal upper respiratory infection, and mouth and eye inflammation usually herald and accompany the major form. Even without treatment, the major disease runs a 6-week course. The minor disease has a 2- to 3-week course.

The abrupt onset and constitutional symptoms that are typical of erythema multiforme bear some resemblance to other major blistering eruptions. An important differentiating feature, however, is the noninvolvement of the face or trunk in erythema multiforme. This is in contrast to what usually occurs in the generalized blistering diseases.

The *generalized blistering diseases* (i.e., pemphigus, etc.) affect the foot only fortuitously and not primarily. Brief discussion of these disorders individually is nonetheless warranted.

Bullous pemphigoid (BP) usually affects the elderly and is characterized by large, tense bullae on otherwise normal skin. Such lesions are found in the region of the groin, the axillae, and the flexor aspect of the forearms, but a form localized to the lower extremities does occur. This disorder is usually benign, self-limiting, and tending to heal spontaneously. Association with internal neoplastic disease has been reported.

The coexistence of bullous pemphigoid and ulcerative colitis has been reported. The absence of basement membrane zone antibodies to colonic mucosal cells makes this occurrence more incidental than "etiopathologic" (26). BP has also been reported in association with other diseases which exhibit alterations of the immune system: rheumatoid arthritis (RA), systemic lupus erythematosus (SLE), pernicious anemia, polymyositis, and factor V inhibitor deficiency (26). Immunoelectron microscopy, however, has cast doubt on the coexistence of BP and SLE; instead, a bullous form of SLE has been proposed (27). Blood eosinophilia has also been reported. When connected with the reported elevations of IgE and "eosinophilic chemotactic factor of anaphylaxis (ECF-A) in serum and blister fluid," bullous pemphigoid deserves inclusion in the list of bullous diseases with associated eosinophilia (28). A few investigators have reported patients with prurigo nodularis who subsequently developed bullous pemphigoid (29).

Dermal-epidermal separation in BP has been shown to require not only antibody but complement as well (30). IgG deposition occurs at the level of the basement membrane, and lesions are subepidermal (31).

Since the advent of immunofluorescent studies, clinicians should be cautious in making the diagnosis of localized (pretibial) bullous pemphigoid when inflammatory findings and immunofluorescence are absent on biopsy. Instead, some investigators contend that simple hydrostatic factors are the probable cause of bullous pemphigoid, and they extend this hypothesis to bullous morphea and diabetes bullosus (31).

Pemphigus, which has four subtypes, is a rare pedal disease, characterized by relapsing bullae which arise without trauma at sites unrelated to friction. They occur in an irregular distribution, ungrouped, on otherwise normal skin or mucous membrane. When the feet are involved, bullae are usually accompanied by a foul odor (32). Cells of the epidermis are so loosely attached to one another that gentle rubbing of the skin removes superficial epidermal layers, leaving a raw, moist base. Lateral pressure against existing vesiculobullae will result in effortless extension of the lesion. These clinical findings are examples of the so-called Nikolsky sign.

Porphyria cutanea tarda (8, 9), a disorder of porphyrine metabolism, is manifested by vesicles and bullae that develop in light-exposed areas. This photosensitivity often occurs on the feet and/or hands, forehead, and nasal bridge. Hyperpigmentation of the skin together with hypertrichosis also occurs. Vesicles and bullae may rupture and heal with scarring. In some instances, bullae may rupture, only to heal with milia formation. Wood's light examination of the urine in these patients reveals a pink or coral red fluorescence (also seen in lead poisoning). Alcohol, barbiturates, griseofulvin, oral contraceptives, and liver toxins are to be avoided since they may exacerbate the eruption.

Lichen planus will lose its characteristic appearance when it involves the sole of the foot. In this location, lesions take on a yellowish hue, resembling deep-seated vesicles (as in dyshidrosis), or they may develop into bullae which ulcerate. This ulcerobullous form of pedal lichen planus is also associated with loss of toenails and cicatricial alopecia of the scalp.

Subcorneal pustular dermatosis of Sneddon-Wilkinson (9) presents with chronic sterile pustules in middle-aged women on the abdomen, axilla, and groin in an annular or serpiginous configuration. In extensive cases the feet may become involved.

Dermatitis herpetiformis (9), also known as Duhring's disease, presents with chronic and relapsing clusters of symmetrical vesicles in the sacral region, buttocks, elbows, and posterior axillary folds accompanied by overwhelming pruritus and burning. These lesions do not occur on normal-appearing skin and do not present a Nikolsky sign upon tangential pressure. Histologically, blisters are subepidermal, and immunofluorescence studies reveal granular (sometimes linear) IgA depositions at the dermoepidermal junction. Gluten-free diets appear to have some effect on the gastrointestinal lesions of this disorder (31).

Scabies patients complaining of nocturnal itching, which is often generalized, should be examined for the vesicles and burrows caused by Sarcoptes scabiei, the mite responsible for scabies (33). The toewebs, fingerwebs, and penis are favorite sites of infestation (8). It is important to remember that this is not presently an uncommon problem in nursing homes. Microscopic examination of a recent vesicle or burrow will reveal either the mite or its pathognomonic red fecal compactions.

Recently, vesicles on the feet have been reported as heralding *pityriasis rosea* in two patients (34). Pityriasis rosea usually begins with a red, scaly "herald patch" which is soon followed by many smaller rose-colored scaling macules that often follow the rib lines. These lesions may be pruritic but are often of only 6 to 8 months duration.

Uremic patients may present with varying types of bullous eruptions. Undialyzed patients on high doses of furosemide and dialyzed patients ("bullous dermatosis of dialysis") can develop bullous photosensitivity. Oral lesions usually do not occur in these mild, self-limiting dermatoses. The mouth, face, trunk, and limbs have been affected in one reported case of chronic renal allograft rejection. IgG and C3 immunofluorescence along the dermoepidermal junction was found, and only after nephrectomy did the bullous lesions resolve (35).

In infants, bullous disease of the extremities must bring to mind *incontinentia pigmenti* (8), a sex-linked dermatosis in which vesicles and bullae may affect the foot. Pigmentary disturbances accompany the blistering eruption in the form of a reticulated pattern.

Acrodermatitis chronica enteropathica (8) also affects infants. It is a comparatively rare disorder with gastrointestinal symptoms, as well as periorificial and acral bullae. A similar presentation has been reported in a patient who suffered from zinc deficiency during total parenteral nutrition for idiopathic intestinal pseudoobstruction (36).

Urticaria pigmentosa (8) also affects the pediatric age group. The condition frequently demonstrates brownish macules on the trunk region. Its bullous form is less common and may even affect a single toe. A cobblestone appearance of the plantar aspect is a notable finding. Lesions characteristically "urticate" or itch when rubbed. Histologically, infiltrates of mast cells in the cutis are found. In cases of visceral involvement, urticaria pigmentosa is known as mast cell disease.

Pachyonychia congenita (8) is a congenital and familial disorder which presents with diffuse keratoses of the palms and soles, thick distorted nails, fine hair, and white patches on the tongue and buccal mucosa. These patients are often born with teeth and exhibit bullae of the soles beneath their keratoses, especially during hot summer months.

Chronic bullous dermatosis of childhood (CBDC) is a benign, uncommon disorder without genetic pattern. It invariably occurs before the age of 10. Initial lesions affect the proximal extremities, then spread to the trunk and genitalia, sparing the mucosa. Tense subepidermal bullae are the presenting lesions. The acute stage may be followed by years of remission with exacerbation with clearing at puberty. A Nikolsky sign is absent. Linear IgA and C3 immunofluorescence at the basement membrane occurs, while serum remains negative for circulating antibodies. Dapsone-corticosteroid combinations seem to be the most effective remedy (37).

Neoplastic disease, such as blistering diseases, have been associated with internal neoplasia.

Dermatitis herpetiformis-like disease may occur in association with choriocarcinoma, malignant tumors of the ovary, uterus, prostate, bladder, rectum, and breast.

Bullous pemphigoid may erupt in cases of melanoma, gastric, and lung carcinoma.

Erythema multiforme can develop in primary cancers and may be secondary to deep irradiation for internal neoplasia. Such occurrences are thought to be an allergic response to necrotic tumor tissue.

Bullous eruptions may be associated with leukemias and lymphomas. In chronic lymphocytic leukemias, the T-type phenotype is considered rare (38).

Braverman (39) recommends that any vesiculobullous disease that presents an atypical appearance or course, or develops in an elderly patient, should alert the clinician to search for an underlying neoplasm.

DIAGNOSTIC AIDS

There are five basic laboratory tests that can assist in making the correct diagnosis: (*a*) the Gram stain; (*b*) KOH prep; (*c*) Tsanck smear; (*d*) the patch test; and of course, (*e*) biopsy.

When performing the Tsanck smear, an early lesion should be selected, its top removed with a scalpel and the fluid contents blotted away in order to avoid contact with the base of the lesion. The lesion is then pinched firmly to prevent bleeding while the floor is scraped with a sharp curette. These scrapings are then spread on a clean glass slide, allowed to air dry, and then stained with Giemsa solution. In pemphigus patients, acantholytic cells with pyknotic nuclei will be seen, whereas in cases of herpes zoster or simplex or in varicella, giant cells with inclusion bodies will be noted (9).

Treatment for all the vesiculobullous diseases that affect the foot includes the prevention of sepsis, soaking to dry the lesions, and incision with drainage of large bullae that interfere with proper function. The entire roof of a vesicle or bulla should probably never be completely removed.

General treatment will vary according to the specific disease. It is wise for the podiatrist to seek the aid of a good dermatologist, internist, or oncologist.

Steroids are sometimes used to minimize the inflammatory components of vesiculobullous disease, whether the foot alone is involved or other body surfaces are affected.

ACKNOWLEDGMENT

A special word of thanks is extended to Ms. Pamela Schlesinger for her review and editing of the manuscript.

References

1. Kiistala U, Mustakkalio KK: Dermo-epidermal separation with suction. Electron microscopic and histochemical study of initial events of blistering on human skin. *J Invest Dermatol* 48:466–477, 1966.
2. Grove GL et al: Effect of aging on the blistering of human skin with ammonium hydroxide. *Br J Dermatol* 107(4):393–400, 1982.
3. Lazaro-Medina A et al: Limitations in the diagnosis of vesiculobullous diseases. *Am J Dermopathol* 5(1):7–10, 1983.
4. Horiguchi Y et al: A case of trophoneurotic bullae. *Dermatologica* 166(4):212–214, 1983.
5. Spanos NP et al: Hypnotically 'reliving' a prior burn: effects on blister formation and localized skin temperature. *J Abnorm Psychol* 91(4):303–305, 1982.
6. Deitch EA et al: The effects of blister fluid from thermally injured patients on normal lymphocyte transformation. *J Trauma* 23(2):106–110, 1983.
7. Bergan T et al: Penetration of cefotaxime and desacetyl-cefotaxime into skin blister fluid. *J Antimicrob Chemother* 10(3):193–196, 1982.
8. Costello MJ, Gibbs RC: *The Palms and Soles in Medicine.* Springfield, IL, Charles C Thomas, 1967, p 576.
9. Domonkos AN: *Andrew's Diseases of the Skin.* Philadelphia, W.B. Saunders, 1971, p 870.
10. Noojin RO: *Dermatology for Students.* Springfield, IL, Charles C Thomas, 1961, p 228.
11. Weismann K et al: Microbiol eczema of the feet. *Br J Dermatol* 107(3):333–337, 1982.
12. Lazzarini S: Contact allergy to benzyl alco-

hol and isopropyl palmitrate, ingredients of topical corticosteroid. *Contact Dermatol* 8(5):349–350, 1982.
13. Shornick JK et al: Herpes gestationis: clinical and histologic features of twenty-eight cases. *J Am Acad Dermatol* 8(2):214, 1983.
14. Bercovitch L et al: Pustular herpes gestationis. *Arch Dermatol* 119(1):191–193, 1983.
15. Ginsburg CM: Staphylococcal toxin syndromes. *Pediatr Inf Dis* 2(Suppl 3):523–527, 1983.
16. Bernstein JE et al: Reduced threshold to suction-induced blister formation in insulin-dependent diabetics. *J Am Acad Dermatol* 8(6):790–791, 1983.
17. Bundino S et al: Infantile acropustulosis. *Dermatologica* 165(6):615–619, 1983.
18. Findlay RF et al: Infantile acropustulosis. *Am J Dis Child* 137(5):455–457, 1983.
19. Brauner GJ: Cutaneous diseases in black children. *Am J Dis Child* 137(5):488–496, 1983.
20. Krinsy WL: Dermatoses associated with the bites of mites and ticks (arthropoda:acari). *Int J Dermatol* 22(2):75–91, 1983.
21. Bhargava RK et al: Seasonal blistering dermatitis. *J Indian Med Assoc* 79(7):98–99, 1982.
22. Bauer EA, Briggaman RA: The mechanobullous diseases (epidermolysis bullosa). In Fitzpatrick TB (ed): *Dermatology in General Medicine*. New York, McGraw-Hill, 1979, pp 334–347.
23. Gompel A et al: Bullous dermatosis associated with dysglobulinemia. *Biomed Pharmacother* 36(4):199–203, 1982.
24. Walton S et al: Trauma-induced bullae: the presenting feature of systemic amyloidosis associated with plasma cell dyscrasia (letters). *Br J Dermatol* 108(5):628, 1983.
25. Holden CA et al: Trauma-induced bullae: the presenting features of systemic amyloidosis associated with plasma cell dyscrasia (case reports). *Br J Dermatol* 107(6):701–706, 1982.
26. Ahmed AR et al: Bullous pemphigoid and ulcerative colitis. *Int J Dermatol* 21(10): 594–598, 1982.
27. Olansky AJ et al: Bullous systemic lupus erythematosus. *J Am Acad Dermatol* 7(4): 511–520, 1982.
28. Bushkell LL et al: Bullous pemphigoid: a cause for peripheral blood eosinophilia. *J Am Acad Dermatol* 8(5):648–651, 1983.
29. Massa MC et al: Bullous pemphigoid with feature of prurigo nodularis. *Arch Dermatol* 118(11):937–939, 1982.
30. Naito K et al: The pathogenic mechanisms of blister formation in bullous pemphigoid. *Invest Dermatol* 79(5):303–306, 1982.
31. Person JR: Hydrostatic bullae and pretibial pemphigoid. *Int J Dermatol* 22(4):237–238, 1983.
32. Steinberg MD: Dermatology in podiatry. In Weinstein F (ed): *Principles and Practice of Podiatry*. Philadelphia, Lea & Febiger, 1968, p 43.
33. Faust EC, Beaver PCV, Jung RC: *Animal Agents and Vectors of Human Diseases*, ed 3. Philadelphia, Lea & Febiger, 1968, pp 330–332.
34. Garcia RL: LTC Letter to the ed. Vesicular pityriasis rosea. *Arch Dermatol* 112:410, 1976.
35. Feehally J et al: An antibody-mediated bullous skin eruption caused by chronic renal allograft rejection. *Transplantation* 34(5): 295–296, 1982.
36. Welsman K et al: Bullous acrodermatitis due to zinc deficiency during total parenteral nutrition: an ultrastructural study of the epidermal change. *Acta Derm Venereol* (Stockh) 63(2):43–46, 1983.
37. Tomecki KJ: Chronic bullous dermatosis of childhood. *South Med J* 76(5):651–653, 1983.
38. Cote J et al: T cell chronic lymphocytic leukemia with bullous manifestations. *J Am Acad Derm* 8(6):874–878, 1983.
39. Braverman IM: *Skin Signs of Systemic Diseases*. Philadelphia, W.B. Saunders, 1970, p 20.

CHAPTER 15

Ulcers of the Lower Extremity

ROBERT G. O'KEEFE and IRVING PIKSCHER

INTRODUCTION

The diagnosis and management of ulcerations of the lower extremity are common and vexing problems in the clinical population of today. The physician must establish a diagnosis and treatment program for an extremity lesion which may be a manifestation of either underlying local or systemic disease. Thus, differential diagnosis, an adequate history, clinical examination, and laboratory tests are necessary to provide the information needed to arrive at a proper assessment and avoid therapeutic problems (Table 15.1).

The diagnostic dilemma can be circumvented by clearly determining certain characteristic features of the lesion when establishing a history. The clinician should attempt to determine the original appearance of the ulcer prior to examination. The ulcer may manifest secondary infection or may have been previously treated by the patient (1). Thus, the appearance of the lesion at the time of examination may be quite different from its initial manifestation. The skin surrounding the ulcer must be examined for dermatologic clues such as stasis pigmentation, edema, petechiae, hemorrhage, color, granulation, and focal necrosis (Fig. 15.1). Precipitating causes of ulceration must also be reviewed. Lesions may develop from self-induced injury (factitial), phlebitic phenomenon, injection, trauma, inappropriate medication, or thermal injury. A family history can establish underlying disorders such as sickle cell anemia, lupus, diabetes, and vascular disease. A current history of hematologic disorders, connective tissue disorders, and other diseases may provide the information needed to make the correct diagnosis. Further clinical clues are the rapidity of ulcer development and pain. Rapidly developing ulcers with little associated clinical pain suggest venous insufficiency, while slowly developing painful lesions suggest arterial insufficiency. Location of the ulcer may also aid in the diagnosis of the lesion. Venous stasis

Table 15.1
General Causes of Extremity Ulcers

Hematologic disease
Sickle cell anemia
Thalassemia
Dysproteinemia
Granulomatous disease
Fungal (maduromycosis, blastomycosis, coccidioidomycosis)
Atypical mycobacteria
Leprosy
Tuberculosis
Syphilis
Metabolic disease
Diabetes mellitus
Gout
Miscellaneous
Chemical burn
Thermal injury
Radiation burn
Malignant disease
Factitial
Decubitus
Vasculitis
Rheumatoid arthritis
Lupus erythematosis
Necrotizing vasculitis
Allergic vasculitis
Vascular disease
Arterial
Arteriosclerosis obliterans
Hypertensive
Venous
Chronic venous insufficiency
Thrombophlebitis

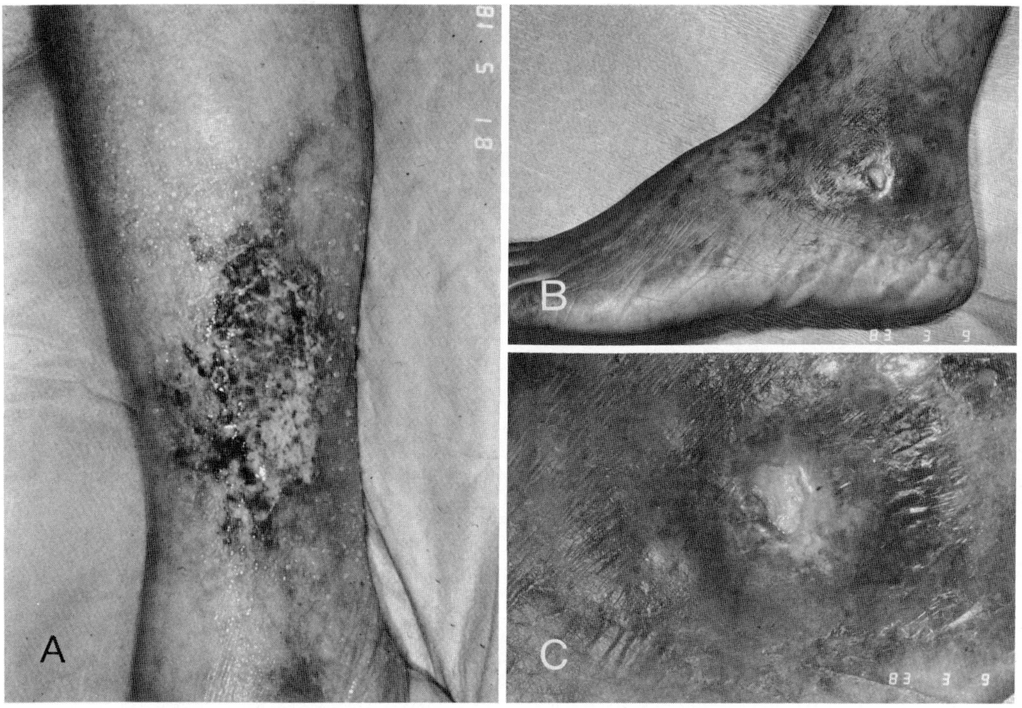

Figure 15.1. (*A*) This ulcerative lesion is complicated by local infection and excoriation from patient abuse. (*B*) This lesion demonstrates surrounding stasis pigmentation. (*C*) Note focal necrosis and absence of tissue granulation, as observed with this ulcer.

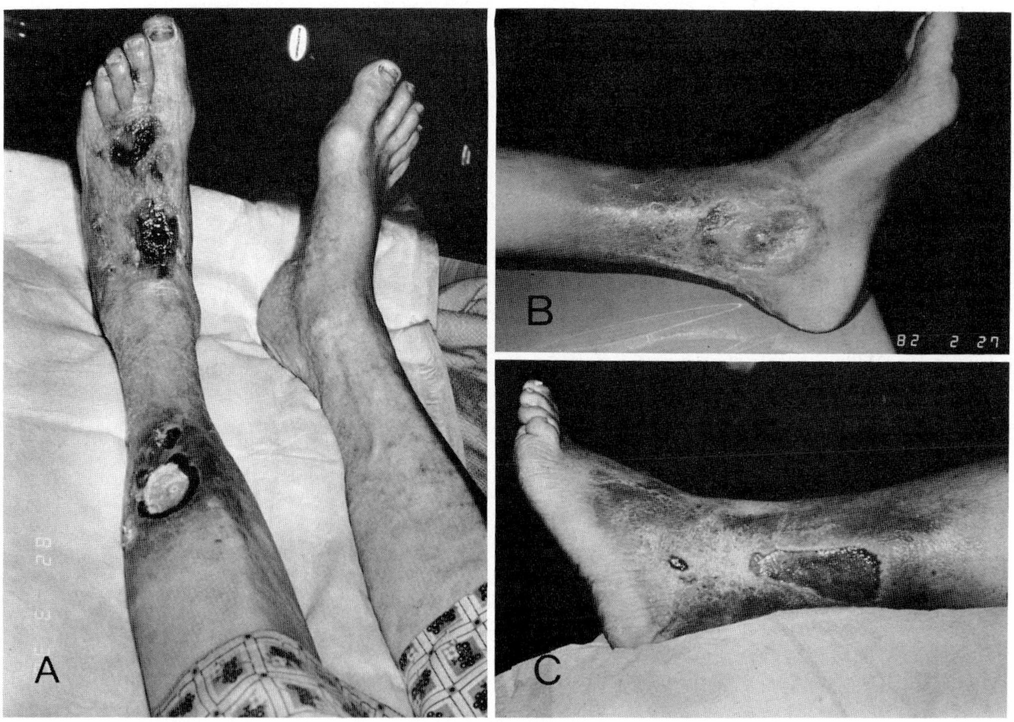

Figure 15.2. Arteriosclerosis obliterans with typical advanced extremity ulceration. (*B*) Longstanding venous insufficiency with stasis and ulcer approximating the medial malleolus. (*C*) Patient with hypertension and venous stasis involving an ulcerative lesion in the posterolateral aspect of the leg.

ulcers often occur over the medial malleolar area, a region drained by the great saphenous system. Ulcers associated with arterial insufficiency occur distal to the region of vessel occlusion. These lesions develop about the toes or dorsum of the foot. Ulcers associated with hypertensive disease usually occur proximal to the level of the lateral malleolus and may extend around the circumference of the limb (Fig. 15.2). Appropriate laboratory analysis can not be understated (2). Suspected underlying local and systemic disease can be further delineated with the diagnostic aid of hematology, blood chemistry, serology, mycology, bacteriology, and pathology (Table 15.2).

Table 15.2
Frequency of Ulcerations of the Lower Extremity

Common
Venous insufficiency
Arteriosclerotic occlusive disease
Neurotrophic disorder involving diabetes mellitus
Uncommon
Vasculitis
Hematologic disease
Granulomatous disease
Hypertensive disease
Rare
Factitial
Malignant disease

HEMATOLOGIC EXTREMITY ULCERS

A variety of hematologic disorders will result in ulceration of the lower extremity. Sickle cell anemia is the most common blood dyscrasia that manifests cutaneous lesions such as indolent ulceration and scars in the lower leg (3). Ulcers are observed in homozygous individuals afflicted by this genetically transmitted disease. Approximately 75% of adolescents and surviving adults will develop indolent ulcers. There is no distinctive clinical feature of these lesions. However, the lateral malleolar area of the extremity is usually affected. The ulcer may be isolated as a single punched out lesion. The ulcer progresses to subcutaneous tissue and may extend to deep fascia and tendons. Pain is usually unremarkable in the locale of the defect. The ulcer is recurrent, and local pigmentation and induration of the cutaneous tissues is observed. These ulcers develop or are aggravated by hematologic crisis (Fig. 15.3).

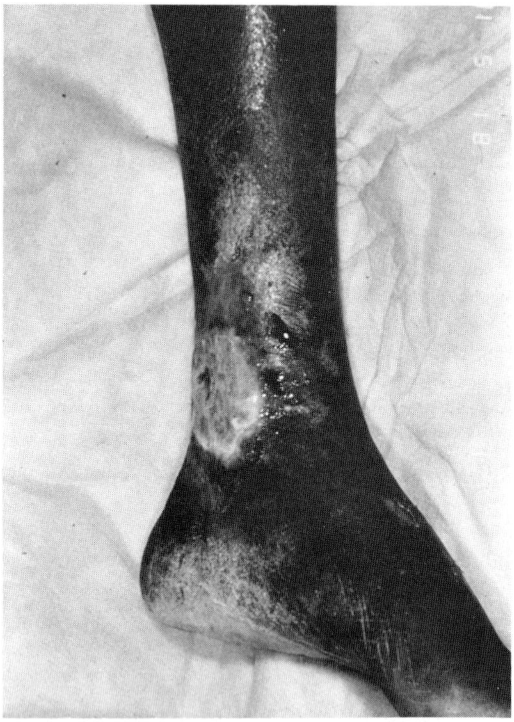

Figure 15.3. The ulcer has a sharply defined border. There is no distinctive feature other than an indolent lesion with regional scars from previous hematologic crisis.

Other hematologic disorders that may produce leg ulcers are thalassemia, polycythemia vera, and the dysproteinemias such as macroglobulinemia and cryoglobulinemia (4). Ulcers uncommonly develop in these disorders but must be considered. Painful necrotic ulcerative lesions rarely develop in thalassemia and polycythemia. However, Raynaud's phenomenon, purpura, necrotic ulceration, and gangrene in the extremities are aggressive clinical cutaneous manifestations of the dysproteinemias. These disorders must be considered in the differential diagnosis in ulcer manifesting disease.

GRANULOMATOUS DISEASE

Deep fungus infections develop cutaneous manifestation which initially appears as papulopustular nodules that enlarge to ulcerative verrucoid granulomatous lesions. These lesions commonly occur in the distal extremity and foot. Infections involving fungi such as blastomycosis and coccidioidomycosis eventually develop typical verrucal plaque or draining abscesses (1). However, coccidioidomycosis may present a cutaneous form of disease which develops chancriform lesions. Atypical mycobacteria, leprosy, tuberculosis, and syphilis also develop granulomatous ulcers of the leg and foot (Fig 15.4). These ulcers appear clinically atypical and are obviously resistant to conservative therapy (4). A localized invasive lesion may develop a mycetoma or apparent tumor produced by fungi. Inoculation of the foot and ankle region by *Nocardia, Actinomyces, Madurella* sp., etc., have heralded maduromycosis, an extremely destructive lesion. Biopsy, mycology, and appropriate bacteriology as well as serology should be considered to ascertain the proper diagnosis.

METABOLIC DISORDERS

Diabetes Mellitus

Cutaneous disorders are often observed in the pathogenesis of diabetes mellitus. The lower extremity tissues are afflicted with vascular disease, neuropathy, and sepsis. In the chronic diabetic state the cutis is susceptible to infection, traumatic pigmentation, xanthomatous lesions, dermopathy, and devastating peripheral neuropathy (5). The combination of macro/microvascular disease and neuropathy profoundly affects the guarded vitality of the tissues of the lower extremity as well as that of other organ systems. The foot may be incapable of sustaining the incident of weight-bearing and every day trauma. Defective sensorium coupled with the trauma of pedal locomotion and vascular impairment may herald mal perforans ulcers (6). Neurotrophic joint disease may develop, creating tarsal joint destruction and ulceration (Fig 15.5).

These diabetic lesions commonly affect weight-bearing structures of the foot, primarily the metatarsophalangeal area. The ulcers may be obscured by a thick keratotic cover (callus) which is manifested by local debridement. Local fibrosis, necrosis, infection, and tissue destruction are observed. Localized infection of ulcerative lesions may develop deep tissue sepsis in neglected cases. Neurotrophic ulcers may penetrate through deep fascia and extend along fascial planes (7). Bone infection is not uncommon with deep mal perforans lesions.

Extremity leg ulcers in diabetes may be associated with ischemia secondary to compromised vascularity. Minor incidence of trauma to the impaired tissue precipitates the development of focal necrosis and ul-

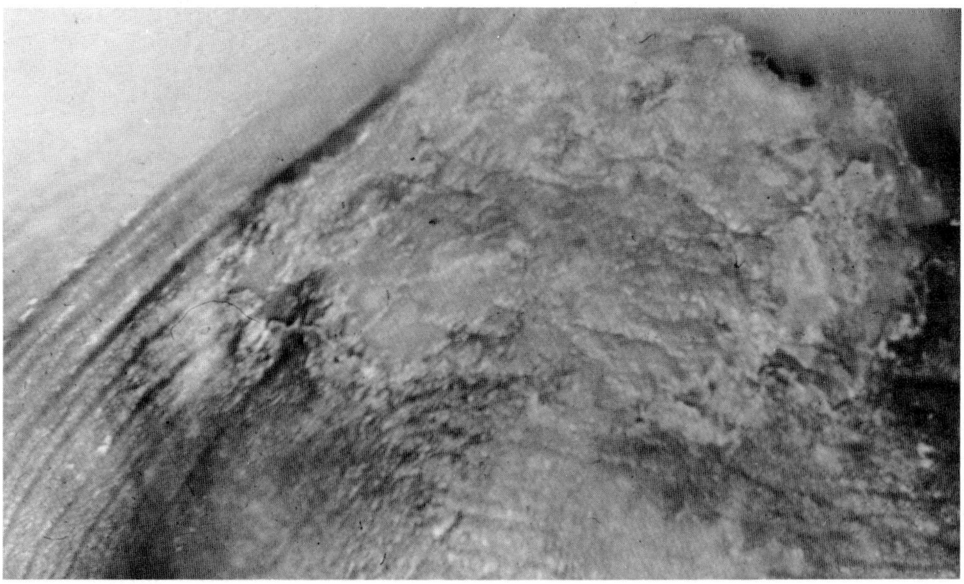

Figure 15.4. Deep fungus infection of the skin. It appears as a verrucoid granuloma. The initiating lesion was a papulopustular nodule, *Viet Nam.* Courtesy of Dr. G. Curin.

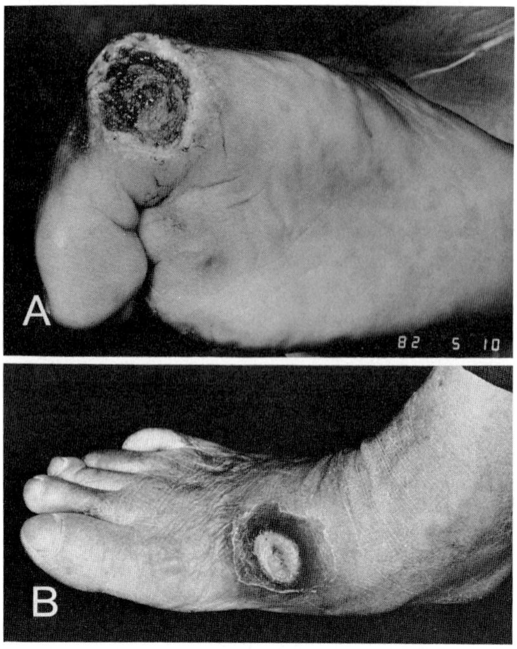

Figure 15.5. (*A*) Neurotrophic ulcers associated with diabetes mellitus. Uncomplicated mal perforans ulcer of the metatarsophalangeal joint. (*B*) Midtarsal ulcer complicated by diabetic neuropathy and development of neuropathic arthropathy.

ceration (8). These lesions may appear as indolent ulcers observed in arteriosclerosis obliterans.

Gout

Hyperuricemia associated with primary gout or secondary to high purine disease states or defective excretion may eventually lead to ulcerative lesions (1).

Prolonged unrecognized hyperuricemia will result in monosodium urate crystal deposition in joints and subcutaneous tissues. Although commonly observed as tophaceous deposits in the hilar of the ear, hands, and elbows, the lower extremities may be affected. Nodules may be present around the malleolar area of the leg and digital areas of the foot. Further deposits and local irritability will precipitate tophaceous ulcer (4). Skin biopsy with preservation of urate crystals will aid in a definitive diagnosis. Surgical debridement and control of the disease state will resolve the lesion.

MISCELLANEOUS LESIONS

Miscellaneous causes of lower extremity ulcers should be assessed in evaluating lower extremity lesions. Causes ranging from factitial insult to melanoma can be associated with unusual ulcerative lesions of the lower extremity. Proper assessment can effect the morbidity and mortality of patients in the aforementioned examples.

Burns to the cutis may be precipitated by chemical, thermal, or radiation injury (1). Extravasation of certain vasopressor drugs and application of nitrogen mustard have created local tissue necrosis and ulceration. Thermal burns and frostbite have caused full-thickness tissue necrosis and localized tissue loss requiring skin grafting and local amputation in some cases. Antiquated use of ionizing radiation for the treatment of benign skin lesions may manifest its destructive effect years later as an ulcerative lesion.

Unrecognized malignant skin lesions may present themselves as atypical ulcerative lesions (4). Malignant melanoma may appear as a purple-to-black pigmented nevus with a central bleeding ulcer. Thus, a discolored bleeding ulcer (late stage melanoma) may be the first precipitating concern of a patient seeking treatment (Fig 15.6). A less aggressive lesion, the epithe-

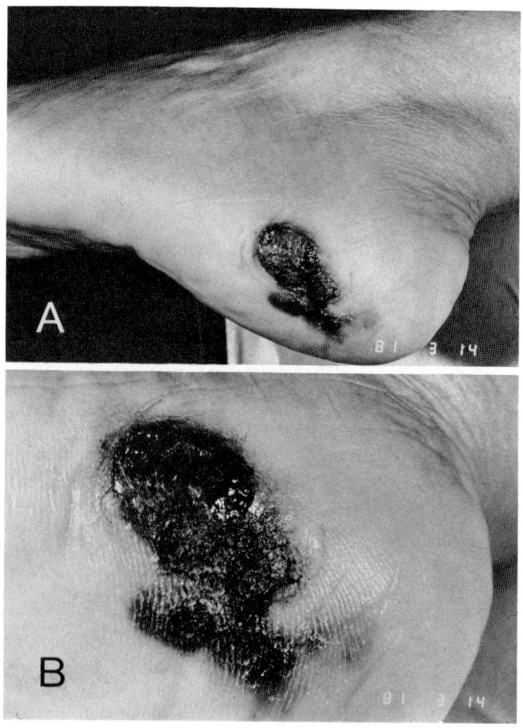

Figure 15.6. (*A*) Malignant melanoma of the heel. (*B*) The melanoma has spread, and a hemorrhagic ulcer has developed in the upper extent of the lesion.

lioma may appear as a caseous furrowing ulcer of the foot.

Factitial or self-inflicted cutaneous wounds may assume an ulcerative process (9). The lesions may appear in bizarre patterns produced by picking, probing with a sharp object, chemicals, cigarettes, etc. Occlusive dressings aid in resolving these masquerading lesions by protecting the skin from self-inflicted trauma.

In chronically debilitated patients, decubitus ulcers are an unfortunate occurrence. These lesions develop from prolonged application of pressure on a dependent body part, disrupting capillary circulation and leading to tissue damage and necrosis (8). The heel of the foot is a common area of decubitus ulcer development. The elimination of prolonged focal pressure and simple ulcer management aids greatly in the eradication of this lesion (Fig 15.7).

VASCULITIS

The most frequently encountered form of vascular inflammation is necrotizing vasculitis. This lesion may be mild and affect the small blood vessels of the skin in the leg, or it may be more aggressive, producing vasculitis of internal organs (4). The end stage of cutaneous lesions is necrosis, ulceration, and occasional focal gangrene (Fig 15.8).

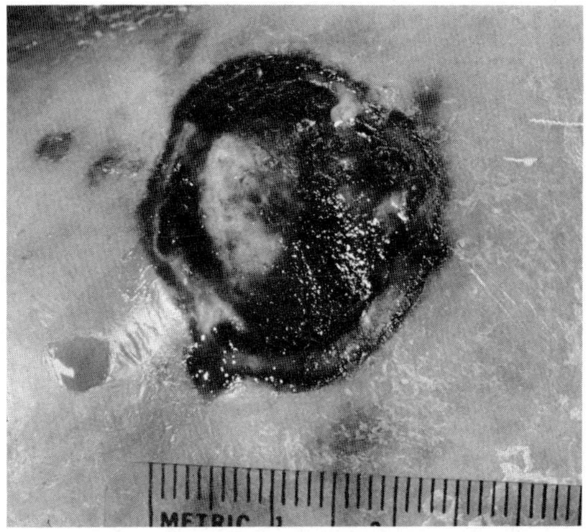

Figure 15.7. Healing decubitus ulcer of the ankle. Local debridement and elimination of focal pressure has reversed the destructive process of tissue necrosis.

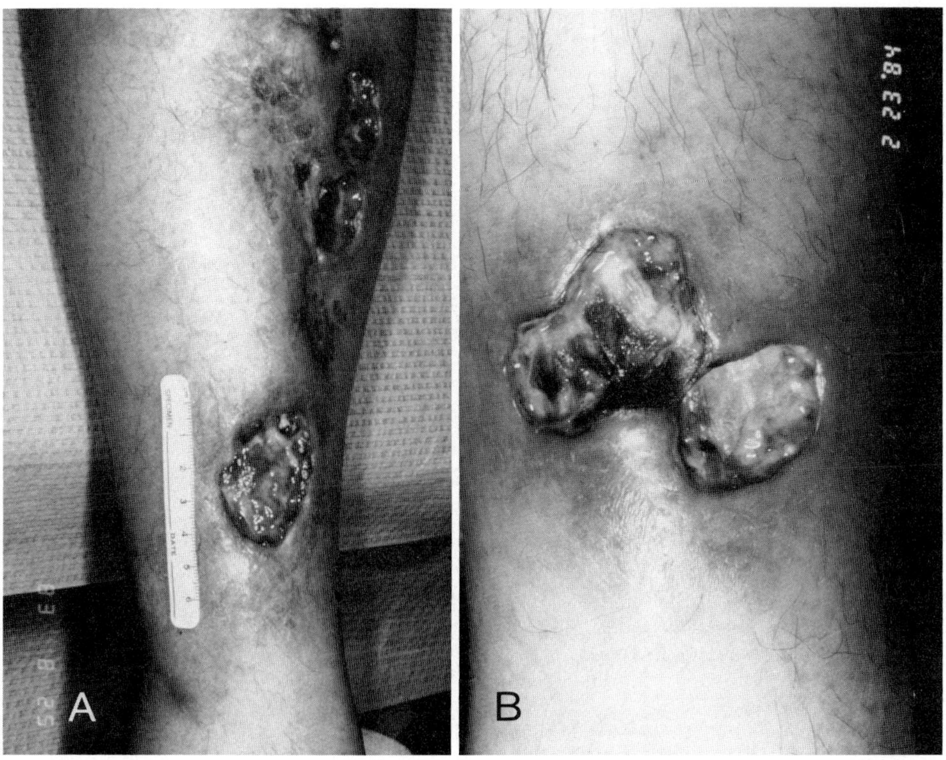

Figure 15.8. (*A*) Necrotizing vasculitis of the lower extremity. (*B*) Necrotic lesions associated with vasculitis. Courtesy of Dr. J. Vanore.

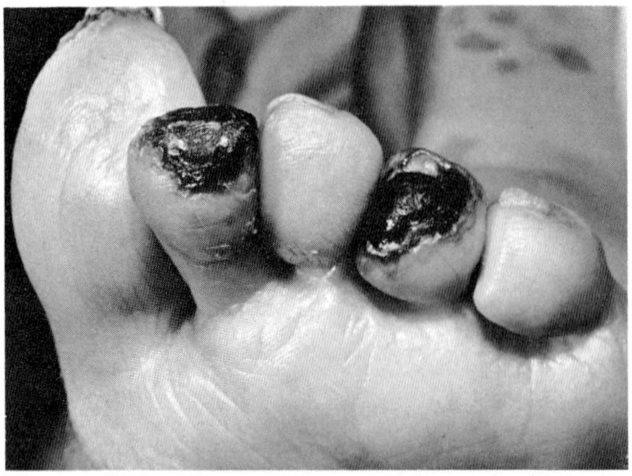

Figure 15.9. Segmental necrotizing vasculitis may cause artery infarction and peripheral gangrene of the toes, as this photograph demonstrates (periarteritis nodosa).

Usually, the tips of the digits are the site of tissue breakdown. The lesion may appear small and involve subcutaneous tissue but may extend to affect the entire digit. Local gangrene of the digits may occur (Fig 15.9). Aggravation or progression of the lesion is associated with exacerbation of the primary disease.

Confirmation of diagnosis is established by skin biopsy (2). Endothelial degeneration and thickening of small vessel walls as well as fibrinoid degeneration of perivascular tissue is observed as well as inflammatory cell infiltrate and leukocytoclasis. Further confirmation of the disease process involves appropriate hematology, lupus erythematosus (LE) prep, antinuclear factor, renal function studies, and immunofluorescence of lesions.

TREATMENT OF VASCULITIS

The treatment of vasculitis ulcerations of the lower extremity necessitates treatment of the underlying systemic disease. As in the case of allergic vasculitis the accompanying precipitating disease may involve drug allergy, infection, or neoplasm (1). Exacerbation of diseases such as systemic lupus erythematosus must be confronted. Systemic antibiosis, eradication of sensitizing drugs, steroid therapy, and immunosuppressive agents play a major role in management of specific vasculitis (10).

VASCULAR DISEASE

Arteriosclerosis Obliterans

Arteriosclerosis obliterans is a progressive occlusive disease of the arterial system. The initial clinical symptom of the disease is usually intermittent claudication or severe pain with activity in the affected extremity. With progressive stenosis of the vessels via intimal fibrous arteriosclerotic plaque and thrombosis, ischemic ulcers will develop in the leg and foot. The severity of ischemia will mirror the extent of disease and is dependent upon adequate collateral circulation and metabolic demands (11). The occlusive disease process becomes more advanced and tissue ischemia more severe, heralding regional ulceration of the extremity.

Ulceration in arteriosclerosis obliterans will appear in the terminal portions of the digits; however, lesions may involve the dorsum of the foot, heel, malleolar area, and leg (Fig 15.10). The rate of progression of the ulcer is insidious and is dependent upon local collateral arterial flow (1, 4). Local skin changes demonstrate typical pallor, dependent rubor, and decreased regional temperature. Unfortunately, minor trauma invariably initiates ulcerative lesions in the vascular impaired extremity.

Ischemic ulcers initially appear to be rather small, round, and punched out, but

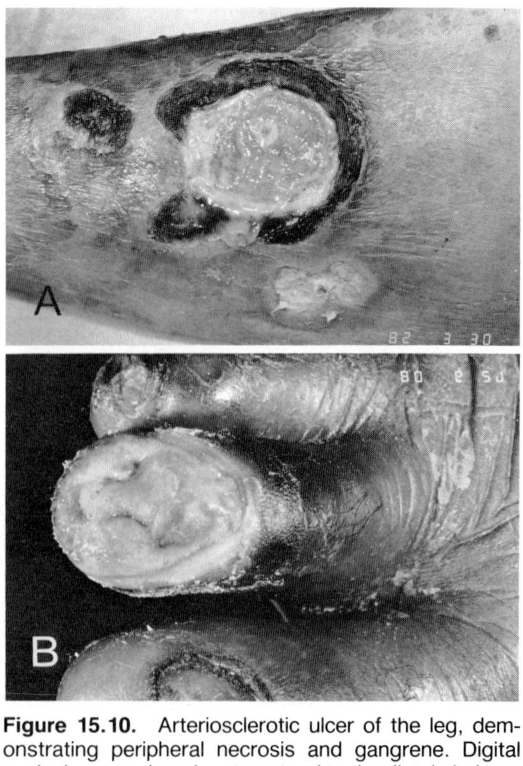

Figure 15.10. Arteriosclerotic ulcer of the leg, demonstrating peripheral necrosis and gangrene. Digital occlusion, causing ulcer to extend to the distal phalanx.

they gradually increase in size. The base of the ulcer is observed as a pale gray or black lesion covered by necrotic debris or yellowish crusted exudate. These lesions demonstrate little evidence of granulation and no tendency for peripheral epithelialization. Ischemic ulcers may extend to the deep tissue layers, communicating with fascia and tendon. Wound infection and osteomyelitis may complicate deep ulceration.

Treatment of arteriosclerosis obliterans is focused on revascularization of the region of arterial occlusion (12). Confirmation of the disease is aided by noninvasive diagnostic procedures such as Doppler ultrasound and ultrasonic arteriography. Definitive diagnosis of the extent of arterial occlusion and the amount of collateral circulation is determined by invasive angiography.

HYPERTENSIVE ULCERS

Patients who have had essential hypertension for an extended period of time may develop ulcers. These lesions share the same characteristics as ischemic ulcers (13). The lesions are bilateral and affect the lateral malleolar area and posterior lateral aspect of the leg. Hypertensive ulcers are typically large and irregular with bridging necrotic areas of tissue. These ulcers remain superficial but are painful and may extend the circumference of the leg. Periulcerative cyanosis, purpura, and local skin slough are common. Arteriosclerotic occlusive disease should be investigated; however, control of essential hypertension appears to be important in the treatment of these aggravating lesions (1).

VENOUS ULCERS

Venous stasis ulcers constitute the most common variety of lower extremity lesions associated with vascular disease. Chronic venous insufficiency features extremity edema, superficial varicose veins, dermatitis, and pigmentation changes. The inability of the extremity venous system to function against gravity allows abnormal retrograde blood flow in the compromised superficial venous network precipitating tissue stasis (12). Intrinsic valve failure or thrombosis produce venous system incompetence and superficial venous hypertension. Subsequent rupture of venules allows extravasation of hemoglobin into the local tissues, causing hemosiderin hyperpigmentation of the area. Tissue capillary fluid exchange is diminished by increased capillary bed venous pressure, creating ultimate ulceration (Fig 15.11).

Ulcers usually occur in the region of the ankle in the vicinity of the malleoli, especially the medial malleolar area (1). These ulcers may develop spontaneously or secondary to traumatic insult. The base of the ulcer is moist with evidence of abundant granulation tissue. Secondary infection is common and is usually confined to the lesion; however, cellulitis may develop in the surrounding skin. Pain may be associated with venous ulcers which are not as intense as those lesions associated with arteriosclerosis obliterans.

The diagnosis of venous insufficiency ulcers can be made on clinical grounds. Confirmation of the competency of the superficial venous system is established by the multiple-tourniquet test or the Trendelenburg test (12).

TREATMENT

The goal of ulcer treatment is the resolution of the lesion via granulation tissue stimulation and restoration of peripheral epithelial growth (4, 12). Local ulcer management aids greatly in the stimulation of granulation and epithelialization. Clearing local dermatitis, infection, edema, and necrotic debris establishes an excellent environment for wound healing (12). The relative success of local ulcer management still remains dependent upon the etiology of the lesion and ability to control contributing factors (Table 15.3).

DRESSINGS

A variety of dressings can be utilized in the management of ulcer disease. These dressings are biologic and nonbiologic, depending upon their physical characteristics and ability to directly stimulate granulation and revascularization of the lesion.

The most common of the nonbiologic dressings that are nonsynthetic are the Betadine and Unna boot varieties. Light Betadine compression dressings are used in routine local wound management (14).

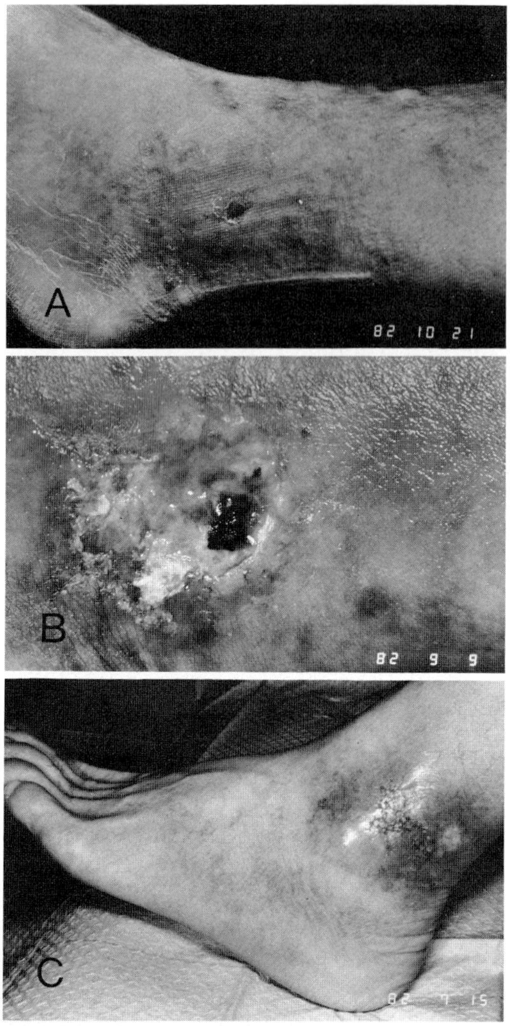

Figure 15.11. (*A*) Venous stasis ulcer with local hyperpigmentation. (*B*) Irregularly shaped venous stasis ulcer, demonstrating moist ulcer base. (*C*) Chronic venous stasis with increased pigmentation. This patient had several episodes of ulcer breakdown.

These dressings are usually changed 2 to 3 times daily and aid in ulcer management. With wet-dry Betadine dressings, local mechanical debridement and inhibition of bacterial surface colonization are obtained. The Unna paste boot is an impregnated dressing of zinc oxide, gelatin, glycerin, and calamine. This dressing is ideal in the treatment of stasis ulcers. The Unna boot inhibits dermatitis, removes edema, and protects the ulcer from repeated local trauma. The Unna boot is applied to clean lesions and may be changed weekly.

Table 15.3
General Treatment of Leg Ulcers

1. Establish etiology
2. Control contributing factors
   - Dermatitis: Compresses, local corticosteroids, antibiosis.
   - Edema: Elevation and bed rest.
   - Occlusive disease: Rest with head of bed elevated, revascularization of extremity via surgery.
   - Sepsis: Local/systemic antibiosis.
   - Systemic disease: Control disease state.
   - Venous insufficiency: Compression stockings, surgery.
3. Stimulate granulation and epithelialization of ulcer.
   - Debridement of necrotic tissue and eschar
     - Surgical
     - Chemical (Enzyme)
     - Physical (Dextran)
   - Dressings
     - Betadine dressings
     - Unna's boot (stasis)
     - Synthetic (2nd skin, polyurethane)
     - Biologic (amnionic membrane, porcine xenograft)
4. Skin coverage for resistant defects
   - Autogenous skin grafting

DEBRIDEMENT

Local wound care and tissue stimulation are instituted by debridement of all necrotic tissue and central eschar. Debridement can be established by surgery, enzyme application, or utilization of hydrophilic polymers. In isolated cases surgical debridement may not be practical where local anesthesia is difficult in areas of regional inflammation. Enzyme debridement is an excellent adjunct to surgical treatment and is preferred by some clinicians (15). In the absence of frank flocculent infection, enzyme debridement aids in the removal of crusty exudate, necrotic tissue, and eschar. Enzyme ointment is applied to the ulcer, avoiding contact with normal epithelial tissue (16). Saline wet-dry dressings are then utilized following adequate granulation of the ulcer bed. In uncomplicated wounds dextran polymer may be utilized (17). These highly hydrophilic polymer beads absorb exudate, bacteria, and necrotic residue from the ulcer surface. Thus, crust formation, bacterial colonization, and degrading metabolite accumulation are greatly inhibited, creating a good environment for granulation.

BIOLOGIC DRESSINGS

Porcine Xenograft

Porcine xenografts are prepared skin tissue from swine that have been employed in the treatment of various cutaneous ulcerations (Fig 15.12). The similarity of dermal and epidermal structures of the porcine graft and human cutis enhances the xenografts efficacy as a biologic dressing (18). The anatomic structure similarity between the biologic dressing and host enhances granulation, revascularization, and epithelialization of the ulcer (Fig 15.13). This biologic covering inhibits bacterial colonization in clean lesions (19). The removal of the porcine graft effects mechanical debridement over the course of therapy, reducing the need for surgical therapy. These biologic dressings are applied to clean ulcerative defects and are ideally changed every 72 hr. Needed local ulcer therapy can be instituted at the time of dressing change.

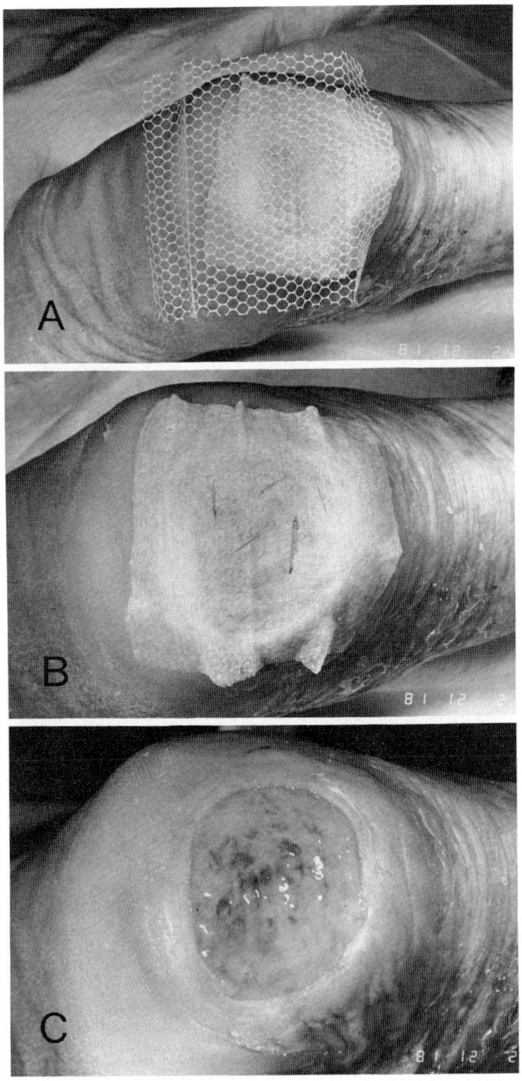

Figure 15.12. (*A*) Decubitus ulcer of the heel. (*B*) Application of porcine skin graft following debridement. (*C*) Graft is maintained with mild compression dressing after contact with lesion.

SYNTHETIC DRESSINGS

Synthetic polyurethane (Op-Site, Medical Products Division, Acme United Corporation, Bridgeport, CT) is an occlusive dressing which has recently been used in therapeutic management of lower extremity dermal ulcers. This material is impervious to fluids but permeable to air and water vapor. Op-Site has had previous wide application as a sterile barrier and dressing in surgery, burn therapy, and autografting.

Applied to clean ulcerative lesions polyurethane dressings discourage exogenous wound contamination and encourages reepithelialization at the wound site (20).

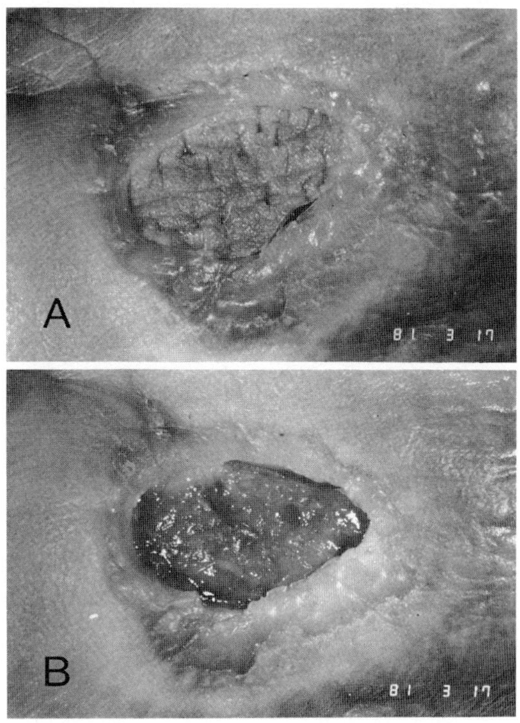

Figure 15.13. (*A*) Porcine graft applied to ulcerative defect. (*B*) Base of ulcer is observed with clear granulation bed and peripheral epithelialization.

These dressings are usually changed every 3 to 10 days. Excessive exudation can be easily removed via sterile aspiration. The transparent polymer membrane allows for easy examination of the wound margins and base through the dressing. Continued local therapy and debridement can be performed as needed between dressing changes. If clinical signs of infection are evident, dressings are changed daily, and proper local antimicrobial therapy is instituted. Contrary to dry occlusive therapeutic modalities, polyurethane maintains a moist environment about the ulcerative lesion. Dehydration is limited, and tissue viability is maintained. This type of oxygen-permeable dressing protects clean serous exudates which enhance migratory cellular elements and, ultimately, epithelialization.

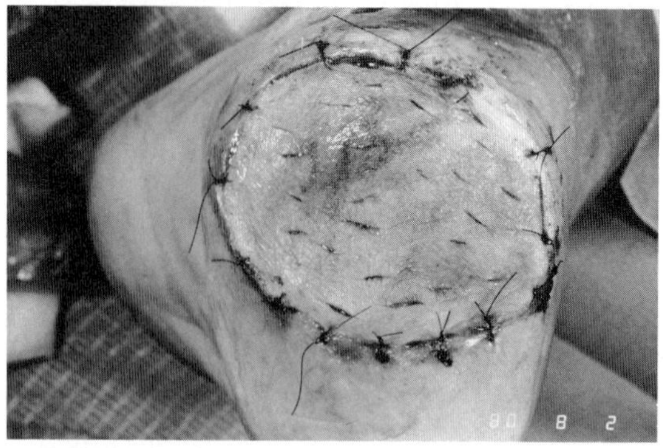

Figure 15.14. Skin graft utilized to correct tissue defect in a patient that had undergone a transmetatarsal amputation.

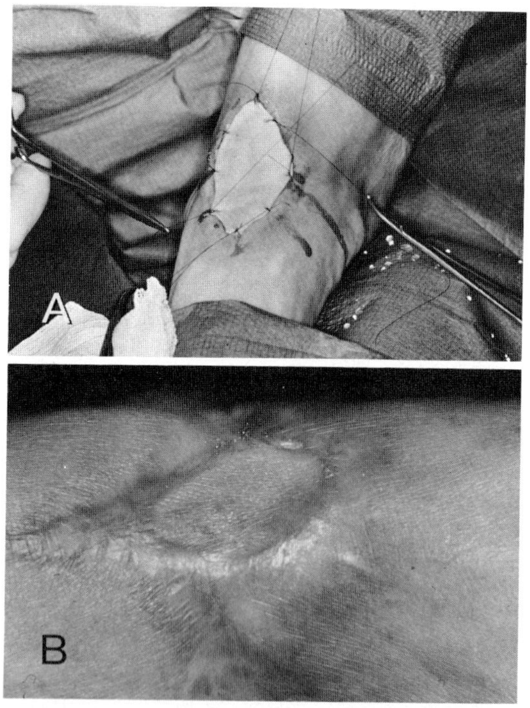

Figure 15.15. (*A*) Split-thickness skin graft applied to chronic ulcerative defect. (*B*) Successful graft in 6 months. The patient suffered from venous hypertension; previous conservative therapy had failed.

SYNTHETIC DRESSINGS

Synthetic colloid dressings have recently been utilized in local management of ulcerative lesions. Spenco 2nd Skin (Spenco Medical Corporation, Waco, TX) commonly referred to as "synthetic skin," is a colloid of a hydrogel dispersion medium of 96% H_2O and 4% polyethylene oxide. This dressing allows transmission of fluids as well as vapors. Absorption of serosanguinous extravasate and necrotic debris can be obtained with little interference with topical medication (21). Spenco 2nd Skin dampens shear forces, making it an ideal covering for ulcerative lesions which may be subjected to friction or rubbing. This hydrophilic colloid reduces local irritability and increases the rate of healing as well as granulation tissue formation.

BIOLOGIC DRESSINGS

Amniotic Membrane Grafting

Although uncommonly utilized, amniotic membranes have proven to be a satisfactory adjunct to the treatment of lower extremity ulcerative lesions.

Amniotic membranes are utilized as temporary allograft dressings which are significantly bacteriostatic (22). Fluid and protein loss from the wound site are discouraged. These biologic dressings are obtained from prepared placental human membranes.

Prior to applications of the temporary graft, the ulcerative lesion must be clinically devoid of infection. The membrane is secured with gauze and changed every 2 to 4 days under sterile technique. Local debridement may be performed as needed between changes. Granulation and epithelialization are enhanced within 2 to 3 weeks in small defects.

AUTOGENOUS SKIN GRAFTING

If conservative methods of ulcer treatment fail to establish closure of cutaneous defects and ulceration reoccurs, skin grafting is an excellent alternative (Fig 15.14). Arterial blood supply must be adequate, and a clean granular bed must be established prior to split-thickness skin grafting of cutaneous defects (23). Resistant venous stasis ulcers usually respond well to autogenous grafting (Fig 15.15). A preferred guide to follow in establishing graft viability is the use of a porcine xenograft. Adherence of the porcine biologic dressing for 24 to 72 hr affords a good prognosis for success in autografting.

References

1. Samitz MH: Cutaneous lesions of the lower extremities in the diagnosis of systemic disease. *J Am Podiatry Assoc* 65:556, 1975.
2. Roenigk HH Jr, Young JR: *Leg Ulcers—Medical and Surgical Management.* Hagerstown, MD, Harper & Row, 1975.
3. Roenigk HH: *Office Dermatology.* Baltimore, Williams & Wilkins, 1981, pp 227–241.
4. Samitz MH, Dana AS: *Cutaneous Lesions of the Lower Extremity.* Philadelphia, J.B. Lippincott, 1971.
5. Arenson DJ, Sherwood CF, Wilson RC: Neuropathy, angiopathy, and sepsis in the diabetic foot. *J Am Podiatry Assoc* 71:618, 1981.
6. Arenson DJ, Sherwood CF, Wilson RC: Neuropathy, angiopathy, and sepsis in the diabetic foot. Part 2. Angiography. *J Am Podiatry Assoc* 71:661, 1981.
7. Levin ME: The diabetic foot. *J Am Podiatry Assoc* 66:825, 1976.
8. Brenner, MA: An ambulatory approach to the neuropathic ulceration. *J Am Podiatry Assoc* 64:862, 1974.
9. Dockery GL: Psychocutaneous disorders: some lower extremity presentations. *J Am Podiatry Assoc* 72:388, 1982.
10. DeLauro TM: Pedal autoimmune dermatologic disease. *J Am Podiatry Assoc* 72:396, 1982.
11. Samitz MH: The tell-tale foot: a unique opportunity to study systemic disease. *J Am Podiatry Assoc* 70:126, 1980.
12. O'Donnell TF: Diagnosis and management of ulcerations of the lower extremity. Hosp Med 2:53–74, 1977.
13. Gohil P, Young JR, Clarke TH: Hypertensive ischemic ulcers of the leg. *J Am Podiatry Assoc* 71:363, 1981.
14. Brenner MA: Another approach to the management of lower extremity ulcerations. *J Am Podiatry Assoc* 72:79, 1982.
15. Gorman JB, Helfand BM, Mazer RS: Topical enzymatic treatment of lower extremity ulcers. *J Am Podiatry Assoc* 70:287, 1980.
16. Altman MI, Goldstein L, Horowitz S: Collagenase: an adjunct to healing trophic ulcerations in the diabetic patient. *J Am Podiatry Assoc* 68:11, 1978.
17. Pace WE: Dextran polymer beads in the local treatment of cutaneous ulcers. *J Dermatol Surg Oncol* 4:678, 1978.
18. Culliton P et al: The efficacy of porcine skin grafts for treating non-healing cutaneous ulcers. *J Am Podiatry Assoc* 68:1, 1978.
19. McCarthy DJ, Axler DA: The efficacy of porcine skin grafts for treating non-healing cutaneous ulcers. Part II. Microanatomical studies. *J Am Podiatry Assoc* 68:86, 1978.
20. McCarthy DJ, Montgomery B: Polyurethane in the management of ulcerating lesions of the lower extremities. *J Am Podiatry Assoc* 73:1, 1983.
21. Cangialosi PC: Synthetic skin: a new adjunct in the treatment of diabetic ulcers. *J Am Podiatry Assoc* 72:48, 1982.
22. Rudnick SS: The use of amniotic membrane grafting in podiatric office practice. *J Am Podiatry Assoc* 71:679, 1981.
23. Tuerk D: Skin grafts of the lower extremity. *J Am Podiatry Assoc* 67:28, 1977.

CHAPTER 16

Unusual Ulcerations of the Lower Extremity

DAMIAN TURSKI, DOUGLAS TAYLOR, and DERRICK WHITTAKER*

INTRODUCTION

Many pathological processes manifest themselves, in part, as ulcerations in the lower extremity. These ulcerative lesions can present special difficulties in diagnosis. It is the intent of this chapter to give an overview of the most unusual acute and chronic lower extremity ulcerations that the physician may encounter (Table 16.1).

ULCERS HAVING VASCULAR ETIOLOGY

Arteriosclerosis obliterans, hypertensive disease, and venous insufficiency as the etiologic basis of ulcerations have been discussed in the previous chapter.

Thromboangiitis Obliterans

This disease is characterized by chronic inflammation of both arteries and veins which most often occurs in young males between 20 and 40 years of age. Characteristically the involvement is segmental, with normal portions interspersed between sites of inflammation. This inflammatory process often extends to the perivascular tissues, leading to fibrosis and scarring that firmly binds together the artery, vein and nerve (1). The medium and small arteries are commonly involved, producing thrombosis of these vessels.

Almost all of the patients have been or are heavy smokers. The most predominant feature of this disease is mild to severe pain. This pain develops because of the ischemic changes which can ultimately lead to ulceration, necrosis, and gangrene occurring in the lower leg and foot. The toes tend to be most commonly effected by thromboangiitis obliterans. The fingertips and fingers are the second most common site for development of lesions. The digit may be pale and cold, or there may be rubor that remains and does not blanch when dependent. When the extremity is elevated, the skin will blanch. Vascular changes tend to be asymmetrical, so not all toes are effected.

Livedo Reticularis

Livedo reticularis is an arteriospastic disorder that produces ulceration through ischemia of the lower extremity. This disease brings about narrowing of the arterioles through vasospastic activities or organic changes. Secondary dilation of capillaries and venules may occur. Blood flow may actually cease or even reverse direction and thrombose the involved vessel. This disease occurs mainly among women between 20 and 40 years of age. The disorder presents as a purplish, mottled vascular pattern somewhat "fishnet" in appearance. Lesions usually appear in the lower extremities, but they can also occur in the buttocks, arms, and trunks (2). A few patients will complain of coldness, numbness, and paresthesia of the involved areas. When the ulcers occur, they begin in the dark infarcted areas that break down into irregular ulcerations.

---

* *Disclaimer:* The content of this paper does not represent the opinions of the Battle Creek Veterans Administration Medical Center. The authors are solely responsible for its content.

The authors present a literature review concerning ulcers of the lower extremity. Various etiologies, pathologies, and pathogenesis of the lower extremity ulcers are discussed. The following causes of leg ulcers are summarized: arterial, venous, lymphatic, vasculitis, hematologic, infections, metabolic, tumor, and miscellaneous.

Table 16.1
Causes of Lower Extremity Ulcers

Arterial	Arteriosclerosis obliterans, thromboangiitis obliterans, hypertensive and livedo reticularis
Venous	Chronic venous insufficiency
Lymphatics	Lymphedema praecox, congenital lymphedema, acquired lymphedema, and elephantiasis nostras
Vasculitis	Necrotizing vasculitis, periarteritis nodosa and systemic lupus erythematosus
Hematologic	Sickle cell, hereditary spherocytosis, thalassemia, polycythemia vera, leukemia, dysproteinemia
Infections	Fungus, superficial and deep. Deep: blastomycosis and sporotrichosis. Syphilis, bacterial and tuberculosis. Tuberculids—erythema induratum and papulonecrotic
Metabolic	Pretibial myxedema, lichenamyloidosis, pyoderma gangrenosum, and diabetes mellitus
Tumors	Basal cell carcinoma, squamous cell carcinoma, kaposis hemorrhagic sarcoma and malignant melanoma
Miscellaneous	Halogens-bromide and iodide. Ergotism, methotrexate, burns, levophed, radiopaque dyes, nitrogen mustard, thermal burns, radiation, decubitus ulcers, lichen planus, erythema nodosum, Weber-Christian disease, rheumatoid arthritis, and factitial (or self-induced)

LYMPHATIC ULCERS

Ulceration is an uncommon complication of lymphedema. Stasis of lymphatic fluid usually occurs due to obstruction of lymphatic vessels. Lymph pressure increases, the lymph vessels dilate, and subsequently the valves become incompetent. This increases lymph stasis; protein content of tissue fluid increases; and fibroblasts proliferate (3). If there is a breakdown of skin, the protein content is a good medium for bacteria to grow, and cellulitis and lymphangiitis results.

Etiology of lymphedema can be divided into primary and secondary causes. Primary lymphedema is due to an inherited defect in the lymphatic system. Secondary lymphedema is a result of infection, carcinoma, radiation, surgery, filariasis, or local tissue injury. Lymphedema praecox is the most common type and affects women 10 times more frequently than men. Congenital lymphedema is a primary type of lymphedema usually present at birth. When it is a hereditary process, it is known as Milroy's disease. With lymphedema, after the age of 40, one must suspect carcinoma. In the male, carcinoma of the prostate is a common tumor type producing obstruction of lymphatics. Lymphomas or carcinoma of the genital tract are common in females as a cause of lymphedema. Nephrosis, nephritis, congestive failure, idiopathic cyclic edema, deficient proteinemia, or myxedema are differential diagnosis for bilateral lymphedema. Edema from venous insufficiency may be difficult to differentiate from unilateral lymphedema.

There is nothing characteristic about ulceration of lymphedema which differentiates it from venous stasis ulcer. These are moist, not painful, with extensive granulation and are usually traumatic in origin. Recurrent lymphangiitis usually is insidious in onset, with an occasional dull pain. There may be fever, malaise, headache, nausea, and vomiting. Red streaks are frequently found along the lymph vessels. Ulceration with lymphangiitis is usually due to trauma. Lymphangiosarcoma may also ulcerate, and biopsy is indicated in such instances. Split thickness grafts are usually necessary to close the skin defect.

In addition to the more common causes of acquired lymphedema, a new variety has appeared. Drug addicts, whose unsterile injections are followed by subcutaneous chronic sepsis with fibrosis and lymphatic obliteration, are now presenting with lymphedema. According to Ger, this condition can lead to ulceration (4).

Elephantiasis nostras is a condition in which venous insufficiency and lymphatic fibrosis are combined. There is gross thickening of the dermis with special exaggeration of the papillary system. Consequently, there is polypoidal granulation which is convered by a thick hyperkeratotic epithelium. Some areas of dermis are composed of hard fibrous tissue, and the surface of the skin is sclerosed and nodular (4). Filariasis is commonly involved in the inflammation and obstruction of lymphatic channels characteristic of elephantiasis. The scrotum may be involved, along with the lower extremities.

SPECIAL ULCERATIVE CONDITIONS INVOLVING VASCULITIS

Vasculitis

Fauci et al have described vasculitis as a clinicopathological process characterized by inflammation and necrosis of blood vessels (5). Vasculitis as seen in the skin may appear with a variety of reaction patterns in one person at the same time, although the basic pathogenesis may be similar in all cases. Cutaneous lesions of vasculitis vary from erythematous macules to purpura, hemorrhagic vesicles, and nodules. Eventually, necrotic lesions and ulcerations occur (Fig. 16.1). Involvement of the lower extremity is quite frequent.

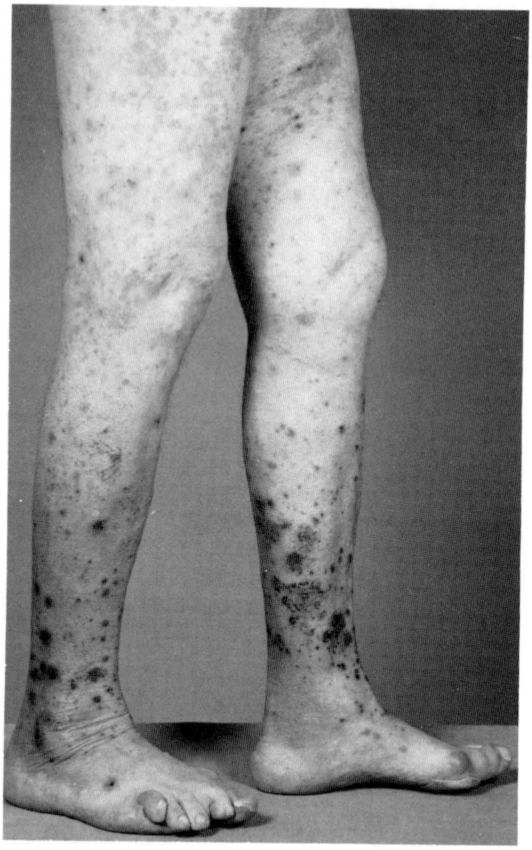

Figure 16.1. Vasculitis: purpura, urticaria, hemorrhagic vesicles, and ulceration characterize acute necrotizing vasculitis.

NECROTIZING VASCULITIS

This disorder is one of the most frequently encountered varieties of vasculitis. In the mild form it can affect the cutaneous tissue of the leg and, when severe, can produce systemic vasculitis of the kidney, malignant hypertension, and even death. Typically, necrotizing vasculitis presents as erythematous maculopapular lesions and eventually evolves to form urticarial papules, raised purpuric lesions, or hemorrhagic vesicles. The most common clinical features are palpable petechiae with necrosis of the overlying epidermis and, finally, ulceration. The lesions usually appear on the lower legs and ankles and are typically painful.

PERIARTERITIS NODOSA

Another entity which manifests lower extremity ulcerations is periarteritis nodosa. The cause of periarteritis nodosa is unknown, and diagnosis of the disease is made through excisional skin biopsy of the lesion. It is characterized by focal or segmental lesions of blood vessels, notably arteries of small to medium size. A variety of clinical presentations, depending on the blood vessel involved, results.

Roenigk noted that the disease occurs in all age groups but is most common in the fifth and sixth decades and affects men more often than women (1).

The pathological hallmark of the disease is acute necrotizing inflammation of the arterial media, with fibrinoid necrosis and extensive inflammatory cell infiltration of all coats of the vessel and surrounding tissue (6). There are a variety of cutaneous lesions that occur, such as livedo recticularis, purpura, urticaria, and subcutaneous nodules, which may ulcerate from infarction.

SYSTEMIC LUPUS ERYTHEMATOSUS

Recurrent lower leg ulcerations have been known to occur in patients with systemic lupus erythematosus (Fig. 16.2). Dubois noted that 5.6% of his patients had ulcerations, most commonly in the malleolar area (7). Systemic lupus erythematosus is an inflammatory connective tissue disorder that may affect multiple organ systems. The disease is 4 or 5 times more common in women and appears most often during the second and third decade of life.

The etiology of the disease is unknown. a wide assortment of skin lesions have been found in systemic lupus erythematosus, among which are malar rash, discoid lesions, purpura, urticaria, nodules, and bullae (8). Many times livedo reticularis may be a prominent finding and is often associated with skin infections and recurrent indolent painful ulceration especially above the ankle.

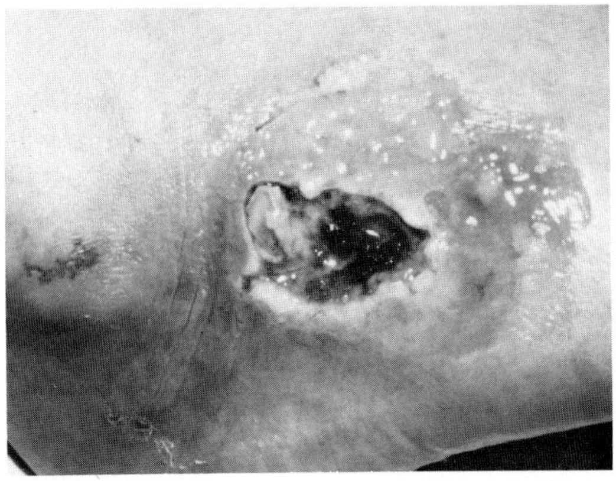

Figure 16.2. Systemic lupus erythematosus. Sharply defined ulceration frequently just above the malleoli are characteristic of systemic lupus erythematosus.

UNUSUAL HEMATOLOGIC ULCERS

Hereditary Spherocytosis

The red cell membrane in this condition is abnormal. Leg ulcers are uncommon. Patients are usually pale, anemic, and have splenomegaly and mild jaundice. Diagnosis is made by the presence of spherocytes and a negative direct combs reaction.

Thalassemia

Leg ulcers occur in less than 5% of intermediate forms of thalassemia but are relatively uncommon. These ulcers are probably due to inadequate tissue oxygenation secondary to lower than normal concentrations of hemoglobin A. Gand et al. raised the question of the connection between thalassemia and glucose-6-phosphate dehydrogenase deficiency (9). Hemoglobin is usually 9 mg or less. Pathogenesis of these ulcers probably involves inadequate tissue oxygenation due to lower than normal concentrations of hemoglobin A.

Polycythemia Vera

This condition involves an increased viscosity of blood and platelets. There is an increase in thromboembolism among patients. Venous stasis and venous thrombosis are not uncommon, and stasis ulcers may occur. Other hematological conditions are *leukemia*, in which leg ulcers are secondary to trauma, and *dysproteinemia*, in which patients demonstrated cryogiobulinemia stasis, hyperpigmentation, and superficial skin ulceration with necrosis.

INFECTIOUS ULCERS

Fungal infections may be superficial or deep. Superficial involvements usually occur only in stratum corneum and epidermis. Deep fungal infections can produce granulomatous ulcerative lesions on the infected skin. Superficial fungal infections that affect the leg usually begin at the web spaces of the feet. Superficial fungal infections that commonly cause tinea pedis include candidiasis species *Trichophyton mentagrophytes* or *Epidermophyton floccosum* and *Trichophyton rubrum* (Fig. 16.3). Deep fungal infections that produce ulceration include blastomycosis, coccidioidomycosis, histoplasmosis, and sporomycosis (Fig. 16.4).

Syphilis in its tertiary stage may present as leg ulcers (Fig. 16.5). It first develops as a deep subcutaneous fixed nodule or plaque that may be singular or multiple. Causative organism is *Treponema pallidum.*

Bacterial infections are not usually the primary cause of leg ulcers. Freidman and Gladstone (10) state that the most common significant bacteria in inflamed ulcerations are *Staphylococcus aureus* and *Escherichia coli.* Louie (11) found that of 20 diabetic foot ulcers, the primary isolates were *Bacteroides*, *Proteus*, *S. aureus*, and *Clostridia* sp., as well as *E. coli. Mycobacterium leprae* is the etiologic basis of ulcerations in leprosy. The condition is uncommon but exists in the United States (Fig. 16.6).

Tuberculosis, so-called tuberculids, were

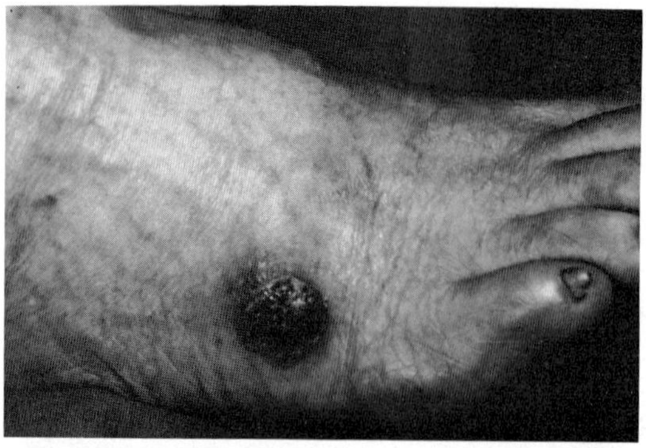

Figure 16.3. Candidiasis may produce a granulomatous lesion which can ulcerate. Special stains such as mucicarmine demonstrate the diagnostic hyphae, mycelia, and spores. (From McCarthy DJ: *Management of Dermal Ulcerations and Wound Complications.* Evanston, IL, Arthur Retlaw, 1981.)

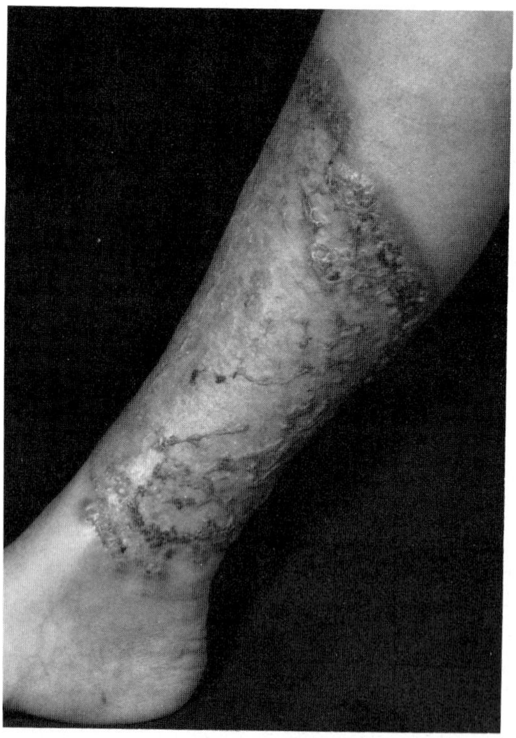

Figure 16.4. Deep fungal infection: large plaques with advancing verrucal borders characterize North American blastomycosis which may procede on to ulceration.

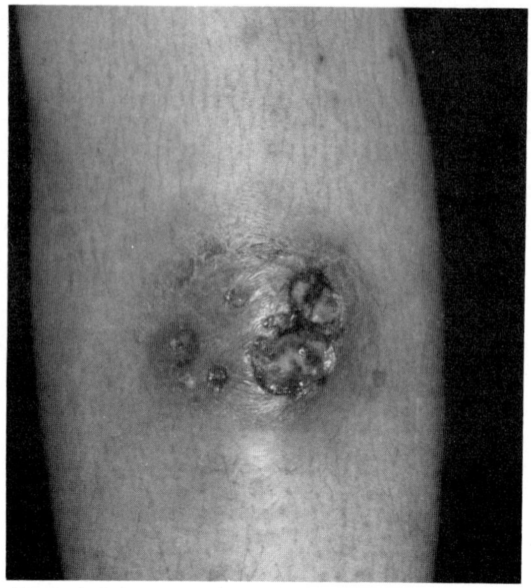

Figure 16.5. Syphilis. Nodules and ulceration characterize leuetic gumma, which can occur in the lower extremities.

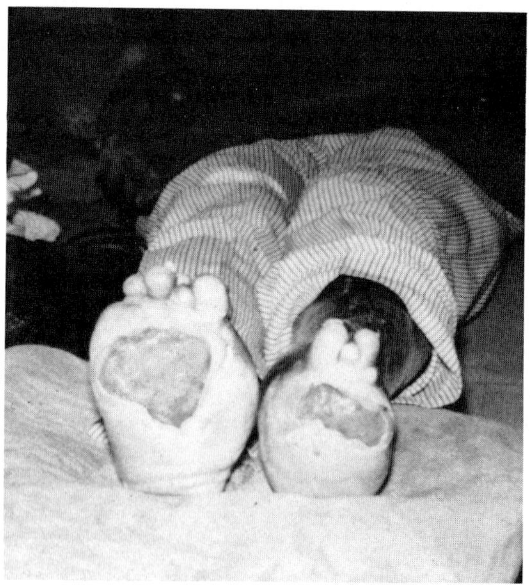

Figure 16.6. Leprosy or Hansen's disease produces a painless ulceration of the lower extremities. (From McCarthy DJ: *Management of Dermal Ulcerations and Wound Complications.* Evanston, IL, Arthur Retlaw, 1981.)

a common cause of leg ulcers (1). Primary tuberculosis appears on the skin, as well as demarcated reddish brown patches containing papules which may ulcerate. Tuberculosis verrucosa cutis usually presents as a single verrucous plaque with an inflammatory border and superficial pustules. Erythema induratum, papulonecrotic tuberculid, lichen scrofulosorum, and lupus miliaris disseminatus faciei are disorders classified as tuberculids thought not to be different diseases. *Erythema induratum* presents as lesions on the lower extremity with chronic subcutaneous plaques of bluish red nodules that may ulcerate. *Papulonecrotic tuberculid* is characterized as indolent papules or nodules that appear on the cutaneous surface of the lower extremity. Papules undergo central necrosis and gray ulceration. Lichen scrofulosorum is a lichenoid eruption of small papules occurring in children with tuberculosis that usually does not ulcerate.

METABOLIC ULCERS

Many metabolic conditions can develop ulcerations and must be considered in the differential diagnosis of lesions. The present discussion deals with unusual metabolic disease manifested in some form of ulcerations.

Pretibial Myxedema

The condition is a metabolic disorder which typically occurs in about 3% of patients with toxic goiters (1). In approximately 50% of patients, the lesions appear during the active hyperthyroid state. Characteristically, the lesions appear as firm, nonpitting, irregular nodules or plaques which may be flesh-colored or yellow and waxy. The overlying epidermis is thin and stretched and has a pigskin appearance. The lesions tend to appear bilaterally on pretibial areas. At times these lesions will ulcerate. Acropachy will occur in 1% of patients with hyperparathyroidism. This syndrome demonstrates clubbing of digits.

Lichen Amyloidosis

This disease is a rare metabolic disorder which may develop ulcerations. This condition can be identified by an eruption of discrete, firm papules which vary in color from red to reddish-brown and occasionally are translucent. It has been noted that a high incidence of lichen amyloidosis is seen in the Oriental population as well as in Ecuador.

Pyoderma Gangrenosum

This clinical metabolic entity has been noted to develop into lower extremity ulcerations. Pyoderma gangrenosum at one time was considered pathognomonic of an underlying chronic ulcerative colitis. At this time, other conditions, such as regional enteritis, gastric ulcers, empyema, and chronic debilitating infections, may be associated with it (12). The skin lesions usually begin as erythematous papulonodules that enlarge into plaques up to 12 mm or more in diameter. The active border is deeply violaceous red, and the central portion is necrotic and ulcerative. The lesions are extremely painful and may be found on other parts of the body and lower leg.

Gout develops as a result of irregularities of purine metabolism and is a systemic disorder with considerable podiatric significance. Localized depositions of monosodium urate in and about joints and tendons result from supersaturation of uricacidemic body fluids. The first metatarsophalangeal joints of mature males are most commonly affected. Other joints of the foot can, however, be affected (Fig. 16.7).

TUMORS

Almost any type of tumor, either primary to the skin or metastatic from some other source, may occur on the lower extremities. Such lesions may ulcerate and have the appearance of a stasis ulcer, which fails to respond to the usual modes of treatment. The reader is referred to Chapter 18 for additional information relative to metastatic skin lesions.

Basal Cell Carcinoma

This low grade malignancy is a common and invasive skin tumor arising within the epidermis. It comprises about 83% of all skin malignancies (13). Basal cell carcinoma occurs frequently in Caucasians who are of fair complexion. These lesions are

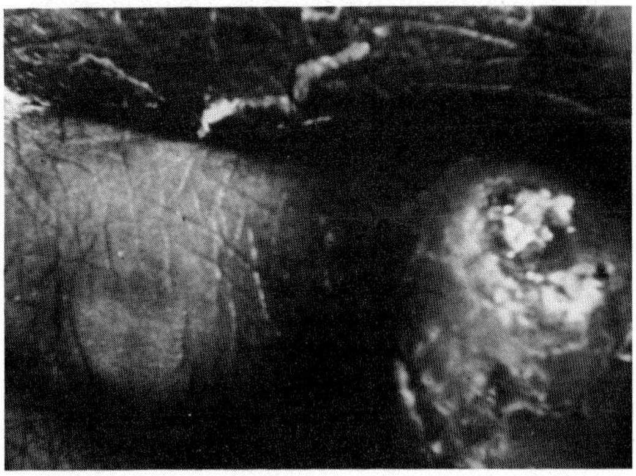

Figure 16.7. Tophi or urate crystals may devitalize and erode the skin, thus producing ulceration. (From McCarthy DJ: *Management of Dermal Ulcerations and Wound Complications.* Evanston, IL, Arthur Retlaw, 1981.)

commonly found on the head and neck and less frequently on the feet. The first reported case of basal cell carcinoma of the foot was reported by Shreiner and Wehr in 1933 (14).

Basal cell carcinoma is thought to be caused by an overexposure to ionizing radiation, chemical carcinogens, or genetic predisposition. Cruik and Campbell believed that the lesion may arise from chronic ulcers, sinus tracts, or hypertrophic scar tissue (15).

The lesions are skin colored in appearance and are papular with slight telangiectasia. They vary in size from 1 to 2 mm to several centimeters in diameter when they have ulcerated. They tend to run a chronic course without any symptoms other than occasional bleeding. If an ulcer is present, the floor will generally be covered by viscous, necrotic material, crusts, and a serosanguinous discharge. Metastasis is less than 0.01% but must be ruled out if the lesion recurs.

Squamous Cell Carcinoma

This epidermal malignancy is another common tumor that may occur anywhere on the extremities, but mucocutaneous junctions are most commonly involved. The majority of these lesions consist of a shallow ulcer surrounded by a wide, elevated, and indurated border. They can also be dome shaped, hard, and infiltrated without ulceration. The tumors are relatively slow-growing lesions composed of irregular masses of epidermal cells that tend to be dyskeratotic and parakeratotic. Squamous cell carcinoma may metastasize, and excessive radiation therapy predisposes the patient to this invasive tumor.

Kaposi's Hemorrhagic Sarcoma

This malignant disease is commonly seen in the legs and feet. The upper extremities and even the face may, however, be involved. It occurs predominately among Jewish, Italian, and Bantu races. It is far more frequent in men than women, and occurs between 50 and 70 years of age. The earliest lesions may be reddish-brown nodules and plaques that are bluish-red (Fig. 16.8). They are usually seen bilaterially and symmetrically and are associated with

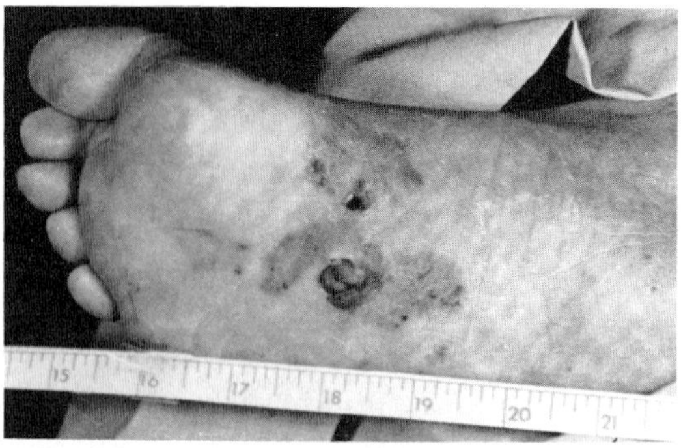

Figure 16.8. Kaposi's hemorrhagic sarcoma. Courtesy of Harcourt, Brace, & Jovanovich: Managing age-related lesions. *Geriatrics*, 1975.

edema. Eventually, purpura and ulceration of the lesions will result. These tumors tend to grow slowly, with old lesions becoming involuted, leaving atrophy and pigmentation in the involved skin.

Malignant Melanoma

This malignancy is a most serious type of neoplasia. It is a cancer of the pigment-producing cells of the skin, eyes, and mucous membrane. This potentially fatal disease does have special predilection for the foot and, left untreated, can spread widely within the body.

There are three principle clinical varieties of melanoma: those arising in the melanotic freckle of Hutchinson, nodular melanoma, and superficial spreading melanoma (16). A study done by Cosman revealed that the lower limb was and continues to be the most frequent site of melanoma (17). This malignancy can occur in males and women with equal frequency and at all ages. The patient may first notice a freckle darker than others which increases in size in an irregular centrifugal fashion. Some display erythema and depigmentation (18). Melanomas have coloration varying from red to white to blue. Occasionally, this lesion will ulcerate and bleed. If noted early, these melanoma can be treated by adequate excision. Survival rates are highest among the very young and very old (see Chapter 18).

MISCELLANEOUS LEG ULCERS

Halogens, bromide, and *iodide* compounds can produce anterior tibial leg ulcers. Iodides produce acneiform follicular pustular, bullous, late fungating, and hemorrhagic ulcers. These lesions can become gangrenous ulcers.

Methotrexate overdoses can produce painful ulcerations of plaques of psoriasis. *Burns, levophed, radiopaque dyes,* and *nitrogen mustard* can cause local necrosis and ulceration. *Thermal burns* may cause ulceration as well as radiation.

Radiation ulcers are characterized by a punched-out appearance, dirty granulating base, undermining of the borders, and extreme pain. Such lesions demonstrate erythema, induration, desiccation of blood vessels, and telangiectasia prior to ulceration.

Decubitus ulcers or pressure sores result from significant pressure to compress the capillary circulation, causing tissue damage and necrosis. They are typically slow to heal.

Erythema nodosum is a common cause of nodules on the lower leg which may on rare occasions ulcerate. These lesions tend to be very painful. *Weber-Christian disease* is a relapsing febrile nodular nonsuppurative panniculitis which can ulcerate. *Rheumatoid arthritis* may be associated with ischemic ulceration. Lesions may occur primarily on the lower leg, associated with a subcutaneous rheumatoid nodule which undergoes necrosis and ulceration.

Necrobiosis Lipoidica Diabeticorum

Focal regions of necrosis within depositions of subcutaneous fat may result in ulceration. Such lesions may occur anywhere within the body. They are known as necrobiosis lipoidica diabeticorum. While these ulcerations often occur among diabetic patients, they are by no means limited to diabetics. The lesions may occur anywhere in the body but are frequently seen on the lower leg (Fig. 16.9). Small vessel microangiopathy produces tender pale centralized plaques having violaceous margins. Necrosis eventually occurs, and definitive diagnosis is usually dependent upon biopsy since the condition is relatively uncommon and can be easily missed.

Scleroderma can resemble Raynaud's disease in that the hands and feet are edematous, erythematous, smooth, and shiny. It is a disease of connective tissue, with a potential for affecting vital organs. Fibrosis and thickening of tissues may terminate the patient's life. In this condition, trophic ulceration can occur, especially near joints and weight-bearing points (Fig. 16.10).

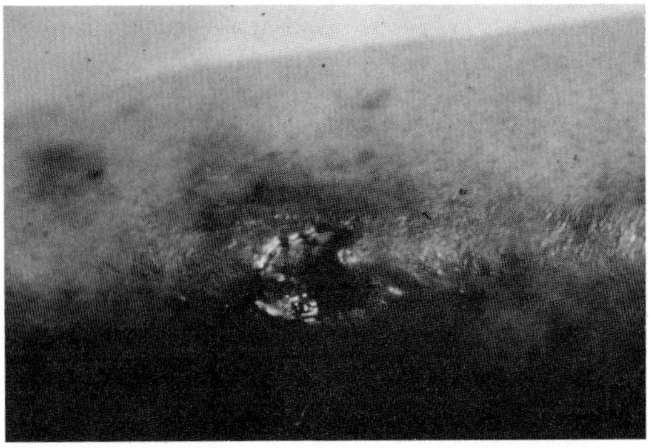

Figure 16.9. Microangiography of small blood vessels within subcutaneous fat may produce ulcerations. Such lesions are called necrobiosis lipoidica diabeticorum. (From McCarthy DJ: *Management of Dermal Ulcerations and Wound Complications.* Evanston, IL, Arthur Retlaw, 1981.)

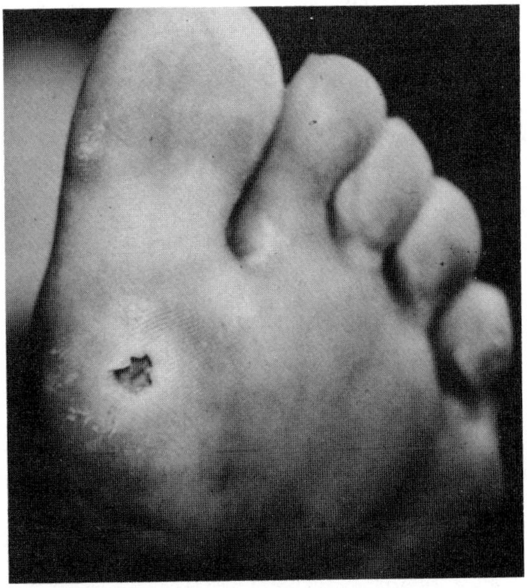

Figure 16.10. Edema and erythema precede the trophic ulcerations of the connective tissue disorder, scleroderma. (From McCarthy DJ: *Management of Dermal Ulcerations and Wound Complications.* Evanston, IL, Arthur Retlaw, 1981.)

SUMMARY

Despite a thorough history, careful physical examination, and critical evaluation of data obtained, the physician may have difficulty ascertaining the precise etiology of lower extremity ulcerations. For this reason it is important for the physician to be aware of the many causes of leg ulcerations. Some have obvious etiologies, but others have obscure causes.

References

1. Roenigk JR, Young HH: *Leg Ulcers, Medical & Surgical Management.* Hagerstown, MD, Harper & Row, 1975.
2. Copeman, PWM: Livedo reticularis: signs in the skin of disturbance of blood viscosity and blood flow. *Br J Dermatol* 93:S19, 1975.
3. Ryan TC: *The Management of Leg Ulcers.* New York, Oxford University Press, 1983.
4. Ger R: Chronic ulceration of the leg. *Surg Ann* 4:123–149, 1972.
5. Fauci AD, Haynes BF, Katz P: The spectrum of vasculitis—clinical, pathological, immunologic and therapeutic consideration. *Ann Intern Med* 89(1):660, 1978.
6. Krupp MA, Chatton MJ: *Current Medical Diagnosis and Treatment.* Lange Medical Publications, Los Altos, CA, 1982.
7. Dubois EL: *Lupus Erythematosus,* ed. 2, New York, McGraw-Hill, 1974, pp 265–285.
8. Brogradir SP, Myers AR: Chronic lower leg ulcerations in systemic lupus erythematosis. *J Rheumatol* 6:2, 1975.
9. Gand S, Cohen T: Thalassaemia and glucose-6-phosphate dehydrogenase deficiency. *Br J Dermatol* 95:203, 1976.
10. Friedman SA, Gladstone JL: The bacterial flora of peripheral vascular ulcers. *Arch Dermatol* 100:29, 1969.
11. Louie TJ: Aerobic and anaerobic bacteria in diabetic foot. *Ann Intern Med* 85:461–463, 1976.
12. Perry HO, Bronsting LA: Pyoderma gangrenosum. *Arch Dermatol* 75:380, 1957.
13. Robins P, Amonette R: Basal cell carcinoma: treatment by the Mohs technique. *Laryngoscope* 82:965, 1972.
14. Shreiner BF, Wehr WH: Primary malignant tumors of the foot. *Radiology* 21:513, 1933.
15. Cruikshank AH, Campbell JA: Cancer in scars, ulcers, and sinus. *J Clin Pathol* 16:573, 1963.
16. Fields LS, Delavro T, Scholl S: Malignant melanoma. *J Am Podiatry Assoc* 68–78, 1978.
17. Cosman B, Heddle SB, Crikelair GF: The increasing incidence of melanoma. *Plast Reconstr Surg* 57:50, 1976.
18. Fields, LS, Delauro T, Scholl S: Malignant melanoma. *J Am Podiatry Assoc* 68(8):1978.

CHAPTER 17

Benign Neoplasia of the Foot

WILFRED LAINE

GENERAL INTRODUCTION

Benign epidermal neoplasia constitutes a complex and sometimes perplexing group of superficial lesions of the foot. Moreover, tumors arising from the deeper mesodermal tissues manifest themselves as "skin tumors."

The present study will be confined to the benign neoplasia of the foot utilizing the classification of skin tumors of the lower extremity used by Samitz and Lewis (1). The histological classification of soft tissue tumors employed will be that advocated by Enzinger and Weiss (2).

Certain categories not pertinent to the foot will, for obvious reasons, be eliminated, e.g., tumors of autonomic ganglia, etc. Osseous cartilaginous lesions, while common in the podiatric field, are inappropriate in a text on podiatric dermatology.

Superficial fibrous tumors, mechanically induced hyperkeratoses, disorders of keratinization, and visual growths will be covered in other chapters.

Soft tissue tumors are currently classified according to cytoplasmic differentiation, i.e., the neoplasm recapitulates the normal structure to varying degrees, as opposed to histogenesis, i.e., the origin of the cells (3). Additionally, they may be further divided into benign and malignant forms. Benign tumors, which more or less resemble normal tissue, usually are not invasive locally. They demonstrate a limited ability for proliferation and tend not to recur locally following excision.

INCIDENCE

It is almost impossible to determine the incidence of cutaneous and soft tissue tumors, and the relative frequency of benign vs malignant lesions. Many of them go unreported, unbiopsied, and unrecognized. This is particularly true of private practice, and the application of hospital data is invalid for the general population.

In Berlin's (4) opinion, slightly more than 2% of the neoplasms found on the human body are located on the foot.

This view was supported by a laboratory review of 67,000 foot tumors from April 1979 through December 1983 (Table 17.1) (5). This study was primarily limited to 25 most common benign lesions of the foot excised in the office setting.

The data suggest that cutaneous malignancies appear to be rare in the foot.

DIAGNOSIS

The evaluation of any cutaneous or soft tissue tumor dictates a complete history and physical, augmented by laboratory studies. The age and sex of the patient, and the evolutionary history and location of the lesion can be very productive for precise diagnosis.

Biopsy provides the histological means by which soft tissue tumors are differentiated. Precise diagnosis may require additional testing such as special stains, histochemistry, immunofluorescence, and ultrastructural studies. It is important to rule out metastatic disease or local extension of a malignancy and reactive processes that may simulate soft tissue tumors and malignancies such as nodular fasciitis.

The most useful and common method for treatment of pedal cutaneous biopsy is the excisional method, in which the entire lesion and a small surrounding area of nor-

Table 17.1.
Twenty-Five Most Common Benign Lesions[a]

	No. of lesions	% lesions
1. Verruca	32,139	47.9
2. Morton's neuroma	11,331	16.9
3. Porokeratosis	7,639	11.4
4. Neuroma	5,097	7.6
5. Inclusion cyst	2,136	3.2
6. Ganglion cyst	1,800	2.7
7. Exostosis	1,382	2.1
8. Squamous cell papilloma	804	1.2
9. Fibroma	582	.8
10. Pyogenic granuloma	481	.7
11. Dermatofibroma	481	.7
12. Nevi	412	.6
13. Digital mucous cyst	277	.4
14. Plantar fibromatosis	262	.3
15. Junctional nevi	255	.3
16. Lipoma	196	.2
17. Hemangioma	147	.2
18. Leiomyoma	138	.2
19. Neurofibroma	124	.1
20. Rheumatoid nodule	111	.1
21. Eccrine poroma	104	.1
22. Gouty tophi	101	.1
23. Digital fibrokeratoma	95	.1
24. Giant cell tumor tendon sheath	85	.1
25. Nodular subepidermal fibrosis	83	.1

[a] From Berlin SJ: *Journal of the American Podiatry Association* 74:341, 1984.

mal tissue is excised. It is ideal for the small lesions seen in the foot.

The incisional or punch biopsy is utilized for a large tumor or lesion, particularly if it is dermal in origin. It is a partial excision of the mass and normal tissue. Disposal punches are available in sizes from 2 to 8 mm in diameter. However, most dermatopathologists would prefer a tissue specimen at least 3 mm in diameter.

Needle biopsies are not indicated for cutaneous lesions of the foot.

Frozen sections are acceptable only in medical centers with experienced pathologists who have been apprised of the clinical picture.

Radiological studies in the form of soft tissue films, CT scans, angiograms, etc., may assist in localizing the mass and defining its boundaries and may aid the surgeon in planning the excision. An effective technique for identifying the extent of cystic masses in the foot is the injection of the sac with equal parts of lidocaine, lypaque, and air to offer contrast with the surrounding tissues and without obliterating the boundaries of the mass with the dye on the radiograph.

The reader is referred to the chapter on diagnostic techniques for additional information.

HISTOLOGICAL CLASSIFICATION OF BENIGN SOFT TISSUE TUMORS OF THE LOWER EXTREMITIES

I. Tumors and tumor-like lesions of fibrous tissue
   A. Benign (including inflammatory and reactive etiologies)
      1. Fibroma (fibroepithelial papillomas ("skin tags")
      2. Proliferative fasciitis
      3. Fibroma of tendon sheath
      4. Keloid and hypertrophic scars
   B. Fibrous tumors of infancy and childhood
      1. Infantile myofibromatosis (generalized and localized)
      2. Infantile digital fibromatosis
      3. Calcifying aponeurotic fibroma
      4. Hyalin fibromatosis
   C. Fibromatoses
      1. Superficial fibromatoses
      2. Plantar fibromatosis
II. Fibrohistiocytic tumors (composed of cells resembling fibroblasts and histiocytes)
      1. Fibrous histiocytoma
         a. Cutaneous (dermatofibroma) histiocytoma cutis, nodular subepidermal fibrosis, sclerosing hemangioma
         b. Deep
      2. Juvenile (anthogranuloma)
      3. Xanthoma (reactive)
         a. Tuberous
         b. Tendinous
         c. Cerebrotendinous xanthomatosis
         d. Plane
      4. Miscellaneous histiocytic reactions resembling neoplasm
         a. Infectious
         b. Granular cell reaction
III. Tumors and tumor-like lesions of adipose tissue

1. Lipoma (cutaneous, deep and multiple)
2. Lipoblastoma and lipoblastomatosis
3. Intramuscular and intermuscular lipoma
4. Lipoma and tendon sheath and joints

IV. Tumors of muscle tissue
1. Smooth muscle
   a. Leiomyoma (cutaneous and deep)
   b. Angiomyoma (vascular leiomyoma)

V. Tumors and tumor-like lesions of blood vessels
1. Hemangioma
   a. Capillary (juvenile, strawberry, nevus)
   b. Cavernous
   c. Arteriovenous
   d. Venous
   e. Granulation tissue type (pyogenic granuloma)
2. Hemangiomatosis
3. Glomus tumor
4. Vascular ectasias (nevus flammeus (port wine stain), Klippel-Trenaunay-Weber syndrome, arterial spiders, angiokeratoma)
5. Papillary endothelial hyperplasia

VI. Tumor and tumor-like lesions of synovial tissue
1. Giant cell tumor of tendon sheath
   a. Localized (nodular tenosynovitis, pigmented nodular synovitis, fibrous histiocytoma of synovium).
   b. Diffuse (proliferative synovitis, florid synovitis, extra-articular, pigmented villonodular synovitis).
2. Tendosynovial cyst (ganglioma, synovial cyst, bursal cyst, cyst of tendon sheath, etc.).

VII. Tumors and tumor-like lesions of peripheral nerves
1. Morton's neuroma
2. Traumatic neuroma
3. Nerve sheath ganglion
4. Neurilemoma (benign schwannoma)
5. Neurofibroma, solitary
6. Neurofibromatosis (von Recklinghausen's disease)
   a. Peripheral
   b. Central

VIII. Cartilaginous tumors
1. Extraskeletal chrondroma

IX. Miscellaneous cutaneous and subcutaneous pedal tumors and tumor-like lesions.
1. Eccrine poroma
2. Clear cell acanthoma
3. Cutaneous myxoid cyst
4. Epidermal inclusion cyst
5. Porokeratosis plantaris discreta
6. Chronic radiodermatitis
7. Rheumatoid nodule
8. Tophaceous gout
9. Epidermal nevus
10. Nevus cell nevi—junctional, compound, and intradermal
11. Blue nevus

The present study will follow the outline just mentioned with the intent to be complete and brief. In some cases, duplication of material mentioned in other chapters is inevitable.

ADIPOSE TISSUE

Lipoma

Solitary lipomas, whether cutaneous, deep, or multiple, probably represent the most common skin-related neoplasms of mesenchymal origin. The cutaneous or superficial lipomas are the most common, but such masses are seldom found in the face, scalp, lower legs, and feet. Deep-seated lipomas are even more rare. They are found late in development and tend to be larger than the cutaneous type. In the extremities they may be found in the subperiosteal tissues or juxtaarticular regions (6), or deep in the hands and feet (7), where they are often mistaken for ganglia.

Lipomas are asymptomatic, unless they cause nerve compression because of their size. Such lesions are slow-growing, ovoid, and have a doughy consistency. They are difficult to differentiate clinically when they are deep in the foot and are only identified upon excision.

Multiple lipomas have been associated with hypercholesterolemia (8) and in diabetic patients at the site of insular injections (9).

Lipoblastoma and Lipoblastomatosis

Lipoblastoma and lipoblastomatosis occur in infancy and early childhood. These lesions are the counterpart of the circumscribed and diffuse forms of lipoma and lipomatosis but differ in their cellular maturity. They occur primarily in the upper and lower extremity as an asymptomatic mass (10).

Intramuscular and Intermuscular Lipoma

The majority of lipomas associated with skeletal muscle occur in adults between 30 and 60 years of age, in the large muscles of the extremities (11). They are normally slow-growing and asymptomatic and become apparent upon muscle contraction.

Lipoma and Tendon Sheath and Joints

Sullivan et al (12) reviewed the pertinent literature in 1956 and described this condition as occurring in both sexes between the ages of 15 and 35. Such lesions usually affect the wrist and hand and, less commonly, the ankle and foot. Many are painful, and 50% are bilaterally symmetrical.

MUSCLE TISSUE LESIONS

Smooth Muscle

LEIOMYOMA (Fig. 17.1)

The more common type of the cutaneous leiomyomas arises from the pilar erector muscles of the skin and appears in adolescence or early adulthood, and some are familial.

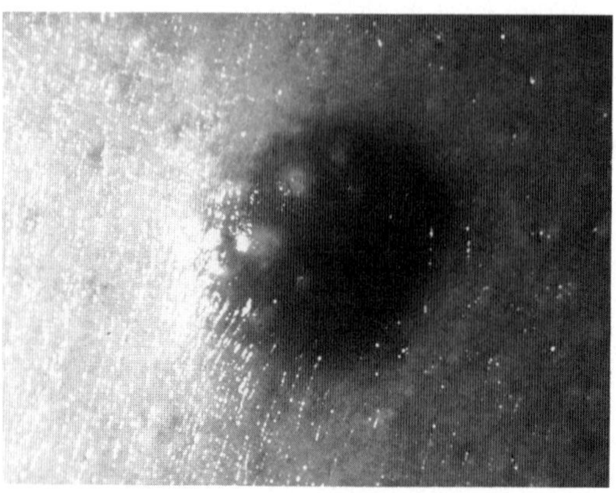

Figure 17.1. Cutaneous leiomyoma.

Such lesions develop as small discrete papules. They eventually form nodules 1 to 2 cm in diameter that may coalesce into a linear pattern following a dermatome. The exterior surfaces of the extremities are most commonly affected, and the lesions may produce significant pain.

Leiomyoma can be problematic to excise because of the number. Moreover, 50% develop recurrences or new lesions (13).

Deep soft tissue leiomyomas are uncommon and are located in the deep muscles of the extremities. These lesions tend to be significantly larger than the cutaneous type. They tend to be discovered later because of their deep location. Many are calcified, leading to incorrect diagnoses.

ANGIOMYOMA (VASCULAR LEIOMYOMA)

Angiomyomas are solitary tumors that develop between 40 and 50 years of age and occur primarily on the lower leg (14). Such lesions usually occur in the subcutaneous tissue without change or modification to the epidermis. They appear as glistening grayish nodules. Angiomyomas are composed of numerous thick-walled vessels, are relatively slow growing, and are painful more often than most.

They respond well to surgical excision.

BLOOD VESSELS

Hemangioma

Hemangioma is defined as a nonreactive process characterized by an increase in the number of normal and abnormal-appearing blood vessels. Two types are recognized. Localized lesions are the most common. The angiomatoses are more extensive and involve large segments of the body. The following types can occur in the lower extremity.

CAPILLARY HEMANGIOMA

Hemangiomas involving capillaries are the largest single group of blood vessel lesions. They are located in the skin or subcutaneous tissue and appear in infancy (Fig. 17.2). Red-purple, elevated capillary-sized vessels lined by flattened endothelium

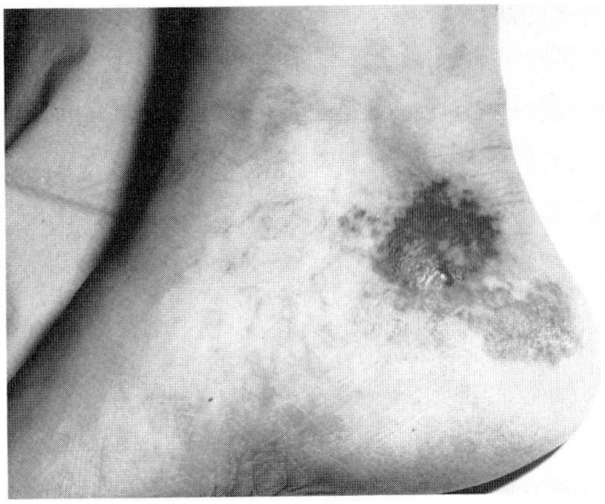

Figure 17.2. Capillary hemangioma.

are characteristic features. Variants of such lesions include juvenile hemangioma or strawberry nevus.

Juvenile hemangiomas are immature forms of capillary hemangiomas. They are very common in infancy, when they demonstrate the characteristic color and elevated appearance of a strawberry. The majority of such lesions gradually regress spontaneously.

VERRUCOUS HEMANGIOMA

Verrucous hemangiomas undergo reactive hyperkeratosis, acanthosis, and papillomatosis. Consequently, they may be confused with a wart (Fig. 17.3). Such lesions tend to recur upon excision. They also tend to develop satellite lesions until completely excised.

CAVERNOUS HEMANGIOMA

Some hemangiomas have a deeper engorged capillary component. The superficial cavernous portion tends to be larger. Such lesions seldom regress, and most require surgery.

ARTERIOVENOUS HEMANGIOMA

Deep and superficial forms of arteriovenous hemangiomas are recognized. The deep type is most commonly found about the head, neck, or lower extremity and is considered to be a malformation (15). Its proximity to the skin determines whether an arteriovenous shunt will be palpated. Arteriography is best used for precise diagnosis.

The superficial form is a painless solitary module, blue to red in color, and does not demonstrate the shunt.

VENOUS HEMANGIOMAS

Hemangiomas involving veins develop as large masses in the muscles of the extremities and are best diagnosed by venography.

GRANULATION TISSUE TYPE OF HEMANGIOMAS (PYOGENIC GRANULOMA)

Pyogenic granulomas are tumors which frequently follow trauma or infection. They are relatively rapid growing, pea-sized to cherry sized, bluish-red lesions with a constricting epithelial collar (Fig. 17.4). These granulomatous masses are usually moist, eroded, smooth, and bleed easily. They sometimes become necrotic or ulcerated (16). Treatment is excision or curettage and electrocautery.

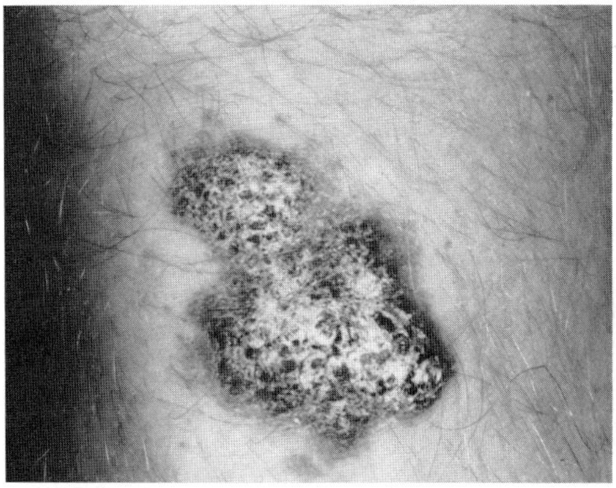

Figure 17.3. Verrucous hemangioma.

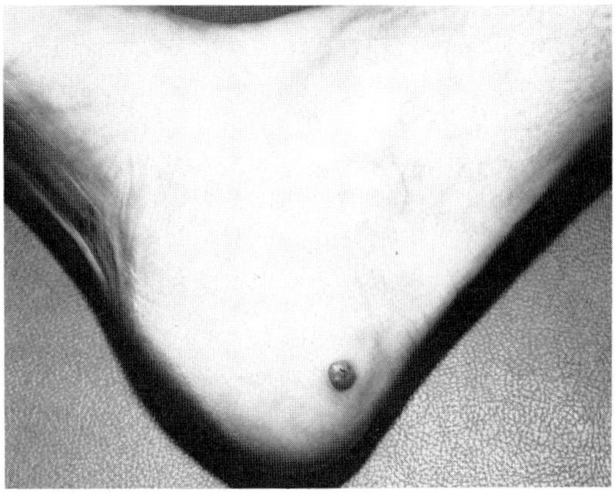

Figure 17.4. Pyogenic granuloma.

Hemangiomatosis

The majority of hemangiomatosis cases present in infancy or childhood as a swelling, with induration of the involved limbs. Discoloration of any extremity, along with hypertrophy of the limb in some instances, may suggest the presence of hemangiomatosis.

Glomus Tumor

The glomus tumor is a soft or firm, small, bluish-red papule of the skin and subcutaneous tissues (Fig. 17.5). They frequently occur on the hands and feet and are often subungual in location. Such lesions give rise to severe paroxysms of pain which are initiated by pressure, trauma, and vasomotor response to cold.

The tumor is an expansion of the structure of a normal glomus, together with an increased number of nerve fibers and vessels.

The degree of color change is dependent on the depth of the lesion. Since some lesions are clinically invisible, whenever the characteristic lancinating pain is experienced, it is valuable to employ a small probe to locate the pinpoint area of sensitivity.

When the lesion is near bone, radiographs are indicated because of possible cortical erosions.

Excision of glomus tumor is the treatment of choice.

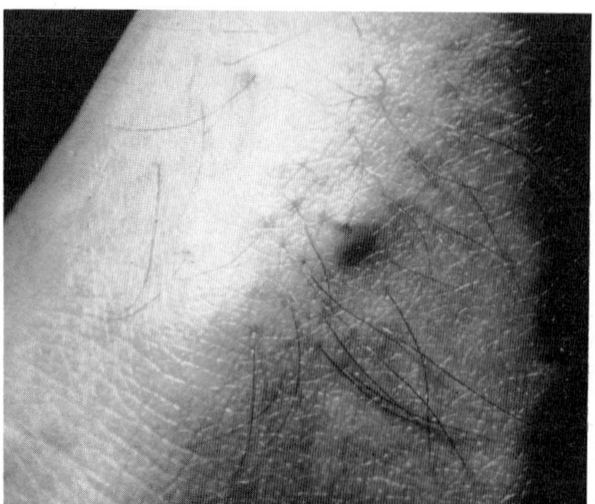

Figure 17.5. Glomus tumor.

Vascular Ectasias

These are a group of lesions that share a common feature of localized dilatation of preformed vessels. While they share this feature, the etiology and clinical picture are different (17).

NEVUS FLAMMEUS (BIRTHMARK)

Most birthmarks are dull pink and are referred to as "salmon patches." Most occur in the region of the head, and they gradually regress over time.

PORT WINE STAIN (NEVUS VINOSUS)

This is a specialized form of nevus flammeus but has no tendency to fade and grows proportionally with the child. It often develops an elevated thickened surface (Fig. 17.6).

KLIPPEL-TRENAUNAY-WEBER SYNDROME

This syndrome includes a port wine stain which is associated with varicosities and hypertrophy of an extremity (18).

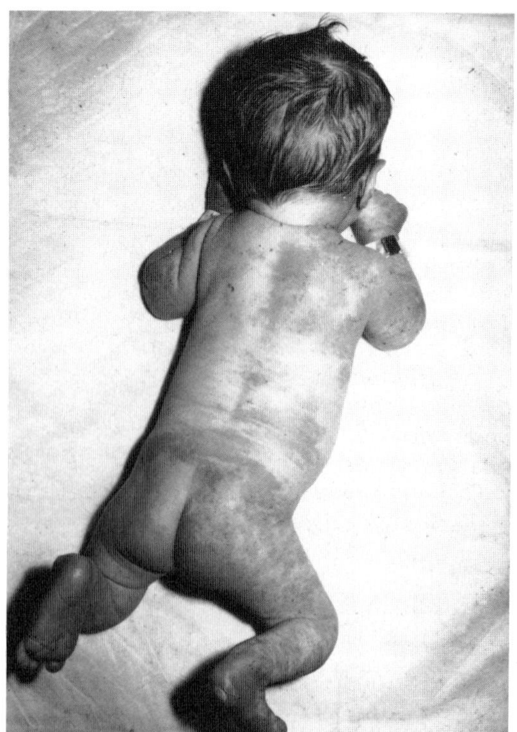

Figure 17.6. Port wine stain.

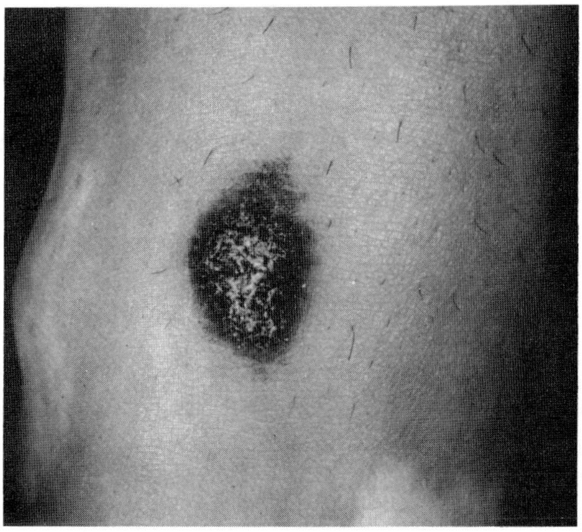

Figure 17.7. Angiokeratoma.

ARTERIAL SPIDER (NEVUS ARANEUS)

Spider nevi are acquired probably through altered physiological states, such as pregnancy. They are characterized by a small central arteriole from which smaller vessels emanate radially. The lesion blanches upon pressure over the central arteriole.

ANGIOKERATOMAS

Angiokeratomas are a group of disorders characterized by dilatation of the superficial vessels of the dermis and an overlying hyperkeratotic epidemis. Such lesions all have asymptomatic vascular regions that demonstrate dark red to black firm papules. They are up to 1 cm in diameter, with varying degrees of hyperkeratosis (19).

Solitary or multiple angiokeratomas may be seen on the lower extremities (Fig. 17.7). They originate as an area of telangiectasia, which is followed by hyperkeratotic and angiokeratotic changes which are probably due to trauma.

Other lesions in this group include angiokeratoma circumscription and angiokeratoma of Mibelli.

Papillary Endothelial Hyperplasia

Papillary endothelial hyperplasias are 2-cm, purple-red, multifocal masses containing clotted blood. The involved regions are surrounded by a fibrous pseudocapsule containing residual smooth muscle or elastic tissue of the preexisting vessel wall. Most evidence indicates that the lesion is an unusual form of organizing thrombus (20).

Endothelial hyperplasias are frequently confused with angiosarcoma. Since the prognosis of this lesion is excellent with adequate excision, differential diagnosis is important.

SYNOVIAL TISSUE

Localized Giant Cell Tumors of Tendon Sheath

Giant cell tumors as they affect tendon sheaths have been described as nodular tenosynovitis (21), pigmented nodular synovitis (22), and fibrous histiocytoma of synovium (23). The diversity of nomenclature indicates the considerable disagreement concerning the origin and nature of such tumors.

Giant cell tumors occur most commonly between the ages of 30 and 50. They are localized in the hand, and sometimes in the feet, ankle, or knee. On fingers, they appear adjacent to the interphalangeal joint in association with either flexor or extensor tendons. Such lesions develop gradually, and are fixed to deep structures but not to the skin unless the tendon is closely related to the skin.

Fletcher and Horn (24) suggest that giant cell tumors of the feet more frequently produce cortical erosions because the dense ligaments of that region are more likely to prevent outward growth of the tumors.

The tumors of tendon sheaths are circumscribed lobulated masses with shallow grooves created by underlying tendons. They tend to be relatively small, but those on the feet are usually larger and more irregularly shaped than those occurring on the hands (25) (Fig. 17.8).

The earliest lesions observed are villous structures that project into the synovial space of the tendon sheath. Limited space prevents continued growth into the cavity so that ultimately the tumor grows outward in a cauliflower fashion and compresses synovial-lined clefts into its substance (25). When such tumors are surgically excised, they appear as exophytic masses attached to tendon sheath, with smooth lobulated contours.

Postoperative recurrences occur between 10 and 44%, depending on the author cited.

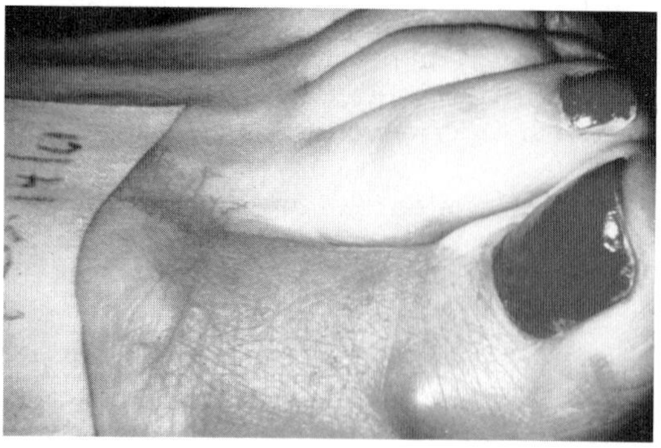

Figure 17.8. Localized giant cell tumor of tendon sheath.

However, Wright (25) feels that the higher figure is more accurate because of extended follow-up on outpatients that was employed by those investigators.

Diffuse Giant Cell Tumor of Tendon Sheath (Proliferation Synovitis, Florid Synovitis, Extraarticular Pigmented Villonodular Synovitis)

Diffuse giant cell tumors are the soft tissue counterparts of diffuse pigmented villonodular synovitis of the joint space. It probably represents an extraarticular extension of the joint process.

This tumor type is rare compared to the localized form and occurs in a younger age group. Symptoms are of long duration and include pain and tenderness in the affected extremity. Anatomically, the distribution is most common in the hand, followed by the ankle and foot. All other locations are relatively uncommon (26).

Tendosynovial Cyst (Ganglion, Synovial Cyst, Bursal Cyst, Cyst of Tendon Sheath, etc.)

Ganglions are thin-walled, tumor-like sacs filled with clear viscous fluid found in direct continuity with the tendon-sheath, capsule, or bursa (Fig. 17.9). They most commonly occur in hands, wrists, and feet. The most popular theory for the development of such lesions assumes that any condition capable of producing synovial effusion can produce synovial cyst (27, 28).

While ganglions occur more frequently in the hand, they are probably more common in the foot than previously reported in the early literature (4) (Table 17.1).

In general, the treatment of tumors associated with tendon sheaths, joint capsules, and bursa is careful complete excision of the tissue mass.

PERIPHERAL NERVES

Morton's Neuroma

The neuroma as described by Morton is not a true tumor but rather a hypertrophy of the affected plantar digital nerve sheath through fibrosis. It is probably an entrapment neuropathy of the plantar digital nerves, most often located plantar to the interspaces between the third and fourth metatarsal heads and/or the bases of the respective proximal phalanges. While this region is the most common location observed, they occur in any of the digital interspaces of the foot. The basic etiology is thought to involve a biomechanical fault of the foot, i.e., flaccid pronation, etc., resulting in compression of the nerve through maldistribution of ground reactive forces.

Characteristically, the patient describes a burning, lancinating pain about the involved digits, necessitating the removal of the shoe and massaging the foot. The only objective sign that is exceptionally reliable is the Muldor's sign. This test involves the lateral compression and alternate relaxation of the metatarsal heads while alternately pushing in a dorsal direction from the plantar surface with the thumb of the contralateral hand, which produces an audible click in the affected interspace.

When the Muldor's sign is present, the neurofibrous lesion should be excised (Fig. 17.10).

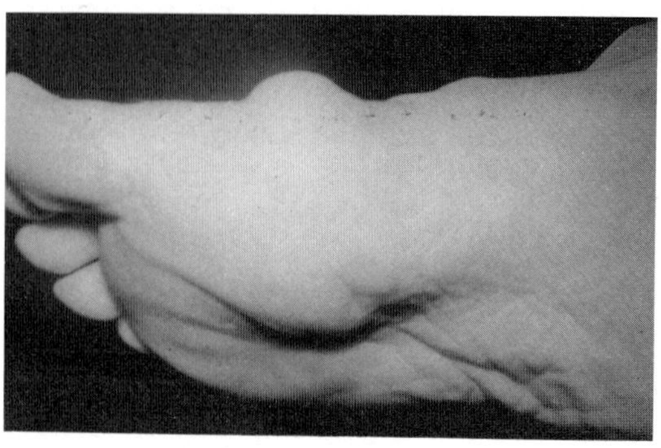

Figure 17.9. Plantar ganglion with dorsal exostosis.

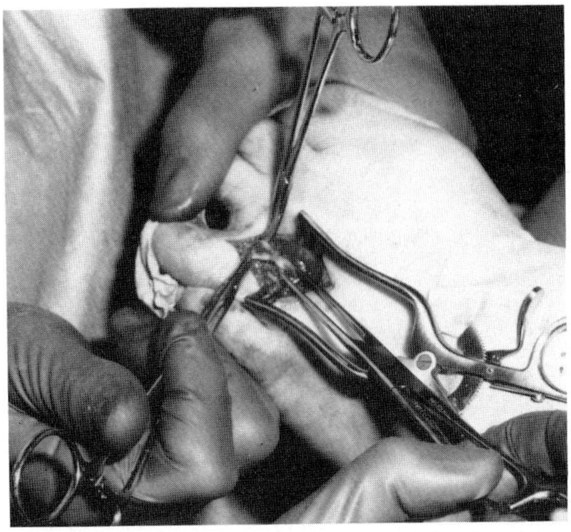

Figure 17.10. Excision of characteristic fusiform Morton's neuroma.

Traumatic Neuroma

The traumatic neuroma is an exuberant proliferation of the end of a nerve in response to surgery, as in excision of a Morton's neuroma, or to some other form of injury. Normally, the ends of a severed nerve reestablish continuity by an orderly growth of axons from proximal to distal. This event occurs through tubes of proliferating Schwann cells. However, if proximity of nerve endings is not established (or is not possible), a disorganized proliferation of the proximal nerves ensues which may produce a neuroma. Strangulation of this proliferating nerve by scar tissue, irritation, infection, etc., may also produce pain at the sites of these firm nodules.

Conventional treatment is directed at excision of the mass and burying the proximal nerve stump in tissues removed from the previous scar.

Attempts have been made to prevent traumatic neuromas by attaching nerve caps to the proximal nerve stump, and coagulating the severed nerve with CO_2 laser or the Bovie. However, no convincing studies on this matter have been described, except anecdotally.

Nerve Sheath Ganglion

The majority of nerve sheath ganglions occur at the head of the fibula in association with the common peroneal nerve (29) and present as tender masses with pain and numbness along the distribution of the nerve. The ganglia are essentially intraneural and represent a degenerative process rather than a true neoplasm.

Neurilemoma (Benign Schwannoma)

Neurilemoma is also referred to as a neurinoma or perineural fibroblastoma. Such lesions are encapsulated nerve sheath tumors consisting of two components: a cellular (Autoni A area) and a myxoid (Autoni B area).

These nerve sheath involvements occur at all ages, but especially between 20 and 50. They have a predilection for the head, neck, and flexor surfaces of the upper and lower extremities (30). Lesions are usually solitary, except when they are in association with von Recklinghausen's disease (30).

In the case of small nerve involvements, the tumor is freely movable, except at a single point of attachment. It may or may not be painful.

Excision is indicated whenever painful lesions are encountered (Fig. 17.11).

Neurofibroma: Solitary (Fig. 17.15)

Solitary neurofibromas are localized lesions that occur in patients not demonstrating von Recklinghausen's disease. They tend to develop in persons between ages 20 and 30, are superficial lesions of the

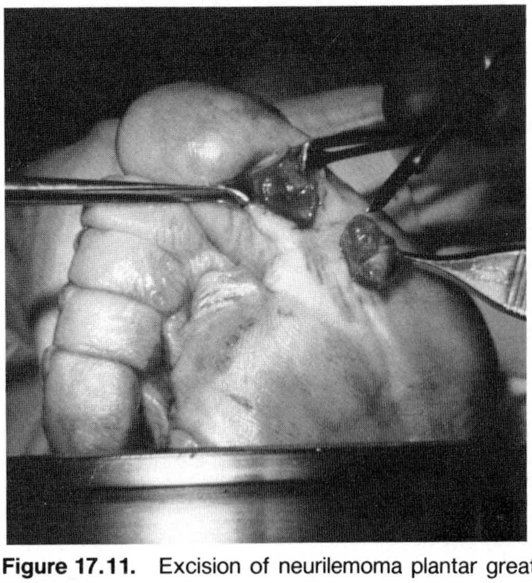

Figure 17.11. Excision of neurilemoma plantar great toe.

dermis and subcutis, and occur with wide distribution throughout the body. Such lesions are slow growing and produce painless nodules. There are several unusual variations of neurofibromas, such as Pacini, pigmented, and granular cell types. However, they are of no interest to the clinician. An exception to this statement is the myxoid form of neurofibroma that usually occurs on the extremities and is easily confused with mylomas.

Neurofibromatosis (von Recklinghausen's Disease)

PERIPHERAL NEUROFIBROMATOSIS

Whenever café au lait spots develop, von Recklinghausen's disease usually may be expected to manifest itself within a few years. The characteristic spots become larger than freckles and tend to occur on the unexposed areas of the body, such as the back (Fig. 17.12). Another characteristic location is the axilla. Crowe et al suggested that only lesions greater than 1.5 cm be considered café au lait spots for diagnostic purposes (31). Since the spots increase with age and 90% of patients with the disease have these lesions, their number can serve as a guide to diagnosis. Patients with more than six spots (greater than 1.5 cm) can be presumed to have the disease without any other stigmata (31).

The neurofibromas of von Recklinghausen's disease make their appearance after the appearance of the café au lait spots and can be found virtually anywhere (Fig. 17.13). The tumors are slow growing. Forty percent of patients have skeletal abnormalities which include erosive defects, scoliosis, bowing of long bones, etc. (31).

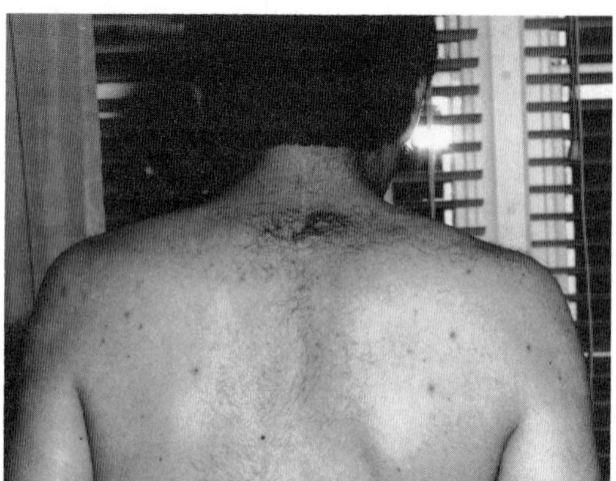

Figure 17.12. Café au lait spots herald the onset of von Recklinghausen's disease.

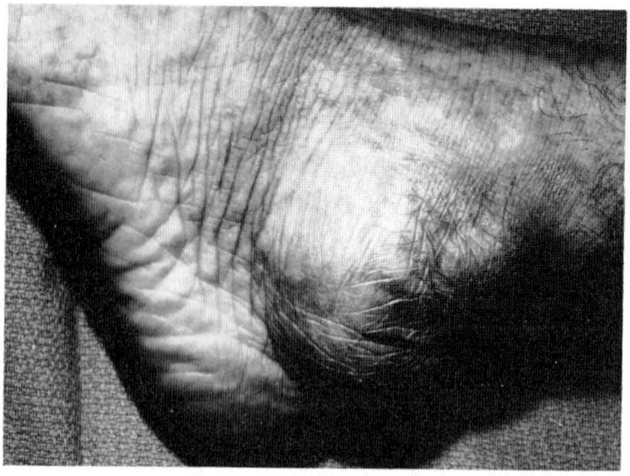

Figure 17.13. Neurofibromatoses of the heel.

CENTRAL NEUROFIBROMATOSIS

In this form of von Recklinghausen's disease, the peripheral manifestations are absent or are very few. Symptoms will be a reflection at the level of nervous system involvement. Bilateral acoustic neuromas are pathognomonic of the disease.

Several types of neurofibromas may occur and are differentiated by gross and microscopic appearances. The localized neurofibroma is the most common. In contrast to the solitary neurofibroma, central localized forms are much larger. The plexiform type is a convulated mass that has been described as a "bag of worms."

In most cases the large number of lesions make surgery impractical. Surgery is reserved for lesions that are large, painful, or in instances in which further expansion would affect organ function. Recurrences occasionally develop and other complications may ensue. In one case, a painful neurofibroma developed plantar to a metatarsal head. Upon excision, the mass was revealed to be a plexiform neurofibroma. The patient subsequently developed neuropathic arthropathy of the ankle and subtalar joints 4 weeks postoperatively. The most important complication of such lesions is malignant transformation and occurs in between 2 and 13% of patients (32).

Cartilaginous Tumors

EXTRASKELETAL CHONDROMA

Extraskeletal chondromas occur primarily in the soft tissues of the hands and feet.

The slowly enlarging mass does not cause pain and is associated with tendon, tendon sheath, or the joint capsule. Such tumors are located outside the periosteum (33).

MISCELLANEOUS CUTANEOUS AND SUBCUTANEOUS PEDAL TUMORS AND TUMOR-LIKE LESIONS

Eccrine Poroma

Eccrine poroma was first described by Pinkus et al in 1956 (34). Such lesions proved to originate from the distal and intraepidermal portions of the eccrine sweat ducts. The site of predilection is the plantar surface of the foot, but the lesion can occur anywhere. They are usually solitary growths which appear on patients over 40 years of age with no sex preference demonstrated. Eccrine poromas are essentially painless, reddish, soft, pedunculated masses which form a shallow cup-like invagination (Fig. 17.14). Samitz et al reported 2 cases of the plantar surface of the foot and toe in 1968 (36). The following aspects of diagnosis and treatment are illustrated: (*a*) the clinical appearance of the lesion, which may be quite specific and permit accurate diagnosis; (*b*) the lesion may be of long duration: (*c*) the tumor is benign; and (*d*) excision is effective as the mode of treatment.

Clear Cell Acanthoma

In 1962, Degos described a slow-growing solitary lesion of the leg of late middle age having a characteristic microscopic picture. Typically the Malpighian cells appear larger and paler than those of the surrounding epidermis (36).

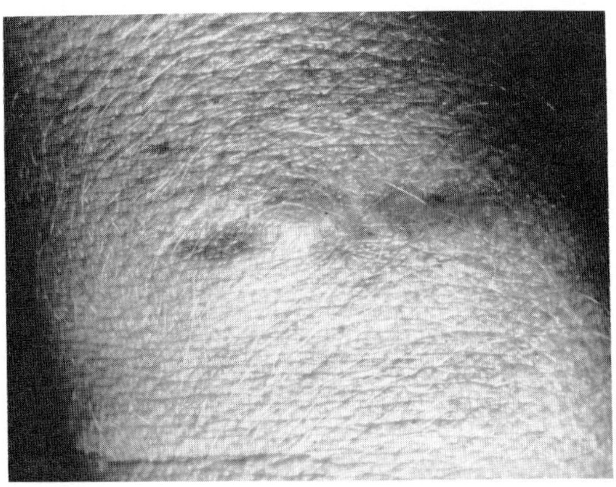

Figure 17.14. Eccrine poroma.

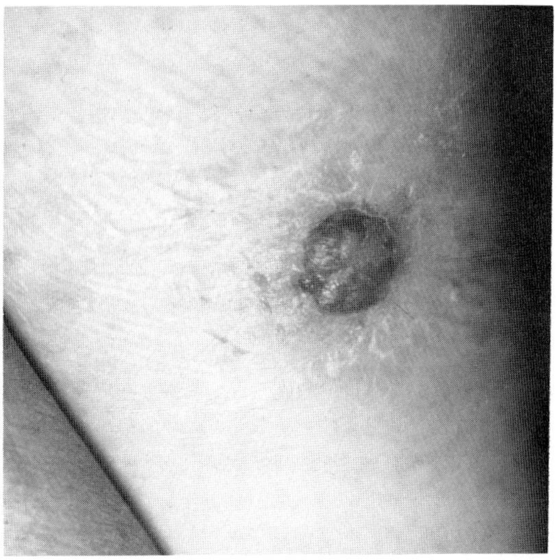

Figure 17.15. Clear cell acanthoma.

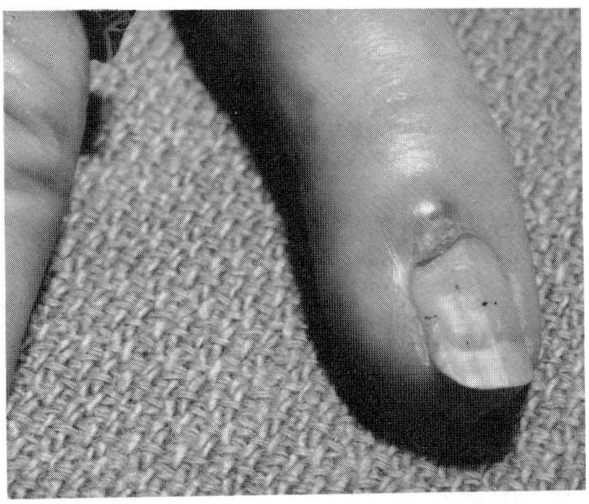

Figure 17.16. Cutaneous myxoid cyst of the finger.

The characteristic lesion is an elevated dome-shaped nodule which is pinkish to reddish-brown in color. Such nodules demonstrate a tendency to bleed (Fig. 17.15). They appear to be "stuck on," look vascular, have a peripheral "wafer-like" scale, a surface exudate, and an advancing rounded border.

Treatment of clear cell acanthoma is excision.

Cutaneous Myxoid Cyst

The majority of cutaneous myxoid cysts occur in the late middle years as oval, fluctuant, translucent masses ranging in size to 1.3 cm in diameter (Fig. 17.16). They occur on either side of the midline at the distal interphalangeal joints of the fingers and toes. Such cysts are filled with a straw-colored viscous fluid.

Considering the resistance of this lesion to many forms of therapy, it has been the author's personal experience with three cases that radical excision is the preferred treatment. Transverse elliptical incisions are employed to excise the digital cyst. Additionally, the head of the underlying intermediate phalanx is resected. Since the lesion has to be excised completely, wound closure is difficult unless the tissues are collapsed by excision of the bone. Despite the present consensus of investigators that myxoid cysts are independent of the joint, the success achieved with these three cases might indicate otherwise.

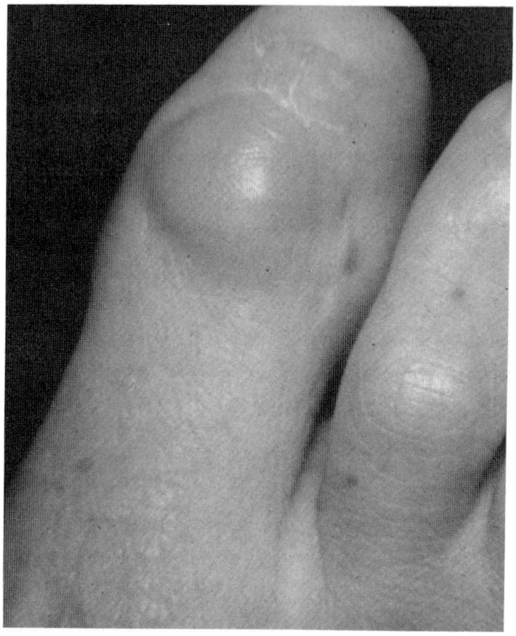

Figure 17.17. Epidermal inclusion cyst following nail surgery.

Epidermal Inclusion Cyst

As the name implies, the majority of epidermal inclusion cysts are acquired by the invagination of a portion of the epidermis by trauma, foreign body, etc. (Fig. 17.17) The epidermis becomes an "inclusion." It is an occasional complication following nail surgery.

Such cysts are somewhat fluctuant, skin-colored, and ovoid shaped. Some lesions may extend to several centimeters in size.

Recurrence of epidermal inclusion cysts are common unless excision is complete (Fig. 17.18*A* and *B*).

Porokeratosis Plantaris Discreta

Porokeratosis plantaris discreta is discussed elsewhere in connection with hyperkeratotic lesions.

This lesion is thought to develop from

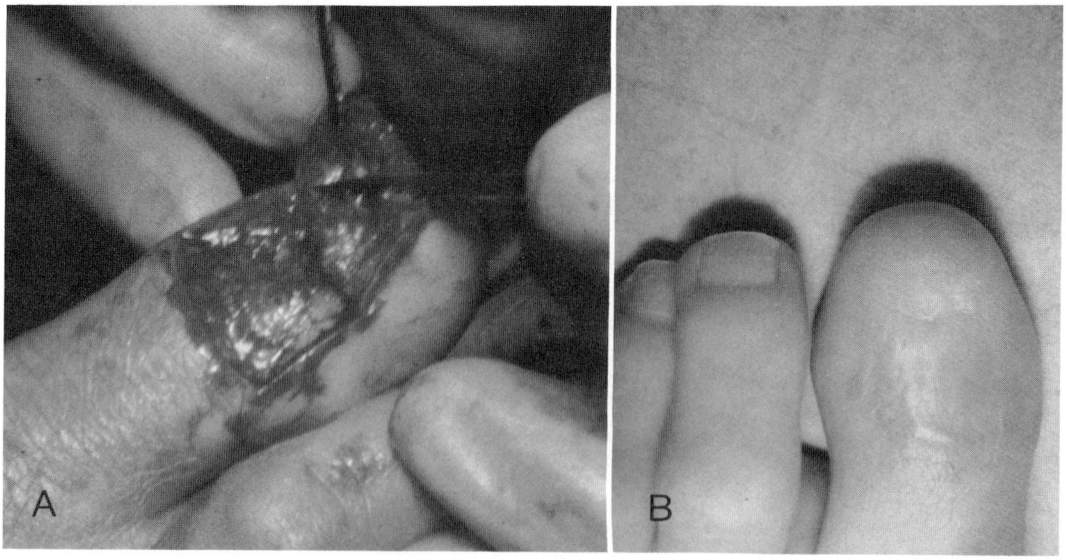

Figure 17.18. (*A*) Surgical correction of epidermal inclusion cyst involving the great toe. (*B*) Postoperative results.

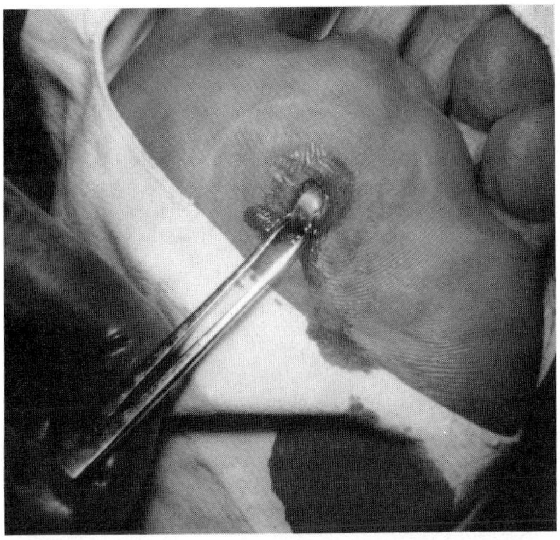

Figure 17.19. Porokeratosis plantaris discreta.

hyperkeratotic plugging of the sweat duct apparatus. Treatment is directed towards the modification of weightbearing abnormalities by surgical and biomechanical means. In addition, with resistant lesions, the author uses a biopsy punch to "punch" out the lesion, particularly when it occurs around the heel. This approach has proven to be remarkably effective (Fig. 17.19).

Chronic Radiodermatitis

Many years ago, the use of ionizing radiation for the treatment of such diverse conditions as poison ivy, tinea pedis, diphidrotic eczema, hyperhidrosis, plantar warts, and intractable plantar keratoses misdiagnosed as plantar warts was popular. The sequelae of this irradiation did not necessarily manifest itself in many cases for up to 20 years. The results of radiation were often a chronic radiodermatitis, a precancerous lesion, consisting of punctate, waxy, atrophic, well-demarcated lesions surrounded by telangiectasis (Fig. 17.20). This lesion was exquisitely painful and ultimately led to hyperkeratosis, ulcerations, and squamous cell carcinoma in many cases. Steinberg recommended wide excision of such lesions until normal yellow adipose tissue was evident. Resection of the underlying metatarsal head whenever the lesion was adherent to the bone was required. If the resultant wound was difficult to close, relaxation incision on either side of the wound, with undermining, was utilized to approximate the margins of the defect.

Rheumatoid Nodule

Rheumatoid nodules appear in approximately 15% of patients with rheumatoid arthritis and are manifest at a late stage in the disease (Fig. 17.21). Such lesions should be excised if they are painful; however, recurrence is high. Rheumatoid arthritis is known to be a chronic autoimmune disorder.

Tophaceous Gout

Gout is an inborn error of metabolism which results in hyperuricemia. Monosodium urate depositions may develop in articular cartilage, the helix of the ear, the skin, and the bursae of elbow and knees, toes, etc. (Fig. 17.22). These deposits tend to occur in relatively avascular tissues such as tendons and cartilage and are variable

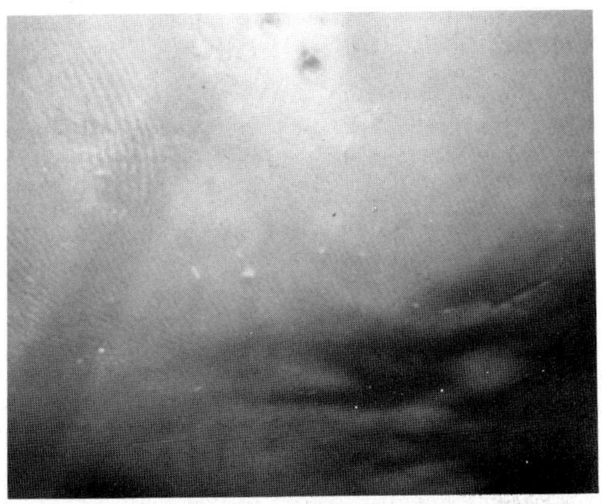

Figure 17.20. Chronic radiodermatitis.

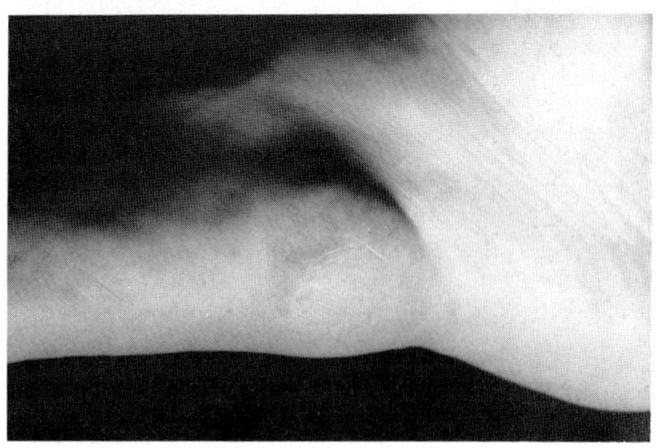

Figure 17.21. Rheumatoid nodule ace of fifth metatarsal.

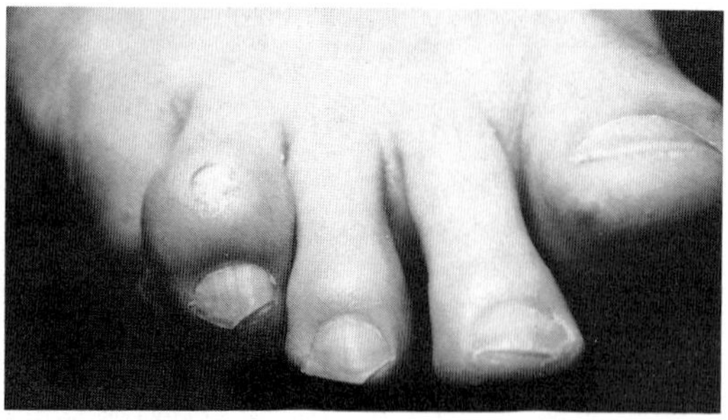

Figure 17.22. Tophaceous gout of the fourth toe.

in size. The overlying skin tends to be shiny, thin, and reddish in color. Ulcers form with injury or when confined tissues become taut with tophaceous deposits.

Acute gouty arthritis is treated with rest, elevation, indomethacin, and nerve blocks. Chronic gout is treated with allopurinol (Zyloprim), a xanthine oxidase inhibitor. Surgery can complicate tophaceous gout and should not be contemplated unless absolutely necessary.

Epidermal Nevus

Epidermal nevi are due to hyperplasia of epithelial cells which are present at birth or soon after. Such lesions vary in size and may be single or multiple. They are frequently seen on the extremities, and their surfaces are often verrucous in appearance. They vary in color, depending upon the amounts of pigment involved (Fig. 17.23). Microscopically, nevus cells may be epithelioid, fibroblast-like, or similar to the sheath of Schwann cells. Cytoplasm tends to be homogeneous and light staining. Nuclei are large and vesicular, and they may coalesce to form multinucleated giant nevus cells. Inflammatory infiltrates are rare, except when folliculitis is coexistent.

Nevus Cell Nevi

Nevus cell nevi constitute a group of lesions which can be subdivided into three types: junctional, compound, and intradermal (39). The histologic location of the nevus cells is the distinguishing feature of each. Junctional nevus cells are usually smaller and flatter and lie in the epidermis, at the dermoepidermal junction, or high in the dermis (Fig. 17.24). It is usually brown-black, smooth, slightly raised, and hairless. Junctional nevi are common on the plantar surfaces of feet and are important because the majority of melanomas arise from the junctional nevus.

The compound nevus lies both at the dermoepidermal junction and intradermally and presents initially as a raised, pigmented nodule. The intradermal nevus is the common mole and does not undergo malignant transformation. It is a pedunculated, lightly pigmented, or flesh-colored lesion.

Connective tissue elements are not pres-

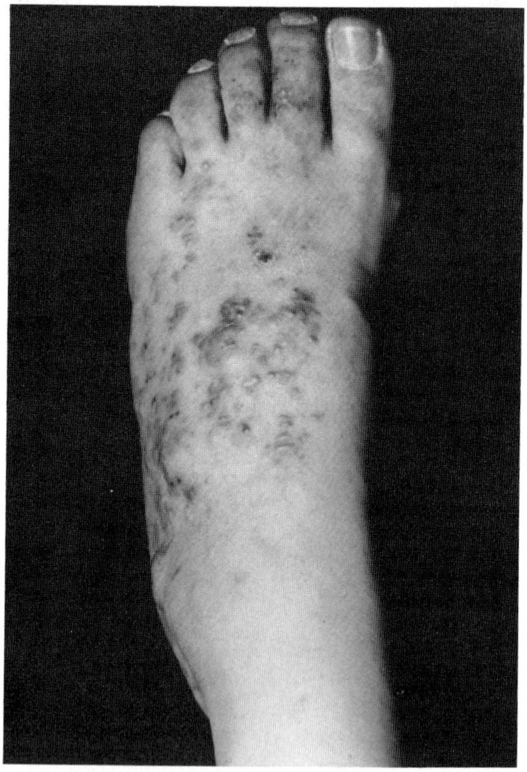

Figure 17.23. Epidermal nevus.

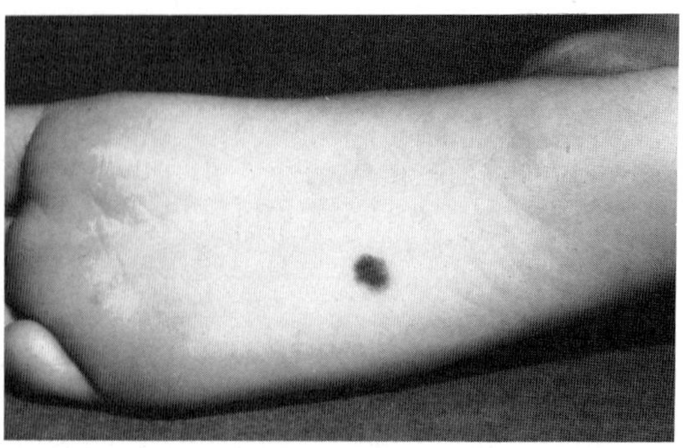

Figure 17.24. Junctional nevus.

ent between keratinocytes and nevus cells in junctional nevi. Electron microscopy has demonstrated an absence of the basement membrane at the epidermal-dermal junction at the lower polls of epidermal nests. This phenomenon is important for an understanding of transformation of junctional nevi into the compound form.

Epidermal nevus cells do not migrate into the dermis in forming compound nevi. Rather, connective tissue elements envelop and pinch off epidermal nests bulging from the epidermis into the dermis. Compound nevi situated deep in the dermis often relate to follicular epithelium. They are, therefore, representative or neuroectodermal and mesodermal elements.

Intradermal nevi are those in which the formation of theques subsides, and nests become distinctly intradermal. It is probable that a thorough examination of all sections of intradermal nevi demonstrate some junctional activity. However, no unusual cytological activity occurs at this higher level.

Junctional nevi which are undergoing changes in color, distribution, or shape should be excised. Pigment leakage, which forms a pigmented halo, and areas of infiltration or nodule formations are signs of change. Bleeding and ulceration of such lesions are ominous occurrences. Subungual pigmented lesions should be excised prophylactically (40).

HALO NEVUS

Halo nevi are those which demonstrate a pigmented central zone surrounded by a halo-like depigmented zone. Such lesions frequently herald spontaneous resolution. Lymphocytic infiltrates are not uncommon in these nevi.

BLUE NEVUS

Blue nevi occur most frequently on the dorsum of the hands and feet and on the face. Such lesions develop after birth and are hairless, smooth, and blue-black in color (Fig. 17.25). These papular lesions may resemble melanomas (41). Differential diagnosis relies heavily on the patient's history: Blue nevi will remain morphologically unaltered for many years, while melanomas change in size, shape and color with some rapidity (41). The margins of these lesions are poorly defined and they do not demonstrate encapsulation.

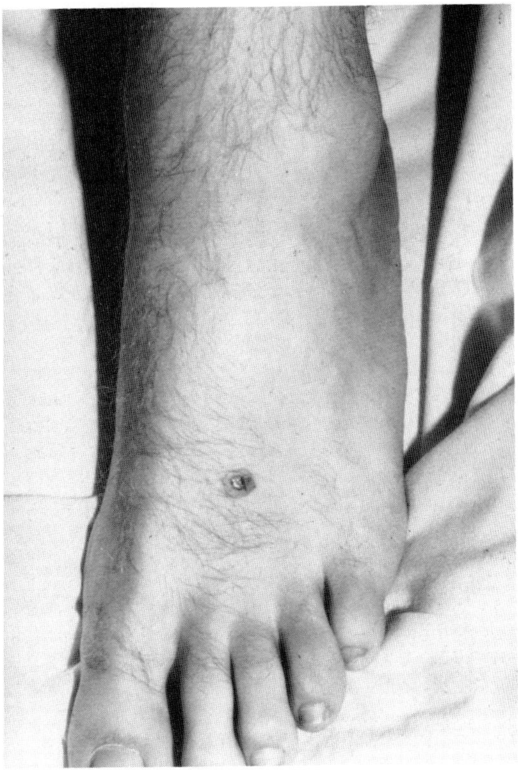

Figure 17.25. Blue nevus.

Microscopic examination reveals few, if any, mitotic figures. Fibrous portions of the dermis are increased. Dermal melanocytes are stellate or fusiform, rich in melanin and are dopa positive. Other constituents of the dermis include plump, short melanophages heavily laden with melanin, but these cells are dopa negative. Blue nevi meet the classic definition of nevi in that they are localized stable excesses of normal skin constituents.

References

1. Samitz MH, Lewis JE: Skin tumors of the lower extremities. *Int J Dermatol* 17:558, 1979.
2. Enzinger FM, Weiss SW: *Soft Tissue Tumors.* St. Louis, C. V. Mosby, 1983, pp 6–7.
3. Hendrickson M: Pathology Lecture Notes. Stanford, CA, Dept. of Pathology, Stanford University School of Medicine, 1984.
4. Berlin SJ: *Skin Tumors of the Foot: Diagnosis and Treatment.* Mount Kisco, NY, Futura Publishing, 1974, p 3.
5. Berlin SJ: A laboratory review of 67,000 foot tumors and lesions. *J Am Podiatry Assoc*

74:341, 1984.
6. Fairbank HAT: A periosteal lipoma. *J Bone Joint Surg* 35B:589, 1953.
7. Booker R: Lipoblastic tumors of the hands and feet: review of the literature and report of 33 cases. *J Bone Joint Surg* 47:727, 1965.
8. Kurzweg FT, Spencer R: Familial multiple lipomatosis. *Am J Surg* 82:726, 1957.
9. Tranguada RE: Subcutaneous lipomas at sites of insulin injection. *Diabetes* 15:807, 1966.
10. Enzinger FM: Benign Lipomatous Tumors Simulating a Sarcoma. In *Management of Primary Bone and Soft Tissue Tumors.* M.D. Anderson Hospital and Tumor Institute. Chicago, Year Book Medical Publishers, 1977.
11. Greenberg SD, Isensee C, Gonzalez-Angulo A et al: Infiltrating lipomas of the thigh. *Am J Clin Pathol* 39:66, 1963.
12. Sullivan CR et al: Lipoma of the tendon sheath. *J Bone Joint Surg* (Am) 38:1275, 1956.
13. Fisher WC, Helwig EB: Leiomyomas of the skin. *Arch Dermatol* 88:510, 1963.
14. Duhig JJ, Ayer JP: Vascular leiomyoma: a study of 61 cases. *Arch Pathol* 68:424, 1959.
15. Reid MR: Abnormal arteriovenous communications acquired and congenital. *Arch Surg* 10:996, 1925.
16. Samitz MH: *Cutaneous Disorder of the Lower Extremities.* Philadelphia, J.B. Lippincott, 1981, p 212.
17. Johnson WC: Pathology of cutaneous vascular tumors. *Int J Dermatol* 15:239, 1976.
18. Letts RM: Orthopedic treatment of hemangiomatous hypertrophy of the lower extremity. *J Bone Joint Surg* 59A:777, 1977.
19. Samitz MH: *Cutaneous Disorders of the Lower Extremities.* Philadelphia, J.B. Lippincott, 1981, p 134.
20. Fitzpatrick TB, Eisen AZ, Wolff K et al: *Dermatology in General Medicine*, ed 2. New York, McGraw-Hill, 1979.
21. Baes H, Tanghe W: Nodular tenosynovitis. *Dermatologica* 149:149, 1974.
22. Mason ML, Woolston WH: Isolated giant cell xanthomatic tumors of the fingers and hand. *Arch Surg* 15:499, 1927.
23. Jones FE et al: Fibrous histiocytoma of Synovium (giant cell tumors of tendon sheath, pigmented nodular synovitis.) *J Bone Joint Surg (Am)* 51A:76, 1969.
24. Fletcher AG, Horn RC: Giant cell tumors of tendon sheath origin. *Ann Surg* 133:374, 1951.
25. Wright CJE: Benign giant cell synovioma. *Br J Surg* 38:257, 1951.
26. Enzinger FM, Weiss SW: *Soft Tissue Tumors.* St. Louis, C.V. Mosby, 1983, p 510.
27. Hajdu SI: *Pathology of Soft Tissue Tumors.* Philadelphia, Lea & Febiger, 1979, p 168.
28. Bowerman JW, Muhletaler C: Arthrography of rheumatoid synovial cysts of the knee and wrist. *J Can Assoc Radiol* 24:24, 1973.
29. Barrett R, Cramer F: Tumors of the peripheral nerves and so-called ganglia of the peroneal nerve. *Clin Orthop* 27:135, 1963.
30. Stout AP: The peripheral manifestations of specific nerve sheath tumor (neurilemoma). *Am J Cancer* 24:751, 1935.
31. Crowe FW, Schall WJ, Neel JV: *A Clinical, Pathological and Genetic Study of Multiple Neurofibromatosis.* Springfield, IL Charles C Thomas, 1956.
32. Enzinger FM, Weiss SW: *Soft Tissue Tumors.* St. Louis, C.V. Mosby, 1983, p 615.
33. Chung EB, Enzinger FM: Benign chondromas of soft parts. *Cancer* 41:1414, 1978.
34. Pinkus H et al: Eccrine poroma. *Arch Dermatol Syphilol* 74:511, 1956.
35. Morris J, Wood MG, Samitz MH: Eccrine poroma. *Arch Dermatol* 98:162, 1968.
36. Samitz MH: *Cutaneous Disorders of the Lower Extremities.* Philadelphia, J.B. Lippincott, 1981, pp 205–206.
37. Taab J, Steinberg M: Porokeratosis plantaris discreta: a previously unrecognized dermatopathological entity. *Int J Dermatol* 9:83, 1970.
38. Weisfeld M: Understanding porokeratosis plantaris discreta. *J Am Podiatry Assoc* 63:138–144, 1973.
39. Gordon M: *Office Dermatology*, Roenigk HH Jr (ed). Baltimore, Williams & Wilkins, 1981.
40. Samitz MH: *Cutaneous Disorders of the Lower Extremities.* Philadelphia, J.B. Lippincott, 1981, pp 218–219.
41. Berlin S: *Skin Tumors of the Foot: Diagnosis and Treatment.* Mount Kisco, NY, Futura, 1974.

CHAPTER 18

Cutaneous Malignancies of the Human Foot

DANIEL J. McCARTHY

Malignant involvement of the integumentary system as it pertains to the human foot is a relatively uncommon podiatric diagnosis. However, it is important to recognize that skin cancer is the most frequently observed cancer in man. It is estimated that as many as 600,000 individual cases of skin cancer are recognized each year in the United States. These statistics do not include an even larger occurence of premalignant skin lesions.

The recent podiatric literature suggests that pedal malignancy may well be on the rise. This chapter will discuss basal cell and squamous cell carcinoma in the human foot, as well as malignant melanoma. In addition, special variants of these basic skin tumors, such as verrucous carcinoma, Bowen's disease, and amelanotic melanoma, will be reviewed.

MALIGNANT MELANOMA

Malignant melanoma (melanocytoma, melanocarcinoma) is a malignant neoplasm of ectodermally derived tissues resulting from tumorigenic activities of melanocytes. Melanocytes normally are pigment-producing cells derived of neural ectoderm which are migratory to the region of the epidermal-dermal interface, where their stellate processes interdigitate with cells of the stratum basale (1).

It has been estimated that about 25 to 50% of such neoplasia results from preexisting, benign pigmented lesions, although many authorities now question these high figures. The average adult ordinarily has about 100 such lesions, and it would appear that the incidence of malignant melanoma should be extremely high. However, it is estimated that only one growth in 100,000 actually develops malignant changes. It is for this reason that pigmented nevi are not to be indiscriminately removed.

Survival rates for patients with malignant melanoma can be as high as 90% when the lesion is detected early and is properly managed. An educated public, alert to the fact that pigmented enlarging lesions demonstrating changes are typical for malignancy, is the best defense against melanoma which might otherwise be life threatening (2).

The usual appearance of malignant melanoma is that of a blackish irregularly marginated growth which usually has a palpable depth (Fig. 18.1). However, it may occur atypically as a translucent gray or reddish tumor; the amelanotic variant of the growth can be even more deceptive. These atypically pigmented lesions have been characterized as being among the most unpredictable tumors in all of oncology. Many if not most cases on the foot (including the subungual site) start as a flat, nonpalpable pigmented spot.

Its most common occurrence involves the skin, but other tissues of ectodermal origin such as the eye are occasionally implicated. Historically, the prognosis for malignant melanoma has been poor: It has a potential for rapid and extensive metastasis, but it is also one of few cancers known to undergo spontaneous remission (2). Lesions having identical histopathological appearance may demonstrate totally different prognosis.

The relationship of age to prognosis has been of interest in recent years. Formerly, melanoma in young patients was thought to be as life threatening as those tumors observed in older patients. However, some

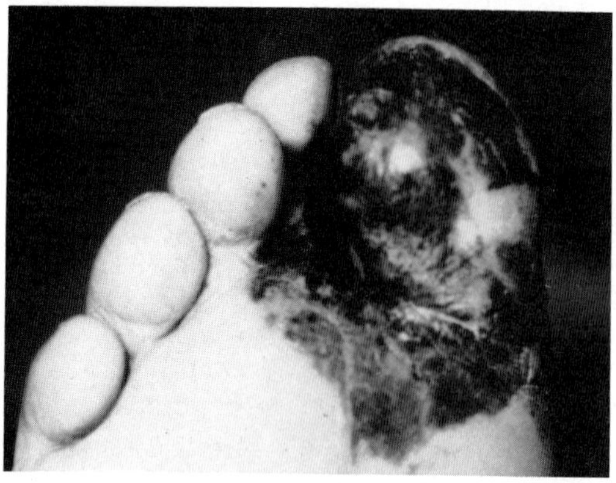

Figure 18.1. Clinical appearance of superficial spreading malignant melanoma. The lesion is fairly typical, demonstrating a bluish-black pigmentation. Courtesy of Dr. Martin Port, Tampa, FL.

authorities feel that statistical studies show that this type of neoplasia was relatively nonaggressive. Similarly, in elderly patients, malignant melanomas may behave in a relatively benign fashion.

Statistical data, however, can be misleading. Rabinowitz of Columbia-Presbyterian Hospital Dermatopathology Department (personal communication) feels that data concerning age and morbidity need to be correlated relative to the types of tumors involved. For example, the elderly have a high percentage of lentigo maligna melanoma with a lower mortality rate. Similarly, it is necessary to know if benign juvenile melanomas are included in the data for the young. Such lesions are actually benign nevi which simulate melanoma but are not metastatic. It is probable, therefore, that true melanomas of young adults may be as life-threatening as for any age group.

The variation in the behavior of melanoma in the prepubertal age group, as compared to that in the middle-aged adult, suggests the possibility of endocrine processes as being active in modulating the expression of malignant melanoma. These tumors can occur at any time of life, but 75% occur between the ages of 30 and 70 (4). The incidence of malignant melanoma ranges from 1.8 to 2.6 individuals among a population of 100,000. Its overall distribution is essentially equal among the sexes, although its occurrence on the lower extremities is higher among females.

Of reported cases, 90% involve Caucasians while only 1% affect blacks. The index of suspicion should be especially high when dealing with red-haired and fair-skinned individuals. The middle-aged population in the United States is increasing rapidly. This may account for the fact that deaths due to malignant melanoma rose from 2500 to 3500 in the decade ending in 1975 in this country. *The Journal of the American Podiatry Association* ordinarily reports one case of malignant melanoma each year (5–13).

Malignant melanoma is definitively diagnosed on the basis of biopsy, often employing special histochemical stains at the light microscopic level. Occasionally, transmission electron microscopy can be used to substantiate pathological findings. Treatment will be discussed at the close of this chapter in relation to the several other cutaneous malignancies.

Melanoma can be classified according to several systems. For example, one of them might be the ability of the neoplasia to kill. The nodular form is most devastating, while lesions differentiating from Hutchinson's freckle, i.e., lentigo malignant melanoma, are most benign (14). Superficial spreading melanoma is an intermediate grade which constitutes 60% of recorded occurrences. Acral lentiginous melanoma accounts for most melanomas of the foot.

Most crucial to assessing prognosis is the determination of the invasiveness of tumor cells into the deeper structures and the degree of metastasis. A complex system of tumor classification is available to oncologists which includes the invasive characteristics of the tumor, the presence of satellite lesions, in-transit metastasis, extent of nodal involvement, and metastasis to distant body locations. This is the so called TNM classification (2).

Clark's levels for the classification of melanocytomas of the skin are currently used by many pathologists.

Level I

This comparatively rare entity assumes that all melanoma cells are above the basement membrane. Its rarity, however, may be more apparent than real since all cases may, at some time, evolve through this precursor stage.

Level II

Melanoma tumor cells in this level have eroded the basement membrane but are limited to the papillary dermis. About 92% of patients falling into this category can be expected to survive.

Level III

Tumor cells fill the papillary dermis, at least focally, and impinge on the reticular dermis. Survival rate is 65%.

Level IV

Tumor cells involve portions of the reticular dermis as well as the papillary portion. About one half of patients in this classification survive.

Level V

Melanoma tumor cells extend into the subcutaneous tissues of the skin. The survival rate for this classification is about 48%. More recently, an increasing number of pathologists prefer the use of an ocular micrometer, as advocated by Breslow, to measure the depth and extent of the tumor. Such findings are thought to be less subjective than Clark's levels and to yield a precise value measured in millimeters. Breslows' method (as do other methods) assumes that tissues are properly oriented and embedded for sectioning and that the specimen is accurately representative of the tumor.

The reader is referred to the chapter on podiatric diagnosis for a more complete review of methodologies which may further assist in assessing malignant melanoma. Such techniques may include electrometric testing and radionucleotide imaging.

The diagnosis and treatment of malignant melanoma is a complex matter, and the podiatric surgeon, who may be the first specialist to observe this potentially lethal neoplasm, is well advised to utilize all of the medical resources which are available.

Pathology

LIGHT MICROSCOPIC HISTOPATHOLOGY

Several cytological variants of malignant melanoma are recognized. Occasionally, well-differentiated malignant melanoma undergoes spontaneous regression. These and other factors make microscopic diagnosis both complicated and confusing. In general, tumorigenesis begins with atypical melanocytic clusters at the epidermal-dermal junction. Pleomorphic melanocytes become involved and pseudovilli (villous-like processes) are frequently seen to interdigitate with contiguous epidermal cells. Intraepidermal nests of tumor cells are frequently observed. Tumor cells are often closely packed, and intercellular spaces are usually narrow as mass penetrates the subjacent dermis. Nuclei of tumor cells are usually hyperchromatic.

The most frequently recognized cells of malignant melanoma are characterized as being of epithelioid type. Their nuclei tend to be large and vesicular; the cytoplasm is abundant, and the cell boundaries are well defined (Fig. 18.2).

Spindle-shaped cells are also common and occur in groups or singly. The arrangement of these cells is fasciculated and in parallel array. Occasionally, these cells are randomly dispersed. The nuclear chromatin pattern is compact, and the cytoplasm often demonstrates bipolar extensions.

Malignant melanoma may mimic a benign nevus: In such cases, small nevoid cells are in evidence. Their nuclei are more compact and the cytoplasm of nevoid melanotic tumor cells is sparse and poorly defined.

A most unusual cell type, the balloon cell, has recently become associated with malignant melanotic tumors. They resemble foam or xanthoma cells but do not contain lipids or cholesterol. Such cells are pale staining and large with a granular, foamy, or structureless cytoplasm.

Lymphocytic infiltrate of the subjacent

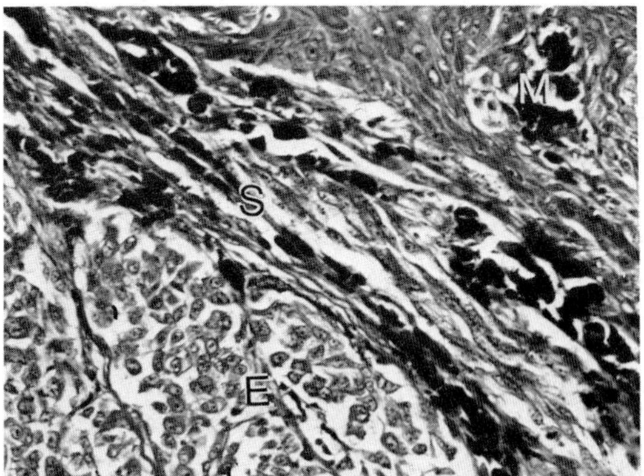

Figure 18.2. Malignant melanoma demonstrating epithelioid-type tumor cells with large vesicular nuclei and abundant cytoplasm (*E*). Spindle-shaped cells (*S*) are present in fascicular array. Good examples of nevus and balloon cells are not present in this section. Light microscopy, medium magnification. *M*, melanin.

dermis is a common feature of melanoma. Melanization of these tumors is highly variable. Indeed, amelanotic melanoma may require special techniques to demonstrate pigment. Melanotic inclusions in tumor cells may be small and well dispersed, or pigment may appear as large irregular granular clumps.

Multinucleated giant cells and large mononuclear cells may also be observed among tumor cells, in addition to the others just described.

ELECTRON MICROSCOPIC FINDINGS

Subcellular organelles such as Golgi apparatus, mitochondria, rough endoplasmic reticulum, and free ribosomes appear much the same as they do within intraepidermal nevus cells. Fibroblast-like tumor cells of spindle shape have been described, and it is thought they might have been dedifferentiated tumor cells which assumed fibroblast-like qualities. Alternatively, they have been described as being the result of a fibromatosis-like reaction masquerading as an atypical fibrous histiocytoma in skin-bearing hosts (15). Such cells demonstrate bizarre hyperchromatic nuclei: They cluster in an epithelial arrangement within regions of lymphocytic infiltrates within a collagenized matrix.

Pigment-producing bodies, the melanosomes and premelanosomes, can be identified in the cytoplasm of tumor cells: However, they do not relate to rough endoplasmic reticulum or Golgi apparatus as they do in nevus cells (Fig. 18.3). Such cells demonstrate an abundance of free ribosomes, but they tend to demonstrate varying degrees of degeneration.

Melanophages are frequently seen in association with melanin-producing cells. Such cells are responsible for degradation of the pigment melanin: Engulfed melanosomes can be seen enclosed within these phagocytic cells in single membrane-limited vacuoles. This type of cell contains organelles rich in acid phosphatase, and

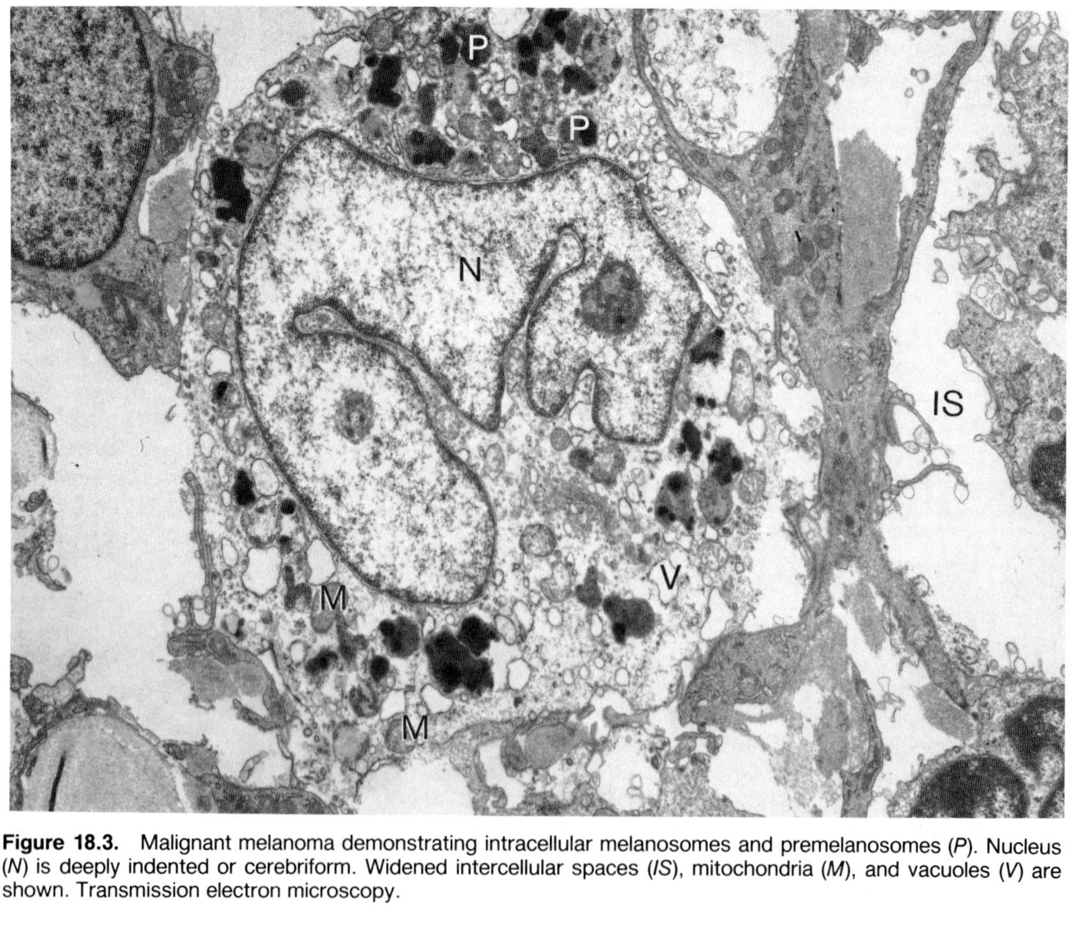

Figure 18.3. Malignant melanoma demonstrating intracellular melanosomes and premelanosomes (*P*). Nucleus (*N*) is deeply indented or cerebriform. Widened intercellular spaces (*IS*), mitochondria (*M*), and vacuoles (*V*) are shown. Transmission electron microscopy.

they appear in lysosomes of variable size and irregular shape.

Epidermal keratinocytes associated with malignant melanoma may demonstrate additional degenerative changes. Nuclei may be pleomorphic and indented with chromatin finely dispersed about the periphery, intercellular spaces are irregularly widened, and desmosomes are frequently disrupted.

Those cells which become invasive extending into the dermis tend to be any shape. Most are cuboidal or polyhedral and anaplastic. Spindle-shaped cells are less commonly observed. The arrangement of tonofilaments is variable; they may relate to desmosomes, but the tonofilament-desmosome complex (TDC) is most often disrupted. Endoplasmic reticulum and Golgi apparatus are usually sparse and poorly developed whenever they are seen. Some cells show an abundance of mitochondria, vesicles, and glycogen accumulation. Cytoplasmic dendritic processes are extensively involved in tumorigenesis.

Desmoplastic melanoma is a rare histologic variant of melanoma. The electron microscopic findings for this lesion are frequently dissimilar to those observed for most common melanomas.

Juvenile melanoma, which is a benign nevus, must be clearly separated from any discussion of melanoma. Juvenile melanoma is a pseudomelanoma which is a histologic simulant of malignant melanoma. These lesions, presently known as Spitz's nevus, demonstrate deceptive tumor cells of spindle or epithelioid type. Tumor cells may, on occasion, project beyond the epidermal-dermal junction into the dermis.

AMELANOTIC MELANOMA

Amelanotic melanoma is a melanotic neoplasm which is essentially free of pigment. The lack of pigment, however, may be more apparent than real: It may actually be present, although in sparse amounts or diffusely spread about the tumor. Special stains such as Masson's ammoniacal silver nitrate solution may localize melanin, and tyrosinase reaction may be helpful if fresh tissue is available (1). Transmission electron microscopy and radionucleotide imaging provide still more sophisticated means of diagnosis (see Chapter 4 on diagnostic procedures).

Since the appearance of amelanotic melanoma is so deceptive, a differential diagnosis must rule out keratosis, granuloma pyogenicum, fibrosarcoma, squamous cell carcinoma, lymphosarcomas, and neural tumors and verrucae.

It is axiomatic in the treatment of all malignant disease that recognition and treatment of cancers be instituted as early as possible. However, the appearance and even light microscopic findings may be confusing and misleading in dealing with amelanotic lesions of the lower extremities. Some suspicious lesions may be precancerous neoplasms, or malignant transformation may be in progress to further cloud the issue.

Limited biopsy or too conservative an excision of suspected malignant on transforming lesions that are enlarging, pigmenting, itching, or burning is an unacceptable practice. Such intervention may initiate metastasis by inducing proliferation and "seeding" of contiguous and remote tissues (16).

The present discussion cites an amelanotic melanoma which was initially diagnosed as squamous cell carcinoma on the basis of its clinical appearance. The lesion involved the nailbed and the skin contiguous to it (Fig. 18.4). The hallucal nail had been previously avulsed by a physician thinking it to be a simple infected ingrowing toenail. The toe was edematous, painful, and produced a purulent discharge, along with some bleeding, over a long period of time. There was no attempt to heal this lesion, and the patient was hospitalized for radical amputation of the hallux with nodal dissection to the level of the inguinal ligament.

The diagnostic dilemma characteristic of the diagnosis of amelanotic melanoma is the focus of the present discussion.

Pathology

DERMATOHISTOPATHOLOGY (LIGHT MICROSCOPY)

Tissues sectioned from the amputated hallux revealed the usual parakeratosis and acanthosis which are typical of many skin lesions. Rete pegs invaded the dermis irregularly, often assuming bizarre configurations. The dermal stroma of collagenic and reticular fibers tended to be loosely structured in regions where tumorigenesis was active. An inflammatory lymphocytic infiltrate with occasional plasma cells could be identified. Tumor nests in junctional arrangement were commonly observed (Fig. 18.5).

Cells at the epidermal-dermal junction were of variable size and shape: The basement membrane was frequently disrupted. Additionally, some poorly differentiated clear cells and foam cells were seen. Individual tumor cells tended to be large, with nuclear anisochromasia a common finding. Occasional blood vessels of small caliber and clumps of erythrocytes invaded the tumor area. Mitotic figures were sometimes visible.

Amelanotic melanoma frequently demonstrates dense clumping of tumor cells, which may be superimposed one upon the other in heaps and whorls. For this reason, it is sometimes useful to make a smear to demonstrate cytological features necessary for diagnosis of unpigmented melanotic tumors. Such criteria may include large and pleomorphic nucleoli, loose orientation of nuclear chromatin, anaplasia of individual cells, and melanotic pigment which might otherwise be masked. Not uncommonly, a dust-like pigmentation is present in the cytoplasm of tumor cells.

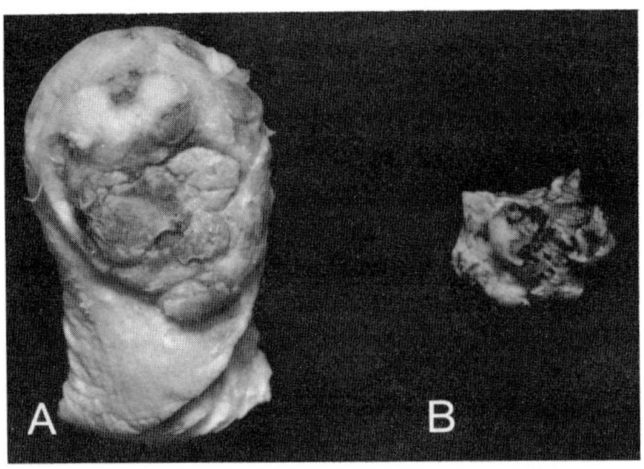

Figure 18.4. Amelanotic melanoma involving the hallucal nailbed. Typical pigment deposition is not immediately obvious. Dissection of the inguinal lymph nodes (right side) revealed metastatic extension of tumor cells.

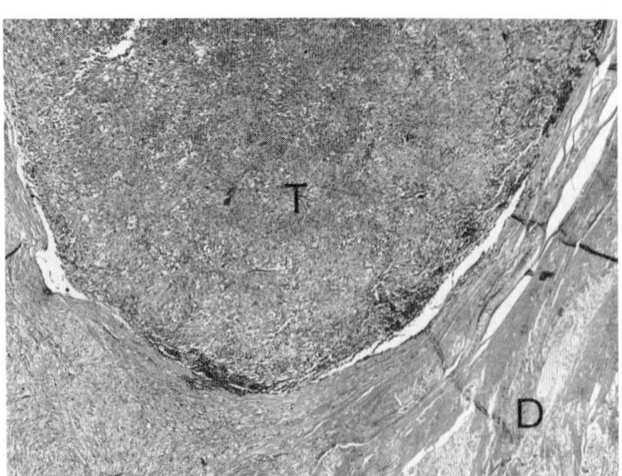

Figure 18.5. Amelanotic melanoma demonstrating tumor cell nests (*T*). Light microscopy, low magnification. *D*, dermis.

Dermatohistopathology

TRANSMISSION ELECTRON MICROSCOPY

Keratinocytes in the amelanotic melanoma tumor examined in our study demonstrated small clusters of somewhat irregular polyhedral cells. Nuclei were relatively large and occasionally were deeply lobulated or indented: Euchromatin was generally finely dispersed, but occasional clusters of interchromatin could be demonstrated. Nucleoli were also typically large, often multiple, reticulated, and segregated.

The intercellular spaces were widened, and the attenuated cytoplasm demonstrated moderate amounts of poorly formed mitochondria. Endoplasmic reticulum and Golgi complexes were occasionally in evidence. Clusters of small lipid droplets were seen with relative frequency.

Some high magnification fields examined revealed the occasional presence of melanophages, and small electron-dense bodies suggestive of melanin could be seen in the limited cytoplasmic regions of keratinocytes. Magnifications near 40,000 times best confirmed the suspected melanogenic activity in tumor cells: Melanosomes and premelanosomes in various stages of melanization were clearly defined (Fig. 18.6).

In addition, phagocytic vacuoles containing residues of melanosomes were demonstrated. Whorl bodies could be identified within the cytoplasm, which was also rich in free ribosomes and cytofibrils. The plasma membranes were generally intact, although small gap junctions were present at some points.

SQUAMOUS CELL CARCINOMA

Carcinomas are malignant new growths made up of cells of epidermal origin. Such

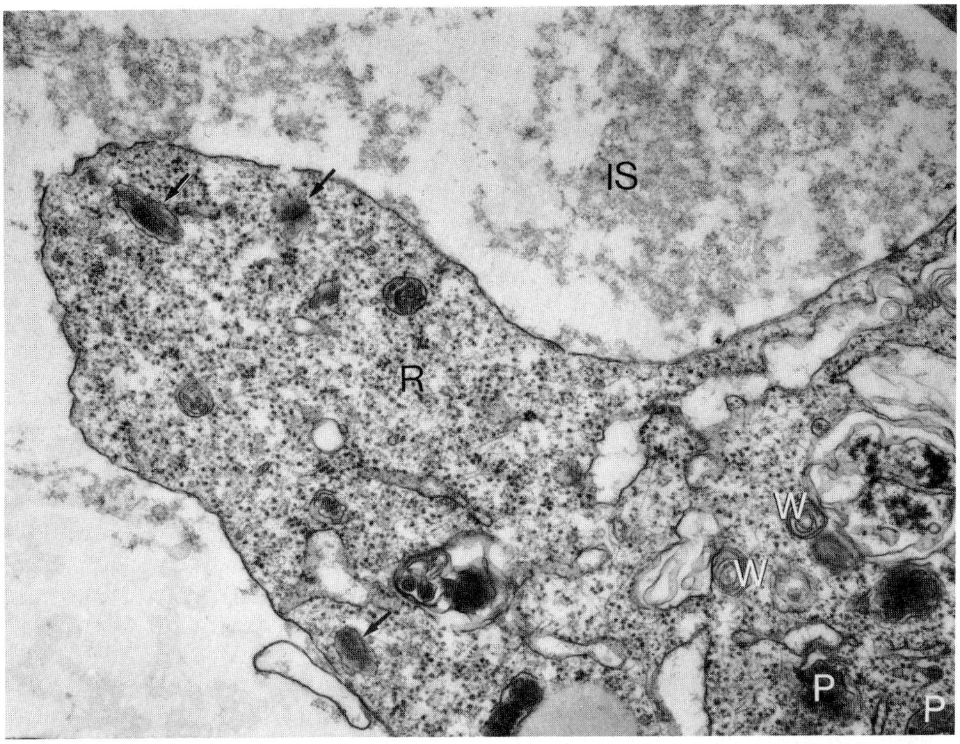

Figure 18.6. High magnification of a portion of a tumor cell in amelanotic melanoma confirmed by the presence of melanosomes and premelanosomes (*arrows*). Intercellular spaces filled with necrotic material (*IS*), free ribosomes (*R*), premelanosomes (*P*), and whorl bodies (*W*) are shown. Transmission electron microscopy.

neoplasms infiltrate the contiguous tissues and give rise to varying degrees of metastasis which may extend to bone. Squamous cell carcinomas (epithelioma, spinalioma, epidermoid carcinoma, prickle cell cancer, spinuous cell cancer, and carcinoma spinocellulaire) arise from low cuboidal cells of the stratum spinosum (1). Some authorities feel that such neoplasia may arise from keratinous cysts. The adnexal structures of the skin may also contribute to tumor development.

Squamous cell carcinoma characteristically appears as a keratotic, scaly slightly elevated lesion. It presents an irregular serpiginous border with a shallow ulcerated center. These ulcers develop scabs that fail to heal. Squamous cell carcinoma as it affects the human foot is often atypical in appearance (Fig. 18.7). *The Journal of the American Podiatry Association* has reported it variously as erythematous, verrucoid, granulomatous, and ulcerative. These neoplasms have appeared on the toes (17), the region of the fibular malleolus (18), the nailbed (19), and the plantar arch region of the foot (20). The author experienced a case of epithelioma of the nailbed in 1955 just 6 months after initiating private practice. This patient expired within 9 months of the initial diagnosis since the inguinal glands had already become involved.

Squamous cell carcinoma has a 3:1 predilection for males. Its incidence is far less than that observed for basal cell carcinoma (21).

The stratum spinosum normally is about the business of keratinization. Its normal metabolism, however, is interrupted in maligancy, and the cells often demonstrate a degree of dyskeratosis. Organelles involved in the biosynthesis of keratin, such as the tonofilament-desmosome complex and the organization of keratohyaline granules, are adversely affected. It is possible that whatever derangement of prickle cells exists may have been present from birth: The expression of malignant disease requires time or some external environmental insult to activate a pre-existing disposition to tumorigenesis. External factors such as radiation or unknown internal factors have

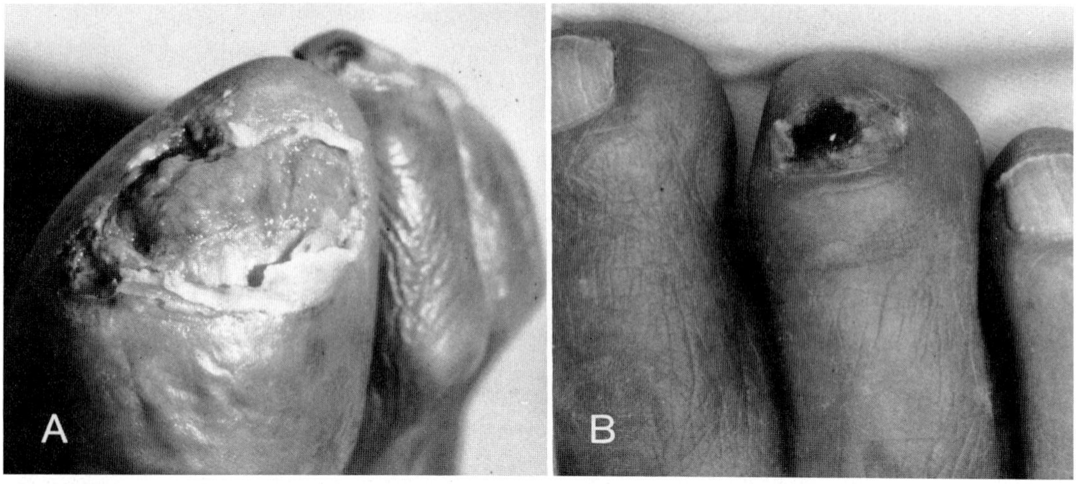

Figure 18.7. Atypical appearance of squamous cell carcinoma of the foot: erythematous scaling lesion of the right hallux with exudation (*A*). Pigmented lesion of the nailbed of the third toe, right foot (*B*). Courtesy of Drs. Dale and Simon, VA Medical Centers, Mountain Home, TN, and Little Rock, AR.

been implicated as inducers of disease. Once a malignant change occurs in the skin, that change must be regarded as permanent since all progeny of malignant cells can produce only other deranged cells.

Diagnosis of squamous cell carcinoma may be difficult at times because the line between that which is benign and that which is malignant is not always clear. Malignant transformation is a stepwise process which occurs over time and may vary at different loci within the same lesion at any given point in time.

The spinaliomas are characterized as tumors with excessive numbers of spinosal cells which have failed to "mature" in a normal way (16). It is a truism in dermatohistopathology that terms applicable in general pathology do not necessarily apply in describing skin disease in a precise way. For example, pathologists may speak of "maturation" of cells in a given tissue. Developmental anatomists refer to cells becoming "determined" as a specific tissue type is formed. Squamous cells which normally are undergoing keratinization are in a process of differentiation. In a sense, they can be said to be "maturing" while basal cells moving up into the spinosum are becoming "determined" (1).

Tumor cells in squamous cell carcinoma appear to be immature or undifferentiated, but are these terms truly applicable to the malignant situation? It was stated earlier that malignant cells can produce nothing other than other malignant cells. Consequently, such cells are determined and more highly differentiated than normal spinosal cells (22).

Epidermal cells may be evaluated according to nine metabolic properties (1). Normal epidermis, benign neoplasia, and low grade malignancy demonstrate normalcy of intracellular respiratory and hormonal controls. In highly malignant lesions, normal hormonal controls are lost: Intracellular respiratory activities may or may not be interrupted.

Intracellular cohesion is patent in normal skin and benign epidermal neoplasia. Intracellular cohesion may or may not characterize malignant skin lesions (1).

Normal enzymatic activity is characteristic of all well-developed keratinocytes. Such activity may or may not persist in benign neoplasia and in skin malignancy of both low and high grade types. Growth control factors are normally present in spinosal cells. They may or may not be present in benign neoplasia and low grade malignancy. However, growth control factor is totally lacking in high grade skin malignancy (1).

Contact inhibitory factors are present in normal and benign neoplasia, but they are absence in malignancy.

Protein constituency of the stratum spinosum has a certain normal profile in the normal epidermis and in benign neoplastic cells. Proteins are altered both in kind and amount in malignant tumors (1).

Interdependence of epidermal cells relative to the underlying dermis is well known in the normal integumentary system. This interdependence is found in benign neoplasia, but it does not exist in the presence of high grade malignancies of the skin. Epidermal cells always demonstrate polarity in the normal situation. However, this feature is lacking in malignancy of the skin. These nine metabolic features of normal skin, as compared with benign and malignant neoplasia, are summarized in Table 18.1.

Pathology

DERMATOHISTOPATHOLOGY: LIGHT MICROSCOPY

Tumor cells of squamous cell carcinoma are heritably deranged keratinocytes which have escaped the usual regulatory influences which control cutaneous metabolism[1]. The tumor grows destructively and invasively into contiguous deep mesodermal tissues. The surface proliferates in an irregular manner, and the Malpighian layer is acanthotic.

The stratum corneum is typically hyperkeratotic and demonstrates parakeratosis. However, it is not unusual for the surface of the lesion to become ulcerated and encrusted.

The dermal inflammatory infiltrate is usually of the lymphocytic or round cell type.

Tumor cells of the involved epidermis may demonstrate wide variations of differentiation. When the epidermis is more or less well differentiated, keratinization may occur among individual cells, along with the appearances of the typical "pearl formation" (Fig. 18.8).

When the epidermal cells of squamous cell carcinoma are anaplastic and mitotic figures are numerous, the lesion can be expected to have a greater tendency for metastasis. Retraction spaces characteristic of basal cell epitheliomas are not seen in squamous cell carcinoma. However, acantholytic processes may lead to the formation of irregular suprabasilar cavities. Clearly, degenerating elements and obviously dyskeratotic atypical cells are associated with these cavitations.

No normal basal cells are identifiable in

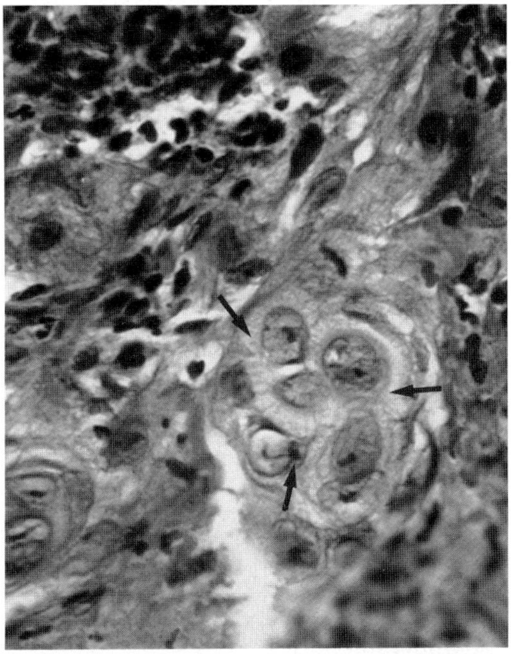

Figure 18.8. Squamous cell carcinoma demonstrating typical intraepidermal "pearl formations" with anaplasia of cells (*arrows*). Light microscopy, high magnification.

Table 18.1.
Intracellular Factors Altered in Cutaneous Malignancy

Intraepidermal factor	Normal integument	Benign neoplasia	Low malignancy	High malignancy
Hormonal control	N[a]	N	N	X
Intracellular respiration	N	N	N	E
Cellular cohesion	N	N	E	E
Enzymes	N	E	E	E
Growth crontrol	N	E	E	X
Contact inhibition	N	N	X	X
Protein normalcy	N	N	X	X
Stromal dependence	N	E	E	X
Polarity	N	E	X	X

[a] N, normal; E, equivocal (may or may not occur); X, always abnormal.

the active tumor. Palisading of the stratum basale is almost never seen. Neoplastic squamous cells organize into nests and tend to be large and pale staining. A total or partial deletion of the basement membrane is usual in these tumors: This loss is best confirmed by the absence of PAS-sensitive substances at the dermoepidermal junction using the periodic acid-Schiff reaction.

Dermatohistopathology

TRANSMISSION ELECTRON MICROSCOPY

Prickle cells implicated in squamous cell carcinomas are arranged in clusters or nests which are loosely immersed within the connective tissue stroma. These cellular aggregates are usually closely packed so that the intercellular spaces are typically narrow. Individual cells tend to be polygonal and irregular in outline.

Nuclei of tumor cells are large relative to the cytoplasm and often present an irregular cerebriform outline (Fig. 18.9). Chromatin occurs clumped and is often seen in relationship to a dense inner nuclear membrane. Nucleoli are generally prominent and demonstrate chromatin and parachromatin material of varying density.

The cytoplasm of neoplastic squamous cells demonstrates an abundance of tonofilaments which appear dense and clumped. Tonofilaments are associated with ribosomes which are irregularly dispersed or in clusters.

The comparatively reduced perinuclear cytoplasm of tumor cells demonstrates relatively substantial amounts of subcellular organelles. Rough endoplasmic reticulum is abundant, and the cisternae are often dilated. Glycogen granules which appear to be membrane bound and occasional lipid bodies can be identified in some sections. Mitochondria are usually seen as edematous and rounded, with their internal cristae imperfectly formed.

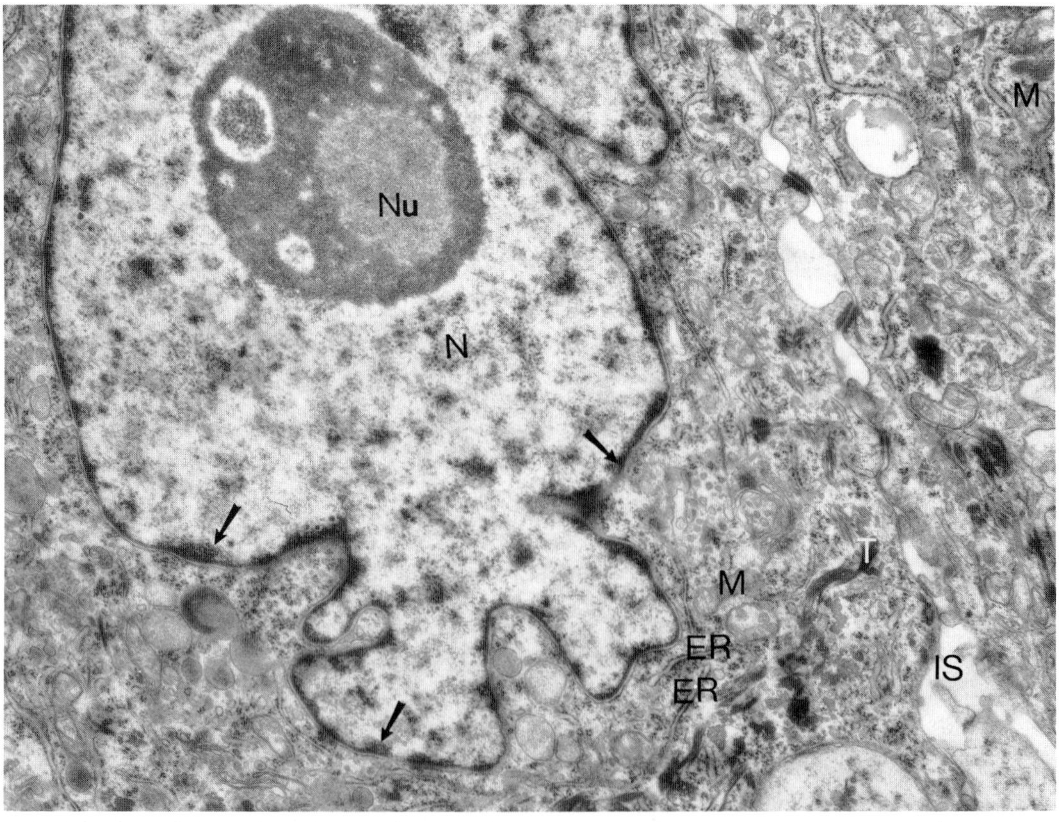

Figure 18.9. Squamous cell carcinoma demonstrating deeply indented cerebriform nucleus (*N*), nucleolus (*Nu*), intercellular space (*IS*), rough endoplasmic reticulum (*ER*), mitochondira (*M*), tonofilaments (*T*). There is margination of chromatin (*arrows*). Transmission electron microscopy.

The typically closely approximated plasmalemma of tumor cells are often characterized by many interdigitating folds or pseudovilli. Occasionally the intercellular spaces near these points are wider than usual. Desmosomes are usually abundant in the neoplastic cells of squamous cell carcinoma. The fields examined by the author revealed some damage to the tonofilament-desmosome complex (TDC). Tonofilaments did not necessarily converge on hemidesmosomes, and in this respect our findings varied from those of some other investigators.

EPITHELIOMA CUNICULATUM (VERRUCOUS CARCINOMA PEDIS)

Epithelioma cuniculatum pedis is a neoplastic variant of squamous cell carcinoma which is peculiar to the plantar surface of the foot. It has been identified in the literature as spinous cell carcinoma, spinalioma, squamous epithelioma, prickle cell carcinoma, epidermoid carcinoma, cutis carcinoides, epithelioma cuniculatum pedis, carcinoma cuniculatum, and verrucous carcinoma (22–25).

The designation "cuniculatum" makes references to the maze-like structure of a rabbit's earthen warren which can be likened to the intermeshed tracts, crypts, and sinuses which traverse the lesion. The term epithelioma is well applied to this tumor because, while it is a locally aggressive mass involving prickle cells, its ability for metastasis is absolutely minimal (22).

The Armed Forces Institute of Pathology reported that over a 3-decade period ending in 1980, 1500 cases of squamous cell carcinoma were identified. Of these, 46 reportings were consistent with a diagnosis of verrucous carcinoma or epithelial cuniculatum.

The first report of verrucous carcinoma occurred in 1948 when Ackerman identified the lesion in the oral cavity (26). The British were first to designate a foot lesion as verrucous carcinoma in 1954 (27). Over the years, the British have gone on to describe a number of instances of verrucous carcinoma of the foot which were so grotesque and deforming to the part that amputation was considered to be the treatment of choice. In no case, however, was metastasis ever involved with this variant of squamous cell carcinoma.

The instance of epithelioma cuniculatum reported here was observed by Dr. Lee Sanders at the VA Medical Center, Lebanon, PA. The verrucous appearing lesion was especially large and interfered with comfortable ambulation (Fig. 18.10). Wide deep excision of the mass was successful in this situation, although the patient subsequently expired because of malignant involvement of the lung. It is important to emphasize that the lung cancer had no relationship with the foot tumor.

Pathology

DERMATOHISTOPATHOLOGY: LIGHT MICROSCOPY

The histopathologic appearance of verrucous carcinoma is doubtless modified by mechanical influences inherent to the function of the foot. The vegetative growth is exceedingly acanthotic, and the rete ridges balloon into the dermis and literally squeeze the dermal papillae into thin strands or trabeculae.

The free surface of the lesion demonstrates considerable desquamation (Fig. 18.11). The stratum Malpighii is invaded by keratin-filled crypts which may interconnect with microabscess and cysts. These

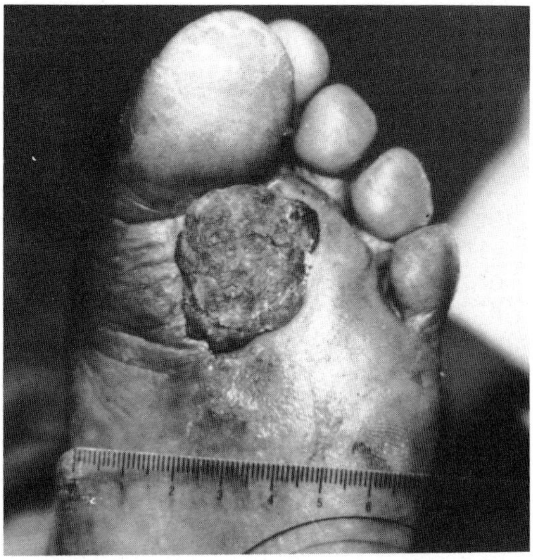

Figure 18.10. Epithelioma cuniculatum (verrucous carcinoma) of the plantar surface of the left foot, demonstrating its verrucoid appearance. Courtesy of Dr. Lee Sanders.

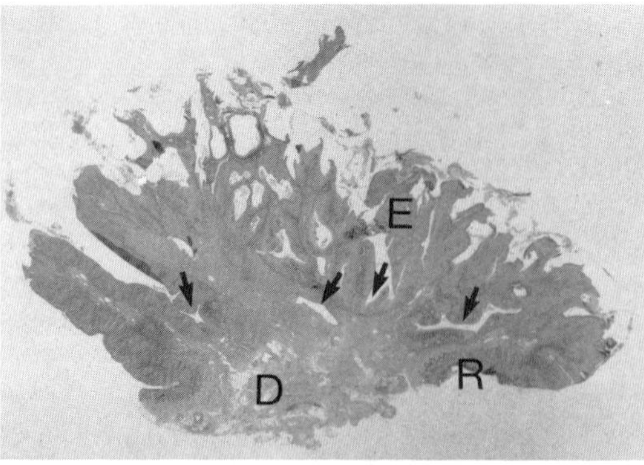

Figure 18.11. Cross sectional semimicroscopic appearance of epithelioma cuniculatum, demonstrating crypts, sinuses, and microabscesses (*arrows*). *E*, epidermis; *R*, ballooning rete pegs; *D*, dermis.

involvements are responsible for the malodorous nature of the tumor. The stratum corneum is typically parakeratotic, and nuclear remnants are frequently caught up into the external layers of the tumor. Individual squamous tumor cells are atypical, anaplastic, and occasionally dyskeratotic. They are usually moderately well differentiated and demonstrate a clear cytoplasm: Nuclei are often large, hyperchromatic, and pleomorphic.

Blood vessels of variable caliber appear to penetrate the epidermis in verrucous carcinoma. In this respect, they resemble verrucae plantaris.

The epidermal-dermal junction usually demonstrates disruption of the basement membrane, and there is clear evidence of invasiveness of tumor cells. Mitotic figures may be frequently observed in the cells of rete peggs which extend deep into the dermis.

The dermis associated with verrucous carcinoma of the foot demonstrates coarse thickened collagenic fibers, and the inflammatory infiltrate is of the round cell or lymphocytic type. Plasma cells, histiocytes, and other infiltrative cell types have also been identified. Vascularity of the dermis in the region of the tumor is typically increased.

DERMATOHISTOPATHOLOGY: ELECTRON MICROSCOPY

Transmission electron microscopy for epithelioma cuniculatum is essentially that of squamous cell carcinoma. It is important to note, however, that viral particles are not associated with the lesion as would be expected in verrucae.

BOWEN'S DISEASE OR SQUAMOUS CELL CARCINOMA IN SITU: VARIANT OF SQUAMOUS CELL CARCINOMA

Bowen's disease has been characterized as squamous cell carcinoma, grade ½. The basement membrane remains intact in this tumor type, and it is, therefore, a squamous cell carcinoma in situ. Bowen's disease does not metastasize and is not truly a malignancy, although it is classified as such.

The original lesion described by Bowen in 1912 was s single well-circumscribed papulonodular growth characterized by a dull erythema and superficial crusting (16). Later, a multiple type having nonelevated scaly or crusted plaques were described. Most lesions have been present over a period of years, and oozing and encrustation with little tendency to heal are characteristic. The podiatric appearance of Bowen's disease is often atypical (Fig. 18.12).

Heredity may play a role in tumorigenesis since there is a statistically clear predilection for its appearance among Anglo-Saxons with fair skin.

Exposure to arsenical compounds and to sunlight (actinic influences) have been suggested as etiologic agents for the develop-

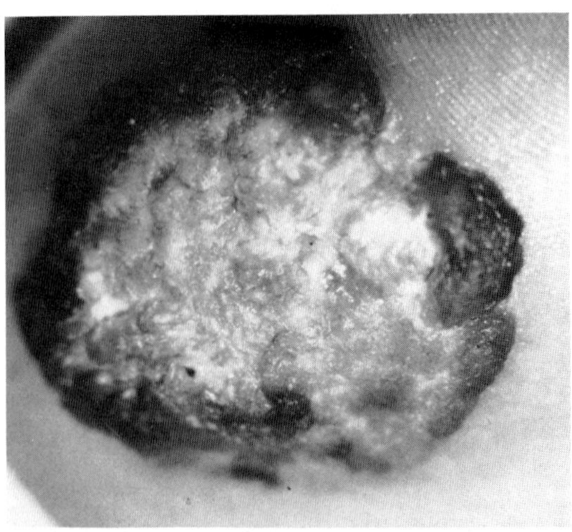

Figure 18.12. Clinical appearance of Bowen's disease of the medial aspect of the heel. The lesion is erythematous with oozing and encrustation. Courtesy of Dr. James Black, VA Medical Center, Tampa, FL.

ment of Bowen's disease. Transmission electron microscopy has demonstrated virus-like particles in the cytoplasm of some prickle cells in this tumor type. These particles appear to arise by budding from the plasma membranes of cells or from tubules closely associated with the plasma membranes (16). Further evidence implicating a viral etiology stems from observations that implantation of filtered and unfiltered homogenates of Bowen's disease specimens into chick embryos produce histologic changes essentially identical to Bowen's disease. Moreover, injection of serum produces similar changes.

Some authorities feel that there is an apparent relationship between Bowen's disease (which is by definition localized and not metastatic) to internal primary malignancy of different types. Just what the relationship is, however, is still unclear. Graham and Helwig's study of 35 cases demonstrated that 80% of patients presenting with Bowen's disease subsequently expired with internal cancers of many types within 9 years of the initial appearance of Bowen's disease (16).

Rabinowitz and Brownstein of the New York Medical College feel that the most recent data do not support the view that Bowen's disease increases the risk of internal malignancies, however. Consequently, they do not feel that exhaustive evaluations for internal malignancy are indicated for such patients (17).

Pathology

DERMATOHISTOPATHOLOGY: LIGHT MICROSCOPY

Histopathologic findings for Bowen's disease are essentially those of intraepidermal squamous cell carcinoma. The epidermis is acanthotic with varying degree of hyperkeratosis and parakeratosis. Most noticeable, however, is the disorder which characterizes keratinocytes of the Malpighian layer. Dyskeratotic changes are common, and the cells of the spinosum are often unusually large with hyperchromatic nuclei. The cytoplasm of cells tends to be markedly eosinophilic (1). Rete pegs are elongated and broadened to the extent that the dermal papillae may be reduced to mere strands (Fig. 18.13).

The dermis usually demonstrates a lymphocytic inflammatory infiltrate.

DERMATOHISTOPATHOLOGY: TRANSMISSION ELECTRON MICROSCOPY

Ultrastructural evaluation of squamous cell carcinoma in situ reveals the cells of the stratum basale and those spinosal cells immediately contiguous to be essentially normal. In those regions of the Malpighian layer which appear to be dyskeratotic, the plasma membranes of cells demonstrate considerable irregularity. The tonofilament-desmosome complex (TDC) are also poorly defined. Desmosomes are reduced in numbers, and tonofilaments appear clumped and fasciculated (16). Membrane-coating granules and keratohyaline granules are sparse or totally absent in the higher spinosal cells in Bowen's disease.

Spinosal cells attempting mitotic division have noticeably widened intercellular spaces, and the densely packed tonofilaments at this level interfere with the mitotic spindle apparatus.

BASAL CELL CARCINOMA

It has been said that basal cell carcinoma (basal cell epithelioma, basalioma) represents the most common of all malignancies in man (28). It is, however, very uncommon with respect to the human foot. Such neoplasia has historically been related to ac-

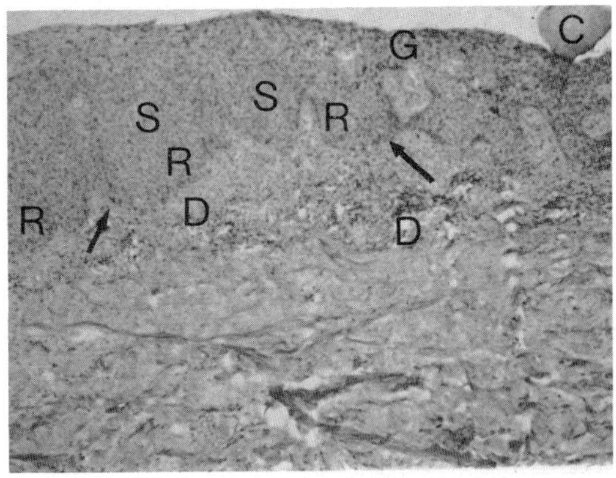

Figure 18.13. Squamous cell carcinoma in situ (Bowen's disease). Rete ridges (*R*) are elongated and broad. The basement membrane is intact (*arrows*). Sloughing stratum corneum (*C*), agranulosis of the stratum granulosum (*G*), stratum spinosum (*S*), and dermis (*D*) are shown. Light microscopy.

tinic activity, which is to say that light rays beyond the violet end of the spectrum seem to excite oncogenicity (28). This factor functions in concert with other environmental factors and genetic influences so that fair-skinned individuals who reside in sun-drenched areas are most likely to develop basal cell carcinoma.

The typical lesion varies in size from millimeters to centimeters. Morphologically, there is usually a central depression which is surrounded by an elevated pearly border (1). Crusting of the skin, ulceration, and telangiectasis are also frequently observed in basal cell epitheliomas. The present discussion identifies a podiatrically relevant lesion submitted by Dr. Gary Dockery. This lesion was on the medial aspect of the heel (Fig. 18.14).

Basal cell carcinomas are not aggressive skin tumors in terms of their ability to metastasize to distant organs. They tend to grow by direct extension, however, and may be locally invasive. In earlier times, such lesions were the cause of much disfigurement and were the cause of the so-called rodent ulcers capable of destroying large portions of patients' faces. Death could result by extension of the mass so as to destroy such vital structures as blood vessels.

A number of variants of basal cell epitheliomas have been observed (29). The most common form is the noduloulcerative type. The primary lesion is a small papule which enlarges slowly. While these lesions are usually flesh tone, they may be bluish, tan, or erythematous. As this tumor enlarges, the umbilicated central portion often ulcerates, and the translucent pearly border, which is somewhat diagnostic, emerges.

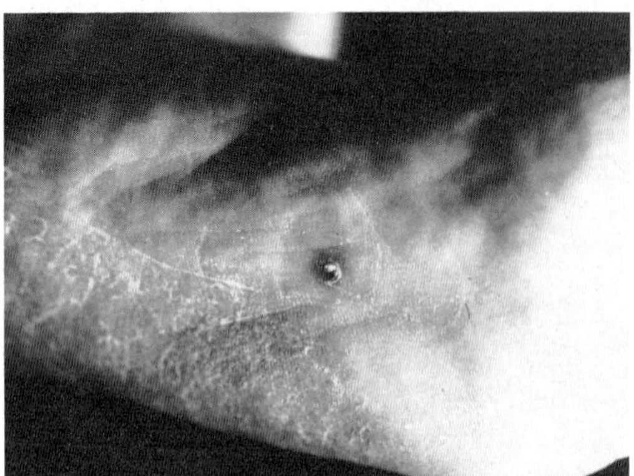

Figure 18.14. Atypical clinical appearance of basal cell carcinoma involving the plantar surface of the foot. Courtesy of Dr. Gary Dockery, Seattle, WA.

Nevoid basal cell epitheliomas represents an unusual inherited type of tumor. They are rare autosomal dominant traits which, when expressed, cause a basalioma which becomes progressively destructive in adult life; they are far more aggressive lesions than those of actinic origin. The onset occurs in childhood with multiple widespread distribution of small pitted lesions on the palms and soles (16). However, these pits are not basal cell carcinomas.

Pigmented basal cell carcinoma resembles malignant melanoma since the lesions are light to dark brown in color. This tumor type may be a variant of the noduloulcerative type, except that considerable melanin pigment is present (26).

Sclerosing basal cell carcinoma is a variant form which resembles a scar or scleroderma. The surface is white to yellow with a smooth firm consistency and may be depressed or flat. The borders of the lesion as seen in the oral cavity are poorly defined, and it is less invasive than most other forms (26). It is possible to confuse sclerosing basal cell carcinoma with morpheaform basal cell carcinoma. The latter variant is much more resistant to treatment, and a misdiagnosis may lead to undertreatment of the condition.

A final variant is superficial basal cell carcinoma which appears as an inflammatory erythematous or scaly lesion which is frequently misdiagnosed. These growths rarely develop nodular components, but small superficial ulcerations may be seen around the irregular thread-like border of the superficially disposed mass. Such lesions are frequently multiple and are more often found on the trunk or extremities as opposed to the other variants which are usually associated with the head and neck.

Basal cell carcinoma (epithelioma) has been characterized as being the least mature member of the tribe of organoid adnexal tumors. Actually, there is serious question as to whether or not basalioma is truly malignant since such tumors do not metastasize (1). For this reason, it might be prudent to call basal cell carcinoma an epithelioma or more simply, basalioma (1).

Basalioma may grow aggressively by direct extension. It has been suggested that a single microscopic cord is responsible for extension of the tumor (29). This occurs by a continuity of cells growing alongside nerves and fascial planes, or by lymphatics or blood vessels. Tumors which appear to be multicentric might actually be a single mass loosely interconnected by tumor cells.

The Swedish authority Isser Brody points to the confusion that exists relative to the cellular origin of basal cell epithelioma (30). He sites six references which state that the lesion arises, in the main, from basal cells. This is, however, a minority view. The adnexa, particularly the outer follicular root sheath, the infundibulum, and other parts of the hair follicles, were implicated by several other investigators. Sudiferous, sebaceous, and pilosebaceous origins have also been suspect (28, 31).

Krompecher and von Hansemann have theorized that the cells of basal cell epithelioma are anaplastic, dedifferentiated cells (32, 33). In this sense, they simulate embryonic cells and fail to differentiate into keratinizing adult epidermis. Pinkus et al proposed the most attractive theory that basaliomas (their preferred term) originate from pleuripotential adult cells which become directed towards tumorigenesis (1).

Brody's study on the histogenesis of basal cell carcinoma identified two main cell types of the epidermis from among the 17 cases he examined. One type did, in fact, have embryonic characteristics while the other demonstrated adult human epidermal cell characteristics. Both cell lines were subdivided into dark, intermediate, and light cell types. The latter differentiation was based on differences in opacity and density of the nuclear matrix and cytoplasm (30).

Pathology

DERMATOHISTOPATHOLOGY: LIGHT MICROSCOPY

Basal cell epitheliomas demonstrate nests of polyhedral cells which contain very large basophilic nuclei. Since the cytoplasm of the cell is reduced, the tumor may appear blue because of the nuclear dominance at the light microscopic level. Cells at the periphery of the nest frequently demonstrate palisading, which is to say that they present a "picket fence" appearance. Nuclei in this situation are elongated and orient at right angles to the epidermal-dermal junction (Fig. 18.15). Tight junctions, sometimes incorrectly termed intercellular bridges at the light microscopic level, are not often seen in diseased cells. PAS positive membranes are usually well-defined, enclosing individual tumor nests.

Mitotic figures are often present, but they need not be especially numerous. Pigment may or may not be present in tumor cells. Abrupt changes can occur as the basal cell epithelioma mass terminates and normal skin appears. Pyknotic nuclei are also common features of the basaliomas.

Basal cell epitheliomas seldom form keratinous cysts which resemble the "pearls" typical of squamous cell carcinoma.

Dermal fibrosis underlying the lesion may be observed with or without an inflammatory infiltrate. The infiltrate is typically of the round cell type. Fibroblasts are usually abundant in the dermis implicated in basalioma.

Ulceration frequently characterizes the central portion of the surface topography in basal cell epithelioma. Peripheral extension of reactive ulcerating tissue below the level of the epidermis is responsible for the pearly border which is observed clinically.

Retraction spaces, which are artifacts of fixation, may develop in basalioma. These halo-like, apparently empty spaces form during fixation and dehydration of tissues in the laboratory: These regions were sites

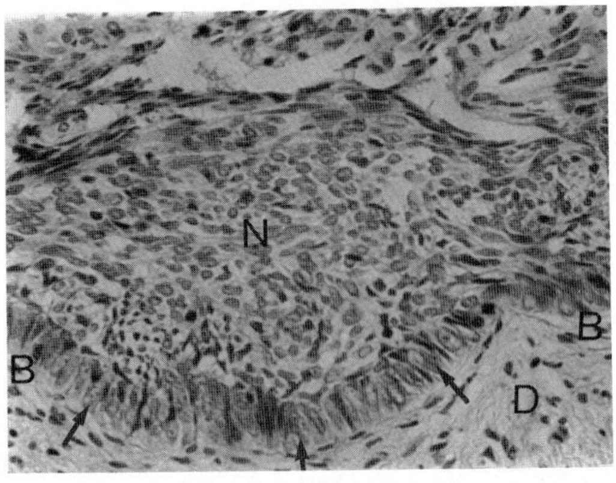

Figure 18.15. Basal cell carcinoma demonstrating palisading of the stratum basale (*arrows*). The basement membrane is intact. There is nesting (*N*) of intraepidermal cells. Light microscopy. *D*, dermis; *B*, basement membrane.

of mucinous deposition which had formerly surrounded the epithelial nests.

One of the features characterizing basal cell epipheliomas is the presence of basal cell "cords" which penetrate down into the dermis. It may be helpful diagnostically to identify such structures, and it is more than likely that examination of a number of serial sections will be necessary to demonstrate this feature.

The dermis of basal cell epitheliomas consists of a stroma which acts as a solid shield in which epithelial nests are embedded. It replaces the papillary portion of the dermis and is situated superficial to the reticular portion. The dermis is often well vascularized, and normal glandular elements of the integument can be observed peripheral to the lesion proper.

DERMATOHISTOPATHOLOGY: TRANSMISSION ELECTRON MICROSCOPY

The predominant cell in basalioma is the adnexal basal cell. Such cells were found to be essentially polyhedral but more pleomorphic than those observed in the normal epidermis. The nuclei were predominating features of the basal cells observed in the present study (Fig. 18.16). The cytoplasm of such cells was relatively reduced. The nuclear membranes appear moderately cerebriform (undulating), and some demonstrated deep indentations. Nuclear chromatin granules were fine and tended to be dispersed peripherally. Those cells containing nucleoli revealed this structure to be quite large and reticulated. The scant cytoplasm reveals some rough endoplasmic reticulum as well as an abundance of free ribosomes. Melanin granules are occasionally seen also.

The cell membranes of the basal cells tended to be undulant with villous projections. Some desmosomal junctions could be observed, and the plasma membranes of adjacent cells were frequently widened and extremely irregular. This alteration did great violence to the tonofilament-desmosome complex. Tonofilaments did not often

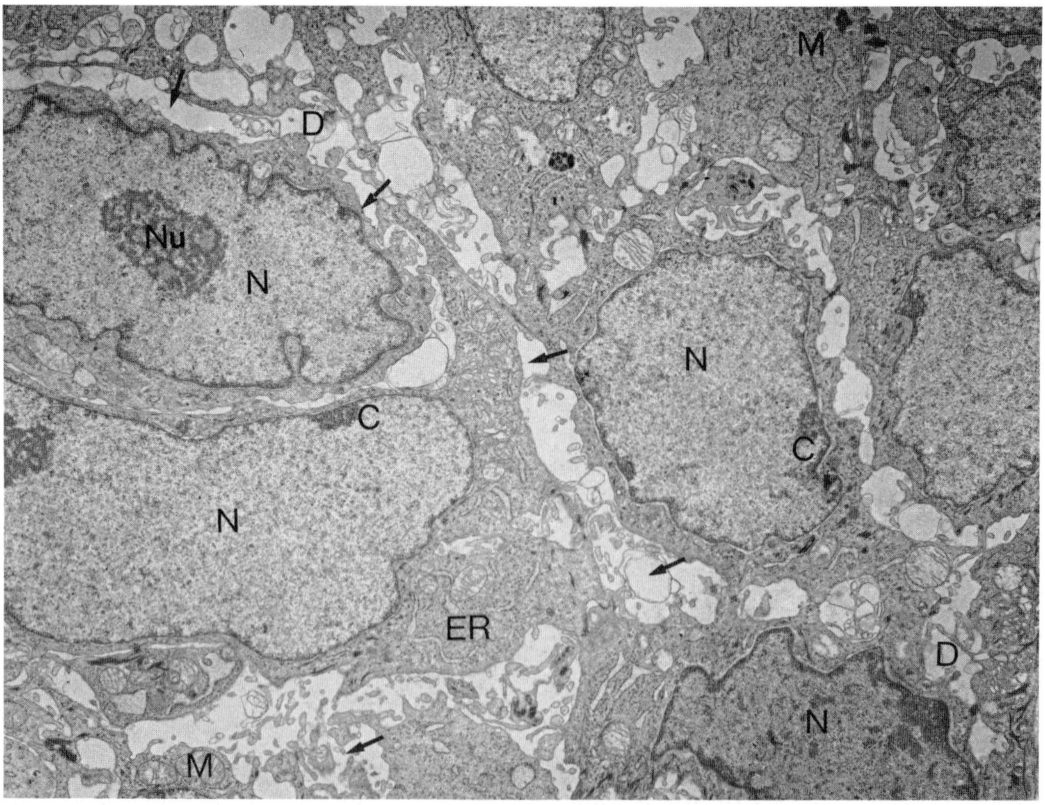

Figure 18.16. Basal cell carcinoma demonstrating prominent cerebriform nucleus (*N*) with large reticulated nucleolus (*Nu*). Chromatin (*c*) tends to be peripherally dispersed. Desmosomes (*D*), rough endoplasmic reticulum (*ER*), mitochondria (*M*) are shown. *Arrows* mark the intercellular spaces. Transmission electron microscopy.

orient perinuclearly nor did they converge upon the hemidesmosomes in the usual manner. Rather, they tended to orient randomly. Desmosomes were usually disrupted, with the component hemidesmosomes hanging limply into the widened intercellular spaces.

Mitochondria were abundant organelles in the specimens examined for the present study. Inner and outer membranes, as well as the cristae, were well formed, but the mitochondria often assumed a well-rounded, edematous shape.

Basal cells are by no means the only cell observed in basal cell carcinoma. A number of so called "intruder cells" are identifiable. Melanocytes and particularly the Langerhans cells, were often in evidence. Merkel cells and the so-called "indeterminate" dendritic cells are also found in basaliomas, and their presence should increase the index of suspicion whenever they are detected.

TREATMENT PLANS IN CUTANEOUS MALIGNANCY

The treatment plan selected in the management of the cutaneous malignancies just discussed should reflect the aggressiveness of the tumor. Melanoma of Clark's level V will require more heroic intervention than squamous cell carcinoma in situ.

Surgical excision is recommended for all malignant diseases of the human skin, but the efficacy of other modalities can be debated. In the present discussion, Fields, DeLauro, and Schall excised a malignant melanoma measuring 3 × 5 cm, but included the tumor in an area measuring 9 × 18 cm with a depth of 8 mm in order to ensure normal tissue at all margins. Dr. Sanders case of epithelioma cuniculatum measured about 2.5 × 5 cm.

The wide deep excision of neoplasia of the skin may require skin grafting, but in most cases, primary closure can be accomplished, or healing by second intention can be permitted. There is a time and place in which amputation is indicated, and nodal dissection may or may not be employed. Certainly, dissection of lymph nodes should not be done indiscriminately.

Recent therapeutic approaches include a variety of modalities, and these will be discussed shortly. One of the very precise surgical approaches for malignant skin disease is Mohs' chemosurgery.

Mohs first described his microscopically controlled method of cancer excision in 1941 (34). Tromovitch and Stegman popularized the fresh tissue modification of the procedure in 1974 (35).

Verrucous carcinoma of the foot was first treated by chemosurgical means by Mohs himself in 1979 (36). A fixed tissue technique was initially employed: The first mass so treated was extensive, and measured 7 cm in diameter. One year later, Swanson and Taylor reported on two additional cases of plantar malignancy of the foot using Mohs' chemosurgery. They viewed this therapeutic approach as one of the modern treatments of choice (37).

Mohs chemosurgery requires the surgeon to function as his or her own pathologist. The intent of the procedure is to remove the entire tumor in stages using microscopic control in order to ensure complete removal of the tumor with all of its extensions and ramifications along fascial planes, nerves, bone, etc.

The original fixed tissue technique involves an initial debulking of the keratinized portion of the tumor mass using dichloroacetic acid. Subsequently, a paste of zinc chloride is layered on the lesion and left in place overnight. This established histological fixation to a depth of several millimeters to the involved tissue, thus imparting both anesthesia and hemostasis. Punched out biopsy sections are first made vertically to establish the depth of the lesion using standard light microscopy. Horizontal sections are then made sequentially to ensure total removal of the tumor mass. Normal tissue should always be demonstrable about the periphery. All sections are mounted with their deep sides up in a freezing microtome: As the tissues are removed, they are mapped, and the growth is reconstructed using a color code to match up each section with its mate.

This, the fixed tissue technique is presently used only for larger lesions, and the surgical defect is usually allowed to heal by second intention.

A more recent modification of Mohs chemosurgery is the so-called fresh tissue technique, which omits the use of zinc chloride paste. Local anesthesia and hemostasis are secured by the usual surgical methodologies. This later modification is reserved for smaller skin tumors.

Other anticancer treatment modalities are available for use in a combined approach, for use with surgery, or for use alone if surgery is contraindicated for some reason. Immunotherapy, chemotherapy, and radiotherapy are all presently in use.

Dinitrochlorobenzene (DNCB) is a substance evoking strong immunologic responses in patients with patent immune competence. Individuals with well-developed immune systems have a more favorable prognosis if they are under challenge by malignancy in general and by malignant melanoma in particular (38). Sensitized white blood cells can also be introduced into patients with melanoma with a favorable response. It is well known that blood transfusions from patients who experienced a spontaneous remission of melanoma can induce regression among some victims of the malignancy (39). Humoral antibodies develop in response to challenge by tumor cell antigens. Titers of antimelanoma antibodies have been shown to be highest when the disease is localized. Whenever melanoma is disseminated, these desirable immune factors decrease (40). It is for these reasons that such sensitizers as DNCB are occasionally employed in cutaneous malignancy.

Gutterman et al sited four proofs for cell-mediated immunity processes in melanoma (38): Melanoma patients demonstrate hypersensitivity to extracts of their own tumors. White blood cell migration is inhibited by melanoma membrane antigens. Lymphocytic blastogenic response to melanoma cells and antigens occurs in a degree which is directly proportional to patient survival. Mononuclear cell cytotoxicity against melanoma cells has also been observed. These factors considered together give insight into the general processes of tumorigenesis.

The fact that cytotoxicity decreases with dissemination of disease suggests the presence of serum-blocking factors. Blocking of antigen-antibody complexes must occur at either the mononuclear cell level or at the tumor cell site itself (38). Antigen-antibody complexes can bind directly at the melanoma loci, or binding can occur at the effector cell location.

Other practical applications of the immune responses in melanoma have been made with injections by several challenge substances in addition to those just mentioned. These include certain streptococcal strains, serratia, vaccinia virus, activated lymphocytes, and *Bacillus Calmette-Guérin.*

Chemotherapeutic approaches have been employed despite of the toxicity encountered. Agents employed include cytoxan, hydroxyurea, actinomycin F, and 5-fluorouracil. The later interrupts cell metabolism by the formation of fraudulant RNA's by replacing uracil normally required for protein synthesis.

The most commonly employed drug, however, is dimethyltriazenoimidazole carboxamide (DTIC). Recently, this drug has been used in combination with the vinca alkaloid Vincristine. Perfusion chemotherapy with L-phenylalanine mustard and Actinomycin D has been used to good advantage following surgery in aggressive malignancies of the skin (41).

Surgical intervention, along with intra-arterial isolation perfusion, may arrest "in transit" metastasis. L-phenylalanine mustard is most commonly employed to perfuse limbs isolated with a tourniquet using a pump oxygenator. The technique is often enhanced by elevating the temperature of the perfusing drug to 42°C.

Endolymphatic therapy is useful in early malignant lesions of the skin in which extension to the regional lymph nodes is suspected but not demonstrable. This technique infuses the isotope ^{32}P-lipoidal to destroy minute nodal metastasis (42).

Radiotherapy to a level of 4500 R with a 33-day time framework has been recommended by Sealy and Pearson (43, 44). This modality has been characterized as being the second most effective treatment for dealing with malignant melanoma. This view, however, is open to considerable challenge since some authorities believe that radiotherapy potentially activates otherwise inactive tumor cells.

Research continues to achieve more effective nonsurgical controls for cutaneous malignancies. The interferones continue to hold promise in this regard. Enthusiasm for its use also is variable, particularly in view of its high cost and the difficulty involved in its synthesis.

Postoperative adjuvant chemotherapy and nonspecific immunotherapy also are utilized in support of surgical intervention. Nitrosoureas such as CCNU and BCNU alone or in combination are frequently used agents. BCG vaccination and *Corynebacterium parvum* are the immunotherapeutic modalities most often mentioned. BCG is often injected into the region of primary tumors following excisional surgery (2).

A number of nonsurgical approaches to cancer therapy have been suggested. The more limited the degree of malignancy, the greater the degree of conservatism which can be considered. However, it must be reemphasized that adequate surgical excision is the preferred therapy. This is true not only of melanoma, but probably of other cutaneous malignancies as well.

Clearly, it is presumptuous for any single practitioner to assume total care of patients with cutaneous malignancies. The podiatric surgeon may well be the primary surgeon who makes the initial diagnosis about lesions affecting the lower extremities. However, the patient's best interests are served when the internist, oncologist, radiotherapist, surgical specialist, and dermatologist, as well as psychiatrists and social workers and other qualified personnel are involved in the total treatment plan. When all resources are properly utilized, malignant disease of the skin as well as all other cancers need not be the threat to life that they were in earlier times.

References

1. Pinkus H, Mehregan AH: *A Guide to Dermatohistopathology.* New York, Appleton-Century-Crofts, 1969.
2. Ruben P, Bakemeier RF: *Clinical Oncology.* Rochester, NY, University of Rochester Press, 1983.
3. Allen AC, Spitz S: Malignant melanoma. A clinicopathological analysis of the criteria for diagnosis and prognosis. *Cancer* 6:1, 1953.
4. Knutson C, Horizm K, Spratt JS Jr: Melanoma. *Curr Probl Surg* 12:3–8, 1971.
5. Sears FW: Ulcerated malignant melanoma of the foot. *J Am Podiatry Assoc* 62(4):156–157, 1972.
6. Galinski AW: Moles and malignant melanoma of the foot. *J Am Podiatry Assoc* 63(2):35–46, 1973.
7. Routsaw PD: Infiltrating malignant melanoma of the heel. *J Am Podiatry Assoc* 63(7):319–320, 1973.
8. Sims LJ, George D, Marcus S: Malignant melanoma: a case report. *J Am Podiatry Assoc*:115–119, 1975.
9. McCraw MH: Malignant melanoma, sole of the foot. *J Am Podiatry Assoc* 66(9):699–700, 1976.
10. Gilchrist AK: Malignant melanoma. *J Am Podiatry Assoc* 68(5):317–320, 1978.
11. Page JC: Nodular melanoma. *J Am Podiatry Assoc* 71(10):571–574, 1981.
12. Fields LS, DeLauro T, School S: Malignant melanoma. *J Am Podiatry Assoc* 68(8):547–554, 1978.
13. Sebastian K, Silverman R: Melanoma of the foot. *J Am Podiatry Assoc* 72(6):324–325, 1982.
14. Kopf AW: *Malignant melanoma.* New York, Masson Publications, 1979.
15. Labreque PG, Hu CH, Winkelman RK: On the nature of desmoplastic melanoma. *Cancer* 38:1205–1212, 1976.
16. Andrade R, Fumport SL, Popkin GL et al: *Cancer of the Skin.* Philadelphia, W.B. Saunders, 1976.
17. Galinski AW, Shapiro LJ, Waldman M: Squamous cell carcinoma of the foot. *J Am Podiatry Assoc* 66(7):550–553, 1976.
18. Cangialosi CP: Primary epidermoid carcinoma of the foot. *J Am Podiatry Assoc* 68(10):691–692, 1978.
19. Dale SJ, Simons J: Subungual squamous cell carcinoma. *J Am Podiatry Assoc* (8):421–425, 1980.
20. Steinhart AN: Squamous cell carcinoma of the sole. *J Am Podiatry Assoc* (7):330–332, 1980.
21. Brietstein RJ, Hugar DW: Squamous cell carcinoma. Comparative study and case presentation. *J Am Podiatry Assoc* 65:120–126, 1975.
22. Seehafer JR, Rahman D, Soderstrom SW: Epithelioma cuniculatum: verrucous carcinoma of the foot. *Cutis* 23:287–290, 1979.
23. Kao GF, Graham JH, Helwig ED: Carcinoma cuniculatum (verrucous carcinoma of the skin). *Cancer* 49:2849–2857, 1980.
24. Prioleau PG, Santa Cruz DJ, Meyer JS et al: Verrucous carcinoma. *Cancer* 45:2849–2857, 1980.
25. Brownstein MH, Shapiro L: Verrucous carcinoma of the skin. *Cancer* 38:1710–1716, 1976.
26. Ackerman LV: Verrucous carcinoma of the oral cavity. *Surgery* 23:670–678, 1948.
27. Aird I, Johnson HD, Lennox B et al: Epithelioma cuniculatum: variety of squamous cell carcinoma peculiar to the foot. *Br J Surg* 42:245–250, 1954.
28. Roenigk HH: *Office Dermatology.* Baltimore, Williams & Wilkins, 1981.
29. Robbins GL: *Pathologic Basis of Disease.* Philadelphia, W.B. Saunders, 1974.

30. Brody I: Contributions to the histogenesis of basal cell carcinoma. *J Ultrastruct Res* 33:149–156, 1978.
31. Pinkus H, Mehregan AH: *A Guide to Dermatohistopathology.* New York, Appleton-Century-Crofts, 1969.
32. Hansemann DP von: *Diemikroskopische Diagnose Bosa Schwulste.* Berlin, Hamwald, 1897.
33. Krompecher E: *Der Basalzellenkress.* Jena, Germany, Fisher, 1903.
34. Mohs FE: Chemosurgery: a microscopically controlled method of cancer excision. Arch Surg 42:279–295, 1941.
35. Tromovitch TA, Stegman SJ: Microscopically controlled excision of skin tumors: chemosurgery (Mohs), fresh tissue technique. *Arch Dermatol* 110:231–232, 1974.
36. Mohs FE, Sahl WJ: Chemosurgery for verrucous carcinoma. *J Dermatol Surg Onchol* 5:302–306, 1979.
37. Swanson NA, Taylor WB: Plantar verrucous carcinoma. *Arch Dermatol* 116:794–797, 1980.
38. Gutterman JU: Immunology and immunotherapy of human malignant melanoma: historic review and perspective for the future. *Semin Oncol* 2:149–156, 1975.
39. Bulkley CB: Long term spontaneous remission of malignant melanoma with visceral metastasis. *Cancer* 36:485, 1975.
40. Brodsky I: *Cancer Chemotherapy II.* New York, Grune & Stratton, 1972.
41. Jewell WR: Critical analysis of treatment of stage II and III melanoma patients with immunotherapy. *Ann Surg* 183:543, 1976.
42. Edwards JM: Treatment of melanoma by endolymphatic therapy. *Proc R Soc Med* 67:96, 1974.
43. Sealy A: The treatment of malignant melanoma with cobalt and hyperbaric oxygen. *Clin Radiol* 25:211, 1974.
44. Pearson D: Radiotherapy in malignant melanoma. *Proc R Soc Med* 67:96, 1974.

CHAPTER **19**

Cutaneous Manifestations of Systemic Disease in the Human Foot

ASHER DON RABINOWITZ

CUTANEOUS MANIFESTATIONS IN THE FOOT OF SYSTEMIC DISEASE

Cutaneous signs and symptoms of systemic diseases, as well as of internal malignancy, are numerous (1). This discussion will focus on selected manifestations that may be seen on the feet. Some of these deserve mention because, although they are rare, they are pathognomonic of one specific illness or malignancy, thus placing the podiatrist in the unique position of being able to make the diagnosis of a systemic illness and advise the patient accordingly. In other cases the lesion or complaint is a less specific marker but must still alert the clinician to a limited number of possible systemic associations. The podiatrist may then initiate the appropriate investigations or consultations to confirm or exclude one of these suspected associated conditions.

DIABETIC DERMOPATHY

Diabetic dermopathy occurs commonly on the feet and even more commonly on the pretibial surface as multiple, round, dull red papules which measure less than a centimeter. Individual lesions may persist for a year or more. These spots enlarge slowly, develop a fine scale, and heal with a pigmented depressed scar. They are more than twice as common in men and occur with increasing incidence the longer the diabetes has been present.

Histologically, thickening of the walls of the superficial dermal vessels is noted. The brown pigmentation is probably due to hemosiderin deposition in the dermis.

The lesions appear to represent a manifestation of diabetic microangiopathy. Minor trauma has been suggested as a precipitating factor.

These pigmented patches ("shin spots") are rather characteristic and are unlikely to be mistaken for atrophic lichen planus, disseminated superficial actinic porokeratosis, or Degos' disease (malignant atrophic papulosis). However, they may not be pathognomonic for diabetes (2, 3).

Diabetic dermopathy is asymptomatic and requires no treatment.

DERMATOGLYPHIC PATTERN

One recent study (4) reported a specific dermatoglyphic pattern associated with diabetes mellitus. As compared with a control group, diabetics showed in the dermatoglyphics of their feet fewer medial loops and a lower epidermal ridge count under the first metatarsal head.

This finding will be of considerable interest if confirmed by other investigators.

BULLOSIS DIABETICORUM

Rocca and Pereyra described asymptomatic blisters on the toes and dorsa of the feet of diabetic patients (5). Blisters may also develop on fingers, arms, and legs. Some of the patients have neuropathy. There is no history of antecedent trauma. The blisters heal slowly but without scarring unless complicated by infection or ulceration.

Histologically, some blisters are subcorneal; others are subepidermal. They may be unilocular or multilocular.

These idiopathic bullae of diabetes must

be differentiated from numerous other blisters which may occur on the feet. Friction blisters occur on the soles and histologically show the roof of the blister to be composed of the stratum corneum and stratum granulosum and the floor of the blister to contain individual necrotic keratinocytes. Epidermolysis bullosa is precipitated by trauma in predisposed individuals. Epidermolysis bullosa simplex and epidermolysis bullosa of the hands and feet (Cockayne) show autosomal dominant inheritance.

Histologically the blister forms by dissolution of the basal cell layer of the epidermis. In epidermolysis bullosa acquisita, there is no family history, and the blister forms in the dermis through the region of the anchoring fibrils. Direct immunofluorescence shows linear deposits of immunoglobulins and complement along the epidermal-dermal junction.

Bullous pemphigoid shows subepidermal blisters, commonly in older individuals, generalized on the body. Immunoelectron microscopy shows the IgG and complement deposits to be located above the basement membrane, rather than below, as in epidermolysis bullosa acquisita.

PRURITUS

Pruritus, or itching, is a very common symptom, which may be due to internal or external causes. Itching as a manifestation of systemic illness does not generally show a predilection for the feet, but itchy feet as part of generalized pruritus certainly may be a symptom of systemic disease.

In evaluating pruritus, it is not adequate to simply ask the patient whether or not his lesion itches. Some patients deny itching because they feel guilty about scratching. Conversely, and more commonly, the complaint of itching is exaggerated.

It is helpful to differentiate itching which awakens the patient at night from less severe pruritus, which only appears in the presence of certain precipitating factors, such as rubbing against clothing, and from which the patient's attention may be easily distracted. Pruritus that awakens the patient may be seen in infestations such as scabies, hepatobiliary diseases, lymphomas, other internal malignancies, and renal insufficiency. Examples of less severe pruritus include asteatosis and diabetes.

In diabetes mellitus the most commonly pruritic areas are the scalp and vulva; however, widespread itching is common too. Control of the diabetes regularly offers relief; however, the degree of pruritus in untreated cases does not parallel the severity of the diabetes. Elucidation of the relationship between diabetes and pruritus is complicated by the fact that diabetes may be associated with asteatosis (xerosis, dry skin), which may act as an independent pruritogenic factor. Excoriations are few in the diabetic but are more commonly complicated by secondary infection. Mild pruritus in diabetics may be controlled by emollients and restriction of the use of soap and water.

Pruritus is seen in about one-quarter of patients with jaundice. It may be seen in jaundice due to obstruction of the common bile duct by a neoplasm, stone, stricture, or congenital malformation, as well as following the ingestion of hepatotoxic drugs and, less commonly, in infectious hepatitis. It responds to suberythemogenic doses of ultraviolet light.

Itching is also a prime symptom of leukemia and lymphoma, especially Hodgkin's disease. In these cases, the pruritus may be relieved by chemotherapy or radiotherapy.

Less commonly, itching may be a symptom of a solid tumor. The sudden appearance of intractable pruritus in the older individual cannot simply be ascribed to asteatosis without adequate medical examination to exclude the possibility of an occult malignancy.

Pruritus may occur as a manifestation of uremia. It often responds to dialysis. Itching seen with the dry skin of generalized myxedema (Fig. 19.1) and, less commonly, with pretibial myxedema can be treated with hydrating measures.

Of course, there are also many nonsystemic causes of itchiness on the feet and lower extremities, which must be excluded. These include neurodermatitis, stasis dermatitis, asteatotic dermatitis, tinea infections, and infestations, including scabies, trombiculosis (chiggers), and cercarial dermatitis (swimmer's itch due to avian or mammalian blood flukes).

NEUROPATHIC PLANTAR ULCER

The neuropathic ulcer (mal perforans) will be discussed in detail in Chapter 8 but should be mentioned as a manifestation of systemic disease. The occurrence of such an ulcer mandates a search for diabetes mellitus, chronic alcoholism with neuropathy, Hansen's disease, spina bifida, syphilis, or syringomyelia (Fig. 19.2).

PRURIGO NODULARIS AND PERFORATING DISORDERS

Prurigo nodularis occurs as multiple disseminated papules or nodules anywhere on the body that the patient can reach to scratch. It is generally considered to represent a severe form of lichen simplex chronicus. Although it commonly occurs without any systemic associations, several cases have been reported in patients with chronic renal failure (6).

Similar lesions have been reported under a variety of names, including perforating folliculitis (7, 8), keratotic papules, reactive perforating collagenosis (9), Kyrle's disease, and Kyrle-like disease. These umbilicated keratotic papules are seen in patients with diabetes mellitus and/or chronic renal disease, many of whom were on dialysis. The keratotic lesions show a predilection for the extensor surface; they demonstrate the isomorphic (Koebner) phenomenon and show linear grouping.

Histologically, prurigo nodularis shows epidermal hyperplasia and in some cases hypertrophy of cutaneous nerves. Kyrle's disease, perforating folliculitis, and reactive perforating collagenosis are all characterized by a crater-like nodule which eventually develops a transepidermal perforation through its base. It is interesting to speculate that the prurigo-like lesion might represent a forme fruste of the Kyrle-like lesion in which no perforation has yet developed. The pathogenesis of these disorders is still unsettled.

Some of these lesions have cleared with ultraviolet phototherapy, which decreased the uremic pruritus. Others cleared as the underlying renal disease or diabetes was controlled by dialysis or medical management. Some responded to topical Retin-A.

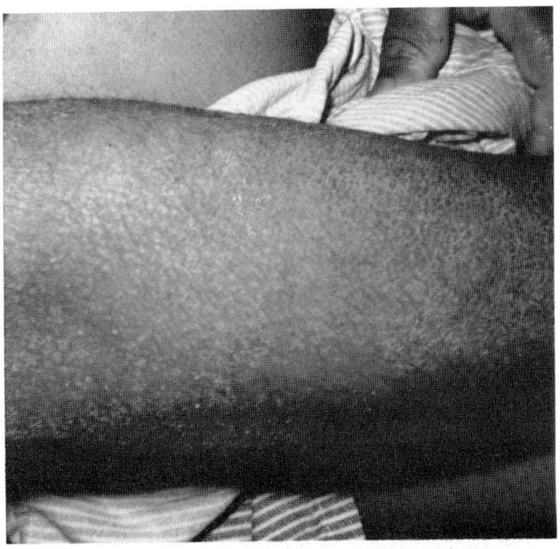

Figure 19.1. Itchy parched skin, simulating eczema craquelé in a patient with thyroid disease.

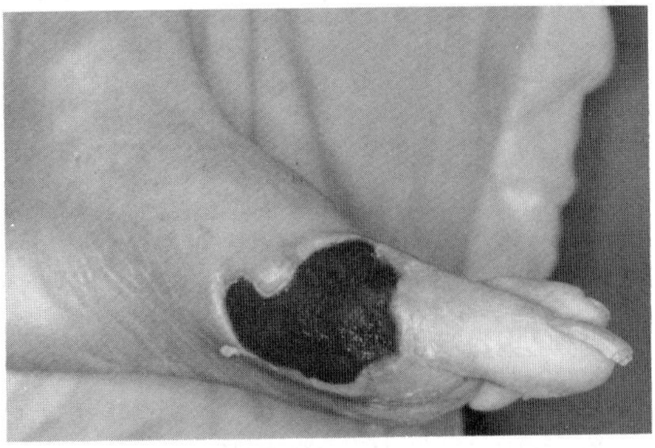

Figure 19.2. This neuropathic ulcer was ignored for many months. Upon hospitalization the patient was found to have diabetes. Note associated thick yellow nails.

MYXEDEMA

Manifestations of both hypothyroidism and hyperthyroidism may be seen in the feet.

Generalized myxedema usually occurs in adult women with fatigue, intolerance to the cold, weight gain and, often, generalized pruritus, as well as cold thickened skin. This cutaneous firm edema is most prominent on the hands, eyelids, and lips. Sweating is reduced; the sodium content of the sweat is increased; and the skin is dry. Hepatic conjugation of vitamin A precursors is decreased, resulting in carotinemia and yellowish skin.

The puffy swelling of the skin is due to deposition of increased amounts of hyaluronic acid between the collagen bundles in the dermis. These changes are quantitatively less than in pretibial myxedema, and special stains for acid mucopolysaccharide (alcian blue, toluidine blue, or colloidal iron) may be needed to demonstrate the mucin deposits surrounding the blood vessels and hair follicles in the dermis. Laboratory tests which help to establish the diagnosis of hypothyroidism include a decreased basal metabolic rate, protein-bound iodine, and I^{131} uptake.

Localized (pretibial) myxedema occurs initially on the shins, toes, and lower abdomen bilaterally as waxy pink or yellow plaques and nodules or as diffuse, firm nonpitting edema of the anterior legs and feet. As the disease progresses, the entire lower limb may enlarge and the skin thicken with a "peau d'orange" appearance. An extreme expression of this thickening of the skin is the development of warty projections over the toes and dorsal of the feet in advanced cases (Fig. 19.3).

Pretibial myxedema is most often a manifestation of hyperthyroidism, but it often only becomes apparent up to three years *after* treatment of thyrotoxicosis with thiouracil or radioactive iodine. It is also seen rarely in euthyroid or hypothyroid patients with chronic lymphocytic thyroiditis. Long-acting thyroid stimulator (LATS) is almost always found in the patient's serum, but the severity of the myxedema does not correlate with the levels of serum LATS. LATS is apparently not the cause of myxedema, as it is detected in about half of the patients with exophthalmic goiter without myxedema.

Pretibial myxedema must be differentiated from chronic lymphedema. Lymphedema, too, is a nonpitting edema and may eventuate in thickened skin with a verrucous surface. Lymphedema itself may follow metastatic carcinomatosis involving the lymph nodes, surgical removal of the nodes, chronic osteomyelitis, chronic lymphangitis, chronic or recurrent cellulitis, and filarial (*Wuchereria bancrofti*) infestation. It may also be hereditary and congenital (Milroy's disease). Elephantiasis merely refers to the gross hypertrophy of a limb associated with chronic lymphedema. Elephantiasis nostras means "elephantiasis of our region," and refers to that caused by common bacterial cellulitis or erysipelas, rather than the more exotic filarial infestation (10). Lymphedema histologically shows hyperplasia of dermal fibrous tissue and its supporting vasculature but no histochemically demonstrable deposition of mucin.

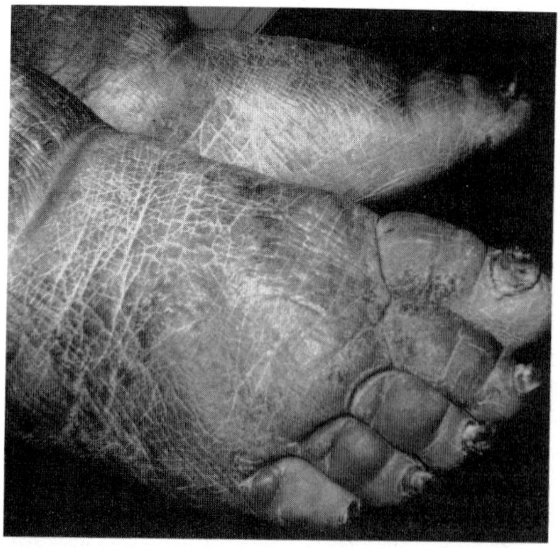

Figure 19.3. Elephantiasis resulting from pretibial myxedema. Note associated onychodystrophy.

Plaques of myxedema may respond to potent corticosteroids under plastic wrap occlusion or to intralesional steroid injection. Lymphedema may respond to specially constructed pressure gradient boots. In myxedema as well as in lymphedema the skin is thrown into rugose folds. The fissures between these folds may become the site of bacterial or yeast infections unless the extremity is soaked daily in a solution such as povidone-iodine.

ACROPACHY

Acropachy or clubbing of the fingers and toes has been known as a manifestation of systemic disease since antiquity. Hippocrates described clubbing in a patient with empyema. Acropachy occurs as bulbous swelling of the terminal phalanges. The nail plate meets the nail fold, forming an angle equal to or greater than 180°. The patient may complain of stiffness in the affected joint.

There is controversy in the literature regarding the relationship of clubbing to hypertrophic osteoarthropathy and pachydermoperiostosis. Some authors consider hypertrophic osteoarthropathy to be a more advanced stage of simple clubbing, in which there is involvement of the proximal parts of the extremities in addition to fingers and toes. Others maintain that in clubbing there is hyperplasia of fibrous tissue but only in hypertrophic osteoarthropathy is there formation of new periosteal bone. In pachydermoperiostosis, clubbing is associated with a family history or similar changes, including thickening of the skin of the face, forehead, and scalp, seborrhea, hyperhidrosis of hands and feet, and effusions of ankles and knees.

Clubbing and hypertrophic osteoarthropathy may have significant systemic associations: about 80% with pulmonary lesions, including tuberculosis, bronchiectasis, malignancy, and empyema; 10% with cardiac lesions; 50% with gastrointestinal and hepatic lesions; and 5% with pretibial myxedema and other less common illnesses, including nasopharyngeal tumors, lymphosarcoma, chronic osteomyelitis with amyloidosis, and pituitary abnormalities.

Conditions to be differentiated include: (*a*) curved nails, which are more common in blacks, and in which the angle at the base of the nail remains about 160°; (*b*) chronic paronychia; (*c*) Heberden's nodes; (*d*) periarticular swelling in arthritis; and (*e*) acromegaly, which results from pituitary secretion of excessive somatotropin.

TOPHI

Tophi occur as chalky white deposits which are extruded through the skin from a periarticular nodule in a patient with gout. Gout occurs both as an inherited disorder of purine metabolism and as an acquired form in a number of circumstances which lead to hyperuricemia and subsequent deposition of monosodium urate in the synovial space. It is much more common in men.

In the acute phase, the metatarsophalangeal joint of the hallux or, less commonly, a joint in the instep, ankle, or knee becomes acutely tender, swollen, hot red, and shiny in the early morning hours. This acute onset is often preceded by trauma, increased alcohol intake, dietary indiscretion, stress, or ingestion of medications such as thiazides (11). The joint swelling lasts a few days. It must be differentiated from cellulitis and erythromelalgia. It is interesting to note that some authors have suggested erythromelalgia as the preferred term to emphasize the redness (ery), the heat (therm), and the pain (algia).

Tophi are the hallmark of the chronic stage of gout which follows increasingly frequent acute attacks. Traumatized tophi may be complicated by cellulitis. Radiographically there are punched out lesions in the subchondral bone. Tophi must be differentiated from ectopic calcification and tendinous xanthomas. Tophi which ulcerate may simulate osteomyelitis or squamous cell carcinoma.

The specific diagnosis is made by demonstrating negatively birefringent urate crystals lying free or within white blood cells in the synovial fluid. In order to demonstrate the urate deposits histologically, the specimen must be submitted in alcohol fixative. Then one may see sheaves of needle-shaped crystals surrounded by granulomatous inflammation.

The acute attacks are managed with colchicine. The chonic stage may be treated with phenylbutazone, intraarticular steroid injections, allopurinol, probenecid, or sulfinpyrazone. Excision of tophi may prevent secondary infection. Steinberg and coworkers have described a method for alleviating the severe pain associated with gouty lesions (12).

PYODERMA GANGRENOSUM

Pyoderma gangrenosum is a cutaneous ulceration first described in 1930, and is characterized by an irregular, elevated, purple, undermined, border surrounded by a zone of erythema (Fig. 19.4). Pyoderma gangrenosum is a misnomer in that it is neither primarily a pyogenic infection nor gangrene. It occurs most commonly between the ages of 20 and 50 but may occur

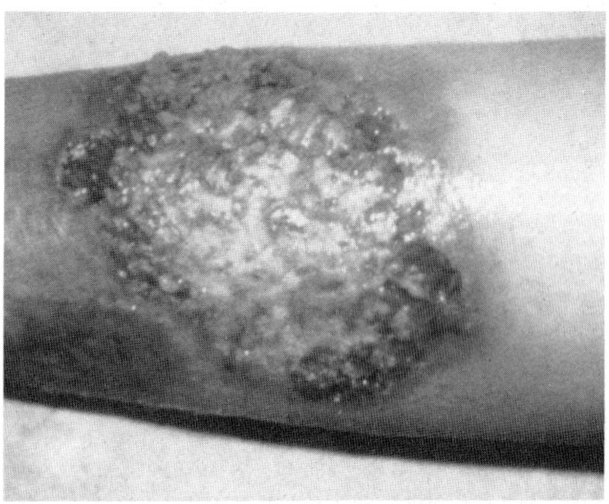

Figure 19.4. Pyoderma gangrenosum with elevated bluish border and a base of exuberant granulation tissue.

at any age. Ulcers are common on the lower extremities but have been reported anywhere on the body, including the mouth and eyes.

Lesions start singly or in crops as small pustules on a red base. The pustules enlarge; the centers become dusky and ulcerate. Neighboring lesions may coalesce to form irregular ulcers many centimeters in diameter. Healing foci develop in the center, while the ulcer spreads centrifugally. A less common variant occurs as diffuse symmetric pustules which simulate dermatitis herpetiformis. Pathergy, the development of new lesions or the exacerbation of existing lesions following minor trauma, is characteristic of pyoderma gangrenosum.

The cause and pathogenesis of pyoderma gangrenosum are unknown, although a variety of immunologic abnormalities have been associated with it. Histologically the ulcer is nonspecific, and many reports suggest that the finding of a leukocytoclastic vasculitis should prompt a search for an alternative diagnosis.

A variety of systemic illnesses may be seen with pyoderma gangrenosum. The most common is ulcerative colitis. Up to half of the patients with pyoderma gangrenosum have ulcerative colitis. Conversely about 5% of patients with ulcerative colitis have pyoderma gangrenosum. The severity of the ulcers often, but not always, parallels the activity of the colitis. About a third of the patients have one of a number of arthritides, including small joint polyarthritis, seronegative rheumatoid-like syndrome, seropositive rheumatoid arthritis, and the arthritis seen with ulcerative colitis. A variant of pyoderma gangrenosum occurring with superficial ulcers and peripheral bullae has been associated with leukemias, lymphomas, multiple myeloma, myeloid metaplasia, and polycythemia vera. If thorough general medical examination fails to reveal gastrointestinal or rheumatologic abnormalities or hematologic malignancy, the diagnosis of pyoderma gangrenosum may still be correct, since about half the cases occur without associated systemic disease (13).

Small early lesions of pyoderma gangrenosum must be differentiated from folliculitis, insect bites, vasculitis, and erythema multiforme. Large ulcers of pyoderma gangrenosum must be differentiated from infectious ulcers, halogenodermas, lupus erythematosus, vasculitis, Behçet's syndrome and factitial ulcers. Chronic ulcerations may simulate squamous cell carcinomas.

The diagnosis is established by typical clinical history and appearance. Laboratory tests aid in excluding clinical simulants. Therefore, biopsy for culture and histology, blood tests, including a serological test for syphilis, serum bromide, liver function tests, hepatitis associated antigen, complete blood count, latex fixation, antinuclear antibodies, and serum protein electrophoresis, as well as sigmoidoscopy and gastrointestinal barium series are indicated.

Therapy includes simple supportive measures including elevation of the involved extremity, astringent compresses, gentian violet, benzoyl peroxide, silver sulfadiazine, and topical sodium cromoglycate. Aggressive debridement and grafting may aggravate the condition by the pathergic response: Intralesional steroids may be helpful. Severe cases may require high dose steroids orally or by intravenous pulse therapy. Other medications reported to be of benefit include dapsone, sulfapyridine, azathioprine, cyclophosphamide, 6-mercaptopurine, and clofazimine. Minocycline and rifampin have also been used.

PARESTHESIAS

It is somewhat curious that while pruritus is generally accepted as a dermatologic symptom, paresthesias are considered to be a neurologic symptom. It should be remebered that the sensation of "pins and needles" in the skin of the toe and the feet may be a symptom of multisystem disease such as diabetes or pernicious anemia (vitamin B_{12} deficiency) (14).

ACRODERMATITIS ENTEROPATHICA

Acrodermatitis enteropathica is a syndrome characterized by diarrhea, failure to thrive, skin lesions, alopecia, paronychia, onychodystrophy, stomatitis, glossitis, and frequent secondary candidal or bacterial infections. The condition was first described in 1936 (15) but not until 1973 (16) was the cause determined to be zinc deficiency. Acrodermatitis enteropathica is transmitted as an autosomal recessive trait with equal incidence in boys and girls. It generally appears after weaning or in formula-fed infants between the ages of 3 weeks and 10 years.

A similar syndrome occurs due to zinc deficiency in the adult, as in patients receiving total parenteral nutrition containing inadequate zinc supplementation, in patients with reduced absorptive capacity following jejunoileal bypass, and in alcoholics as a result of malnutrition and malabsorption.

The symptoms may appear in any order, but often the cutaneous lesions are first. Symmetric, small, vesiculobullous lesions arise, collapse, and coalesce to form sharply marginated plaques on the hands and feet and around the eyes, ears, nose, mouth, and perineum.

Many cases have initially been misdiagnosed as systemic thrush, atypical epidermolysis bullosa, or atypical psoriasis.

The diagnosis is confirmed by finding low serum zinc levels. Therapy is with oral zinc sulphate or intravenous zinc supplementation. Less specific therapy is with diiodohydroxyquin or iodochlorhydroxyquin. These effect remission of the lesions by enhancing zinc absorption.

NECROLYTIC MIGRATORY ERYTHEMA

Necrolytic migratory erythema is a cutaneous sign of a glucagon-secreting α cell tumor of the pancreas. The cutaneous lesions first appear as diffuse erythema with exudation on the dorsa of the feet in women in the fifth to seventh decades. Dull red patches, which over about a week develop a central violaceous hue, or ring-shaped lesions, or collapsed blisters, may be seen and spread from the feet to involve the legs, groin, and trunk (Fig. 19.5).

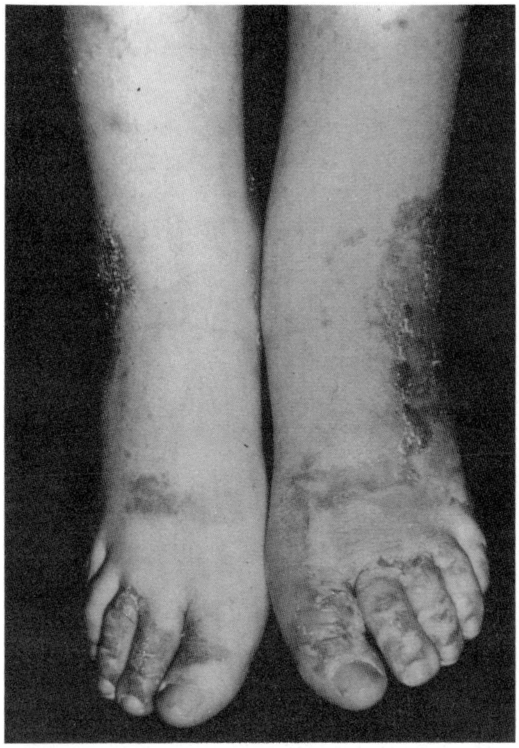

Figure 19.5. Scaly patches of necrolytic migratory erythema.

Histologically, lesions show dissolution of the superficial Malpighian layer and a perivascular mononuclear infiltrate. Most patients have a painful swollen tongue and inflammed lips (17).

Diagnosis is confirmed by elevated serum glucagon levels. Resection of the glucagonoma cures the dermatitis.

ELEPHANTIASIS NEUROMATOSA AND CAFÉ AU LAIT SPOTS

Neither the solitary neurofibroma nor the café au lait spot alone is pathognomonic of systemic disease. But a patient who has over five café au lait spots, each measuring over 1.5 cm has neurofibromatosis (von Recklinghausen's disease).

This condition has protean manifestations involving many organ systems. Of importance to the podiatrist is the possibility of presentation of a previously undiagnosed case with lesions limited to the foot.

Café au lait spots are oval, evenly pigmented tan macules which may occur anywhere on the body. Histologically these spots show hyperpigmentation of the lower epidermis and, in many cases, the presence of giant pigment granules (macromelanosomes).

Neurofibromas are benign tumors of the peripheral nervous system which occur as soft nodules anywhere on the body and can generally be pressed into the underlying skin (buttonhole sign).

Elephantiasis neuromatosa is a soft tissue hypertrophy which may contain hemangiomatous, lymphangiomatous, and neural components, the latter in the form of plexiform neuromas (18).

Therapy consists of conservative local excision of the neurofibroma or hypertrophied tissue.

ERYTHEMA MULTIFORME

Erythema multiforme is one of the most common and at the same time clinically distinctive reaction patterns in the skin. While it may appear anywhere on the body, if frequently occurs on the hands and feet. Lesions are usually multiple and appear "target-shaped" with a ringed, often slightly elevated, and erythematous zone surrounding a macular dusky center, which generally evolves into a bulla.

Histologically, the blister may be intraepidermal or subepidermal or both, and within the epidermis there are necrosis of individual keratinocytes and hydropic degeneration of the basal cell layer. In the dermis there are melanophages and perivascular mononuclear inflammation.

Erythema multiforme may be precipitated by numerous causes. A complete medical review may reveal one of the following:

1. Medications taken up to 2 weeks prior to onset. The more common offenders include barbiturates, penicillin, salicylates, and sulfonamides
2. Vaccines
3. Contact with 9-bromofluorene in a chemistry laboratory
4. Ingestion of the emulsifier in margarine
5. Herpes simplex and less commonly zoster
6. Other infections, e.g., pulmonary: mycoplasma, tuberculosis, coccidioidomycosis, Coxsackie virus, etc.
7. Malignancy

Therapy remains controversial. Severe cases may be managed with systemic steroids. In general, the lesions resolve spontaneously with elimination of the precipitating factor.

CONCLUSION

This discussion has not exhausted the list of conditions on the feet that may be manifestations of systemic disease. Others, such as the ungual fibromas of tuberous sclerosis (19, 20) (Fig. 19.6) and purpura in vasculitis or mastocytosis (21), may be discussed elsewhere in this book. It also behooves the podiatrist to be familiar with lesions that occur slightly higher on the body, such as erythema nodosum and necrobiosis lipoidica (Fig. 19.7), which also serve as important clues to generalized disease and further demonstrate that the skin is, indeed, the mirror of the body's health.

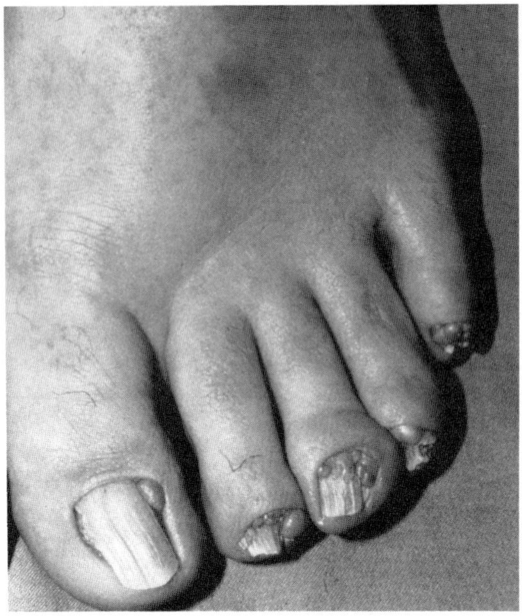

Figure 19.6. Periungual fibromas (Koenen's tumors) in a patient with tuberous sclerosis.

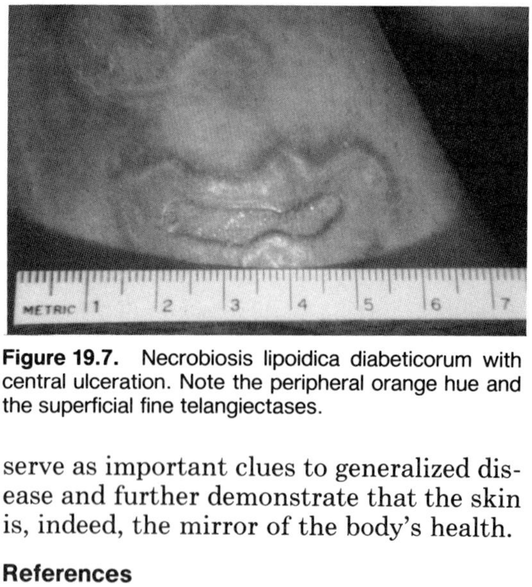

Figure 19.7. Necrobiosis lipoidica diabeticorum with central ulceration. Note the peripheral orange hue and the superficial fine telangiectases.

References

1. Port M: Systemic disease. *J Am Podiatry Assoc* 69:341, 1979.
2. Helfand AE: Hunting diabetics by foot. *J Am Podiatry Assoc* 64:399–406, 1974.
3. Port M: Diabetic dermopathy. A controversy in dermatology. *J Am Podiatry Assoc* 72:418–423, 1982.
4. Erlick NE, Engel ED, Parkers GE, Karpo AS, Davis RH: A dermatoglyphic predictive index for maturity onset diabetes. *J Am Podiatry Assoc* 73:465–474, 1983.
5. Rocca FP, Pereyra E: Phylctenar lesions in

the feet of diabetic patients. *Diabetes* 12:220–223, 1963.
6. Rien BE, Lemont H, Cohen RS: Prurigo nodularis: an association with uremia. *J Am Podiatry Assoc* 72:321–323, 1982.
7. Hurwitz RM, Melton ME, Creech FT III, Weiss J, Handt A: Perforating folliculitis in association with hemodialysis. *Am J Dermatopathol* 4:101–108, 1982.
8. White CR, Heskel NS, Pokorny DJ: Perforating folliculitis of hemodialysis. *Am J Dermatopathol* 4:109–116.
9. Cochran RJ, Tucker SB, Wilkin JK: Reactive perforating collagenosis of diabetes mellitus and renal failure. *Cutis* 31:55–58, 1983.
10. Fields GS, Imanuel H, Marcus S: Elephantiasis nostras. A case report and review of the subject. *J Am Podiatry Assoc* 66:28–31, 1976.
11. Horwitz LR, Liebman JA, Cavolo DJ: Thiazide-induced hyperuricemia and gout. *J Am Podiatry Assoc* 72:511–516, 1982.
12. Steinberg MD, Steinberg LB, Fields GS, Fields LS: Gout and Sudeck's atrophy. A simplified approach to treatment. *J Am Podiatry Assoc* 65:379–383, 1975.
13. Murray JC: Pyoderma gangrenosum with IgA gammopathy. *Cutis* 32:477–486, 1983.
14. Gohil P, Haynie RL, Spencer AM, Clark TH: Vitamin B_{12} Neuropathy with pernicious anemia: Description and a case report. *J Am Podiatry Assoc* 71:73–78, 1982.
15. Brandt T: Dermatitis in children with disturbances of the general condition and the absorption of food elements. *Acta Dermato-Venereol* 17:513–546, 1936.
16. Barnes PM, Moynahan EJ: Zinc deficiency in acrodermatitis enteropathica: multiple dietary intolerance treated with synthetic diet. *Proc R Soc Med* 66:327–329, 1973.
17. Lewis AE: The glucagonoma syndrome. *Int J Dermatol* 18:17–22, 1979
18. Harris WC, Alpert WJ, Marcinko DE: Elephantiasis neuromatosa in von Recklinghausen's disease. A review and case report. *J Am Podiatry Assoc* 72:70–72, 1982.
19. Feinstein MH: Foot pathology associated in tuberous sclerosis and von Recklinghausen's disease. *J Am Podiatry Assoc* 62:336–350, 1972.
20. Scheffler NM, Sheitel PL: Periungual fibromas. *J Am Podiatry Assoc* 65:148–151, 1975.
21. Vega M, Rosenfeld S, Rabinowitz AD: Chronic pigmented purpura. *J Am Podiatry Assoc* 72:412–417, 1982.

CHAPTER 20

Connective Tissue Disorders

MARTIN PORT, MARY L. OTTINGER, and NEIL A. FENSKE

The connective tissue diseases (previously called collagen vascular diseases, collagen diseases, and collagenoses) are acquired disorders of connective tissue with varying degrees of vascular involvement (1). The vascular lesions range from telangiectases through vasospastic phenomena to necrotizing arteritis. As advances were made in immunologic techniques, autoantibodies were recognized in these diseases which resulted in their being labeled autoimmune or immunological diseases. The connective tissue diseases include rheumatoid arthritis (RA), discoid lupus erythematosus (DLE), systemic lupus erythematosus (SLE), progressive systemic sclerosis (PSS) and morphea, polyarteritis, and Sjogren's syndrome. While each has a specific clinical picture, overlap syndromes do occur with combinations of both clinical and laboratory abnormalities of two or more of the disorders. The diseases of most relevance to podiatrists include rheumatoid arthritis, lupus erythematosus (LE), and scleroderma.

CLINICAL SIGNS IMPORTANT IN THE CONNECTIVE TISSUE DISEASES

Certain cutaneous clinical findings, while not unique to the connective tissue diseases, do, when taken into consideration with other clinical and laboratory findings, help to corroborate a presumptive diagnosis or to assess prognosis. Periungual telangiectases (Fig. 20.1) lead one to suspect one of the connective tissue disorders. Raynaud's phenomenon in association with lupus erythematosus (LE) suggests a relatively favorable prognosis. Several of the more important cutaneous reaction patterns seen in association with these diseases are lesions of vasculitis, livedo reticularis, Raynaud's phenomenon, and telangiectases (Table 20.1).

Vasculitis

The often referred to vasculitis of the connective tissue diseases is leukocytoclastic angiitis which affects the small vessels of the skin and internal organs. Histologically, the small vessels (capillaries, venules, and arterioles) show endothelial swelling and fibrinoid deposition in and around the wall. A predominately neutrophilic infiltration invades the vessel wall as well as perivascularly. Scattered nuclear fragments, so-called nuclear dust, which result from nuclear disintegration are characteristically seen (1).

The diagnostic clinical lesions associated with this type of vasculitis are palpable purpura (Fig. 20.2). Also seen are erythematous macules and papules, urticaria, purpuric nodules, hemorrhagic vesicles and bullae, and ulcerations (Fig. 20.3).

Livedo Reticularis

Livedo reticularis is a blotchy bluish-red mottling or reticular pattern of the skin of the extremities (Fig. 20.4). It is the result of insufficiency of the arterial blood supply, with dilatation of the small vessels in the periphery of the cone of distribution of the obstructed arteriole (2). Physiologic livedo reticularis is called cutis marmorata. Other forms are idiopathic (localized), congenital, and symptomatic (secondary).

When the pattern occurs asymmetrically, in patches, or in association with erythematous nodules, ulcerations, or digital gangrene, it is usually caused by vasculitis due to an underlying systemic disease. Among the diseases which cause livedo reticularis are the connective tissue diseases, syphilis, tuberculosis, and intravascular occlusion by atheromatous emboli, thrombocytosis, and coagulopathy.

Raynaud's Phenomenon

Raynaud's phenomenon is an episode of constriction of the small arteries or arterioles of the extremities resulting in intermittent changes in color of the overlying skin (3). A characteristic triphasic reaction of pallor (due to ischemia), cyanosis (due to stasis) (Fig. 20.5), and rubor (due to reactive hyperemia) develops symmetrically. It is often precipitated by exposure to a cooler temperature or by emotional stress. The term Raynaud's phenomenon is used

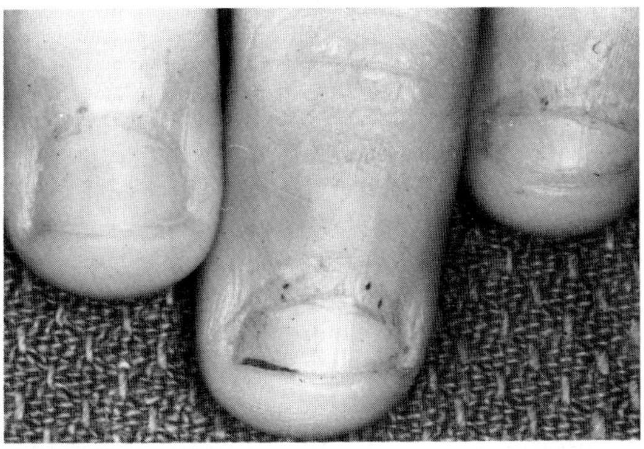

Figure 20.1. Periungual telangiectasias are markers for the connective tissue disorders. Often they are thrombosed, as evident in the middle finger of this patient.

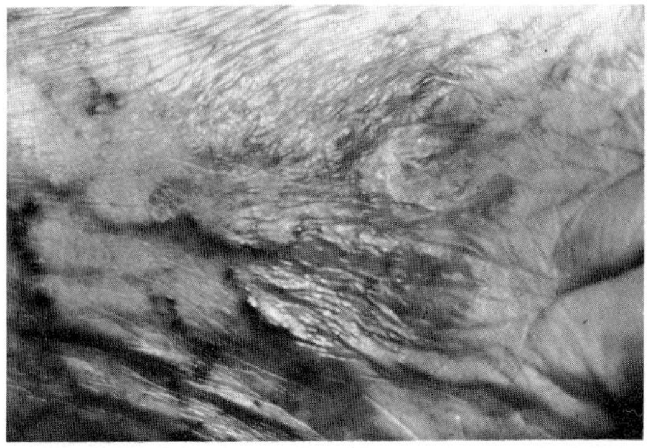

Figure 20.2. Palpable purpura is the clinical hallmark of leukocytoclastic vasculitis of the small blood vessels.

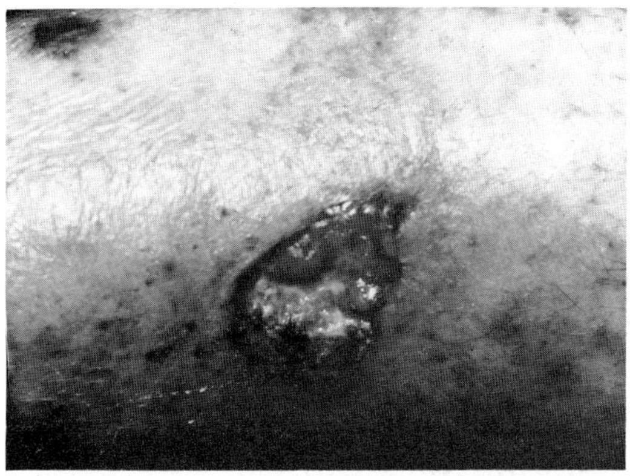

Figure 20.3. Ulceration may occur in areas of extensive leukocytoclastic vasculitis, especially on the lower legs, where increased stasis or hydrostatic pressure may play a provocative role. Note the palpable purpuric lesion superiorly.

Table 20.1.
Cutaneous Signs of Connective Tissue Disease[a]

Sign	Dermatomyositis	Lupus erythematosus	Scleroderma
Calcinosis	+	+	0
Cutaneous vasculitis	0	0	+
Edema	+	+	+
Erythema	+	0	+
Livedo reticularis	0	0	+
Pigmentation	0	+	0
Poikiloderma	+	0	+
Purpura	0	0	+
Raynaud's phenomenon	+	+	+
Sclerosis	+	+	0
Sun sensitivity	+	0	+
Ulceration	+	+	0

[a] Adapted from Winkelman RK: The cutaneous diagnosis of dermatomyositis, lupus erythematosus and scleroderma. *NY State J Med* 63:3080, 1963.

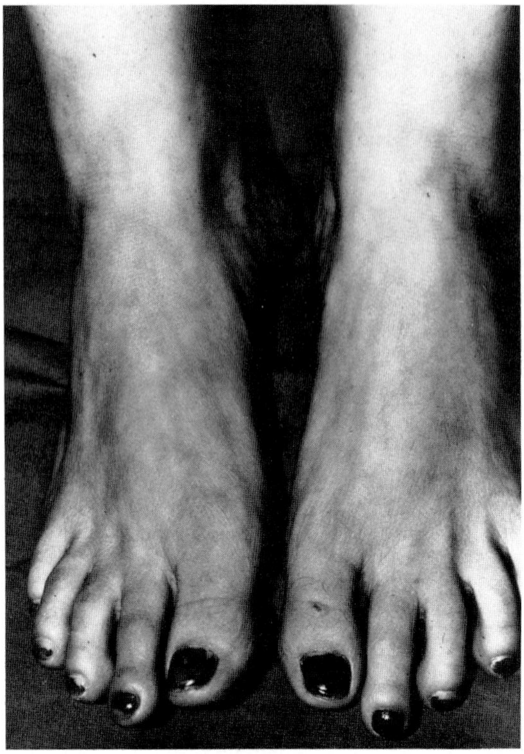

Figure 20.4. Livedo reticularis is a mottled discoloration of the skin due to arterial insufficiency of medium-sized cutaneous arteries.

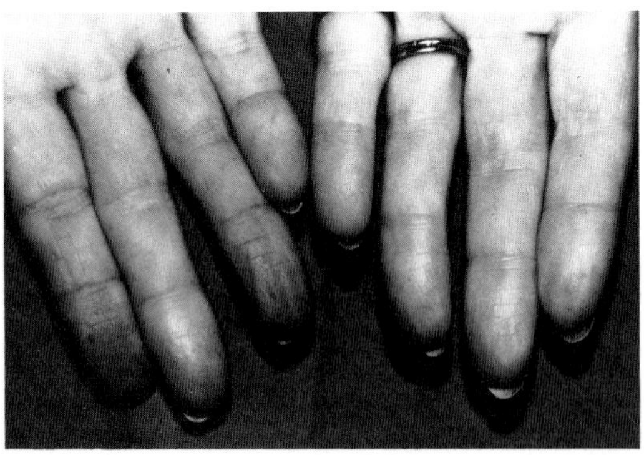

Figure 20.5. Raynaud's phenomenon is characterized by a triphasic response to cold exposure: pallor, cyanosis, and rubor. This patient is experiencing the second phase of cyanosis.

to refer to local changes of a functional nature in the acral arterioles and does not reflect the status of the peripheral vascular system as a whole.

Initially the fingers and/or toes become white as arteriolar constriction produces blanching with pain, numbness, and sometimes increased sweating. Next, cyanosis occurs due to very slow blood flow from the arterioles as their vasoconstriction lessens. Finally, the digits become hyperemic as a result of complete vasodilation of the arterioles and venules. This is often accompanied by a tingling or burning sensation. The triphasic reaction occurs in only two-thirds of the patients. Cyanosis and rubor, or pallor and rubor, may otherwise be expressed (4).

Raynaud's phenomenon occurs predominantly in females, usually bilaterally. Episodes take place from a few times per day to several times per year. As the vasospastic process becomes more severe, attacks may occur in the summer as well as in the winter. Massive gangrene is not a feature of Raynaud's phenomenon; in fact, amputation of the distal phalanx due to necrosis is extremely uncommon.

Differential diagnosis should include acrocyanosis, which is a persistent cyanosis of the hands and feet unrelieved by temperature elevation. Raynaud's phenomenon may occur primarily, as in Raynaud's disease, or it may occur in association with a number of conditions and diseases discussed in this chapter, namely, scleroderma, LE, rheumatoid arthritis (RA), and dermatomyositis (Table 20.2).

Telangiectasia

Telangiectasia is a permanent dilatation of cutaneous capillaries and venules. It may appear as fine bright red lines, heavy cords, or as a spider-shaped macule (5). Telangiectases are common normal findings on the face, especially the malar area, of persons with chronic wind and sun exposure. Linear cuticular telangiectases occur in the skin around the nailbed in LE, dermatomyositis and, occasionally, scleroderma. Mat-like telangiectases occur on the face and trunk in scleroderma. In these connective tisue diseases they are usually associated with other signs of inflammation such as postinflammatory hyper- or hypopigmentation, atrophy, necrosis, petechiae, or purpura (6).

LABORATORY TESTS IMPORTANT IN CONNECTIVE TISSUE DISEASES

While the connective tissue diseases are accompanied by a large array of abnormal

Table 20.2.
Conditions Demonstrating Raynaud's Phenomenon[a]

- I. Without associated and contributing conditions or disease
  - A. Raynaud's disease
- II. With associated and contributing conditions or disease
  - A. After trauma
    1. Occupation related
    2. Following injury or operation
  - B. Neurogenic lesions
    1. Shoulder girdle compression syndrome
    2. Carpal tunnel syndrome
    3. Other nervous system diseases
  - C. Occlusive arterial diseases
    1. Arteriosclerosis obliterans
    2. Thromboangiitis obliterans
    3. Embolism
    4. Thrombosis
  - D. Intoxication
    1. Heavy metals
    2. Ergot
  - E. Miscellaneous diseases and conditions
    1. Scleroderma
    2. Lupus erythematosus
    3. Rheumatoid arthritis
    4. Dermatomyositis
    5. Angiokeratoma corporis diffusum (Fabry's disease)
    6. Paroxysmal hemoglobinuria
    7. Cold hemagglutinins or cryoglobinemia
    8. Primary pulmonary hypertension
    9. Myxedema

[a] Adapted from Fairbairn JF II, Juergens JL, Spittell JA Jr: *Peripheral Vascular Diseases*, ed 4. Philadelphia, W.B. Saunders, 1972, p 388.

laboratory values, several tests are particularly relevant and helpful in the diagnosis of these diseases. Like other tests, their presence or absence is not absolutely diagnostic, but they have such general importance in connective tissue diseases that some amplification of them is given here. The laboratory tests discussed are antinuclear antibodies (ANA), LE cell phenomenon, and rheumatoid factor (RF). A discussion of nail fold capillaroscopy—a new and simple method of examining cutaneous vessels for vasculitis—is also included.

ANTINUCLEAR ANTIBODIES (ANA)

Antinuclear antibodies react with a variety of nuclear antigens and are found especially in the sera of most patients with SLE. Although also present in many other conditions, they are usually of low titer and in a nonspecific homogenous pattern. They are classified as antinucleoprotein, anti-RNA, antiextractable nuclear antigen (ENA), antihistone, antibodies to cytoplasmic antigens, and antinuclear-associated antigens. Most laboratories screen a serum for ANA by the fluorescence technique, and if the assay is positive, then evaluate antibodies to certain subset antigens (1).

Besides the connective tissue diseases, many drugs have been associated with development of ANA and clinical symptoms of SLE. Among them are hydralazine, procainamide, sulfonamides, penicillamine, and chlorpromazine. In most patients the ANA disappears within a few months after the drug is discontinued.

ANA has become an important marker for a variety of connective tissue disorders. There is a marked heterogeneity of these factors, and there is a clinical relevance to individual subsets and clusters of specific ANA.

The antinuclear antibodies are demonstrable in four nuclear staining patterns with fluorescent antibody techniques (1).

These are homogeneous, speckled, nucleolar, and membranous. The homogeneous pattern shows diffuse nuclear staining and is produced by antinucleohistone. The speckled pattern shows minute points of staining all over the nucleus. It is caused by a glycoprotein antibody that is found in patients with connective tissue diseases other than SLE. The nucleolar pattern highlights the nucleolus. The membranous or peripheral pattern demonstrates the periphery of the nucleus and is caused by an anti-DNA histone. In patients with SLE, the homogenous pattern is the most common, whereas the membranous pattern is most specific, and the speckled pattern is seen occasionally. The nucleolar pattern is a marker for scleroderma.

LE Cell

The LE cell phenomenon is found in more than 80% of patients with SLE. It may also be seen, although in lower percentages, in DLE, systemic sclerosis, rheumatoid arthritis, and drug eruptions. To test for LE cells, heparinized blood is incubated for 30 to 60 min. The formation of the cell requires the presence of a 7s IgG antibody which reacts with deoxyribonucleoprotein from damaged leukocytes. The DNA, and immunoglobulin, along with serum complement, form a large homogenous mass that is extruded from the damaged cell. The LE cell is a leukocyte which engulfs one or more of these masses. Alternately, masses of these LE bodies may be found extracellularly and may be surrounded by leukocytes. This test is positive in 75% or more of patients, but the phenomenon may be intermittent and may require repeated examinations. LE cells may also be found in the whole blood or bone marrow of LE patients but are more reliably found *in vitro* as above (7).

Rheumatoid Factor (RF)

Rheumatoid factors are autoantibodies directed against antigenic determinants on the Fc fragment of immunoglobulin G (IgG) molecules. They are found among the IgM, IgA, and IgG classes of immunoglobulin antigen-coated particles (latex fixation) or with sensitized sheep cells.

Rheumatoid factors are not specific for rheumatoid arthritis but are seen in a variable portion of patients with acute and chronic inflammatory diseases as well as in some normal individuals. These conditions include the other rheumatic diseases, viral infections, chronic inflammatory diseases, and neoplasms after chemotherapy or radiation.

In most nonrheumatic conditions, titers of rheumatoid factor are lower than in RA. Thus, the specificity of the RF reaction for RA increases with serum titer. The sensitive sheep cell agglutination test is slightly more specific for RA than is latex fixation, and positivity for both is more specific for RA than either test alone.

Nail Fold Capillary Microscopy

Nail fold capillary microscopy is a simple and useful diagnostic technique for the connective tissue diseases. It utilizes the premise that abnormalities seen in the nail fold capillaries reflect abnormalities in capillaries elsewhere in the body. Maricq and Maize (8) described the technique, using an ophthalmoscope set at +40 which views the nail fold through a drop of mineral oil.

Four specific patterns are described: normal, scleroderma (SD), lupus erythematosus (LE), and nonspecific, which differ on the basis of the morphology of the capillary loops and on the presence or absence of avascular "skip" areas. The normal nail fold capillary pattern, which may be seen in all individuals who are not too darkly pigmented, shows the capillaries as dots in the proximal portion of the proximal nail fold as they are viewed from the end and as regularly spaced hairpin-like loops more distally as they are viewed from the side. In about 5% of the population, the subpapillary venous plexus may also be seen.

The SD pattern shows a characteristic widening of the capillary loop, although normal loops may be present in the same nail fold. Loss of capillaries shows avascular areas adjacent to the capillary loops. Also, the loops may be distorted, showing a disorganized pattern of the nail fold capillary bed, and branched "bushy" formations may be seen, signaling new capillary growth.

The LE pattern shows widened, tortuous loops with little dilatation. Avascular areas are rarely seen; however, there is some disorganization of the pattern. The subpapillary venous plexus is visualized more frequently in LE, although this may be due to an increase in translucency of the skin secondary to steroid treatment. A nonspecific pattern consists of a disorganization of the capillary pattern with or without avascular areas but no specific changes in capillary structure.

To test the specificity of the technique, Kenik et al (9) studied photographs of 24 connective tissue disease patients and five controls, with one of the authors studying them in a blind fashion. He correctly identified the scleroderma-dermatomyositis pattern in 17 of 18 photographs of scleroderma patients and 5 of 5 dermatomyositis patients. Of the lupus patients, six of eight showed the tortuous LE pattern. This pattern is not specific nor unique to lupus patients, but assists in diagnosing a connective tissue disease.

The results of examination of 130 connective tissue disease patients revealed that the nail fold patterns of patients with dermatomyositis and scleroderma were indistinguishable; of the patients with scleroderma, 74% had the SD pattern; of the patients with systemic lupus, 53% had the LE pattern. None of the patients with scleroderma had the LE pattern, and 6% of the systemic lupus patients had the SD pattern. The nail fold technique in patients with Raynaud's phenomenon may have some predictive value with respect to scleroderma. Maricq et al (10) studied 18 patients with Raynaud's disease, half of whom had the SD pattern. Four of the nine eventually developed clinical scleroderma.

LUPUS ERYTHEMATOSUS

Lupus erythematosus (LE) is an inflammatory disease of unknown etiology which may involve any organ system. Discoid lupus erythematosus (DLE) is thought to represent a wholly cutaneous form of LE and presents with lesions characterized by persistent localized erythema, adherent scales, expanded follicular plugs, telangiectasia and atrophy (Fig. 20.6). Healing with scarring, pigmentation and atrophy is typical (Fig. 20.7). Although DLE is supposed to be limited to the skin, a small number of patients with DLE have serum autoantibodies (11). Whether this indicates a subset of patients at risk for later development of SLE is conjectural. Conversely, approximately 15% of patients with SLE also have discoid skin lesions indistinguishable from those occurring in DLE (12).

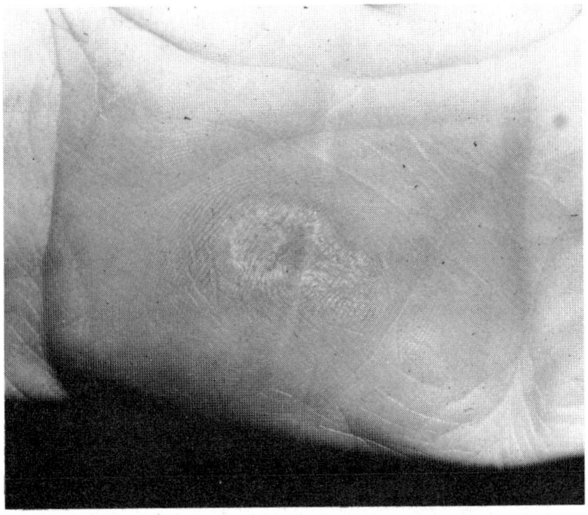

Figure 20.6. Discoid lesions, the hallmark of DLE, may also occur in SLE. Follicular plugging does not occur on the palms and soles due to the absence of pilosebaceous units in these specialized areas of the skin.

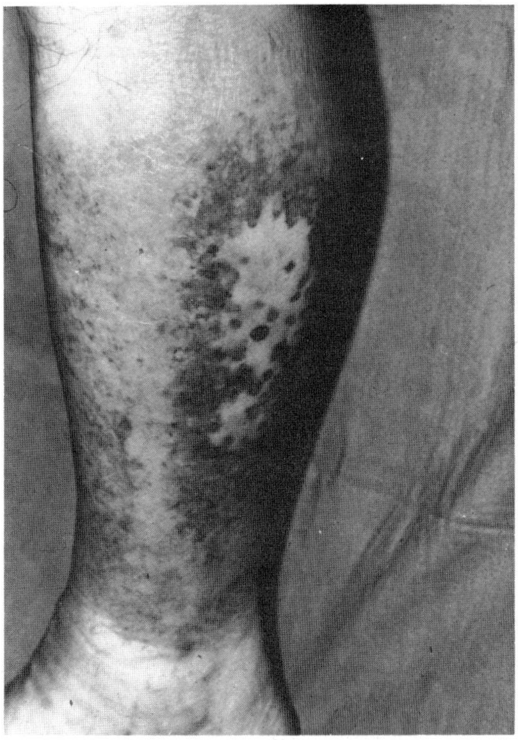

Figure 20.7. Old or "burned out" lesions of DLE typically consist of scarring and hypopigmentation surrounded by a ring of hyperpigmentation.

SLE occurs in 2.6 per 100,000 individuals and favors females in a ratio of 2:1. The age of onset varies greatly, with the majority of patients in the third and fourth decades of life.

Multiple antibodies against the patient's own cells and cell components have led to the classification of SLE as an autoimmune disorder. The presence of antinuclear antibodies, DNA, and serum complement in the glomeruli of patients with SLE suggests that tissue damage results from circulating antibody-antigen complexes.

Clinical Manifestations

One of the most common early symptoms of SLE is fatigue. This may then be followed by a diffuse erythematous maculopapular rash most often manifested in areas of sun exposure. The patients may also demonstrate fever, arthritis or arthralgia, renal disease, lymphadenopathy, pleurisy, pericarditis, seizures, and gastrointestinal symptoms.

Joint manifestations are the most common sign of SLE. Arthritis and arthralgia occur in almost all LE patients. Commonly, arthritis with swelling, tenderness, and erythema is found. The joint symptoms may precede other symptoms manifested after some weeks or months. Morley et al (13) highlighted the articular symptoms of lupus manifesting in the foot and reported three patients with subluxation and contractures of the metatarsophalangeal joints and interphalangeal joints. In all cases the patients had earlier, more severe hand deformities.

Cutaneous Manifestations

Cutaneous involvement in SLE occurs in approximately three-fourths of all patients. The classic butterfly rash of erythema and edema of the cheeks and bridge of the nose occurs in about one-third of patients. The next most common rash is a pruritic maculopapular eruption located usually above the waist. Scattered macules are seen on the palms and rarely on the soles (Fig. 20.8). The classic lesions of chronic DLE as described above may also occur. The discoid lesions may precede the onset of systemic disease by several months to more than 20 years.

Tender, punched-out, slowly healing leg ulcers occur near the malleoli (Fig. 20.9). Hemorrhagic bullae may be seen due to thrombocytopenia. Rarely, gangrene results due to arteritis of medium-sized arteries. Raynaud's phenomenon occurs in 15% of patients and may precede the diagnosis of SLE. Thrombophlebitis may be the first manifestation of SLE.

Telangiectasia is common and may be seen on examination of the proximal nail fold. Squared telangiectatic mats are often present inside the lower lip and on the cheeks, digits, and forearms. Raynaud's phenomenon is often seen with such telangiectases; however, both are more common in scleroderma than SLE (14).

Digital lesions include small periungual infarcts due to vasculitis. If digital arteritis occurs, distal digital necrosis may follow (Fig. 20.10). Rarely, cryoproteins may cause occlusion and gangrene of entire digits.

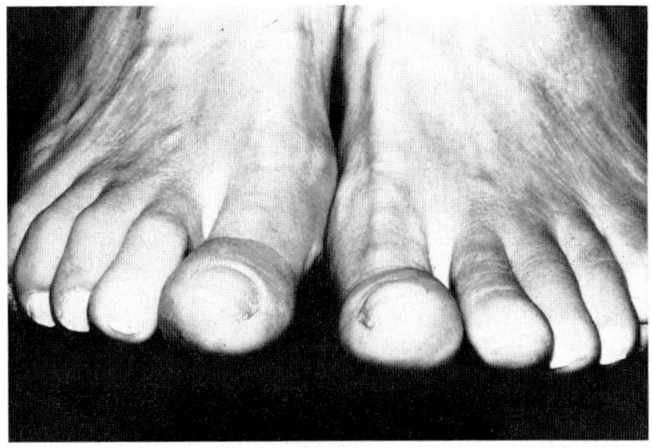

Figure 20.8. Maculopapular, erythematous lesions on the palms and soles occur in SLE.

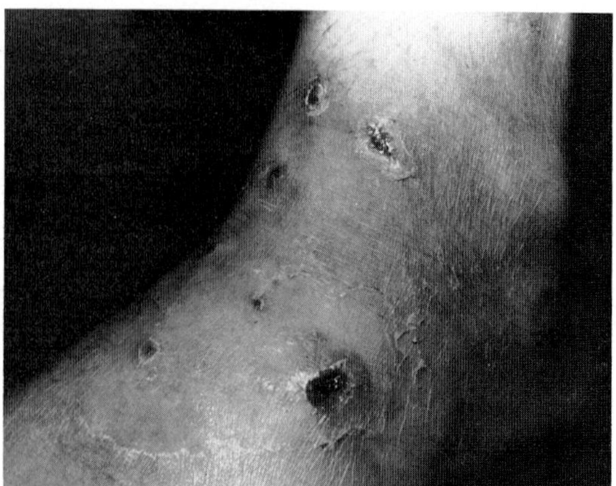

Figure 20.9. Vasculitis in SLE may be manifest as punched-out ulcerations on the ankles.

The type of skin lesion may be a marker of a lupus subset and a predictor of prognosis or systemic involvement (15). Vasculitis may take several forms: nail fold changes, splinter hemorrhages (Fig. 20.11), urticaria, palpable purpura, necrosis, and ulceration. Cutaneous vasculitis is associated with renal involvement and is a sign which reflects disease activity. Patients with SLE who have discoid lesions generally have a more benign course. Similarly, Raynaud's phenomenon is also associated with a more favorable outcome.

Sontheimer et al (16) characterized a clinically distinct form of cutaneous LE which they called subacute cutaneous LE. It presents symmetrically with a nonscarring superficial eruption located predominately over the cheeks, nose, ears, upper trunk, and extensor surfaces of the arm. Morphologically, the papulosquamous eruption may form plaques or annular polycyclic configurations (Fig. 20.12). The pathologic changes are intermediate between those of DLE and SLE. These patients frequently have a mild systemic illness marked by musculoskeletal complaints and serological abnormalities. Thus, these patients are thought to have an illness intermediate in severity between DLE and SLE.

Specific mention of the foot in SLE is rare. Kidawa and Roth (17) reported a 22-year-old black female who presented with extensive areas of hyperkeratosis surrounded by depigmentation. Deep to the keratosis was a yellow-white cheese-like substance which was in turn resting superficial to an erythematous base. These lesions were present for 6 months. Later, the skin lesions spread to include the legs, arms, and neck. An ulcer of the palate formed, and the nephrotic syndrome developed. Ultimately, SLE was diagnosed, and the patient was successfully treated with chloroquine. Mandel et al (18) reported a 34-year-old white female with established

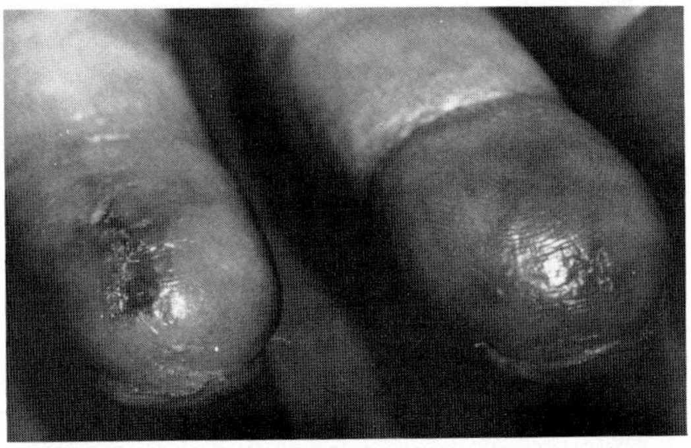

Figure 20.10. Distal digital necrosis, due to digital arteritis, results in irregular pitted scars when healed.

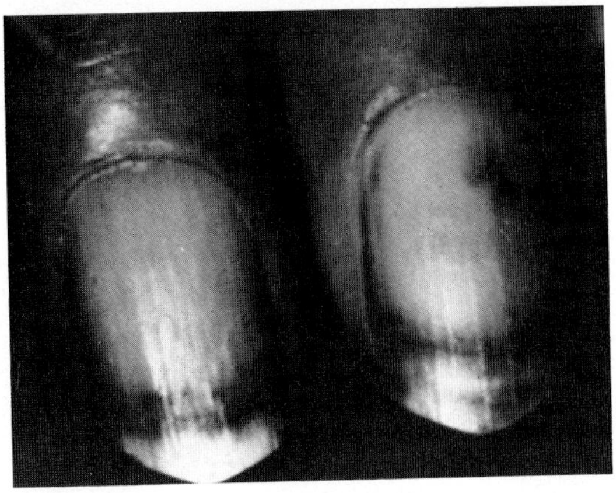

Figure 20.11. Splinter hemorrhages are a sign of vasculitis.

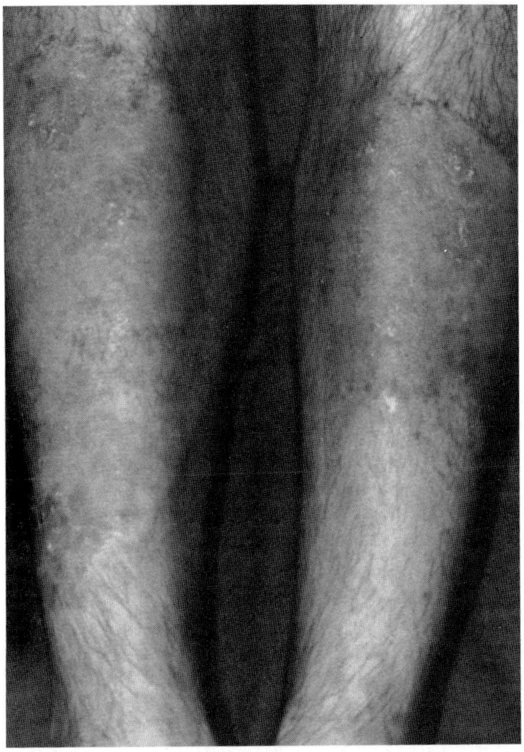

Figure 20.12. Papulosquamous plaques which heal with minimal scar formation are seen in subacute cutaneous LE, a subset of SLE. Typically, concomitant polycyclic lesions are also present.

SLE who developed digital gangrene of the toes secondary to vasculitis. Ultimately, a transmetatarsal amputation was performed.

Treatment

Avoidance of excessive sunlight, cold, and stress is important. As there is no cure, medications are used for palliation, and consideration should always be given to minimizing side effects. For the skin lesions, fluorinated topical steroids under occlusion or intralesional steroid injections are utilized. Recently, total lymphoid irradiation has been tried in eight patients with SLE who had failed to respond to steroids. These patients have improved so far, with 18- to 24-month follow-up (19).

SCLERODERMA

Scleroderma is a disease of unknown etiology and incidence. The term literally means "hard skin," and was originally applied to a condition in which the skin was harder than normal, with reduced mobility on deeper tissues. Through common usage, it is also now applied to diseases in which the skin changes are a prominent feature but which include involvement of other organs (20).

The term scleroderma includes two entirely different processes: (*a*) progressive systemic sclerosis (PSS), or systemic scleroderma, which incorporates symmetrical thickening of the skin with fibrosis and degenerative changes in the synovium, digital arteries, and certain internal organs, notably, the esophagus and intestinal tract, lungs, heart, and kidney; and (*b*) localized or focal scleroderma, which refers to a group of disorders unassociated with systemic disease demonstration circumscribed or patchy fibrosis limited to the skin and, in some cases, immediately subjacent tissues (21, 22) (Table 20.3).

The occurrence of PSS suggests important sex- and age-related factors—it affects females 3:1 over males and occurs more frequently from ages 15 to 44, the childbearing years. There is a higher frequency among black females, with no racial differences found in males (23).

Table 20.3.
Classification of Scleroderma[a]

I. Progressive systemic sclerosis (PSS)
  A. Classical disease: PSS with diffuse scleroderma
    Symmetric diffuse involvement of the skin affecting trunk, face, proximal and distal portions of the extremities; with a tendency toward early appearance of disease of the esophagus, intestine, heart, lung, and kidney
  B. CREST syndrome (formerly known as acrosclerosis)
    Relatively limited skin involvement. Prominence of:
      Calcinosis
      Raynaud's phenomenon
      Esophageal dysfunction
      Sclerodactyly
      Telangiectasia
    Demonstrates prolonged delay in appearance of internal manifestations which are distinctive; pulmonary hypertension and biliary cirrhosis. Many also show evidence of Sjogren's syndrome.
  C. Overlap syndromes
    1. Sclerodermatomyositis
    2. Mixed connective tissue disease (MCTD); combination of PSS, SLE, polymyositis
II. Localized scleroderma
  A. Morphea
    1. Plaque-like
    2. Guttate
    3. Generalized
    4. Less typical forms: subcutaneous, keloid.
  B. Linear scleroderma with or without melorrheostosis
  C. Scleroderma *en coup de sabre* with or without facial hemiatrophy
III. Chemically induced sclerodermoid conditions
IV. Eosinophilic fasciitis

[a] Adapted from Rodnan GP: Progressive systemic sclerosis. *Clin Rheumat Dis* 5:1, 1979.

Progressive Systemic Sclerosis

CLINICAL MANIFESTATIONS

PSS is a generalized disorder affecting both skin and internal organs. It includes a wide spectrum of disease, from diffuse scleroderma with extensive cutaneous changes (Fig. 20.13) and early development of serious systemic involvement, to the CREST syndrome with limited skin changes (24).

Internal organs affected by PSS include the gastrointestinal tract, heart, lung, and kidney. Motility disorders and reflex esophagitis are esophageal signs. Cardiac involvement often is unrecognized, but myocardial fibrosis can result in a major clinical diagnostic sign (25). Pigmentation occurs in 30 to 50% of scleroderma patients; usually there is brown to brown-black discoloration, with involvement primarily of the face, and to a lesser extent, of the abdomen, legs, axillary folds, and dorsal hands (26, 27) (Fig. 20.14).

TREATMENT

There is no cure for systemic sclerosis, so treatment consists of managing the organs involved in an attempt to sustain quality of life. Renal failure is the most frequent cause of death; thus, early aggressive blockade of renin and angiotensin is necessary to protect the remaining function. Irreversible pulmonary fibrosis is the second most frequent cause of death and is unresponsive to therapy. A regimen of prednisone therapy has been shown to give modest improvement in pulmonary function for patients with an inflammatory or vascular lung disease.

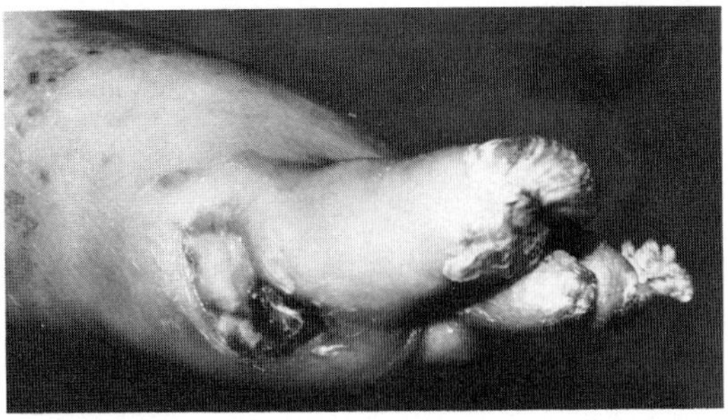

Figure 20.13. Poorly healing ulcerations occurring over bony prominences are a sign of advanced scleroderma. Note the nail dystrophy, a sign of compromised digital vascularity.

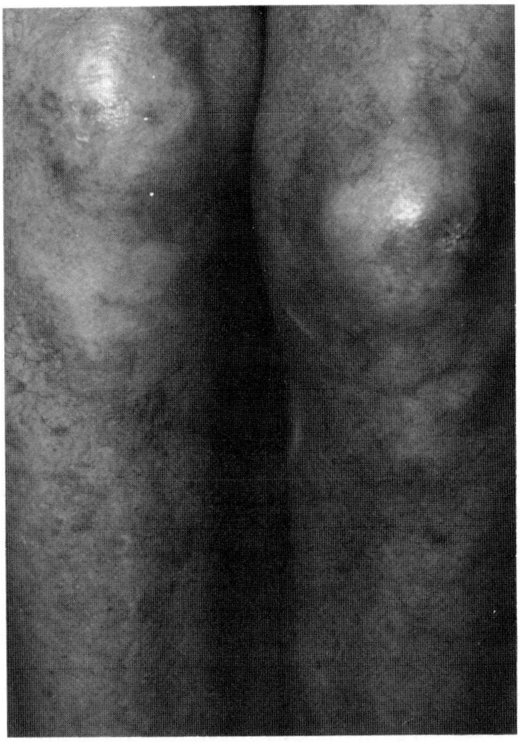

Figure 20.14. Cutaneous dermal thickening, pigmentary alterations, and livedo reticularis are seen on the legs of this patient with scleroderma.

Skin involvement is most troublesome early in the illness. General skin care and avoidance of trauma are important principles to encourage, along with regular movement and exercise to maintain pliability, circulation, and joint mobility (28).

CREST Syndrome

CLINICAL MANIFESTATIONS

The CREST syndrome is one which demonstrates a relatively benign, slowly progressive course of sclerosis (26). Prominent findings include calcinosis cutis, Raynaud's phenomenon, esophageal dysfunction, sclerodactyly, and telangiectasia. It was formerly known as acrosclerosis, due to limitation of the cutaneous sclerotic process to the distal extremities and face. CREST patients have limited internal involvement and, therefore, have a better prognosis than PSS patients. They are not exempt, however, from late visceral disease and may develop trigeminal neuralgia or pulmonary fibrosis with pulmonary hypertension (28). The esophagus is the most frequently involved internal organ, although dysmotility may not be present for many years (29).

CUTANEOUS MANIFESTATIONS

Raynaud's phenomenon is commonly the first manifestation and generally precedes cutaneous involvement by a number of years. Mat-like telangiectases predominate on the face, oral mucosa, and upper extremities (29). Chalky white calcium deposits forming primarily around the peripheral joints are termed calcinosis cutis. It occurs, on the average, 10 years after the onset of the sclerotic process (27). The calcinosis of CREST syndrome tends to be more extensive, and the telangiectasia is more florid than that of PSS with diffuse scleroderma (22). The association of calcinosis and scleroderma was first noted in the early 1900s and is still referred to as the Thibierge-Weissenbach syndrome.

TREATMENT

As with PSS, there is no cure, so the goal is management of manifestations. General skin care should be stressed, and symptoms of esophagitis may be controlled with antacids.

Mixed Connective Tissue Disease

CLINICAL MANIFESTATIONS

Mixed connective tissue disease (MCTD) was first described as a distinct clinical entity in 1972 by Sharp and co-workers (30). It is an overlap syndrome demonstrating features of SLE, PSS, and polymyositis. There is a female preponderance, with a mean age of 37, unknown incidence, but generally good prognosis. The most common symptom is joint pain, followed by symptoms of Raynaud's phenomenon (episodes of color change in the extremities), swollen hands, muscle tenderness, and proximal muscle weakness. There is a high incidence of pulmonary interstitial fibrosis and a low incidence of renal disease.

CUTANEOUS MANIFESTATIONS

Cutaneous manifestations generally include features of both SLE and scleroderma. A diffuse, nonscarring, persistent alopecia occurs in 67% of patients. Laboratory findings demonstrate a high titer of antibody to RNP, a ribonuclease-sensitive form of ENA (extractable nuclear antigen), which is the key diagnostic clue, and a very high ANA titer with a particulate pattern. Rheumatoid factor is present in more than 50% of patients.

TREATMENT

Mild disease is often controlled by nonsteroidal antiinflammatory drugs, or low doses of corticosteroids. With severe major organ involvement, a dose of 1 mg/kg of prednisone is initiated (31). Corticosteroid therapy generally produces a good response (32).

Localized Scleroderma

Localized scleroderma is a disorder of connective tissue limited to the skin, subcutaneous tissue, and muscle. A relatively benign disease, the eruption usually resolves spontaneously after an indefinite period (29). Three times more frequent in women, it favors persons in the second through fourth decades of life and occurs more frequently in Caucasians (33).

Plaque-like morphea is the most frequently encountered type of localized scleroderma. It has a predilection for the trunk and extremities. It consists of a few well-defined, indurated, smooth ivory-colored plaques not bound down to deeper structures (Fig. 20.15). Active lesions have violaceous borders, known as the "lilac ring" which fade as the inflammation sub-

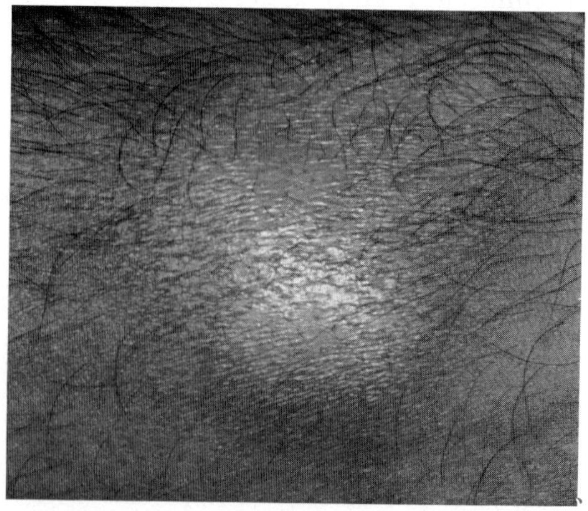

Figure 20.15. Smooth ivory-white plaques surrounded by a lilac-colored border are characteristic of morphea, a localized form of scleroderma limited to the skin.

sides. Loss of hair and absence of sweat are demonstrated in a fully developed lesion. The eruption may heal without sequelae or may result in atrophy and postinflammatory pigmentary changes. Transition to systemic scleroderma seldom occurs.

Guttate morphea occurs infrequently and is characterized by small, round, chalk-white lesions, with a distinctive purplish border (33). They have little tendency to coalesce and gradually undergo atrophy (29). It must be differentiated from lichen sclerosis et atrophicus (white spot disease), which demonstrates comedo-like keratotic plugs, white papules, or macules with angulated edges which may coalesce into plaques (33).

Generalized morphea is rare and is not associated with systemic involvement (33). It may begin in a generalized eruption or may extend from one or more lesions. It favors the upper trunk and thighs and less frequently involves the scalp, face, neck, and lower legs. The lesions are indistinguishable from those of plaque-like morphea, except for the large number of lesions (29). Arthralgia and arthritis are sometimes seen. LE cells and homogenous antinuclear factor have been decribed. The condition usually persists for years, although improvement may be seen in 3 to 5 years (33).

Linear scleroderma is an acute, single unilateral plaque that most frequently affects the lower extremity and less often affects the scalp and face. It is seen chiefly in children, usually under 10 years of age. The eruption consists of a single band-like area of ivory-colored induration affixed to underlying structures (Fig. 20.16). This form of scleroderma may penetrate deeply, even involving muscle and bone. As a result, muscle atrophy and impaired bone growth result in contracture and shortening of the limb (linear hemiatrophy) (29). Linear scleroderma is often associated with congenital anomalies of the vertebral column, namely, spina bifida occulta.

Linear scleroderma occurring on the head is called scleroderma *en coup de sabre*, resembling the scar following a sabre cut. The lesions are linear, sclerotic, ivory-colored depressed plaques that have an irregular hyperpigmented border with telangiectases and linear alopecia. They extend into the scalp and may go as far down as the neck (33). There may be an associated facial hemiatrophy (Parry-Romberg's syndrome), in which one side of the face undergoes sclerodermatous changes with atrophy of underlying subcutaneous tissues and muscles (24).

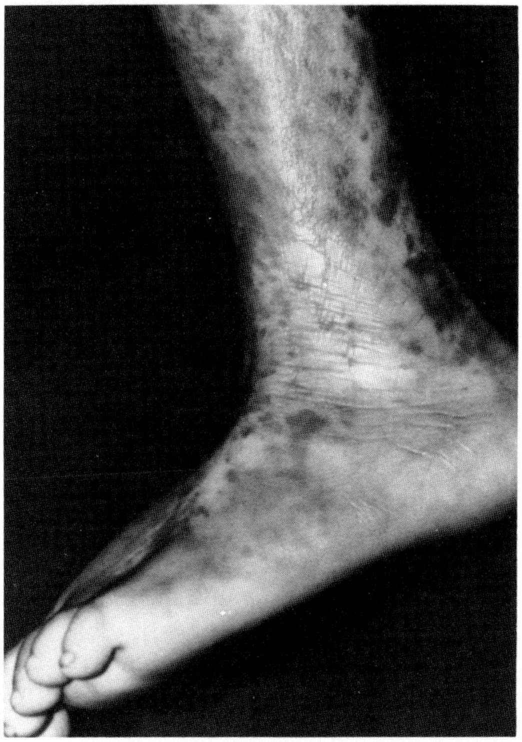

Figure 20.16. Linear scleroderma usually involves the lower extremity and, like morphea, is not a manifestation of systemic scleroderma.

TREATMENT

Localized scleroderma is a self-limiting process, and no specific treatment has been shown to alter its course. Surgical correction of contractures or of disfiguring deformities has been helpful.

Eosinophilic Fasciitis

Eosinophilic fasciitis (Shulman's syndrome) is a scleroderma-like disorder first described by Shulman in 1974 (34). Of the cases reported, there is a 2:1 male preponderance with an age range from 4 to 88 years (22). The etiology is unknown, although a history of recent trauma or unusually strenuous physical exertion is often related. A great majority of the cases have started in either the fall or winter months, but no definitive corollary has been established (35).

The onset may follow a brief prodrome of fever, myalgia, and weakness, and is characterized by pain, swelling, and tenderness of the forearms and legs, occasionally involving the feet and hands. Severe induration of the skin soon develops, with marked limitation of motion of the hands and feet. Flexion contractures may develop within 2 to 3 weeks. The induration may remain confined to the extremities or may spread to involve the trunk, neck, or face. Skin over the indurated areas gives a cobblestone appearance, often described as that of an orange peel, and feels irregularly nodular (34, 36).

Raynaud's phenomenon and internal manifestations of PSS are conspicuously absent. Laboratory studies demonstrate an early transient eosinophilia up to 30%, an increased erythrocyte sedimentation rate (ESR), and hypergammaglobulinemia. Diagnosis is confirmed histologically, utilizing a deep wedge biopsy including skin, subcutaneous tissue, fascia, and muscle. Inflammation and fibrosis may be found in all layers but are greatest in the fascia, which may be thickened as well (22).

TREATMENT

Systemic corticosteroids in small doses provide substantial relief of symptoms, although some cases have involuted spontaneously (23). While most patients appear to undergo full remission after 2 to 4 years of disease, long-term follow-up reveals that some eventually develop scleroderma (37).

DERMATOMYOSITIS

Dermatomyositis is a rare connective tissue disorder affecting both children and adults. It is thought to be primarily a diffuse angiopathy which affects not only the muscles and skin, but also the gastrointestinal tract, adipose tissue, and nervous system (38). When characteristic skin lesions are present, the condition is termed dermatomyositis. Skin is involved in 60% of the cases, although muscle weakness is the key symptom. Females have twice the involvement as do males. The age group most affected is 30 to 60 years old, although a childhood form exists as well. Dermatomyositis shares some features with lupus erythematosus, scleroderma, and rheumatoid arthritis, and is often classified with them under the heading of "collagen vascular diseases."

The etiology of dermatomyositis is unknown, but it appears that hypersensitive immunological mechanisms are involved. Theories suggest abnormalities of the humoral and/or cell-mediated systems which may be triggered by infection, vaccination, neoplasia, or trauma.

Clinical Manifestations

The first symptoms are proximal muscular soreness and weakness. A skin eruption is frequently present when patients become symptomatic. The neck flexors may be severely involved, in which case the patient may not be able to lift his head off the bed. A Trendelenburg gait may be an early finding. The muscles may feel doughy on palpation.

Apart from the musculocutaneous problems, arthralgias and dysphagias may occur. Less commonly, abdominal pain, intestinal ulcers, diffuse cardiomyopathy, and interstitial pneumonitis have been reported.

Cutaneous Manifestations

The characteristic skin lesions are the heliotrope discoloration of the upper eyelids and Gottron's papules overlying the knuckles. The heliotrope rash is often preceded by an edematous phase. Gottron's papules are erythematous violaceous papules and plaques occurring most commonly over the interphalangeal joints of the hands, as well as on the elbows, knees, and ankles (Fig. 20.17). They may resolve, leaving poikilodermatous change. These lesions occur more commonly in dermatomyositis patients but are less specific than heliotrope, as they occur in some LE patients (39).

The lower extremity shows dusky-red poikilodermic patches over bony prominences (Fig. 20.18). As the lesions age and atrophy, they show a "salt-and-pepper" appearance. Ulceration may occur over the malleoli (36).

Laboratory Findings

In acute disease, a moderate leukocytosis may occur. The sedimentation rate is nor-

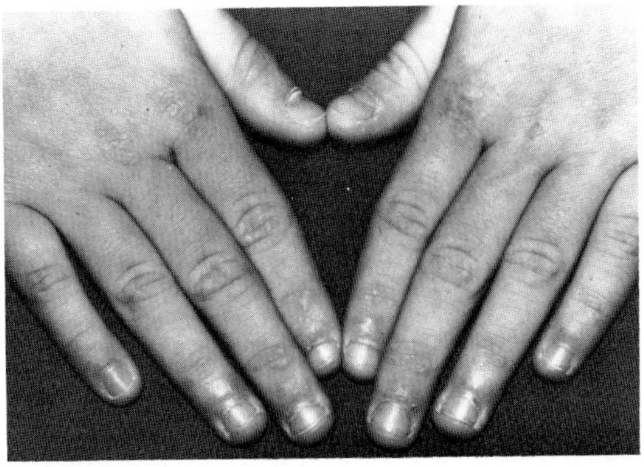

Figure 20.17. Scaling erythematous plaques occurring on the skin, overlying joints of the hands (Gottron's sign) and feet, are characteristic of dermatomyositis.

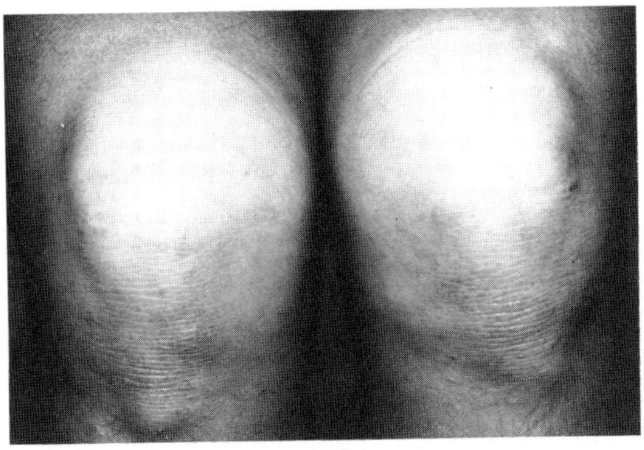

Figure 20.18. Dusky-red poikilodermatous areas are present over the knees of this patient with dermatomyositis.

mal, and anemia may develop in chronic cases. Serum levels of enzymes released from muscle disease, specifically, aldolase, serum glutamic oxaloacetic transaminase (SGOT), and lactic dehydrogenase (LDH), are elevated. Creatine phosphokinase (CPK) is more specific for muscle disease but less sensitive than aldolase (40). Assessment of serum muscle enzyme activity is a useful diagnostic procedure. At the time of diagnosis, the most consistently reliable determination is the SGOT. In charting the clinical response to corticosteroid therapy, it was a common finding that there were differences in the rate of reversal of specific enzyme abnormalities. CPK activity reverted more quickly than SGOT. Aldolase values reacted like CPK but were not as sensitive. Satisfactory disease control did not exist clinically unless normal levels of both SGOT and CPK were maintained (41).

The electromyogram helps to confirm myopathy; however, muscle biopsy is the most definitive method of confirmation. The muscle fibers show irregular areas with loss of cross striations and a waxy type of eosinophilic necrosis. There is variation in fiber size and in the number of sarcolemmal nuclei increases. Early regeneration is evident, and inflammatory cellular infiltrates are present. The pathology of the skin is nonspecific inflammation, with a mononuclear perivascular and scattered infiltrate in the dermis. The serological tests for dermatomyositis, namely, rheumatoid factor, LE cells, and ANA, are not specific and cannot be relied upon to help with the diagnosis. A significant percentage of patients who have the onset of dermatomyositis beyond 50 years of age also have an occult malignancy. A thorough examination for pulmonary, bowel, and kidney tumors should be initiated and performed annually thereafter if a malignancy cannot be found (40).

Childhood Dermatomyositis

Dermatomyositis in children is distinguished from the adult form by early muscle weakness, extensive and early calcinosis, and vasculitis (42). The usual presenting symptoms are muscular weakness, stiffness, easy fatigability, and a skin rash (43). Fever may be the presenting symptom (41). Malignancy is not associated with dermatomyositis in children, while it does affect 20% of adults with the disease (44). Since the adoption of vigorous corticosteroid therapy along with adequate physical therapy and meticulous follow-up, the prognosis for childhood dermatomyositis is much better, and most patients have good musculoskeletal function.

RHEUMATOID ARTHRITIS

Rheumatoid arthritis (RA) is a generalized systemic illness which is characterized by the manner in which it involves joints but also demonstrates many extra-articular signs. It is an autoimmune disorder producing a chronic inflammatory response, with an as yet unproven etiology. Current concept integrates three factors involving etiology: (*a*) genetic makeup of the host; (*b*) the autoimmune response; and (*c*) an inciting agent (45, 46).

Clinical Manifestations

The diagnosis of RA is primarily based on clinical grounds; thus, criteria for diagnosis have been established (Table 20.4). The "typical" rheumatoid arthritic complains of stiffness and pain in multiple joints. Joint swelling is boggy, and the joints are tender to touch, particularly the small joints of the hands and feet. Distal interphalangeal joint involvement is rarely found. The joints are usually not erythematous but often have an elevated temperature. There is a limited range of motion with diminished muscle strength of involved joints. Palmar erythema and prominent veins on the dorsum of the hand, as well as subcutaneous nodules on the extensor surface of the forearm, are often found (47).

Extra-articular complications are found in a number of organ systems. The most common ocular complication of RA in adults is keratoconjunctivitis sicca. Hematologic abnormalities include eosinophilia and thrombocytosis, although the most significant complication is Felty's syndrome (chronic arthritis, splenomegaly, and leukopenia).

Pulmonary disease in RA includes pleuritis, interstitial fibrosis, and pulmonary nodules. Cardiac complications occur in several forms, all of which are related to granulomatous proliferation. They include pericarditis, myocarditis, aortic valve disease, conduction defects, and coronary arteritis.

Vasculitis, although part of the pathology of RA, is also used to group the extra-articular complications which are a result of altered blood supply. There are several forms: (*a*) distal arteritis; (*b*) cutaneous ulceration; (*c*) peripheral neuropathy; (*d*) pericarditis; (*e*) arteritis of the viscera, presenting as claudication or infarction of the organ; and (*f*) acroosteolysis.

Vasculitis may only be demonstrated in a neurovascular disease. One pattern is a mild distal sensory neuropathy with symptoms of paresthesia or "burning feet," together with signs of decreased touch and sharp-dull discrimination. Another pattern is that of a severe sensorimotor neuropathy (mononeuritis multiplex), with a drop foot characteristic of muscle weakness. The symptoms are identical to those of polyarteritis. (See section on polyarteritis.)

Cutaneous Manifestations

Patients with longstanding RA often have skin that is pale, translucent, shiny, and atrophic. It is not bound down to underlying tissue as in scleroderma. The skin changes are most apparent on the hands, fingers, and toes (4, 47, 48). Palmar erythema is also a frequent feature.

Rheumatoid nodules develop in 20% of patients with RA, particularly in those with severe forms demonstrating a positive rheumatoid factor. They tend to occur over pressure points, and the extensor surface of the elbows, and lumbosacral area are the most frequent locations, although they also may be found on the hands, knees, ears, and scapula. Pedal morbidity, in the form of bunions, hammertoes, ulcers, and callosities, has been reported in 85 to 92% of RA patients (49).

Rheumatoid vasculitis is an arteritis that

Table 20.4.
American Rheumatological Association Criteria for Rheumatoid Arthritis[a]

1. Morning stiffness for at least 6 weeks
2. Pain on motion or tenderness of at least one joint for at least 6 weeks
3. Swelling (soft tissue or fluid) of one joint for at least 6 weeks
4. Swelling of a second joint within 3 months lasting for at least 6 weeks
5. Symmetrical or bilateral swelling of metacarpal-phalangeal, proximal interphalangeal, and metatarsal-phalangeal joints for at least 6 weeks
6. Subcutaneous nodules over bony prominences or extensor surfaces
7. X-ray changes (at least decalcification in periarticular bone)
8. Positive test for rheumatoid factor
9. Poor mucin precipitate from synovial fluid
10. Characteristic histologic evidence of synovitis
11. Characteristic histopathology from rheumatoid nodule biopsy

[a] Adapted from Koffler D: Immunology of rheumatoid diseases, *Clin Symp* 31 (4):25, 1979.

involves the small arteries. Features include peripheral neuropathy, digital gangrene, nail fold infarcts, and cutaneous ulcers (Fig. 20.19). A common form of necrotizing vasculitis involves the venules of the skin. Cutaneous venulitis most often appears on the lower extremity or over dependent areas. It is seen as erythematous papules (palpable purpura) which do not blanch upon pressure. The venular lesions are not related to duration but rather to the severity of the arthritis.

Treatment

There are three primary areas involved in management of a patient with RA: (*a*) supportive measures; (*b*) drugs; and (*c*) surgery (50).

Supportive measures are indicated throughout all phases of the disease. They include education of the patient and family, rest, physical exercise and therapy, occupational therapy, and rehabilitation services.

Drug treatment is divided into three phases. Phase I is antiinflammatory agents. Aspirin is still the appropriate drug for initial treatment. Nonsteroidal antiinflammatory drugs (NSAIDs) are indicated if a patient is not able to tolerate aspirin. Local corticosteroid injections are also a valuable part of the therapeutic regimen. Phase II is remission-inducing agents, including antimalarials (i.e., hydroxychloroquine), gold salts, and penicillamine. As knowledge of dosage and toxicity has advanced, there has been a tendency to use these drugs earlier in the course of the disease and no longer to consider them a drug of last resort. Phase III are the immunoregulatory and/or experimental agents, including systemic corticosteroids, azathioprine, cyclophosphamide, and levamisole.

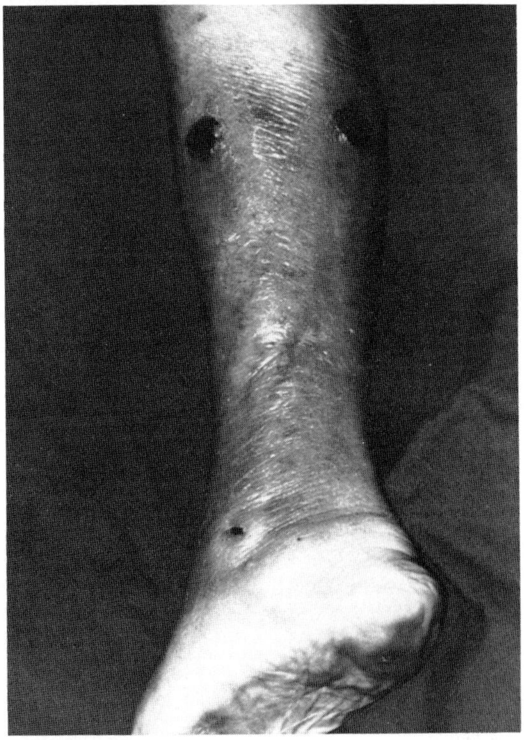

Figure 20.19. Punched-out ulcers due to vasculitis are present in this patient with rheumatoid arthritis.

Surgical procedures include those which are prophylactic and those which are reconstructive or restorative. Prophylactic procedures include synovectomy, release of a trapped nerve, local excision of nodules, and fusion of cervical spine. Restorative or reconstructive procedures include arthrodesis, arthroplasty, and joint replacement.

Arthrodesis was the only procedure available for the arthritic ankle until recent years. Total ankle replacement is now an option for the rheumatoid patient with a stable ankle and whose rearfoot deformity can be difficult due to the softness of the bone and typical valgus rearfoot and abducted forefoot. A metatarsal osteotomy may be indicated for a painful callus over a prominent metatarsal which is not rigidly subluxed. For fixed subluxation, metatarsal head excision is indicated. Multiple metatarsal head excisions (II through V) are often combined with a double-stemmed silicone prosthesis in the first metatarsophalangeal joint for rheumatoids with severe forefoot involvement.

POLYARTERITIS

Polyarteritis is a variable multisystemic disease characterized pathologically by inflammation and fibrinoid necrosis of medium-sized and small arteries. It used to be known as periarteritis nodosa. The term nodosa was dropped, as nodules were not frequently found. Polyarteritis replaced periarteritis because the entire arterial wall is involved. Muscle and joint complaints predominate, and the disease seems to have some relationship to the vascular lesions of

RA, SLE, rheumatic fever and, possibly, adrenocortical steroid therapy (51). Patients develop polyarteritis vascular lesions with serum sickness and allergic reactions to sulfonamides, iodides, thiouracil, dilantin, penicillin, and other drugs. Lesions have been reproduced in experimental animals which have been challenged with a variety of protein antigens. Also, infectious agents have been implicated, namely, β-hemolytic *Streptococcus*. Experimental lesions in animals have been induced by administering carcinogens or creating experimental hypertension.

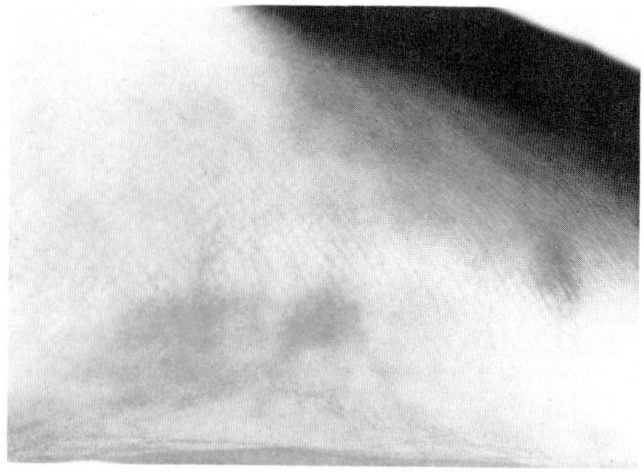

Figure 20.20. Tender nodules occurring in a linear configuration are seen on the foot of this patient with periarteritis nodosa.

Clinical Manifestations

The clinical features are protean, with initial presentations which include fever of unknown origin with weight loss, primary renal disease, hypertension, acute abdominal pain, pulmonary complaints, myocardial infarction or coronary insufficiency, muscular aching, tenderness and wasting, or peripheral neuritis.

Cutaneous Manifestations

Cutaneous changes occur in 25% of the cases. Variably sized tender skin or subcutaneous nodules often occur linearly and in crops along the course of blood vessels (Fig. 20.20). Purpura may occur as well as vesicles and bullae, urticaria, angioneurotic edema, a scarletiniform rash, livedo reticularis, and cutaneous necrosis. Distal necrosis of the fingers and toes has been reported; however, Raynaud's phenomenon and gangrene of the extremities are rare. It has been recently reported that painful feet are the presenting complaint in 4% of the patients with classic polyarteritis (52).

It is felt that there is a relationship between polyarteritis and rheumatoid arthritis because there have been reports of a diffuse arteritis occurring in patients with RA that is clinically and pathologically indistinguishable from polyarteritis. There is some concern that the reason vasculitic lesions are being seen with increased frequency in RA patients may be due to a deleterious side effect of steroid therapy.

GENERAL PODIATRIC CONSIDERATIONS

The feet of patients with connective tissue disease are generally painful, atrophic, and dysvascular. In the case of rheumatoid arthritis, if the vasculature is adequate, surgical procedures may be performed for pain relief and correction of deformities. However, in many cases of lupus erythematosus and scleroderma, the peripheral circulation is diminished, and biomechanical and palliative measures are indicated. Often, pain in the feet is the most troublesome manifestation of connective tissue diseases, and proper podiatric care can be an enormous benefit to the patient's ability to function.

References

1. Moschella SL, Moschella SL, Pillsbury DM, Hurley KJ (eds): *Dermatology*. Philadelphia, W.B. Saunders, 1975, pp 913–959.
2. Moschella SL, Moschella SL, Pillsbury DM, Hurley KJ (eds): *Dermatology*. Philadelphia, W.B. Saunders, 1975, p 837.
3. Spittell JA Jr, Fairbairn JF II, Juergens JL, Spittell JA Jr (eds): *Allen-Barker-Hines Peripheral Vascular Diseases*, ed 4. Philadelphia, W.B. Saunders, 1972, p 388.
4. Braverman IM: *Skin Signs of Systemic Disease*, ed 2. Philadelphia, W.B. Saunders, 1970, p 350.
5. Stewart WD, Danto JL, Maddin S: *Dermatology: Diagnosis and Treatment of Cutaneous Disorders*, ed 4. St. Louis, C.V. Mosby, 1978, p 573.
6. Fitzpatrick RB, Arndt KA, Clark WH, Eisen AZ, Van Scott EJ, Vaughan JH: *Dermatology in General Medicine*. New York, McGraw-Hill, 1971, p 16.
7. Fye K, Matsopoulos H, Talal N, Sudenberg HH, Stites DP, Caldwell JL, Wells JV (eds): *Basic and Clinical Immunology*. Los Altos, CA, Lang, 1976, p 363.
8. Maricq HR, Maize JC: Nailfold capillary

abnormalities. *Clin Rheum Dis* 8:455–478, 1982.
9. Kenik JG, Maricq HR, Bole GG: Blind evaluation of the diagnostic specificity of nailfold capillary microscopy in the connective tissue diseases. *Arthritis Rheum* 24:885–891, 1981.
10. Maricq HR, LeRoy EC, D'Angelo WA, et al: Diagnostic potential of in vivo capillary microscopy in scleroderma and related disorders. *Arthritis Rheum* 23:183, 1980.
11. Prystowsky SD, Gilliam JN: Discoid lupus erythematosus as a part of a larger disease spectrum. *Arch Dermatol* 111:1448, 1975.
12. Rothfield NF, March CH, Fitzpatrick RB, Arndt KA, Clark WH et al: *Dermatology in General Medicine*. New York, McGraw-Hill, 1971, p 1493.
13. Morley KD, Leons A, Rynes RI: Lupus foot. *Br Med J* 20:557–558, 1982.
14. Fries JF, Holman HR: *Systemic Lupus Erythematosus: A Clinical Analysis*. Philadelphia, W.B. Saunders, 1975, p 28.
15. Callen JP, Kingman J: Cutaneous vasculitis in SLE. *Cutis* 32:433–436, 1983.
16. Sontheimer RD, Thomas JR, Gilliam JN: Subacute cutaneous lupus erythematosus. *Arch Dermatol* 115:1409–1415, 1979.
17. Kidawa AS, Roth RD: SLE heralded by pedal cutaneous lesions: report of a case. *J Am Podiatry Assoc* 68:117–119, 1978.
18. Mandell LM, Martin EM, Gudas CJ: Pedal complications of SLE: a case history. *J Am Podiatry Assoc* 68:535–541, 1978.
19. Henahan J: Anticancer treatments can fight arthritic disorders. *JAMA* 250:2096–2097, 1983.
20. Barnett AJ: *Scleroderma (Progressive Systemic Sclerosis)*. Springfield, IL, Charles C Thomas, 1974, pp 31–49.
21. Jablonska S: *Scleroderma and Pseudoscleroderma*, ed 2. Warsaw, Polish Medical, 1975, pp 243–272.
22. Rodnan GP: Progressive systemic sclerosis. *Clin Rheum Dis* 5:1, 1979.
23. Tierney RJ: Rheumatology corner: scleroderma. *Minn Med* 64:475, 1981.
24. Hochberg MC: The spectrum of systemic sclerosis—current concepts. *Hosp Pract*:61, 1981.
25. Spector FC, Kalish SR, Spinner SM: The sclerodermatous foot. *J Am Podiatry Assoc* 72:114, 1982.
26. Fenske NA, Millins JL: Scanning the skin for signs of connective tissue disorders. *Geriatrics* 36:47–86, 1981.
27. Winkelmann RK: The cutaneous diagnosis of dermatomyositis, lupus erythematosus and scleroderma. *NY State J Med* 63:3080, 1963.
28. LeRoy EC, Kelly WN, Harris ED Jr, Ruddy S, Sledge CB (eds): *Textbook of Rheumatology*. Philadelphia, W.B. Saunders, 1981, p 1224.
29. Irgang S: Scleroderma: a comprehensive review. *Cutis* 12:848, 1973.
30. Sharp GC, Irving WG, Tan EM, Gould RG, Holman HR: Mixed connective tissue disease—an apparently distinct rheumatic disease syndrome associated with a specific antibody to an extractable nuclear antigen (ENA). *Am J Med* 52:148–149, 1972.
31. Sharp GC, Kelly WN, Harris ED Jr, Ruddy S, Sledge CB (eds): *Textbook of Rheumatology*. Philadelphia, W.B. Saunders, 1981, p 1151.
32. Chubick A, Gilliam JN: A review of mixed connective tissue disease. *Int J Dermatol* 17:123, 1978.
33. Moschella SL, Moschella SL, Pillsbury DM, Hurley HJ Jr: *Dermatology*. Philadelphia, W.B. Saunders, 1975, p 933.
34. Shulman LE: Diffuse fasciitis with hypergammaglobulinemia and eosinophilia: a new syndrome (abstr). *J. Rheumatol* 1 (Suppl 1):46, 1974.
35. Sills EM: Diffuse fasciitis with eosinophilia in childhood. *Johns Hopkins Med J* 151:203–207, 1982.
36. Samitz MH: *Cutaneous Disorders of the Lower Extremities*, ed 2. Philadelphia, J.B. Lippincott, 1981, pp 121–129.
37. Torres VM, George WM: Diffuse eosinophilic fasciitis. *Arch Dermatol* 113:1591–1593, 1977.
38. Banker BQ, Victor M: Dermatomyositis (systemic angiopathy) of Childhood. *Medicine* 45:261, 1966.
39. Callen JP: *Cutaneous Aspects of Internal Disease*. Chicago, Yearbook Medical Publishers, 1981, p 21.
40. Mills JA, Fitzpatrick RB, Arndt KA, Clark WH et al (eds): *Dermatology in General Medicine*. New York, McGraw-Hill, 1971, pp 1518–1525.
41. Sullivan DM, Cassidy JT, Petty RE, Burt A: Prognosis in childhood dermatomyositis. *J Pediatr* 80:555–563, 1972.
42. Dubowitz V: Muscle disorders in childhood. *Br J Hosp Med* 2:1627, 1969.
43. Goel KM, Shanks RA: Dermatomyositis in childhood. *Arch Dis Child* 51:801, 1976.
44. Schaller JG: Dermatomyositis. *J Pediatr* 83:699–702, 1973.
45. Robinson WD, Hollander JL, McCarty DJ Jr: *Arthritis and Allied Conditions*, ed 8. Philadelphia, Lea & Febiger, 1972, p 297.
46. Bennett JC, Kelly WN, Harris ED Jr, Ruddy S, Sledge CB (eds): *Textbook of Rheumatology*. Philadelphia, W.B. Saunders, 1981, p 887.
47. Harris ED Jr, Kelley WN, Harris ED Jr,

Ruddy S, Sledge CB (eds): *Textbook of Rheumatology*. Philadelphia, W.B. Saunders, 1981, p 928.
48. Gilkes JJ: Cutaneous manifestations of the rheumatic diseases. *Practitioner* 220:68–72, 1978.
49. Black JR, Cahalin C, Germain BF: Pedal morbidity in rheumatic diseases: a clinical study. *J Am Podiatry Assoc* 72:360–362, 1982.
50. Ruddy S, Kelley WN, Harris ED Jr, Ruddy S, Sledge CB (eds): *Textbook of Rheumatology*. Philadelphia, W.B. Saunders, 1981, p 1000.
51. Shulman LE, Harvey AM, Hollander JL, McCarty DJ (eds): *Arthritis and Allied Conditions*, ed 8. Philadelphia, Lea & Febiger, pp 918–939.
52. Cupps TR, Fauci AS: *The Vasculitides*. Philadelphia, W.B. Saunders, 1981.

CHAPTER 21

Pedal Dermatologic Emergencies

THOMAS DELAURO

INTRODUCTION

The human foot is encased in a warm dark moist environment by materials which are often incompatible with health: our feet are constantly bombarded with dermatologic insults which may eventually express as a skin disease. Skin pathology manifests itself with great variability. One must learn to differentiate those which pose a threat to life (Fig. 21.1), vs. those which are of great concern to the patient because of their abrupt appearance but which are relatively benign (Fig. 21.2). Such is the division between the true dermatologic emergency and those disorders which are more startling than life-threatening.

Skin changes need not always be the result of primary dermatologic diseases. Integumentary pathology may occur secondary to underlying vascular, neural, or musculoskeletal pathology. Consider a hypothetical case study of a patient presenting with hyperpigmentation and desquamation about the medial forefoot: Tinea pedis or some other scaling dermatoses might well form a reasonable working diagnosis. This individual, however, could actually be exhibiting signs of a subacute sequelae of a 2-week-old gouty attack (Fig. 21.3). Skin changes in such an instance can be reflective of primary rheumatologic disease. Such examples emphasize the need for ascertaining the true etiologic hosts of the presenting symptomatology. An adequate treatment plan will never be forthcoming until diagnosis is made with precision.

Simply listing dermatologic conditions randomly or by etiology is not always the most clinically helpful approach. Rather, a classification based upon the type of lesion (i.e., macule, papule, etc.) would seem more useful.

Using such a system to categorize especially threatening pedal dermatologic disorders, one may divide the symptomatology into four morphologic groups: vesiculobullae, erythematous macules, purpuric eruptions, and nodular diseases. In each category, only those diseases dangerous to life or limb will be discussed in the present study. Dermatoses that may occur abruptly but without serious consequences will be omitted. They will, however, be discussed elsewhere in this text.

VESICULOBULLOUS DISEASES

Differential Diagnosis

The mechanobullous diseases, cryoglobulinemia, and those vesiculobullae associated with internal carcinoma are representative of this grouping. As they have been more fully discussed in the chapter on blistering diseases, the reader is referred to that chapter.

ANTICOAGULATION NECROSIS (1)

This particular syndrome was originally described in reference to patients taking warfarin sodium. The same disorder, however, has been reported in patients receiving intravenous and low dose heparin sodium therapy. Initial lesions consist of localized erythematous areas that rapidly progress to bullae. These bullae soon become hemorrhagic and progress to true necrosis. While heparin necrosis usually occurs within localized injection sites, its possible occurrence in areas unrelated to injection is quite alarming.

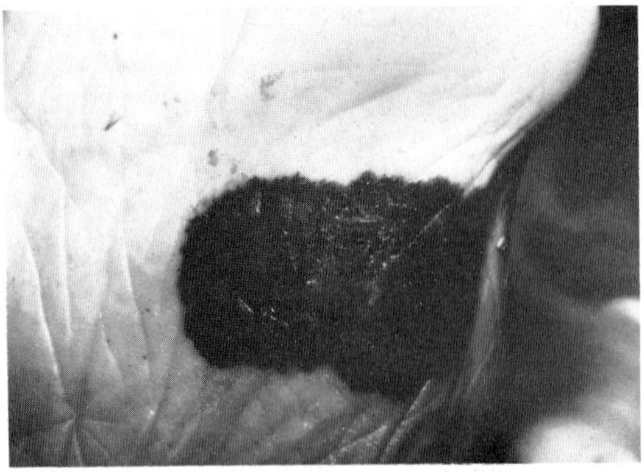

Figure 21.1. Malignant melanoma of the sole.

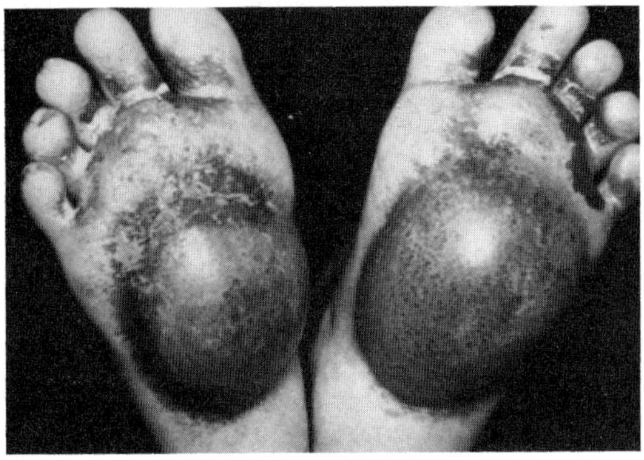

Figure 21.2. Primary irritant contact dermatitis.

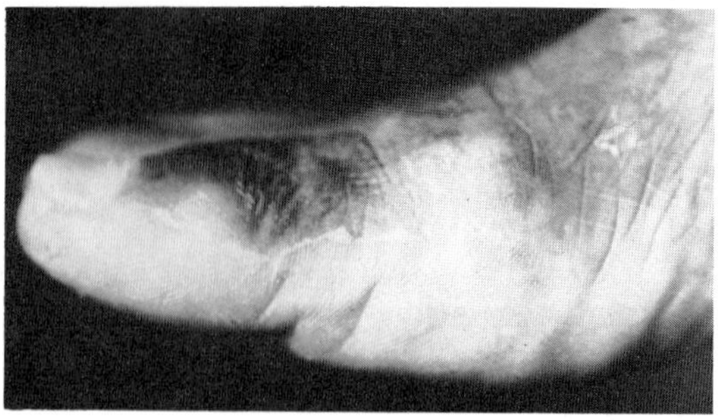

Figure 21.3. Skin changes in a 2-week-old gouty attack.

Heparin necrosis often develops within 6 to 13 days of treatment, whereas warfarin necrosis occurs much sooner (in 3 to 5 days). Beyond this differentiating feature, both conditions are clinically indistinguishable. Dermal and subcutaneous erythrocyte extravasation, the absence of marked inflammatory response, and occlusion of dermal and subcutaneous veins by fibrin thrombi constitute the histopathologic findings. Women appear to be more likely to develop the disease than men.

The delayed onset witnessed in either type of anticoagulation necrosis has suggested an immunologic etiology. Recently, an immunoglobulin platelet aggregating factor that is heparin-dependent has been found; a similar finding in warfarin-treated patients remains to be identified. Such a platelet aggregating factor could account for the combination of thrombocytopenia and thrombosis seen in these patients.

Thrombosis can also be accelerated through withdrawal of broad-spectrum antibiotics (overproduction of vitamin K factors) or through elevations of free fatty acids within the bloodstream (either heparin-induced or as occurs in obese patients). Very often these are associated findings in patients on heparin or warfarin therapy, hence, the increased tendency toward the infarction and thrombocytopenia witnessed in such cases.

ERYTHEMATOUS MACULES

Differential Diagnosis

ROCKY MOUNTAIN SPOTTED FEVER (2)

The causative organism, *Rickettsia rickettsii*, is transmitted to humans by the bite of its arthropod vector, the tick. Disease incidence is greatest during late spring and early summer, when ticks are most active. Usually within 1 week of contact, an abrupt onset of disease occurs which is characterized by severe headache, fever, chills, nausea, and generalized myalgia.

The fourth febrile day is joined by the erythematous macules affecting hands and feet, which is a characteristic of this disorder. Soon these lesions spread centrally to the trunk and face. In 2 or 3 days, macules become papular and then purpuric, a phenomenon consistent with vasculitis (see below). This vessel pathology occurs throughout internal viscera, accounting for the mortality of this illness secondary to shock or renal failure. Ironically enough, the simple administration of tetracycline can prevent death when the disease is recognized early.

MENINGOCOCCEMIA (2)

Meningococcemia may present in the same fashion as Rocky Mountain spotted fever. However, differentiation is possible since the rash of meningococcemia occurs extremely rapidly after the onset of constitutional changes (not after several days, as in spotted fever).

LEUKOCYTOCLASTIC ANGIITIS (3)

The lesions of this disorder begin as erythematous macules, but they are rapidly modified into purpuric lesions. Hence, leukocytoclastic angiitis is more appropriately discussed in the section below on purpuric lesions.

PURPURIC ERUPTIONS

In contrast to erythematous macules, purpuric lesions are the result of actual bleeding into the skin. This represents the deposition of pigment, and therefore lesions will not blanch upon diascopy. Purpura will assume different configurations based upon the dimension of the pathologic vessels. Rupture of small vessels (i.e., arterioles, venules, and capillaries) will result in pinpoint or "petechial" hemorrhages, whereas damage to larger vessels will result in ecchymosis, hematoma, or hemarthrosis (Fig. 21.4).

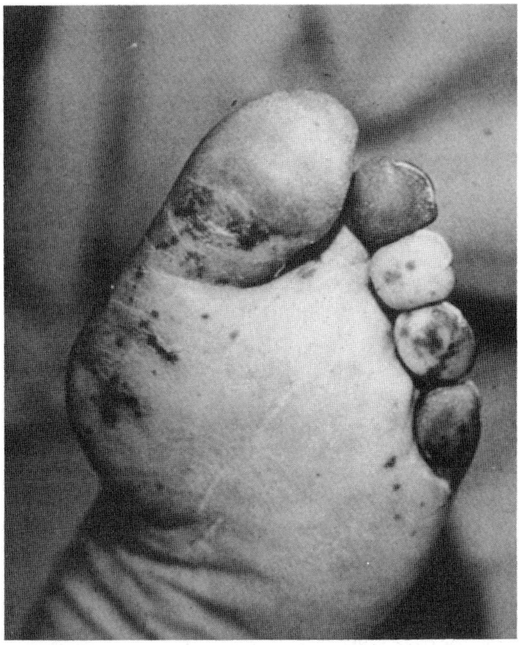

Figure 21.4. Purpuric changes secondary to rheumatoid vasculitis.

Differential Diagnosis

LEUKOCYTOCLASTIC ANGIITIS (LCA) (3)

This autoimmune disease affects arterioles, capillaries, and venules in skin and internal organs. It differs from other forms of angiitis (i.e., macroscopic panarteritis nodosa, Wegener's granulomatosis) both histologically and in its broader clinical manifestations. LCA derives its name from the characteristic appearance of the leukocytes found in involved segments. These cells exhibit nuclear fragmentation, or "nuclear dust", hence, the designation leukocytoclastic angiitis.

The cutaneous changes of LCA are secondary to exudation and hemorrhage rather than to ischemia. Blood vessels within the upper dermis are usually affected, leading initially to the formation of an erythematous macule, as described previously. Edema and subsequent extravascular hemorrhage transform macules into papules and then purpuric papules, respectively. The feet, ankles, and lower legs are characteristically involved in a bilateral fashion. Progression of disease leads to thrombosis and therefore ulceration.

Leukocytoclastic angiitis may appear in two clinical forms (3): (*a*) Henoch-Schoenlein or anaphylactoid purpura, or (*b*) a cutaneous-systemic variant. The former affects mainly young boys, is preceded by an upper respiratory infection with mild constitutional symptoms, and predilects for the late fall and early spring months. In addition to the cutaneous rash, the vasculitis can affect the kidney, gut, and joints, leading to complaints referable to these areas.

The cutaneous-systemic form (a designation selected by Braverman), more commonly affects adults; there is no sex predilection. The form represents a spectrum of disease: It may range from pure cutaneous to purely visceral involvement, with a certain percentage exhibiting both cutaneous and visceral involvement. Signs of cutaneous vasculitis are preceded by mild constitutional changes, as in the Henoch-Schoenlein form. Death can result from vasculitis-induced renal failure. Fortunately, fatality occurs in only a small percentage of patients (in contrast to the rapidly fatal course of macroscopic panarteritis nodosa). Early urinalysis in such patients can detect renal involvement, permitting rapid initiation of therapy directed at halting the process.

Leukocytoclastic angiitis can therefore exist in a relatively benign form, but it may develop serious complications. It can also occur, for unknown reasons, in association with patients afflicted by rheumatoid arthritis, lupus erythematosus, leukemias, and lymphomas.

Diagnosis depends upon recognition of characteristic lesions and histopathology.

BACTERIAL ENDOCARDITIS (4)

Bacterial endocarditis exists in subacute and acute clinical forms, determined by the infectious organism and the presence of pre-existing cardiac disease. The acute type with its rapidly fulminating course results from invasion by true pathogens; a prior cardiopathy is not a prerequisite. Conversely, subacute bacterial endocarditis occurs in patients with congenital or rheumatic heart disease following injection with less pathogenic bacterial species.

In either case, vegetations composed of fibrin and platelets develop at the site of infection. Small fragments may now break free and embolize to any tissue, producing a variable clinical picture (Fig. 21.5). Cutaneous lesions of the extremities are secondary to such vascular change and may be petechial or gangrenous. In the case of petechial lesions, histologic section reveals these to be secondary to an immune vasculitis, and therefore they are probably not embolic in nature.

The combination of fever, cardiac murmurs, and cutaneous lesions of the type to be discussed are certain indicators of bacterial endocarditis. In the subacute type, subungual splinter hemorrhages are often found. Digital pulps may exhibit tender, purple, or erythematous subcutaneous papules known as Osler's nodes. Larger nodules, probably embolic in origin, may develop on the palms and soles. These are known as Janeway lesions. Emboli to larger arteries may create claudication or frank gangrene.

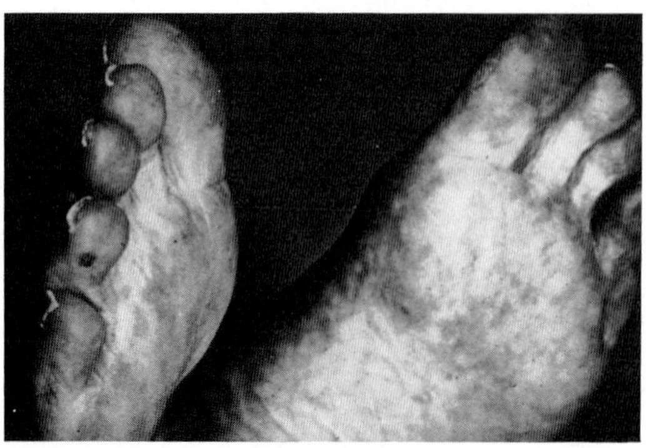

Figure 21.5. Microembolism of the feet.

In contrast, acute bacterial endocarditis demonstrates many petechial and embolic changes, but Osler's nodes and Janeway lesions are absent.

In either case, early diagnosis is imperative since few untreated patients survive. No laboratory tests have been found helpful in the diagnosis of this condition.

OTHER LIFE-THREATENING DISEASES THAT MAY MANIFEST PALPABLE PURPURA

Meningococcemia, leukemia, and rickettsial disease may also manifest with palpable purpura, as described above.

NODULAR DISEASE

Nodules represent masses located beneath the skin. When they approach large dimension, they may be called tumors. Nodules may be either soft or firm, solitary or multiple, tender or nontender, and fixed or nonfixed to the overlying skin.

Differential Diagnosis

LEUKOCYTOCLASTIC ANGIITIS (3)

The identical pathologic process may affect vessels more deeply placed within the dermis. In this location, nodules develop, rather than purpuric papules. These nodules are inflammatory in nature, and tender to palpation. When vessels in this cutaneous location are affected, other presentations include livedo reticularis and atrophie blanche.

BACTERIAL ENDOCARDITIS (3)

The reader should recall that Osler's nodes and Janeway lesions may occur in these patients.

MACROSCOPIC PANARTERITIS NODOSA (3)

Because of the larger-sized vessels afflicted, this autoimmune disease does not primarily affect the skin. According to

Braverman, its only valid cutaneous signs include 5- to 10-mm subcutaneous nodules (which are in actuality small aneurysms). These nodules follow the course of arteries. Ulcerations result from infarction, in addition to gangrene of fingers and toes, and ecchymoses secondary to rupture of aneurysms and weakened arterial walls (Fig. 21.6). As in leukocytoclastic angiitis, visceral blood vessels are also affected. As a result, macroscopic panarteritis nodosa frequently follows a fatal course.

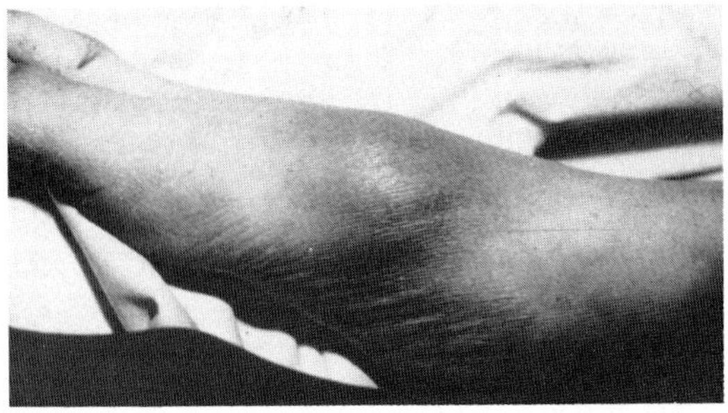

Figure 21.6. Nodose lesions of panarteritis nodosa on the dorsum of the foot.

THE PANNICULITIDES

The panniculitides represent a group of painful disorders involving subcutaneous fat. Factitial and purulent types result from readily identifiable etiologies. The remaining types form the "nodular nonsuppurative" variety.

Nodular nonsuppurative panniculitis may be associated with fever and a synovitis of the distal articulations, including the metatarsophalangeal joints. Females in the third to fourth decade of life appear to be most commonly affected, although an infant form does exist (4). Occasionally single, but more often multiple, tender subcutaneous nodules develop in recurrent crops, which is characteristic of these disorders. Necrosis and drainage of the nodules rarely occurs. Histologically, these nodules form secondary to leukocytic invasion. The postinflammatory healing and fibrosis lead to localized fat atrophy, which is manifest clinically as hyperpigmented depressions in the previously nodular areas. Although they occur most commonly over the shins, dorsal foot nodules have been reported in both the adult and infant forms (5).

Nodular nonsuppurative panniculitis is included because of its association with pancreatic diseases (6), including carcinoma of the pancreas (particularly that of the body and tail of the pancreatic body. Such patients usually present with multiple panniculitic areas of the lower extremities, which in theory are the result of circulating lipases released by the diseased pancreas.

Nodular nonsuppurative panniculitis has been found to be associated with trauma, halogen compounds or other drug ingestions, and infections, especially of a tuberculous nature. Association with histoplasmosis has also been reported (7), as well as dermatomyositis (8), systemic lupus erythematosus (8, 9), and steroid withdrawal. Other conditions, such as ulcerative colitis, jejunoileal bypass surgery (10), erythema nodosum, sarcoidosis, Hodgkin's disease, glomerulonephritis, diabetes mellitus, and α-1-antitrypsin deficiency have been implicated (7). This last occurrence, with α-1-antitrypsin deficiency patients, has resulted in terminal disease. These disorders are generally not immediately life-threatening conditions, however.

CASE REPORTS FOR STUDY

Case 1

An obese female patient in her early 30s was admitted for corrective foot surgery. She was an insulin-dependent diabetic who had been on a course of cephalosporins preoperatively for an ulceration of her right heel which recently closed. Postoperatively, the patient was given low dose heparin sodium injections subcutaneously as a prophylactic measure: The surgeon wished to avoid the development of deep thrombophlebitis while she required total bed rest.

On the third postoperative day, the patient developed painful hemorrhagic bullae on her feet and legs bilaterally. Drug sensitivity eruption was suspected, and all medications discontinued. On the fourth postoperative day, she developed massive chest pain and was immediately transferred to intensive care, where she expired of a myocardial infarction. What is your assessment?

COMMENT

This patient had anticoagulation necrosis, which ultimately led to her death secondary to coronary occlusion. Her sex, obesity, and history of diabetes mellitus, when coupled with her delayed cutaneous response to heparin therapy, point to this possibility.

Case 2 (11)

A male patient in his early 20s presented with a maculopapular rash of both ankles which had spread to the legs as well. In addition to these dermatologic findings, he experienced weakness, recurrent fever, and anorexia, and he gave a history of repeated bouts of pharyngitis and unremitting cough. Laboratory examination revealed the patient to be pancytopenic, with multiple immunologic deficiencies. His rash was diagnosed as neurodermatitis, and appropriate topical steroids were prescribed.

Several months later, this same patient presented with spiking fevers and the residua of the earlier rash (now excoriated and hyperpigmented) on both ankles and legs. He remained pancytopenic. While awaiting consultation he expired from a severe pneumonia which was proven to be the result of opportunistic pathogens at autopsy. What is your impression?

COMMENT

Several clues exist as to the possible presence of vasculitis. They are (*a*) the combination of skin rash with multiorgan disease, (*b*) the synchronous or consecutive involvement of several organ systems, (*c*) the occurrence of common diseases in an atypical setting (*i.e.*, peripheral vascular disease in a young patient), and (*d*) constitutional symptoms that are out of proportion to physical findings.

Some of these clues were observed in the present case study, hence, the suspicion of vasculitis, and a tireless search for its cause should have been initiated. A biopsy of the skin lesions at autopsy demonstrated that they were secondary to vasculitis.

Case 3 (12)

A middle-aged male required hospitalization for undiagnosed abdominal pain. He exhibited mild fever, and while in the hospital, developed chest pain of pleuritic nature. Abnormal blood findings include thrombocytosis and an elevated erythrocyte sedimentation rate. Radiologic examination of the chest had revealed signs indicating pulmonary infarction, for which the patient was treated. Similar studies of the abdomen gave evidence of large bowel obstruction.

On the fifth hospital day, podiatric consultation was initiated because of an erythematous macular rash which had developed on his feet and ankles bilaterally. Some macules had transformed into purpuric papules, which in turn progressed to areas of frank necrosis. What is your impression?

COMMENT

Henoch-Schönlein, or anaphylactoid, purpura is notably a disease of children but can occur in adults. The progression of early lesions into purpuric papules is virtually pathognomonic of leukocytoclastic angiitis. The involvement of internal viscera that is a part of this disorder accounts for the pulmonary and gastrointestinal findings. Once the diagnosis was made, a course of systemic corticosteroids ameliorated the condition, permitting early discharge from the hospital and avoiding a fatal outcome.

Case 4

A 50-year-old agitated, restless female complained of red and purple skin lesions that predominate subungually and periungually. This patient had suffered rheumatic fever as a child and now takes oral penicillin prophylactically as partial treatment for a resulting cardiopathy. She perspired profusely, was in great discomfort, and exhibited a fairly rapid pulse rate. She admitted to some chest pain as well. The skin lesions themselves do not blanch on diascopy. Tender erythematous areas on the digital pulps were also noticed. All of the skin findings occurred within a period of a few days, together with generalized malaise. What is your impression?

COMMENT

This clinical picture is one of subacute bacterial endocarditis. The skin lesions are the splinter hemorrhages and Osler's nodes discussed earlier and represent definite embolic phenomena. Cardiac murmurs heard on chest auscultation, together with this patient's febrile state, form the basis for a medical emergency. Awareness of seemingly unrelated foot lesions in relation to a patient's general condition is paramount in this example.

SUMMARY

Pedal dermatoses worthy of immediate attention because of their life-threatening potential may present as vesiculobullae, erythematous macules, purpuric eruptions, and nodose lesions. They are true dermatologic emergencies, since visible skin changes represent similar visceral pathologic processes. Once these serious conditions have been excluded, the practitioner may begin to assume that his/her patient's problem is purely a local one.

ACKNOWLEDGMENT

A special word of thanks is extended to Ms. Pamela Schlesinger for her review and editing of this manuscript.

References

1. Levine LE, Bernstein JE, Soltani K, Medenica MM, Yung CW: Heparin-induced cutaneous necrosis unrelated to injection sites. *Arch Dermatol* 119:400–403, 1983.
2. Costello MJ, Gibbs RC: *The Palms and Soles in Medicine.* Springfield, IL, Charles C Thomas, 1967, p 422.
3. Braverman IM: *Skin Signs of Systemic Diseases.* Philadelphia, W.B. Saunders, 1970, p 215.
4. Hendricks WM, Ahmad M, Gratz E: Weber-Christian syndrome in infancy. *Br J Dermatol* 98:175–186, 1978.
5. Winkelman RK, Tucker SB: Biopsy in diagnosis of inflammatory nodules of the leg. *Cutis* 21:183–187, 1978.
6. Sibrack LA, Gouterman IH: Cutaneous manifestations of pancreatic diseases. *Cutis* 21:763–768, 1978.
7. Pottage JC Jr, Trenholme GM, Aronson IK, Harris AA: Panniculitis associated with histoplasmosis and alpha-1-antitrypsin deficiency. *Am J Med* 75:150–153, 1983.
8. Winkelmann RK: Panniculitis in connective tissue disease. *Arch Dermatol* 119:336–344, 1983.
9. Izumi AK, Takiguchi P: Lupus erythematous panniculitis. *Arch Dermatol* 119:61–64, 1983.
10. Williams HJ, Samuelson CO, Zone JJ: Nodular nonsuppurative panniculitis associated with jejunoileal bypass surgery. *Arch Dermatol* 115:1091–1093, 1979.
11. Isaacson YA, Greenberg RN: A young man with fever, rash, lymphadenopathy. *Hosp Pract* 17:114K, O, P, 1982.
12. Clark CV, Hunter JAA: Anaphylactoid purpura presenting as a medical and surgical emergency. *Br Med J* 287:22–23, 1983.

CHAPTER 22

Skin Complications in Wound Closure

MICHAEL H. FEINSTEIN

Complications encountered in foot surgery which specifically affect the skin are relatively common but are rarely documented in surgical or dermatologic literature. Any complication which affects the healing of skin and adjacent tissues can adversely alter the outcome of the procedure. Prevention, early diagnosis, and rapid accurate treatment will minimize postoperative problems.

WOUND DEHISCENCE

Dehiscence is defined as a bursting open or gaping of a surgical wound. Many problems inherent in foot surgery contribute to wound dehiscence as a relatively common complication (Fig. 22.1).

The most serious consequences of dehiscence occur in abdominal wounds, which can disrupt as late as 25 days after surgery and cause evisceration. In the foot, wound dehiscence rarely occurs while sutures are in place. When dehiscence occurs prior to suture removal, the usual causes are injury to the part, severe edema, and inappropriately thin suture material which can break or tear through the skin. Premature suture removal is also a contributing factor.

Poor technique with postoperative dressings may cause delayed healing by placing tension on the wound or by restricting the local circulation and venous drainage.

Additionally, traumatic handling of the skin and deep tissues can be a major cause of surgical wound dehiscence. Too vigorous retraction may cause localized tissue necrosis and probably contributes to an increased incidence of delayed healing in certain areas of the foot (Fig. 22.2*A* and *B*).

Infection, hematoma, and seroma are complications which cause wound disruption by fluids taking space deep to the skin and not allowing strong layered tissue union. Moreover, the normal chemical and metabolic environment necessary for normal healing is altered.

Nutritional factors can be a cause of wound dehiscence and delayed healing and are prevalent in a significant segment of our population. For example, hypoproteinemia can cause wound disruption by prolonging the lag phase and preventing the onset of the fibroplastic phase. Vitamin C deficiency prevents hydroxylation of proline by fibroblasts and prevents synthesis of collagen. Patients with low zinc levels, which can be induced by surgical trauma, have less capacity for epithelialization, less gain in wound strength, and less synthesis of collagen and other necessary proteins (1). When suspicion of nutritional deficiencies exists, a careful dietary history must be taken, and proper supplements need to be administered prior to any elective procedure.

The relationship of certain drugs to wound healing should be of great interest to the foot surgeon. The importance of corticosteroids used systemically, injected immediately postoperatively, and applied topically has been well documented. Patients who have been on significant doses of prednisone for extended periods will sometimes demonstrate significant delay in the rate of wound healing. Immediate postoperative injection of short-acting phosphate corticosteroids into the surgical site appears to be relatively insignificant in adversely affecting wound healing. Topical steroids on the surgical scar have caused hypo- or hyperpigmentation of surrounding skin and atrophy of the scar.

Aspirin and other nonsteroidal anti-inflammatory oral medications are used extensively in the postoperative period for analgesia and prevention of thrombophlebitis. Other than a possibility for increased hematoma, there is no evidence of significant effects on the healing wound from this class of drugs.

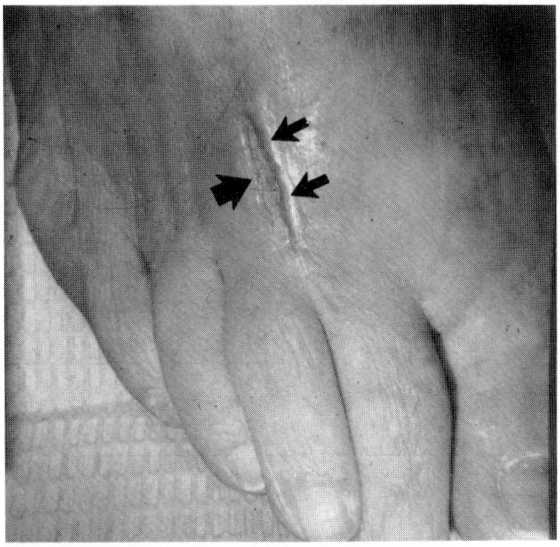

Figure 22.1. Wound dehiscence affecting the skin and subcutaneous tissues (*arrows*). Healing took 3 months. The patient had a history of alcoholism and had identical healing problems when surgery was performed on the other foot.

There are certain sites on the foot which appear to have a higher incidence of predilection for wound dehiscence. The heel and dorsum of the foot over the lesser metatarsophalangeal joints are most prone to wound tension and traction from ambulation.

TREATMENT

If delayed healing is a possibility, every other suture may be removed to check the tensile strength of the wound. Adhesive strips and butterflies may be useful in keeping the wound coapted for an extended period to gain further strength.

When a wound dehisces, there is a danger of infection, and prophylactic antibiotics should be instituted. Cultures of the wound exudates taken as deep as possible are important, as are radiographs taken after an

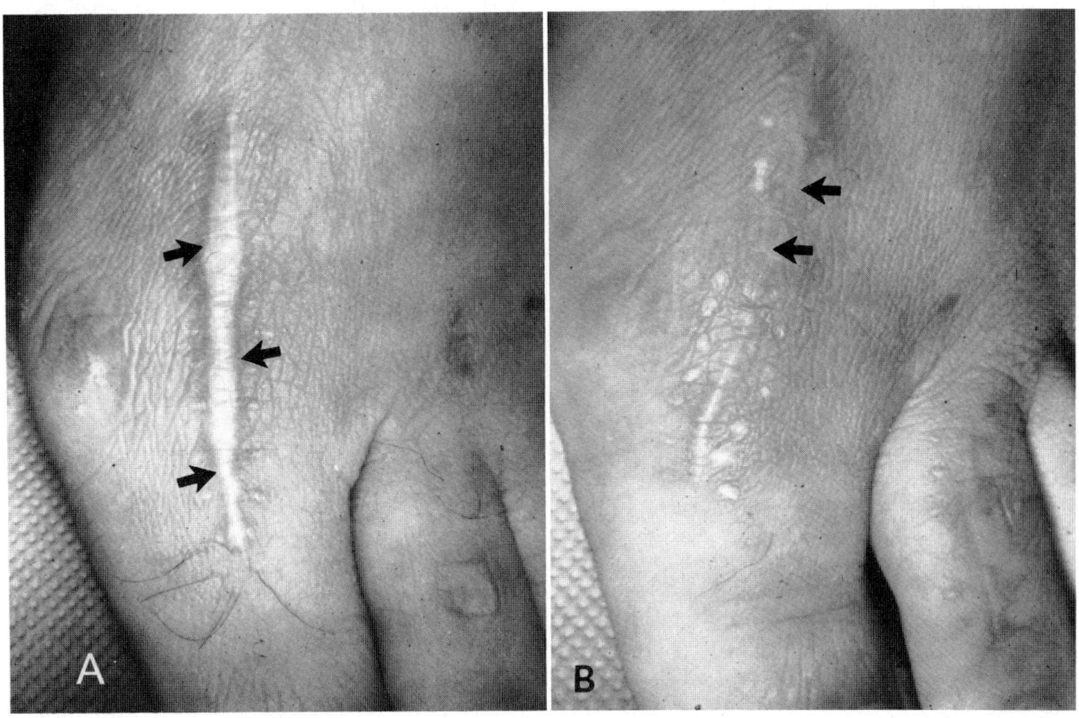

Figure 22.2. (*A* and *B*) Hypertrophic scar on one foot occurring as a result of excessive trauma in wound handling (*A*, *arrows*). Surgery on both feet was performed at the same time 6 weeks previously. A relatively normal scar is seen on the other foot (*B*, *arrows*).

appropriate time period, usually 10 to 14 days, to rule out osteomyelitis.

Local treatment requires debridement of necrotic tissue. Surgeon's preferences vary, but often warm soaks with or without additives are of value. Saline or antiseptic wet compresses are also useful in order to draw wound exudates and act as a protective barrier. The dried compresses when removed debride necrotic tissue and stimulate granulation.

Assessment of any underlying contributory causes should be a vital step in treatment. Generally, the patient should remain nonambulatory to limit tension on the wound, and the foot should be elevated to reduce edema. Hematoma and seroma should be drained from deep tissues. Nutritional factors should be closely checked, and any necessary supplements instituted. When circulatory problems are implicated, appropriate medications, mechanical factors, and possible consultation should be considered.

HYPERTROPHIC SCARS AND KELOIDS

The clinical differentiation of keloids from hypertrophic scars lies in the amount of scar production.

Hypertrophic scars are more scar tissue than the surgeon expected. These lesions may regress spontaneously and remain stable (Fig. 22.3).

Keloids are excessive deposits of collagen which continue to enlarge well beyond the original size and shape of the wound (Fig. 22.4). The initial appearance of the wound may be normal, but over the next 4 to 6 weeks collagenic materials continue to be laid down, making the problem ever more apparent. The lesions may have varied shapes, or may be single or lobulated and sessile or pedunculated. The color and consistency changes from pink with a rubbery consistency to darken and become more firm with age. The lesions are far more frequent in younger age groups. Keloid formers will often discontinue formation of these lesions in later life. Keloids are more common in darker-skinned races. They most often affect the face, ears, and pectoral and deltoid regions. They are only rarely encountered in the foot. The etiology is unknown, but hereditary is thought to be a factor.

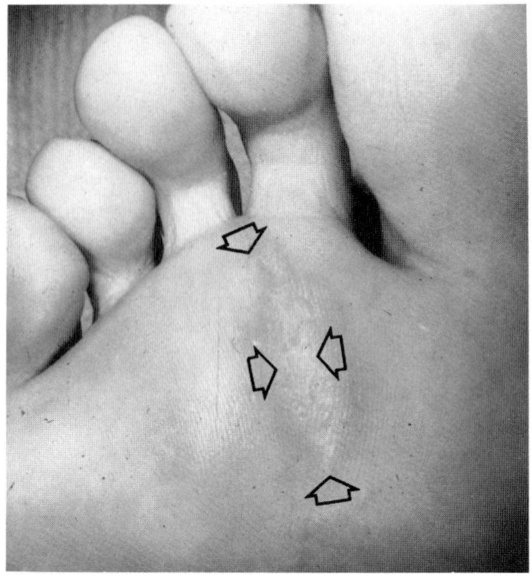

Figure 22.3. Keratosis involved with a plantar scar on a weight-bearing area of the foot (*arrows*).

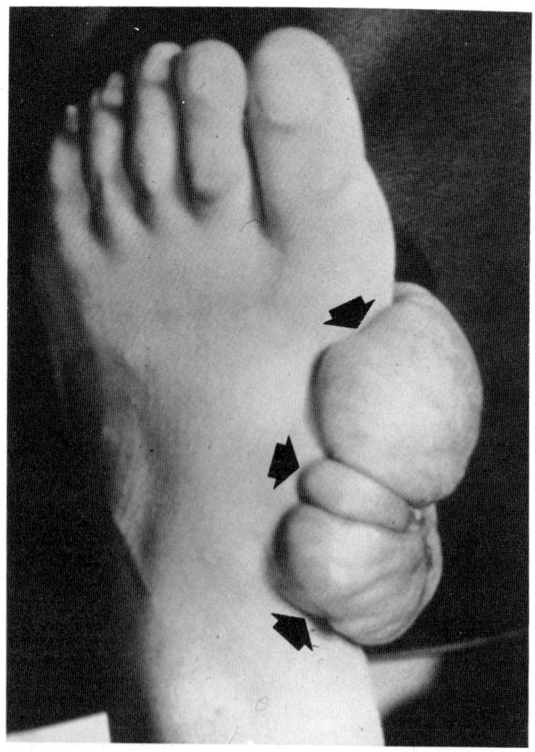

Figure 22.4. Keloid affecting the foot (*arrows*). Courtesy of the Audio-Visual Department of the William Scholl College of Podiatric Medicine.

Treatment involves reduction of collagen formation to the scar. Surgical revision of small lesions usually involves relief of skin tension with total or partial excision of the keloid. One must be prepared, however, for recurrence of these lesions. The use of intralesional steroids, especially triamcinolone acetonide, has been moderately successful. Some advocate the use of freezing modalities. The role of radiation in the treatment of these lesions is highly controversial.

Pressure dressings are often utilized as a part of the prophylactic treatment regimen to compress the developing hypertrophic scar. The rationale is that there is a certain amount of water present which can be compresed by dressings (2).

A severe hypertrophic scar or keloid affecting the foot can be an extremely disturbing complication. These lesions will affect joint mobility and function and render the wearing of shoes impossible. A careful history and meticulous surgery without skin tension at the outset are imperative in high risk groups. The risks and possible benefits of performing surgery at all in these groups must be carefully considered by both the surgeon and the patient.

COMPLICATIONS RESULTING FROM FOREIGN BODIES IN WOUNDS

Local Sequelae

Foreign body granulomas and inclusion cysts are common postoperative complications. These lesions can form from any foreign substance causing a tissue reaction in the wound. Suture materials and starch powder granules are most often implicated in the formation of these lesions. The simple precaution of washing the gloved hands with sterile saline solution before surgery will help prevent this problem.

Absorbable sutures are generally dissolved by the local reaction of phagocytic cells and tissue fluids within a certain time span. When this reaction does not occur, for whatever reason, the suture attracts a layer of macrophages surrounded by fibroblasts, and a thin fibrous capsule is formed.

When these lesions are present in deep tissues, they may be painless but are quite painful in superficial areas. They often appear a month or more after surgery as a hyperpigmented painful nodule within the scar line. They may be raised with a white central area. Sometimes it is possible to curette these lesions under local anesthesia, but at times surgical scar revision is necessary. The author (3) reported the incidence of serious foreign body granulomas in a series of 50 patients in whom Supramid Extra suture material was utilized for skin and deep closure. This material is a synthetic polyfilament polymerized caprolactam, and its apparent lack of tissue response was well documented in the literature. Five patients required additional surgical procedures to resolve their complications (Fig. 22.5*A–D*).

Wire sutures are often utilized in foot surgery for fixation of fractures and osteotomies. There are cases whereby the wire ends loosen and cause pain. Inflammation, ganglion cysts, and ulceration can occur as a result of irritation in the subcutaneous tissue. Care must be taken during surgery to ensure that the wire ends are buried adequately in drill holes. The wire should be excised if it loosens (Fig. 22.6).

Bone wax is commonly used by surgeons at bone ends to provide for hemostasis. Julsrud (4) reported an allergic reaction in the foot following the use of this material. He reported a severe local inflammatory reaction 6 days postoperatively. Serosanguinous fluid was present which cultured *Staphylococcus aureus*. A portion of bone wax had not adhered and was removed after migrating through subcutaneous tissue.

The widespread use of silastic joint implants in foot surgery has led to the increased incidence of wound complications relating to these procedures (Fig. 22.7). Implants of this type are rarely cemented but rely on medullary drill holes, suture in bone, and capsule closure for fixation. Factors which can cause wound problems include improper placement, fracture of the bone cortex, and injury. Wound breakdown can also result from the use of an implant which is too large for the area in which it is used. Local allergic reactions to silastic used in joint replacement are extremely rare. There is, however, some indication that particles of silastic may migrate to other parts of the body, but the possible consequences are not yet clear.

Cutaneous Complications Associated with Dressings and Casts

Complications affecting the surgical wound and surrounding skin may take many forms. There are many reports of

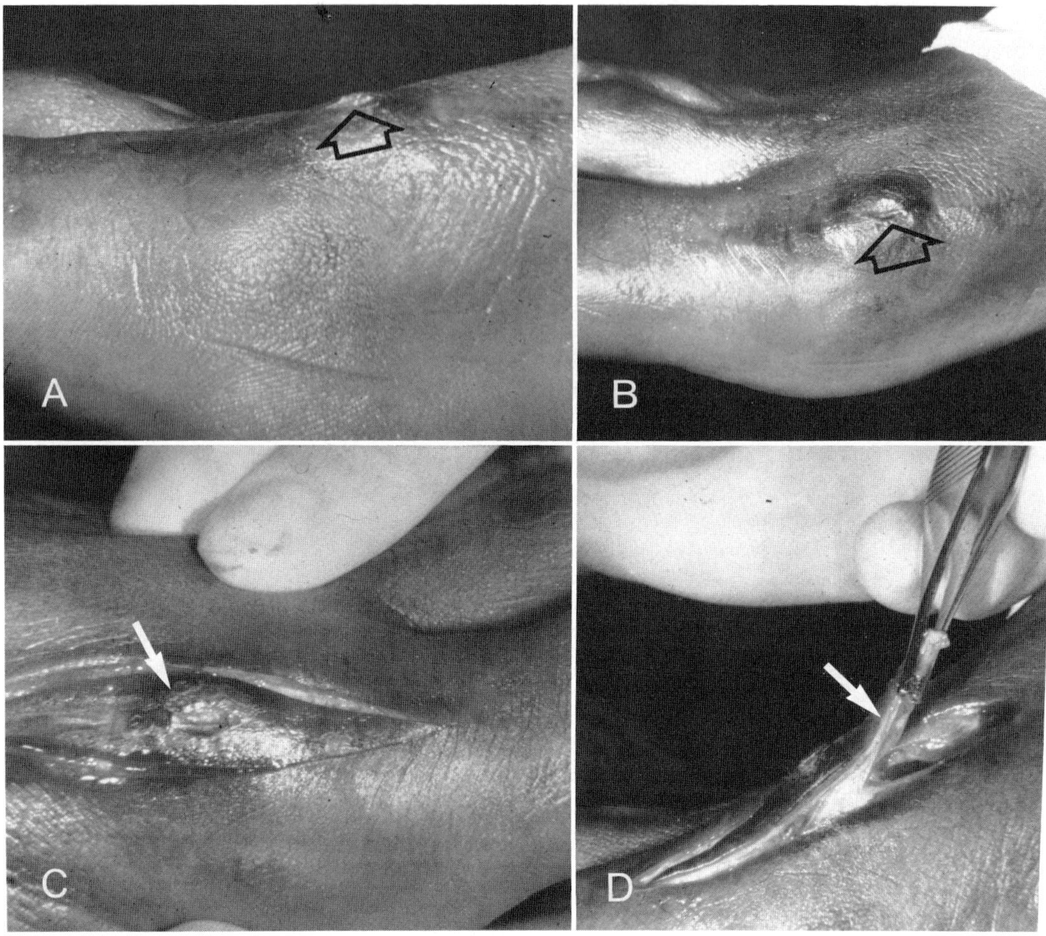

Figure 22.5. (*A* to *D*) Excision of a painful inclusion cyst (*arrows*) in subcutaneous tissue which resulted from a foreign body reaction to Supramid Extra nonabsorbable suture material.

unusual organisms found in dressings causing infections.

Mead and associates (5) reported a case of an unusual contaminant in Elastoplast dressings. They reported a postoperative infection caused by *Rhizopus*, an opportunistic fungus in the class Zygomycetes, following spine surgery. Erythema in the immediate area of the incision which quickly evolved into edema, erythema, bullae, denudation, and pustules was apparent 4 days postoperatively.

A series of *Clostridium perfringens* infections resulting from contaminated nonsterile elastic bandages was reported by Pearson and associates (6). All five cases involved adult onset diabetics who had un-

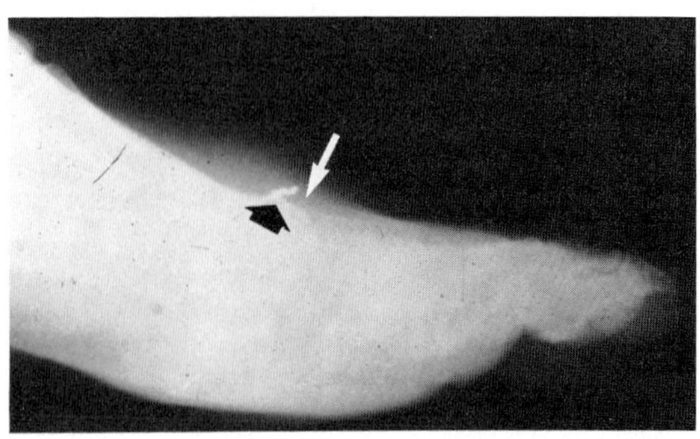

Figure 22.6. Wire suture used for fixation in an osteotomy site. The tail of the wire has loosened from its drill hole (*black arrow*), causing a ganglion cyst of the extensor hallucis longus tendon, as well as severe pain and skin inflammation along the incision area (*white arrow*).

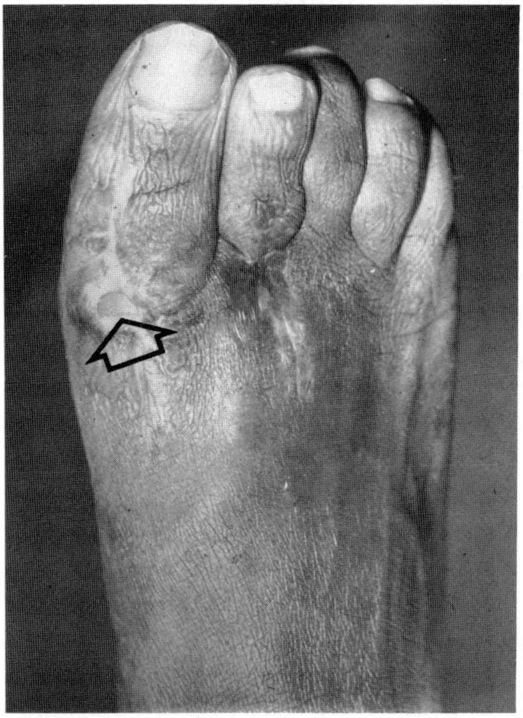

Figure 22.7. Silastic implant visible in wound following injury to the area. The implant apparently loosened, causing tissue breakdown (*arrow*). Courtesy of Max Weisfeld, D.P.M.

dergone lower extremity amputations, whereby elastic bandages were used as outer wraps. They stress the important point that a gauze sterile dressing acts as a protective barrier only as long as it remains dry. Transudates from the wound or fluid from an external source can destroy the protective effect and allow bacteria from outer wrappings to reach the wound.

Another example of wound contamination by this wick effect can occur with the use of plaster dressings. Greenberg (7) reported testing 163 plaster bandages from 14 different manufacturers. He found that all were contaminated by anaerobes, including *Clostridium* species.

The dangers of thermal injuries associated with plaster dressings are documented extensively (8, 9). Temperatures of up to 50°C have been reported following the application of a modified Robert Jones dressing. Third degree burns can occur if these temperatures are sustained for 5 to 15 min.

The thicker the cast or splint, the higher will be the temperature produced in the exothermic plaster reaction. Plaster dries from outside to inside, and the thickness of multiple layers blocks the outward escape of heat. Other factors contributing to heat buildup are the covering of heated plaster with cotton or elastic dressings, placing the part directly on a pillow or mattress, and covering the part with a blanket. All of these factors limit access of air to dissipate heat.

A further important consideration with the use of plaster is the amount of water used. The bandage should be very moist and not excessively squeezed dry prior to application. Water will prevent burns because it has a high capacity for heat absorption.

Plaster of Paris skin burns may be contributed to by other less obvious factors in foot surgery. A possible secondary cause may be the decreased vascular supply to the operated area resulting from the use of hemostatic drugs like epinephrine. Also, certain general anesthetic agents can cause a decrease of thermal regulation at the skin level.

Local Allergic Reactions (Contact Dermatitis)

The surgeon often utilizes numerous agents on the surgical site and surrounding skin preoperatively, intraoperatively, and postoperatively.

Allergic reactions can occur from many external sources and may easily be confused with local irritation or skin reaction to occlusion (Fig. 22.8). Adhesive tape, for example, is often listed by the patient as an allergen but usually has caused mechanical irritation and not a true allergic reaction.

The skin may become more highly sensitized because of the preoperative shave and vigorous scrubbing as part of the sterile prep.

Some of the potential sources of skin allergy include: (*a*) antiseptic prep solutions—Betadine, mercurials, hexachlorophenes, etc.; (*b*) wound coverings—gauze, elastic wraps, Xeroform, Adaptic, Furacin gauze, etc.; (*c*) Adhesive tapes; and (*d*) topical antibiotics.

Minor allergic reactions respond well to topical steroid preparations. Severe allergic reactions may require treatment with sys-

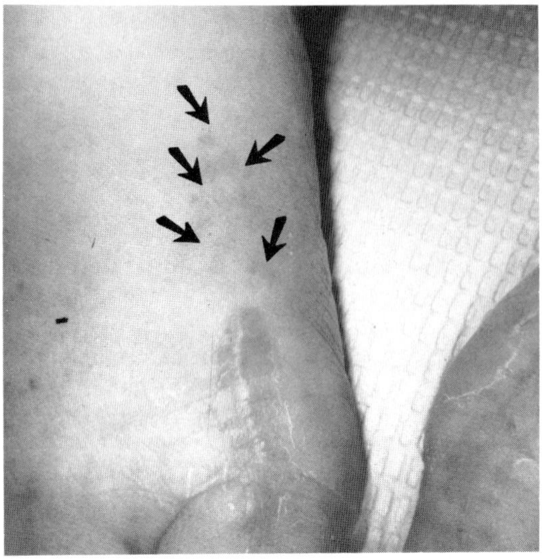

Figure 22.8. Skin irritation present 2 weeks following suture removal as a result of occlusion and mechanical irritation of surgical dressings (*arrows*).

temic steroids and antihistamines. Patch testing may be helpful in isolating the cause of the reaction and ensuring discontinuation of its use.

Fungal Infections

Fungal infections caused by dermatophytes are fairly common postoperative problems affecting the foot. These organisms are often harbored by the patient on their nails or in the web spaces. The most common organisms isolated are *Trichophyton rubrum* and *Trichophyton mentagrophytes.*

Dermatophyte infections are often divided clinically into three main categories: (*a*) intertriginous dermatophytosis—these are red and scaly lesions between the toes which are usually macerated. Fissuring with secondary bacterial infections are common. Differential diagnosis includes monilial infection, *Pseudomonas* infection, erythrasma, and psoriasis. This type of tinea pedis can be a significant source of complication in digital surgery. (*b*) Chronic papulosquamous or hyperkeratotic dermatophytosis—these lesions often affect the heels but can affect the whole plantar aspect of the foot. The lesions consist of layers of keratosis with scaling and, often, adjacent areas of erythema. Differential diagnosis includes psoriasis, pityriasis rubra pilaris, xeroderma, chronic contact dermatitis, and shear calluses of the heel. These lesions are significant in surgery because the keratosis and scaling cause difficulty in rendering the skin sterile preoperatively. (*c*) Acute vesiculo bullous dermatophytosis—characterized by vesicles and bullae filled with a clear or straw-colored fluid. As the lesions rupture and dry, they leave circular areas of scaling and erythema. These lesions may occur anywhere on the foot. Differential diagnosis includes bullous pemphigoid, pustular psoriasis, keratodermia blennorhagica, acute contact dermatitis, dyshidrosis, and dermatophytosis.

The author encountered a case of bullous pemphigoid mimicking acute vesiculobullous tinea pedis affecting the incision line of a bunion surgery one week after suture removal. A single bullous lesion was present and did not respond to antifungal or antibacterial treatment. The lesions quickly progressed to affect the neck, face, hands, and oral mucous membranes. Definitive diagnosis was made by biopsy of the bullous lesions.

The specialized requirement imposed on the skin of the postoperative patient contributes to the presence of increased numbers of dermatophytes. Often the toes are splinted and held together with dressings or casts for extended periods, causing perspiration and moisture buildup. During this time the patient usually cannot bathe or practice usual foot hygiene. Dressings and casts increase perspiration without the ability for evaporation, which may sensitize the skin and act as an excellent environment for multiplication of organisms.

Although there are thousands of species of fungi, only about 55 have been identified as pathogenic in man. Some of these, including *T. rubrum*, *T. mentagrophytes*, and *candida*, commonly affect the skin as well as the deeper tissues of the surgical wound (10).

Rare mycotic infections which have been reported affecting surgical wounds include cryptococcosis (Fig. 22.9), sporotrichosis, aspergillosis (Fig. 22.10), chromomycosis, nocardiosis, and mycetoma (11). Predisposing factors which cause these organisms to overgrow include treatment with long-term corticosteroids, long-term use of antibiotics, diabetes, and immunosuppression by chemicals or disease processes (12).

Diagnosis of mycotic infections is made intuitively clinical appearance, KOH examination, and cultures. Treatment depends on the type of lesions present and the clinician's choice of medications. Caution regarding overtreatment and sensitization is important, especially when a surgical area is involved.

Viral Infections

The wart is the predominant entity in any discussion about viral infections affecting the foot.

Warts are caused by a type of papovavirus in the papilloma group. They are intranuclear pathogens, with plantar warts having the highest number of virus particles present. Plantar warts differ from other warts in the greater amount of keratin present, which is probably the result of pressure.

Transmission of the wart virus is debatable but important in surgery. Most clinicians readily accept the spread of warts to new sites of infection within the patient by autoinoculation. Many also feel that the virus can be transmitted to new areas by inanimate objects, including surgical instruments (13).

Many foot surgeons have experienced the unfortunate complication of having multiple verrucae form in a scar line following semielliptical excision of a single lesion (Fig. 22.11). This can be a serious problem when it occurs on the weight-bearing surfaces of the foot.

The author has had the experience of treating a young girl who had undergone skin grafting procedures of her heel for

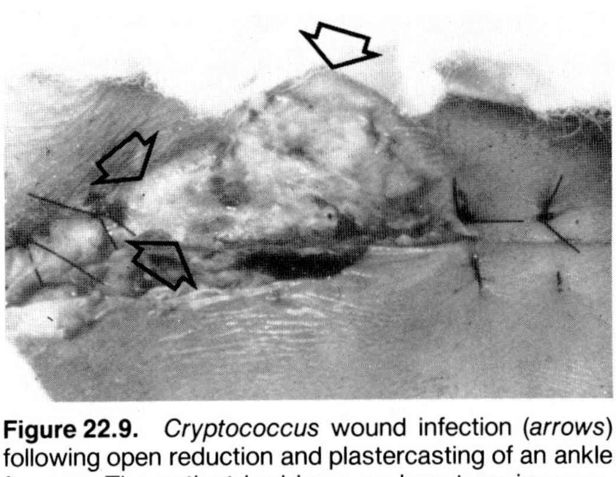

Figure 22.9. *Cryptococcus* wound infection (*arrows*) following open reduction and plastercasting of an ankle fracture. The patient had been on long-term immunosuppressive drugs. Courtesy of Evan Farmer, M.D.

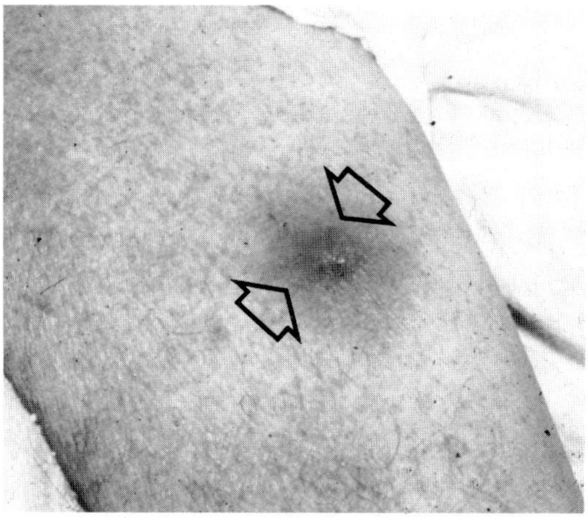

Figure 22.10. Aspergillosis infection at injection site (*arrows*) in a patient being treated with chemotherapy for Hodgkin's disease. Courtesy of Evan Farmer, M.D.

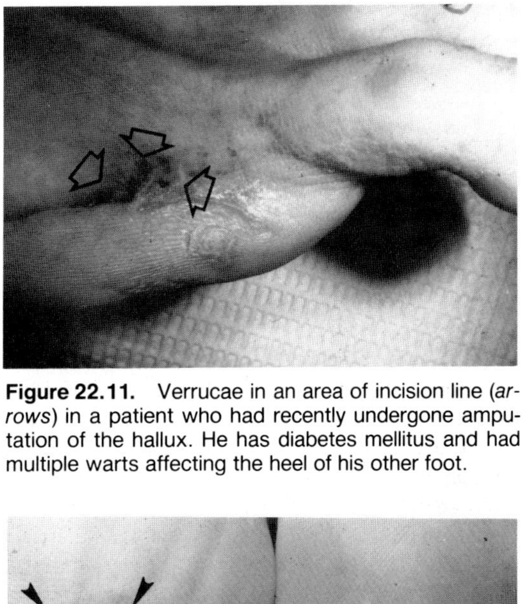

Figure 22.11. Verrucae in an area of incision line (*arrows*) in a patient who had recently undergone amputation of the hallux. He has diabetes mellitus and had multiple warts affecting the heel of his other foot.

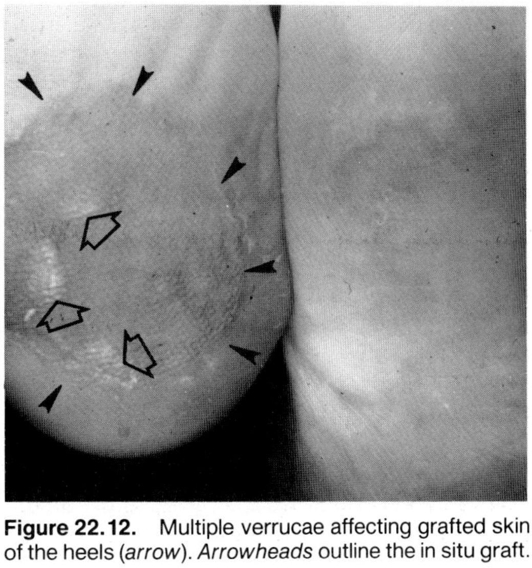

Figure 22.12. Multiple verrucae affecting grafted skin of the heels (*arrow*). *Arrowheads* outline the in situ graft.

treatment of intractable mosaic verrucae and had demonstrated recurrence of lesions on her newly grafted skin (Fig. 22.12).

Other viral infections rarely affect the feet, and reports of their incidence are uncommon.

Parasitic Infestation

Reports of parasites affecting surgical wounds are rare in the United States (14). Cutaneous myiasis, the infestation of tissue by fly larvae, is seen relatively often in emergency rooms in low socioeconomic areas. The parasites enter through ulcers, surgical wounds, or other open lesions. They feed on necrotic tissue, and when this is depleted, on living tissue. Myiasis is generally due to unsanitary conditions whereby flies have laid eggs directly on the wound, on dirty dressings, or on clothing. The eggs then hatch from the warmth of the host's skin and begin to feed (15).

There are numerous species of flies which can cause maggot infestation and are most frequently found in tropical climates.

Although it was once thought to be beneficial for a surgical wound or ulcer to be debrided by maggots, the possibility of destruction of viable tissue and secondary bacterial infection poses a significant threat.

Most treatment involves removal of the larvae, with measures to prevent infection or treat it when it is present. The parasites are best removed under local anesthesia with debridement of all necrotic debris and with copious irrigation. Some clinicians advocate the use of agents which are toxic to the larvae, but these agents may also be toxic to the tissues of the surgical wound or ulcer.

References

1. Peacock EE, VanWinkle W: *Wound Repair*, ed 2. Philadelphia, W.B. Saunders, 1976, pp 231–240.
2. Elkouri ER, Pascente R: Keloids: a review of current clinical evaluation and treatment. *J Am Podiatry Assoc* 69:543–544, 1979.
3. Feinstein MH, Rubin L, Brown HN: Supramid extra: a random in vivo study with a previously reported nonreactive suture material. *J Am Podiatry Assoc* 67:807–810, 1977.
4. Julsrud ME: A surgical complication: allergic reaction to bone wax. *J Foot Surg* 19:152–152, 1980.
5. Mead JH et al: Cutaneous *Rhizopus* infection: occurrence as a postoperative complication associated with an elasticized adhesive dressing. *JAMA* 242:272–274, 1979.
6. Pearson RD, Valenti WM, Steigbigel RT: Clostridium perfringens associated with elastic bandages. *JAMA* 244:1128–1130, 1980.
7. Greenberg L: A bacteriological analysis of plaster of Paris bandages. *Can Med Assoc J* 60:4–7, 1949.
8. Becker DW: Danger of burns from fresh plaster splints surrounded by too much cotton. *Plast Reconstr Surg* 62:436–437, 1978.
9. Kaplan SS: Burns following application of plaster splint dressings. *J Bone Joint Surg* 63A:670–672, 1981.
10. Feldman WE, Hedaya E, O'Brien M: Skin abscess caused by *Candida albicans:* unusual presentation of *C. albicans* disease. *J Clin Microbiol* 12:44–45, 1980.
11. Delacretaz J, Grigoriu D, Duce IG: *Color Atlas of Medical Mycology.* Chicago, Yearbook Medical, 1976.
12. Codish SD, Sheridan ID, Monaco AP: Mycotic wound infections: a new challenge for the surgeon. *Arch Surg* 114:831–835, 1979.
13. Noe JM, Chase RA: Surgical transplantation of warts. *Plast Reconstr Surg* 64:101–103, 1979.
14. Davis E, Shuman C: Cutaneous myiasis: devils in the flesh. *Hosp Pract* (*Dec*):115–123, 1982.
15. Beck JW, Davies JE: *Medical Parasitology*, ed 2. St Louis, C.V. Mosby, 1976, pp 200–201.

Suggested Readings

Abel RB et al: The incidence of isolation of Candida species from the human foot. *J Am Podiatry Assoc* 66:237, 1976.

Arnold HJ et al: *Candida albicans* arthritis in a healthy adult. *South Med J* 74:84, 1981.

Ary KR, Maxwell JR, Printz DW: Erysipeloid of Rosenbach: a postoperative complication. *J Am Podiatry Assoc* 71:40, 1981.

Barker DJ, Cotterill JA: Development of subepidermal bullae in the split-skin graft donor site of a psoriatic. *Dermatologica* 160:311, 1980.

Barrano VP, Soloman H: Eczematous dermatitis from nickel. *JAMA* 220:1244, 1972.

Beck JW, Davies JE: *Medical Parasitology.* St. Louis, C.V. Mosby, 1976, pp 200–201.

Beneke ES: *Scope Monograph on Human Mycoses.* Kalamazoo, MI, Upjohn, 1970.

Kubba R, Taylor JS, Marks KE: Cutaneous

complications of orthopedic implants: a two-year prospective study. *Arch Dermatol* 117:554, 1981.

McKenzie AW, Aitkon CVE, Ridsdill-Smith R: Urticaria after insertion of Smith-Peterson vitallium nail. *Br Med J* 4:36, 1967.

Norton L, Chvapil M: Comparison of newer synthetic and biological wound dressings. *J Trauma* 21:463, 1981.

Page JC, Friedlander G, Dockery GL: Postoperative *Fusarium* osteomyelitis. *J Foot Surg* 21:174, 1982.

Ratanarapee S, Jesadapatarakul S, Mangkalanond K: Spontaneous exit of a gnathastome through a surgical wound. *Southeast Asia J Trop Med Public Health* 12:376, 1981.

Roenigk HH: *Office Dermatology*. Baltimore, Williams and Wilkins, 1981.

Truppman ES, Ellenby JD, Schwartz BM: Fungi in and around implants after augmentation mammoplasty. *Plast Reconstr Surg* 64:804, 1979.

Yamaguchi T: *Color Atlas of Clinical Parasitology*. Philadelphia, Lea & Febiger, 1981.

CHAPTER 23

Fibrous Lesions of the Foot

STEVEN J. BERLIN

The fibroblast is a highly versatile cell; it is the primary cell in the formation of all connective tissue. Consequently, such cells have the potential for developing into a variety of materials necessary for the production of the different forms of connective tissues. Fibroblasts are normally mobilized in reparative and defensive processes of the body, and they are active in granulation and scar tissue formation. Additionally, they are implicated in productive fibroses which accompany invasive neoplastic growths. Moreover, proliferating fibroblasts take an active part in the formation of the stroma and parts of the matrix of palpable "tumors" produced by invading cancers. They may also proliferate in an intimate fashion as parts of other sarcomatous neoplasms (1). Such lesions are usually characterized by a high degree of anaplasia. Fibrous tumors are seen in many varieties. It is the purpose of this chapter to familiarize the student and practitioner with these lesions.

FIBROMAS

Fibromas are benign neoplasms derived from fibrous tissues and are commonly associated with other connective tissue structures. Such lesions are rarely seen in the foot in a pure state. They are, however, frequently seen in the skin in association with other soft tissue structures. Benign fibromas of the foot represent less than 1% of nonmalignant lesions as they are found in the pedal extremities (2). Fibromas have often been described in two forms: fibroma molle is characterized as a soft-type mass, while fibroma durum is a much harder and firmer type of structure or lesion.

Fibrous tumors (fibromas) occur at any age. Certainly, these growths appear anywhere on the foot and even develop within the connective tissue sheaths of nerves, tendons, and periosteal structures of bones. Connective tissues of the dermal structures of the skin may also be tumor-prone. Fibromas generally arise spontaneously and are usually asymptomatic. They may create discomfort when they are in close proximity to nerves. These lesions are most often found to be oval or spherical in shape (Fig. 23.1).

Fibromas are generally encapsulated lesions, usually small, measuring 1 to 4 cm in diameter; their consistency may vary from hard to soft. Their surgical appearance often reveals white glistening masses, and they are generally avascular lesions.

The histological appearance of fibromas is characterized by great numbers of spindle-shaped fibrocytes with elongated nuclei. Varying amounts of collagen are generally found in the matrix between the fibroblasts (Fig. 23.2). These fibrous constituents give the lesion its firm consistency. Anaplasia is not a characteristic of fibrous tumors.

The clinical state of fibromas is that of a firm or semifirm type of lesion. These lesions are generally freely movable, but when they become complicated by association with nerve and tendon, they are less mobile. On clinical examination, these tumors may often appear to be similar to other benign tumors or cysts.

Treatment of fibromas is usually that of simple surgical excision. The recurrence rate is generally minimal when adequate excision is employed. Fibromas are generally benign. However, they may undergo malignant change, but this is a rare instance.

DERMATOFIBROMAS

Dermatofibromas are benign asymptomatic fibrous tissue tumors which have a predilection for the lower extremities. They can occur anywhere and have been described as button-type lesions (Fig. 23.3).

Dermatofibroma is typically seen in middle-aged or older patients. It usually presents as a solitary lesion. Rarely, several lesions may be present. It is a firm, stony-hard nodule which measures up to 1 cm in size. Such lesions are adherent to the skin, but they are movable over the underlying deeper tissues. The surface of dermatofibroma is usually smooth. They can be rounded, slightly elevated, and are occasionally surrounded by a furrow-like depression.

Dermatofibromas belong to a class of lesions known as nodular subepidermal fibrosis. These tumors include sclerosing hemangioma, histiocytoma, including hemosiderin histiocytoma and lipoidal histiocytoma.

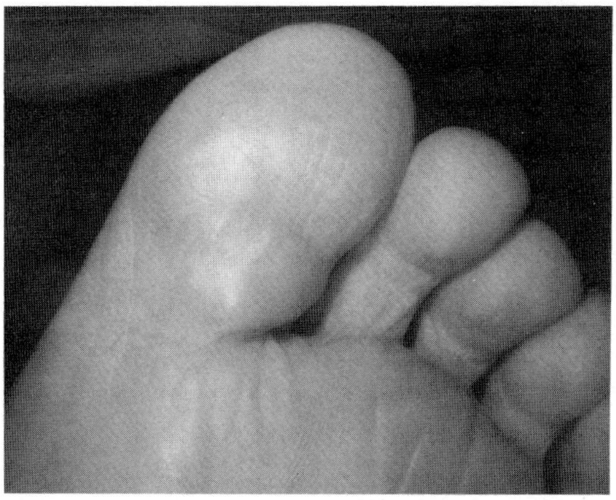

Figure 23.1. Fibroma demonstrating the typical oval or spherical shape.

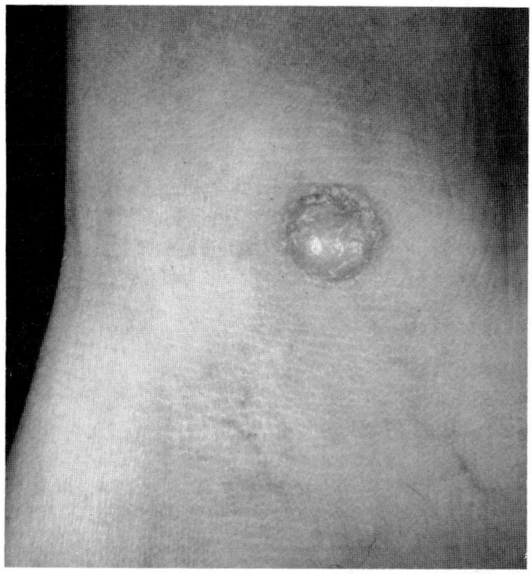

Figure 23.3. Dermatofibroma demonstrating typical button-like appearance.

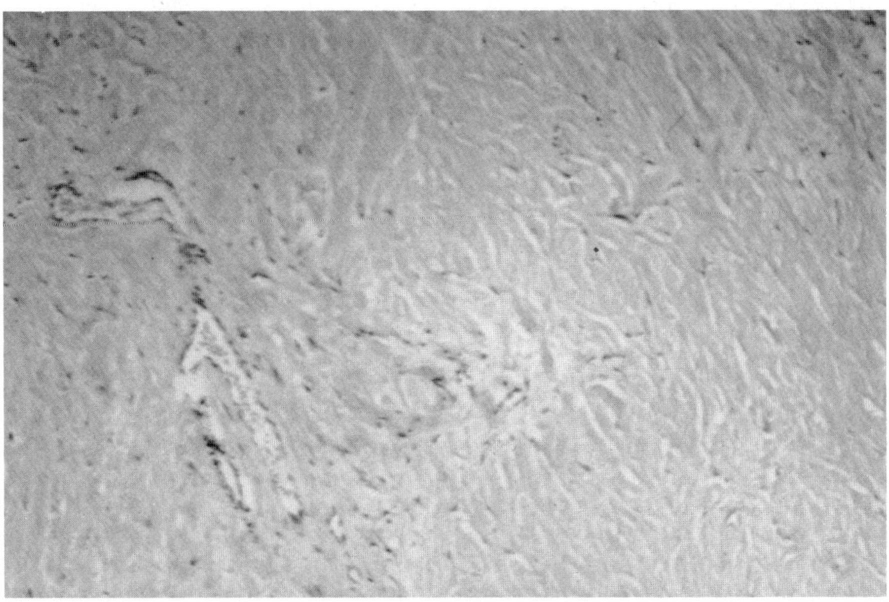

Figure 23.2. Histologic appearance of fibroma (of tendon sheath). *F,* fibroblast; *S*, stroma; *M*, matrix.

The color of the lesion varies from ivory to pinkish, yellow-brown, or bluish-black, depending on the tissue constituencies of the tumor. Blood vessels of sclerosing hemangioma, fibrous tissues of nodular fibrosis, and histiocytes containing lipid or hemosiderin or both are examples of tissue influences on tumor appearance.

Dermatofibroma usually starts as a papule which enlarges to a predetermined size. Spontaneous involution occurs rarely; malignant change almost never occurs (3). Simple surgical excision generally results in a cure.

DERMATOFIBROSARCOMA PROTUBERANS

Dermatofibrosarcoma protuberans is a malignant lesion of fibrous tissue which rarely metastasizes. It is a raised, cutaneous fibrous tumor that characteristically exhibits a marked tendency for recurrence. Hoffman in 1925 first reported the lesion and named it dermatofibrosarcoma protuberans (4). Other terms used to describe the tumor include progressive and recurring dermatofibroma, hypertrophic morphea, sarcomatous tumors resembling keloid, and fibrosarcoma of the skin. O'Brien and Stout, in their review of malignant fibrous xanthomas, include dermatofibrosarcoma protuberans in their group of storiform fibrous xanthomas (5).

Dermatofibrosarcoma usually begins as a firm fibrous plaque or as small raised nipple-like projections. Such lesions may be present for a number of years, but they eventually enter a phase of rapid growth with the formation of multiple nodules (6). In some instances, however, growth can be either progressive or rather rapid from the outset. The growth appears clinically as a raised, firm multinodular tumor (Fig. 23.4). It is fixed to the overlying skin, but the mass is movable over the deeper tissues (7). A reddish to bluish discoloration of the skin frequently precedes the appearance of the definitive lesion. Most lesions on the extremities are situated proximally, involving skin of the upper thigh or arm. In 115 cases studied by Taylor and Helwig, two of the tumors were identified as occurring on the foot or ankle (6). Burckhardt also reported two cases on the foot (7). The age at which most lesions are originally noted occurs

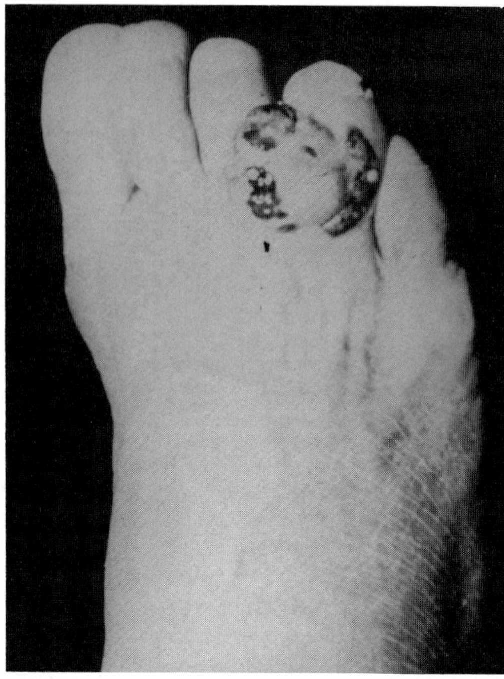

Figure 23.4. Dermatofibrosarcoma demonstrating firm, raised multinodular appearance.

most commonly between the second and fourth decades of life (8). The duration of lesions prior to the initial excision is usually between 3 to 10 years. In some instances dermatofibrosarcomas may become symptomatic in less than 6 months from the date of onset. Lesions are found in male patients four times more frequently than in female patients. About 80% of the patients are Caucasians. Pain or tenderness in a previously asymptomatic nodule is the most common initial complaint (7). In some instances a period of rapid growth may also be the presenting chief complaint. Taylor and Helwig reported 16.5% of their patients as having a history of prior trauma relative to the site of tumorigenesis (6). The rapidity of growth of the tumor can often be associated with some degree of trauma.

Most of the specimens occur as two solitary masses, but they are usually multinodular. Diameter of the lesions averages about 5.0 cm. The tumors are firm, rounded, and well circumscribed. Extension of tumor cells into the subcutaneous fat or skeletal muscle is occasionally evident. Adherence of the fibrous tumor to the overlying skin is also present in most cases.

The lesions are composed of uniformly

spindle-shaped cells which extend from the corium into the subcutaneous fat or beyond (6). The central portions of the lesions tended to be more cellular; the peripheral areas are less cellular and have an abundance of coarse collagen fibers. The tumor may be well-circumscribed, but it more often blends into the contiguous normal skin and beyond. Individual tumor cells tend to be plumper, and their nuclei tend to be rounded in the cellular portions. Such tumors are characteristically quite vascular. The fibroblastic infiltrate is occasionally arranged in broad fascicles which tend to interlace. A striking architectural characteristic of dermatofibrosarcoma is how the tumor cells are arranged about a central hub, producing a pattern resembling the spokes of a cartwheel.

A second, less frequent histological variant more often seen in recurrent tumors is much less cellular and is comprised of small spindle-shaped and stellate cells with pyknotic nuclei (6).

Dermatofibrosarcoma must be differentiated from sclerosing hemangioma, neurofibrosarcoma, fibroma, liposarcoma, Kaposi's sarcoma, lipoma, melanoma, spindle cell melanoma, malignant neurilemmoma associated with von Recklinghausen's disease, malignant melanoma, fibrosarcoma, and malignant fibrous histiocytoma.

The treatment of choice for dermatofibrosarcoma is wide local excision of the tumor. It is important to histologically identify contiguous margins of apparently normal tissue. The option of a regional lymph node dissection should be reserved to selected cases (9). The malignant potential for dermatofibrosarcoma protuberans has remained controversial. Its propensity for local recurrence with infiltration of surrounding tissues and the formation of satellite nodules is well known. Reports of visceral and lymph node metastases have been rarely described (10). In the largest study by Taylor and Helwig, about half of the patients had one or more local recurrences (6). In that same study, no visceral or nodule metastasis occurred. These surgical cases included six instances of radical *en bloc* resection with regional lymphadenectomy. Most required skin grafting to cover the resultant defects. Burkhardt et al, in a series of 50 cases, reported one patient who expired as a result of suspected metastatic spread (7). In a study by McPeak et al, five patients demonstrated visceral metastasis but no tumor cells were demonstrable in the regional lymph nodes (8).

JUVENILE APONEUROTIC FIBROMA

The juvenile aponeurotic fibroma (calcifying fibroma) is of clinical importance since it appears to be a benign tumor having a self-limited growth potential. This tumor was first described by Keasbey in 1953 (1). Such lesions demonstrate a histologic impression of cellularity and invasiveness (11). The lesion may be interpreted by some surgeons and pathologists as an invasive malignant neoplasm and may be treated more aggressively than is justified (1). These fibromas have a tendency to recur after excision, but they do not metastasize. They demonstrate a predilection for occurrence in the hands and feet of children.

It is interesting to note that four cases in patients over 30 years of age had been reported by Lichtenstein and Goldman in 1964 (12). However, the lesion still predominates in children and young adults. In Keasbey's original study, four occurrences of the tumor appeared in children ranging from 2 through 9 years of age. Two occurred in the thenar space, one in the hypothenar space, one midline of the sole of the foot, and one in the fat pad beneath the calcaneus. Since the original reporting, many additional cases have been reported around the world (11). Only 12 cases were identified on the lower extremity in the Keasbey study (1). Of these, five occurred on the foot, three of which were on the plantar aspect.

Clinically, the aponeurotic fibroma has no distinguishing characteristics (11). It usually appears as a poorly circumscribed mass which is firm, rather fixed, asymptomatic and painless (Fig. 23.5). However, it can also be well-defined and have well-circumscribed borders. In either case, the overlying skin is not fixed to the lesion, and there is no dimpling. There is no discoloration of the surrounding skin. If pain exists, it is usually because of the lesions' space-occupying properties and consequent interference with function. Soft tissue contractures have been described in association

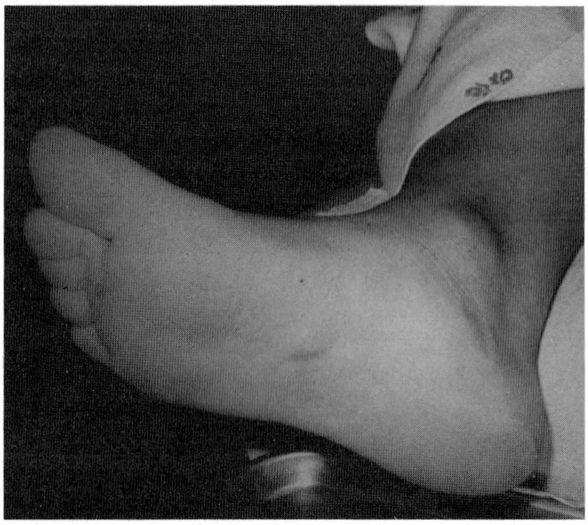

Figure 23.5. Juvenile fibromatosis on the plantar surface of the foot demonstrating well-defined circumscribed borders.

with aponeurotic fibromas. Such occurrences can result in confusing these lesions with plantar or palmar fibromatosis and nodular fasciitis (11). The sex distribution appears to be essentially equal, although there may be a slight preponderance of males with this lesion.

Radiographs show a relatively radiopaque soft tissue mass without bony involvement. Early diagnosis can be facilitated by recognition of a fine stippling of focal calcification of the tumor.

Keasbey states that the hallmark of juvenile aponeurotic fibroma is the morphology of the fibrocyte (1). Most fibromas demonstrate inconspicuous, greatly elongated, fusiform nuclei enclosed in long, fibrillar cell bodies. Conversely, aponeurotic fibromas are dominated by numerous darkly staining, plump, oval nuclei. The second distinctive feature lies in the fact that all the cells seem to be oriented in one direction. They appear to be a sheet of cells all oriented along one plane. This is in sharp contrast to most fibromas, wherein the cells are characteristically haphazard in arrangement.

In more deeply seated fibromas, prominent patterns of intersecting and intertwining fasciculi produce a more or less "herring bone" effect. Keasbey feels the prominence of the characteristic nuclei and their striking parallel orientation are the distinguishing microscopic features of this tumor (1).

Another microscopic characteristic of this tumor is its unique wide infiltration by tumor cells of skeletal muscle, fat, blood vessels, and skin adnexa (13). Lesions such as desmoids tend to destroy muscle fibers by overgrowing and replacing them, but the aponeurotic fibroma moves through skeletal muscle, separating the intact muscle cell from its nuclei. In addition, the fibroma cells may encircle blood vessels and nerve trunks in the tumor's path without appearing to overgrow or destroy these adjacent structures (14).

Keasbey was impressed with nuclear morphology, but more recent authors, including Goldman (1970), site similar nuclear orientation in ordinary palmar and plantar fibromatoses. Moreover, they emphasize chondroid differentiation of the aponeurotic fibroma as its unique feature (15). Lichtenstein and Goldman reported that spindle cells manifest chondroblastic changes. Occasionally, frank hyaline cartilage differentiation occurs at sites of calcification, which distinguishes the lesion from typical fibromatosis. In such instances, the condition is referred to as "the cartilage anologue of fibromatosis" (12).

The treatment of this fibroma must be tempered with patience. In spite of its aggressive histologic appearance, it remains a benign lesion, with no reported tendency to metastasize. Frequent recurrence, especially in young children, appears to be the rule. However, repeated conservative local excision remains the treatment of choice.

Dermal fibromas, such as nodular subepidermal fibrosis, sclerosing hemangiomas, and xanthofibromas, are clearly dissimilar to juvenile aponeurotic fibroma. They all appear in the elderly and are probably related to trauma. Neurofibromas and neurofibromatous malformations may occur in childhood and may resemble aponeurotic fibromas clinically. Whether similar appearing fibromas occur singly or as a part of a generalized von Recklinghausen's neurofibromatosis, their individual microscopic characteristics differentiate them from aponeurotic fibroma.

Aponeurotic fibroma may resemble Dupuytren's type of plantar and palmar fibromatosis in orientation of cell type and hereditary etiology. However, each is unique on microscopic examination. Juvenile aponeurotic fibromas may resemble giant cell tumors of the tendon sheath in that small numbers of multinuclear giant cells occur adjacent to areas of calcification. More mature aponeurotic fibromas concentrate the tumor cells into more solid and discrete cords resembling the formation of a tendon. However, close microscopic inspection distinguishes "calcifying" juvenile aponeurotic fibroma as described by Keasbey from other fibromas (1).

ACQUIRED DIGITAL FIBROKERATOMA

Acquired digital fibrokeratoma are benign, acquired growths usually found on the fingers. However, they can be found on the hands, toes, and feet as well. It usually arises spontaneously; it is asymptomatic, and many cases have been reported in the literature.

Clinically, this tumor type presents as a solitary, firm, and more or less hyperkeratotic projection arising out of a collarette of slightly raised skin. They resemble rudimentary supernumerary digits. Most lesions are present for several months to several years before excision is attempted. They grow slowly and are asymptomatic, unless traumatized (16). No family history is usually present. Digits are usually favored; since both fingers and toes are subject to repeated trauma. In a study of 32 cases by Verallo (1968), six tumors occurred on the toes. They were often situated around the nails but could also be located over joints on their dorsal, medial, or lateral aspects (17). Most patients range in age from 30 to 60.

The tumors were all firm, skin-colored, and varied in height from 5 to 15 mm. In some instances these lesions may become darker with age.

The tumor matrix is composed mainly of somewhat thickened collagenic bundles accompanied by fibroblasts which oriented in the direction of the longitudinal axis of the lesion and are in continuity with the underlying dermal connective tissue stroma. The overlying epidermis is usually acanthotic and hyperkeratotic. Elastic fibers are usually present in the dermis but in varying amounts (16).

Supernumerary digits knuckle pads, subungual fibroma, cutaneous horns, eccrine poroma, pyogenic granuloma, histiocytoma, dermatofibrosarcoma protuberans, verruca vulgaris, and fibromas are lesions to be considered in the differential diagnosis. Fibroma simplex and knuckle pads have a distinct dermal architecture. Both lesions demonstrate an absence of elastic fibers which is quite unlike that of acquired digital fibrokeratoma. Supernumerary digits are present at birth, arising near the bases of the metatarsophalalangeal joints. Such tumors are most often bilateral, and they may be familial. Cutaneous horns are mainly epidermal growths. They may occasionally have a prominent dermal core of quite distinctive architecture (18). Subungual fibroma of tuberous sclerosis may closely resemble acquired digital fibrokeratoma but are unlike it since they are usually multiple and tend to recur (17).

Acquired digital fibrokeratoma may also resemble the garlic clove fibroma. Three such cases were reported by Steel (1965). These lesions were associated with the toenails and fingernails and were projected from the dorsal surface of the nails. The growths were loosely attached by pedicles "resembling garlic cloves with the outer skin peeled away" (19).

Histologic examination reveals a dermal core of interlacing bundles of dense collagenous bundles which contain capillary channels and are covered by hyperkeratotic epidermis. They were painless and did not recur after excision (19). These lesions rarely recur after simple local excision.

RECURRING DIGITAL FIBROUS TUMOR OF CHILDHOOD

Recurring digital fibrous tumor of childhood is a distinct fibrous tumor characterized by the appearance of one or more circumscribed, reddish-pink nodules on the digits of the hands or feet. Many cases have been reported in the world literature.

The tumor is recognized or diagnosed within the first year of life in 80% of cases. Both sexes are affected equally. The tumors occur and recur exclusively on the digits. Following surgical excision, the tumor can be expected to recur in about 60% of the cases (20).

A typical clinical presentation was reported in a 14-month-old girl first seen in April 1975. The tumor appeared as pinkish nodules involving the fourth and fifth toes of the right foot. They had been present for 1 month and had been increasing in size. All lesions were excised in June of 1975 because of their continued growth. However, the lesions recurred in August of 1975, and at the same time an additional nodule appeared on the third toe of the same foot (21).

An almost complete replacement of the dermis by a fibrous mass is characteristic of recurring digital fibrous tumors of childhood. The fibrous tissue extends from the lower epidermal surface deep into the contiguous subcutaneous tissue.

The epidermis is somewhat acanthotic, and the growth replaces the dermis by an infiltrative process. The tumor mass is composed of proliferating fibroblasts and coarse collagen bundles. Such extensions procede from below the epidermis deep into the corium and into the subcutaneous fat tissue. Fibroblasts are typically fusiform and show sweeping fascicles oriented in various directions together with collagen bundles. Small strands of elastic fibers are occasionally seen in the growth. The capillary blood vessels associated with these lesions are thin-walled and rather numerous (21).

Reye (1965) reported six additional cases of recurring digital fibromas of childhood found in infants or young children and confined to the fingers and toes. He distinguished these lesions from other forms of fibromatosis by identification of distinct cytoplasmic inclusions. He considered these to be viral in origin (22). However, the origins of those inclusion bodies are unknown: Attempts to isolate a virus by electron microscopy have failed (20). The presence of these intracytoplasmic inclusion bodies separates this tumor from other fibrous tumors.

Dermatofibroma, benign fibroma, digital mucous cysts, and fibrous hematoma need to be differentiated from recurring digital fibroma of childhood.

Three cases of spontaneous remission of recurring digital fibroma of childhood have been reported (20). Despite the high rate of local recurrence, no cases of distant metastasis have been reported. In the past, surgical excision or amputation have been associated with a recurrence rate of 60%. Presently, observation alone is recommended after the diagnosis has been established. Surgical approaches are appropriately reserved for those cases in which contracture deformities or functional impairment of the digit occur (23).

PERIUNGUAL FIBROMA (KERNAN'S TUMOR)

Congenital generalized fibromatosis, including multisystemic diseases such as tuberous sclerosis and von Recklinghausen's disease, can present unique dermatologic manifestations on the lower extremity. The podiatrist may identify such occurrences as periungual fibroma.

Periungual fibromas, otherwise termed Kernan's tumors, present as firm, smooth, flesh-colored growths protruding from the nail folds (Fig. 23.6). They are "potato-like lesions" of varying yellow and pink coloration. Such lesions can be extensive enough to disrupt the entire nailbed. Kernan's tumors are seen in over 50% of the cases of tuberous sclerosis (24). They usually appear at puberty and continue to develop with age. The periungual tumors can be arranged in an arch around the base of the nail as nail-like multiple, minute, filamentous protrusions. Early lesions can appear as a ridge in the nail or as a "budding seed" with a ridge located distal to the bud (25). Patients usually complain of a dystrophic nail or of an excessive growth of skin over the nail. Shoe pressure may cause pain secondary to growth of the tumor, and splitting of the nail plate may occur. The literature describes most tumors as being essentially asymptomatic.

Schwarzentraub (1978) reports a case in which the patient had a medical history of

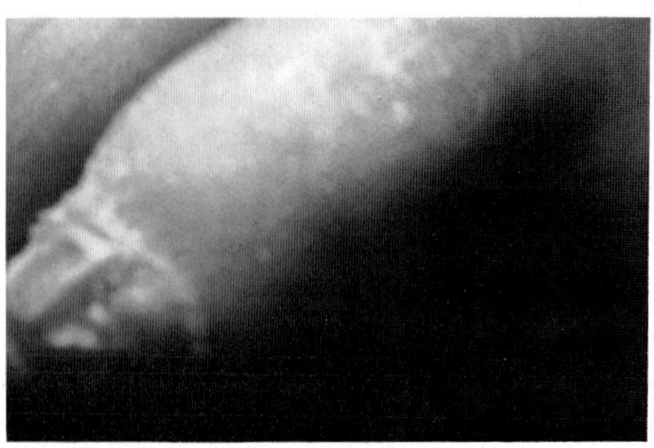

Figure 23.6. Periungual fibroma demonstrating smooth, firm, flesh-colored protrusions.

epilepsy and mild mental retardation. Periungual fibromas developed on all 10 toenails that had been removed several years previously (26). Schwarzentraub concluded that both tuberous sclerosis and the previous nail surgery or trauma had been factors in the etiology of the tumors (26). The author has had similar experiences with this lesion (27).

This tumor may present with a suspicious odor, and discoloration of this lesion often prompts further evaluation. These lesions bleed freely when irritated. Radiographic examination may show projections from or thinning of the distal (ungual) phalanx of the digit. Bony pathology is infrequently encountered.

Since these lesions are generally asymptomatic, they may require no treatment. However, if they become symptomatic or cosmetically unacceptable, a radical excision of the tumor involving the nailbed and nail matrix should be performed because these lesions have a high recurrence rate (28). In rare cases a modified terminal Symes-type procedure was performed with total removal of the distal phalanx (29).

KELOIDS AND HYPERTROPHIC SCARS

A keloid is an indurated brawny elevated lesion with claw-like extensions protruding beyond the original site of an injury (30). It is a benign scar tissue tumor which has been described in the time before Christ and was first identified by name in 1806 by Albert. The lesion "cheloide" from the Greek "shele" meaning crab claw, refers both to the crab-like extension of the lesions and to their tendency to grow laterally into the normal tissue. Addison, in 1854, used the term keloid as it is spelled today. At that time the term meant a mark or blemish, which is better known today as morphea or scleroderma.

The etiology of keloid formation is generally unknown. Most believe that local trauma is the primary precipitating factor. Keloids usually appear within 1 year of the inciting factor. They have also been known to be caused by a variety of injections, vaccinations, and various types of bites. Keloid formation is also associated with various skin tensions and motion on wounds. They may also be formed secondary to poor surgical technique and surgical complications such as infections. A positive family history is also known to be related to keloid formation. Other possible theories as to the cause of keloids include biochemical and biophysical effects, fibroblastic diaphysis, and chemotrophic effects of serum on fibroblasts (30).

Differentiation in sex is generally minimal and usually is equal between males and females. These lesions may occur at any age but seem to be more frequently seen between the ages of 10 and 30 years (31). Most frequent locations for keloid formation include the face, neck, ears, and presternum and deltoid regions. The foot and lower extremity are not nearly as commonly involved, but they, indeed, do occur. Clinically, keloids are firm and tender growths. These lesions generally bring the patient to your office because of their cosmetic disfigurement (Fig. 23.7). It is not uncommon for these lesions to be painful. Racial predisposition is well known: Negroes are more commonly affected.

Hypertrophic scars, on the other hand,

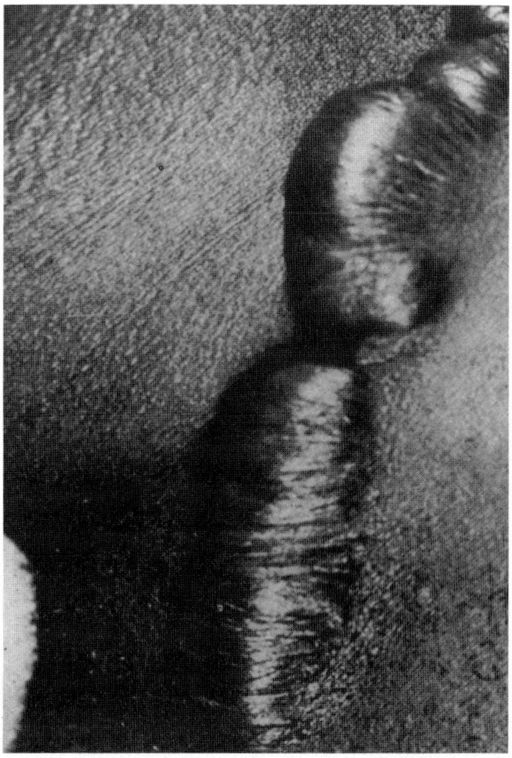

Figure 23.7. Keloid demonstrating disfiguring growth characteristics.

occur with equal frequency in both blacks and whites. Keloids tend to be much larger and firmer than hypertrophic scars. They also have a tendency to grow gradually and rarely regress spontaneously, as do hypertrophic scars. Often keloids can be differentiated from hypertrophic scars by observing the amount of scar formation. Larger formations indicate a keloid while lesser amounts of cicatrization suggest a hypertrophic scar.

Treatment of keloids can be extremely frustrating. Unfortunately, no good method has been developed which consistently provides acceptable results or cure. Intralesional steroid injections have been one of the most frequent forms of therapy. Other types of treatment include radiotherapy as well as radical surgical excision and grafting. These efforts may also develop complications which result in additional keloid formation. Cryotherapy has also been utilized in the treatment of keloid formation. Perhaps the best treatment for keloid formation is to prevent them from forming. One must remember that all skin incisions produce some degree of permanent scarring. A good surgeon tries to minimize this scar formation and, consequently, the complications associated with skin healing. It is important to know the patient's general health, as well as his or her nutritional status prior to performing any surgical procedure. Such understanding can assist in avoiding disfiguring skin lesions such as keloids.

Malignant degeneration of keloid formation is known to exist, but these occurrences are extremely rare. Keloids require great care and skill in treatment. They are highly resistent to both conservative as well as surgical management, particularly in comparison to hypertrophic scars.

PLANTAR FIBROMATOSIS

Plantar fibromatosis is a benign condition most frequently involving the plantar aponeurosis of the foot (Fig. 23.8). Plantar fibromatosis, however, may occur anywhere on the foot and need not be confined only to the plantar fascia. These are reactive lesions and not true neoplasms. Plantar fibromatosis may occur in relation to other conditions, particularly Dupuytren's contractures of the plantar fascia and also Perone's disease.

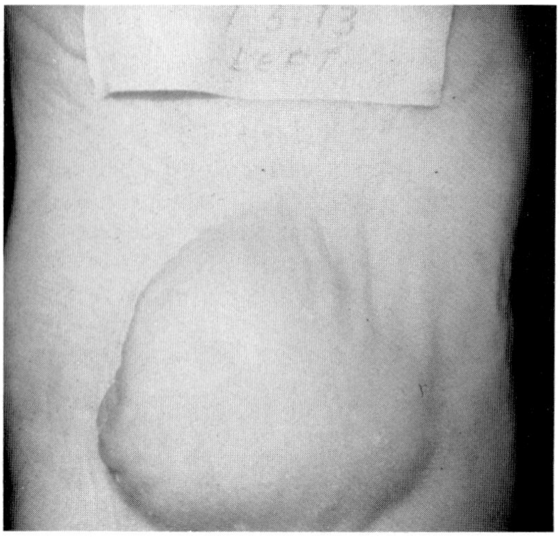

Figure 23.8. Plantar fibromatosis involving the central band of the plantar aponeurosis of the foot.

Plantar fibromatosis was first described by Letterhaus in 1897: The true etiologic factor of this disease is still unknown. They most frequently occur in the central band of the plantar aponeurosis as a solitary lesion, but such lesions may be multiple as well. These growth, are nonencapsulated masses, (Fig. 23.8), and they may infiltrate completely through the plantar fascia. In some instances it may also involve the dermal portions of the skin.

TREATMENT

Curtain advocated a small s-shaped incision on the plantar medial aspect of the foot (32). This incision was meant to reduce the complications involving the vascular structures. The author does not recommend total plantar fascial stripping when excising plantar fibromatosis because the recurrence rate of these lesions is extremely high—75%. One of the greatest surgical errors is that of attempting to strip the plantar fibromatosis from the plantar fascia itself (Fig. 23.9). Plantar fibromatosis generally infiltrates the whole plantar fascia, making its separation impossible.

Generally, these lesions recur in the dermal structures of the skin and subcutaneous structures as well. An interesting relationship exists between certain types of fibromatosis and fibrosarcomas. Some pathologists add that aggressive forms of fibromatosis closely resemble low grades of fibrosarcoma histologically.

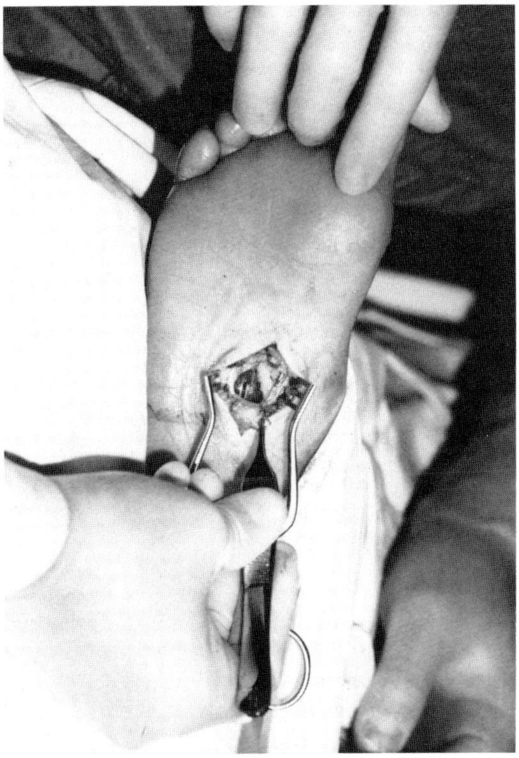

Figure 23.9. Excision of plantar fibromatosis from foot of a 14-year-old Caucasian male. A direct linear midline incision is employed.

FIBROSARCOMAS

Fibrosarcomas are considered rare on the foot. They are probably the most common soft tissue sarcoma. Fibrosarcomas may be differentiated into those that are well differentiated and those that are poorly differentiated tumors. These tumors vary in size and malignant cellularity. The higher the malignancy, the greater the potential of metastatic spread and mortality. Fibrosarcomas on the foot deserve radical surgical excision and in many instances amputation.

CONCLUSION

Fibrous tumors of the foot may present as very unusual, as well as very interesting, types of lesions. The majority of fibrous lesions, as they affect the foot, are benign, but malignancies do occur. When malignant tumors occur, they should be treated aggressively. Overall, fibrous tumors and lesions of the foot represent less than 5% of all tumors that affect the foot (2).

References

1. Keasbey LE: Juvenile aponeurotic fibroma (calcifying fibroma): a distinctive tumor arising in the palms and soles of young children. *Cancer* 6:338–346, 1953.
2. Berlin SJ: A laboratory review of 67,000 foot tumors and lesions. *J Am Podiatry Assoc* 74(7): 341–347, 1984.
3. Samitz MA: *Cutaneous Disorders of the Lower Extremities*, ed 2. Philadelphia, J.B. Lippincott, 1981.
4. Hoffman E: Über das knollentreibende Fibrosarkom dar Haut (Dermatofibrosarcoma Protuberans). *Dermatol Z* 43:1, 1925.
5. O'Brien JE, Stout AP: Malignant fibrous xanthomas. *Cancer* 17:1445–1455, 1964.
6. Taylor HB, Helwig EB: Dermatofibrosarcoma protuberans: a study of 115 cases. *Cancer* 15:717–725, 1962.
7. Burkhardt BR, Soule EH, Winkelmann RK, Ivins JC: Dermatofibrosarcoma protuberans: study of 56 cases. *Am J Surg* 111:638–44, 1966.
8. McPeak CJ, Cruz T, Nicastri AD: Dermatofibrosarcoma protuberans: an analysis of 86 cases, five with metastasis. *Am Surg* 166:803–816, 1967.
9. Hausner RJ, Vargas-Cortes F, Alexander RW: Dermatofibrosarcoma protuberans with lymph node involvement: a case report of simultaneous occurrence with an atypical fibroxanthoma of the skin. *Arch Dermatol* 114:88–91, 1978.
10. Brenner W, Schaefler K, Chhabra H, et al: Dermatofibrosarcoma protuberans metastatic to a regional lymph node: report of a case and review. *Cancer* 36:1897–1902, 1975.
11. Zeichner AM, Uhlman RE: Juvenile aponeurotic fibroma. *J Am Podiatry Assoc* 68(10): 697–702, 1978.
12. Lichtenstein L, Goldman RL: The cartilage analogue of juvenile aponeurotic fibroma. *Cancer* 17:810, 1964.
13. Vatopoulos PK, Garofalakis EE, and Papathanassious BT: Juvenile aponeurotic fibroma. Report of a case. *Acta Orthop Scand* 45:158–1974.
14. Allen PW, Enziner FM: Juvenile aponeurotic fibroma. *Cancer* 26:857–867, 1970.
15. Goldman RL: The cartilage analogue of fibromatosis (aponeurotic fibroma): further observations based on seven new cases. *Cancer* 26:1325, 1970.
16. LoBuono P, Jothikumar T, Kornblee L: Acquired digital fibrokeratoma. *Cutis* 24:50–51, 1979.
17. Verallo VM: Acquired digital fibrokeratomas. *Br J Dermatol* 80:730–736, 1968.
18. Bart RS, Andrade R, Kopt AW, Leider M: Acquired digital fibrokeratomas. *Arch Dermatol* 97:120–129, 1968.

19. Steel HH: Garlic-clove fibroma. *JAMA* 191:1082, 1065.
20. Arundell FD: Proceedings: recurring digital fibrous tumor of childhood. Case I (Beckett) and Case II (Demar L.) *Arch Dermatol* 111:1372, 1975.
21. Cuskey RJ, Nabai H, Homayoon R: Recurring digital fibrous tumor of childhood. *Cutis* 23:359–361, 1979.
22. Reye RDK: Recurring digital fibrous tumors of childhood. *Arch Pathol* 80:228, 1965.
23. Nakavasu K, Maruo M, Ueda K, Ose C: Infantile digital fibromatosis. *J Cutaneous Pathol* 7:431–433, 1980.
24. Morgan E, Wolfort F: The early history of tuberous sclerosis. *Arch Dermatol* 115:1317, 1979.
25. Hugar DW, Rozelle RW: Tuberous sclerosis. *J Am Podiatry Assoc* 73(7):369–371, 1983.
26. Schwarzentraub P: Multiple periungual fibroma (Kernan's tumors): a case report. *J Foot Surg* 17(2):79–80, 1978.
27. Berlin SJ: *Soft Somatic Tumors of the Foot: Diagnosis and Surgical Management, Podiatric Medicine & Surgery, A Monograph Series.* Mt. Kisco, NY, Futura, 1976.
28. Saltzman BS: Periungual fibroma. *J Am Podiatry Assoc* 68(10):696, 1978.
29. Willis WF, Garcia RL: Giant angiofibroma in tuberous sclerosis. *Arch Dermatol* 114:1843–1844, 1978.
30. Helwig EB: Atypical fibroxanthoma. (In) *Tumor Seminar, Proceedings of the 18th Annual Tumor Seminar of San Antonio Society of Pathologists,* 1961. *Tex J Med* 59:664–667, 1963.
31. Enzinger FM, Lattes R, Torloni H: Histological typing of soft tissue tumors. *WHO* 3:1969.
32. Curtin JW: Fibromatosis of the plantar fascia. *J Bone Joint Surg 47A:*1605, 1965.

Suggested Readings

Costello MJ, Gibbs RC: *The Palms and Soles in Medicine,* Charles C Thomas, Springfield, IL, 1967, p 224.

Eder DM, Kirschenbaum SE, Schaffer PE: Benign stromal fibromatosis on the dorsum of the foot. *J Foot Surg* 18(2):83–85, 1979.

Fielding MD, Berlin SJ (eds): *Skin Tumors of the Foot: Diagnosis and Treatment,* vol 3, Mt. Kisco, NY, Futura, 1974, pp 201–205.

Jaffe HL, Lichtenstein L, Sutro CJ: Pigmented villonodular synovitis, bursitis, and tenosynovitis. *Arch Pathol* 31:731, 1941.

Kashuk KB, Pasternack WA: Aggressive infiltrating plantar fibromatosis. *J Am Podiatry Assoc* (9):1980.

Ledderhose G: Zur pathologie der aponeurose des fusses und der hand. Arch Klin Chir SS:694, 1897; cited in Allen RA et al: Soft tissue tumors of the sole. *J Bone Joint Surg* 37A.

Michelson HE: Nodular subepidermal fibrosis. *Arch Dermatol Syphilol* 27:812, 1933.

Novicki DC, Anselmi SJ: Fibrous histiocytoma. *J Am Podiatry Assoc 68* (8):1978.

Soule EJ, Enriquez P: Atypical fibrous histiocytoma, malignant fibrous histiocytoma, malignant histiocytoma, and epithelioid sarcoma: a comparative study of 65 tumors. *Cancer* 30:128–143, 1972.

Spjut HJ, Dorfman HD, Fechner RE et al: *Atlas of Tumor Pathology: Tumors of Bones and Cartilage.* Washington, DC, Armed Forces Institute of Pathology, 1971, pp 400–410.

CHAPTER 24

Podiatric Dermatologic Therapeutics

GARY L. DOCKERY

INTRODUCTION

Podiatric dermatologic therapeutics is applied or clinical pharmacology that is concerned with the use of drugs in the treatment of lower extremity skin disease. The extensive scope of this discipline is obvious when one considers that a drug may be broadly defined as any chemical substance that affects biologic systems.

Skin diseases may be treated by the administration of drugs by several different routes, such as topically, orally, intralesionally, or by direct systemic application. It is not the intent of this chapter to provide a complete and comprehensive list of all drugs that might possibly be used in dermatology therapy. The drugs covered in more detail in this chapter represent a large percent of the medications prescribed by practitioners treating lower extremity dermatological conditions.

The chapter is organized according to therapeutic categories within the classifications of topical, intralesional, or systemic therapy. Although great care has been taken in compiling and editing the information presented in this section, the reader is advised to consult the manufacturer before prescribing or administering any infrequently used or unfamiliar medication to be certain that there have been no changes in the indications or recommended doses. Furthermore, additional precautions must be taken when prescribing medications for children, pregnant women, or nursing women (1, 2). Specific treatments and preferred therapy for different types of dermatological conditions may be found in the chapter devoted to that disorder.

PRINCIPLES OF TREATMENT

Dermatological drugs are chemical substances that are used for the prevention, diagnosis, or treatment of skin conditions. Most of these drugs are differentiated by their ability to act selectively in biological systems to accomplish a desired effect. This selective action with regard to their use is the basis of pharmacotherapeutics.

Vehicles are used to deliver the active ingredients to the skin and hold them there, to absorb water and prevent its evaporation, or to assist the skin in cooling of its surface. An accurate assessment of the type of medication required also includes the appropriate type of vehicle to transport it.

Every podiatric medical student learns the axiom, if the skin is dry, wet it; it it is wet, dry it. If the skin is unresponsive, stimulate it; and if it is inflamed, soothe it. For practical purposes this is true for a majority of cases. For example, to treat a skin lesion that is oozing or moist, the podiatrist should prescribe a wet dressing, followed by a lotion. On the other hand, a dry or chronic scaling patch would be treated with an ointment, since wet dressings may be drying and may worsen the condition.

The following degree of skin change with the corresponding list of appropriate vehicles may be used as a general guide for assessing a treatment plan.

Skin Change		Vehicle
Acute Response	↓	Wet dressings
Edema, erythema		Lotions
Vesiculation, oozing		Aerosols, sprays
Infection pruritis		Powders
Chronic Response	↓	Creams
Dryness, scaling		Emulsions
Lichenification, fissuring		Gels
Erythema, pruritis		Ointments

In other words, the type of skin lesion, rather than the cause, should direct the initial therapy. It must be remembered, however, that the type of skin lesion may show rapid change during therapy, and appropriate adjustments should be made in the treatment approach.

Careful follow-up of the patient is essential since one of the most common problems following skin treatment is overtreatment. This frequently occurs when the patient was given far too much of a given topical medication and he or she continues to use it long after the skin condition has cleared. The other situation involves the patient who has been using an inappropriate medication for long periods of time which has actually been making the skin problem more acute. Therefore, it is wise for the podiatric physician to see the patient at moderately frequent intervals early in the management of a skin problem. As the condition improves, visits can be extended to long intervals.

Because many patients become confused about the time intervals of treatment or simply cannot remember the physician's instructions regarding their part in the therapy, it is wise to provide printed instructions outlining the procedures. Patients often do much better when provided with a printed form setting forth in understandable terms the nature of their skin disorder and a means of correcting it. The printed sheet saves countless hours of repeated instructions to patients who forgot what to do. It is wise to have printed instruction sheets covering such items as how to mix and perform Epsom salt foot soaks, how to care for an eczematous foot dermatitis, or how to manage tinea pedis.

With these principles of treatment in mind, let us now turn to the *prescribing* principles of prescription writing.

PRESCRIPTION WRITING

A prescription is a written order by a physician to a pharmacist. In addition to the name of the patient and that of the physician, the prescription should contain the name or names of the drugs ordered and their quantitites, instructions to the pharmacist, and directions to the patient. The practice of writing long, complicated prescriptions containing many active ingredients, adjuvants, correctives, and various vehicles has been abandoned in favor of using single pure compounds. Even when combinations of several active ingredients are desirable, the pharmaceutical companies often have available several forms of suitable combinations.

Drugs may be prescribed by their official names, which are *United States Pharmacopeia* (USP) or National Formulary (NF); by their nonofficial generic names, which are *New Drugs* (ND), formerly *New and Nonofficial Drugs* (NND), or *United States Adopted Name* (USAN); or by a manufacturer's trade name.

Parts of Prescription

Traditionally a prescription is written in a certain order and consists of four basic parts:

1. The superscription, which includes the patient's name, address, the date, and the symbol R_x, the abbreviation for recipe, the imperative of the recipere, meaning "Take thou."
2. The inscription, which states the names and amounts of the ingredients to be used.
3. The subscription, which contains directions to the pharmacist. Often it consists only of M., the abbreviation for misce, meaning "mix."
4. The signature, which is abbreviated "S" or "Sig," and contains the directions to the patient, such as "Take one teaspoonful three times a day before meals." The signature should indicate whether the medicine is intended for external application and whether it has some special toxic properties. Whenever possible, instructions of a general nature, such as "take as directed," should be avoided since the patient may have misunderstood the verbal directions given by the physician.

Trends in Prescription Writing

The parts of the prescription described in the previous section represent a tradition that is undergoing considerable change. Latin, even in the form of abbreviations, is no longer mandated. At the present time, prescriptions are usually written in English. Even such abbreviations as M. or Sig. may be avoided. It is also advisable to avoid as much as possible the use of the decimal point and state the number of milligrams in a dose instead of using the decimal fraction of a gram.

Much confusion results from the fact that the name of a drug is not spelled out on a label, and therefore, the patient knows only that he is taking some sort of pills or applying some kind of medication having certain physical characteristics. The busy physician wastes much time trying to identify medications given to his patients by other physicians. It may be very difficult to identify a drug by a patient's verbal description.

In traditional pharmaceutic practice, the name of a prescription drug does not appear on the label of the package that the pharmacist furnishes the patient. However, the physician may instruct the pharmacists to put information on the label by including on the prescription the direction, "Label as such," or "LAS," or, merely, "Label." For several years, the American Medical Association has encouraged physicians to follow this practice and to make an exception only when such disclosure would be detrimental to the welfare of the patient. The reasons for believing prescription drugs should be labeled with their names and strength have been set forth repeatedly:

1. The patient has the right to be informed about his illness and the medications prescribed.
2. In emergency situations, such as accidental poisoning, overdose, or attempted suicide, immediate identification of a prescription drug from the label may be lifesaving.
3. The information is valuable when the patient changes doctors, moves to another locality, or contacts the prescribing physician at a time when records are not readily avilable.
4. The information on the label is of value in group practices in which the patient may not always have the same attending physician.
5. It is advisable that the patients with allergies know what is being prescribed.
6. This specific information on the label helps to prevent confusion between two or more drugs being taken concurrently, or between medications being taken by different members of the same family.
7. If it becomes necessary to issue a warning against the use of a particular drug, the name on the label serves to alert those who have been given prescriptions for the product.

The reasons that have been advanced opposing the labeling of prescription drugs with the name and strength are far less persuasive than those just given for labeling. There are, of course, some occasions when such labeling is inadvisable for psychological or other reasons, but in these circumstances, the instructions can be omitted from the prescription.

Restrictions on refills are controlled by law for certain narcotics and drugs subject to abuse. However, it is advisable for the podiatrist to designate the number of refills and the number of doses usually required in any specific condition, and to instruct the patient to take all of the prescribed medication as directed or to destroy the remaining drugs. Prescriptions with open-end authorization for refills, especially if marked "refill prn" or "ad lib," remain valid indefinitely. When this authorization is given in advance (on the prescription at the time of writing), the physician would be well advised to place some time limit on the authorization.

DRUG ADMINISTRATION

Absorption

The intensity and duration of the response to a single dose of a drug of a given concentration will vary depending upon the rapidity with which blood or tissue levels are to be achieved. Factors modifying absorption include the following.

SOLUBILITY

One property of drugs that can be modified to provide a longer duration of effect is their solubility when given by subcutaneous or intramuscular injection. For example, unmodified water-soluble penicillin must be injected as often as six times per day to maintain constant therapeutic levels. If the penicillin is combined with procaine and thus rendered less soluble, its absorption from the injection site will continue for more than 12 hr. Drugs administered orally may, however, be well absorbed even though they are insoluble in water.

Chemical Properties: A drug may be dispensed in different chemical forms suitable for many different routes of administration. For topical use, local anesthetics or antihistamines may be dispensed to better advantage as the lipid-soluble free base rather than the water-soluble salt.

Routes of Administration

The routes of drug entry into a patient can be classified as *enteral* or *parenteral.* Enteral routes are those by which a drug is placed directly into the gastrointestinal tract, from which absorption occurs across the enteric membrane: This includes oral and rectal routes. Parenteral administration bypasses the gastrointestinal tract and includes injections and topical applications.

Enteral Routes

ORAL

Oral administration is relatively safe, painless, convenient, and economical, and is therefore, the most frequently used route. The onset of action after oral administration is delayed in comparison with the effect after parenteral administration. The major limitations of the oral route are that the drug may not be well absorbed from the gastrointestinal tract; that irritating drugs may cause many local side effects; that the taste may be unpleasant; and that some drugs, such as proteins that are digested or certain steroids that are inactivated by the liver, do not reach the general circulation as well after oral administration. In an emergency situation, when rapid onset of action is important, or if the patient is unable to swallow, another route should be chosen.

RECTAL

Certain drugs may be given by suppository or, less commonly, by enema. Drugs that may be irritative when given orally are better tolerated when given by this route, and nausea does not prevent giving the drug.

Those routes of administration listed from this point on are parenteral, by which is meant any route of administration that does not require absorption across an enteric membrane into the portal circulation and immediate transport to drug metabolizing sites in the liver.

Parenteral Medication

Parenteral administration, one of the commonly used methods of giving medications to patients, is also the most dangerous of all administration procedures. It can cause permanent injuries and is, therefore, undertaken only by highly trained and well-informed professionals who fully understand the hazards of this technique. A few precautions which must be considered when introducing drugs parenterally include: (*a*) avoidance of nerve damage; (*b*) location of the injected medicaments; (*c*) concentration of the injected drug; (*d*) sterility; (*e*) the vehicle employed; and (*f*) the volume of injection.

Drugs may be injected into the skin, under the skin, into the muscles, the joints, nerves, veins, and even into the arteries. Drugs may, in fact, be injected into almost any accessible part of the body. Injection is an effective means of providing slow or rapid drug action and can control therapeutic response with great accuracy. Asepsis must be maintained, and errors in dosage cannot be readily corrected.

The major disadvantage of injections, other than complications, is pain, but this can be greatly reduced if the needle is sharp and is inserted and withdrawn quickly, bevel upwards. Injections should never be made where nerves or bone will be struck or where the tissue is dense and nonelastic because the distension produced by the injected fluid is painful, and may cause tissue damage. Isotonic solutions should be used whenever possible, and hypertonic solutions should be avoided.

Whenever possible, sites are chosen that are poorly supplied with sensory nerves, such as the outer side of the arm or the thigh, to minimize the pain of injection. When the thigh area is employed, the precautions against sepsis must be maintained because injections in this region are more likely to be followed by gas gangrene than injections in the upper part of the body. By pinching up the skin or stretching it, the sensitivity of the surface is lessened. For intravenous and intradermal (intracutaneous) injection, the needle is inserted with the bevel at an acute angle, almost parallel with the blood vessel and skin. In other injections the needle is inserted with a quick thrust at right angles to and through the skin.

Parenteral Routes

INJECTIONS

Subcutaneous

Solutions or suspensions of drugs can be injected into the subcutaneous areolar tissue. When small volumes are injected, the skin overlying the muscle is lifted, and the needle enters the tent thus formed. When larger volumes are given, the inner surface of the thigh is preferable. Large volumes of isotonic fluid are absorbed from these sites, and such an injection is often referred to as a hypodermoclysis or just clysis. Irritating solutions are more painful if given by this route than if given intramuscularly or intravenously.

Intramuscularly

Muscle is more vascular and less sensitive than subcutaneous tissue, and irritating solutions or suspensions are better tolerated when given intramuscularly. Absorption from the intramuscular site is somewhat more rapid than from subcutaneous injection sites. Small volumes (2 ml or less) are given into the deltoid muscle. Larger volumes (up to 10 ml) are given into the gluteal mass underlying the upper outer quadrant of one buttock or the other. The vastus muscle underlying the lateral surface of the thigh is an alternate area for injection.

Intravenous

The intravenous route makes possible accurate control of dosage and rapid dilution of more caustic materials. Onset of action is even more rapid than after intramuscular or subcutaneous administration. The volume of fluid that can be injected intravenously is also greater than is possible by other parenteral routes. Even if the volume and rate of injection are carefully controlled, the intravenous route is far more hazardous than other routes of administration because of the initial high local concentration of drugs that can result. Drugs administered intravenously have rapid access to the general circulation and have systemic effects.

Intraarterial

Drugs may be injected into the artery, perfusing a specific area of the body in order to achieve a high local concentration in the area before dilution by the entire plasma volume occurs. Vasodilators may be given intraarterially during the vasospastic state following an acute arterial occlusion. This route is infrequently used in dermatologic therapeutics.

Intradermal

A small amount (less than 0.5 ml) of an isotonic material can be safely injected into the skin. If the injection is properly superficial, a wheal will be formed. Antigens for skin test are injected in this way. Local anesthetics injected in this manner provide an insensitive area through which a larger needle may be passed without pain for deeper injection of local anesthetics.

TOPICAL

This route of drug administration includes application to oral mucous membranes, the skin, and other epithelial surfaces. Topical therapy may be instituted to achieve a local drug effect, such as a locally applied corticosteroid to relieve various localized skin disorders. Topically applied medication occasionally may provide a route by which a systemic blood level is obtained. Most drugs do not penetrate the intact skin well, and this route is generally used for local drug effects. Important systemic drugs, such as penicillin, should not be used topically since sensitization frequently occurs with potentially serious systemic consequences.

We will concentrate our discussion on three main classification categories, which include topical therapy, intralesional therapy, and systemic therapy.

TOPICAL THERAPY

There are two primary considerations to take into account when discussing dermatologic topical preparations, the medication and the vehicle. Both of the variables must be appropriate for the specific condition being treated. The efficacy of topical therapy derives from both the physical actions of the vehicle and the chemical action of the applied medications. These actions, which include wetting, hydration, softening, lubricating, or drying, are designed to return the injured or diseased skin to a stable physiologic state while making the patient comfortable in the process.

Nonmedicated Topical Agents (or Vehicles)

The vehicles used in topical therapy include liquids (wet dressings, tinctures, paints, or lotions), semisolids (emulsions, gels, or creams), or solids (ointments or powders).

WET DRESSINGS

Wet dressings dry oozing secretions, soften scales and crusts, and aid in cleansing purulent lesions. The end result is a drier, cleaner surface for epithelialization to occur. In addition, wet dressings are also beneficial in relieving burning, itching, and paresthesia by the cooling sensation provided by the solution. The foot soak is often preferable to the wet compress because of ease of application. Plain tap water can be used, and I prefer to use aluminum acetate (Burow's solution) diluted 1:10 for soaking. Epsom salt (2 tblsp per pint of water) is also frequently prescribed; however, this may result in overdrying of the skin surface. Because of their tendency to produce maceration, foot soaks should not exceed 20 min. Wet dressings are indicated in vesicular pustulae, bullous, or on ulcerative or exudative lesions.

TINCTURES AND PAINTS

Tinctures and paints are alcoholic or hydroalcoholic solutions which, after being applied to the skin, dry and leave a uniform film of the active medication on the skin. Castellani's paint, gentian bismuth, or gentian violet tincture are used similarly for treatment of intertrigo, interdigital lesions, and fissuring. Sprays and aerosols also act in a similar fashion.

LOTIONS

Lotions are suspensions of powders in a liquid vehicle, such as calamine, or preparations in which the active medication has been dissolved. The main vehicles for lotions include water, propylene glycol, and alcohol or combinations of these liquids. As the vehicle evaporates on the skin, the active ingredients are deposited at the site of application. Lotions have the advantage of being more easily applied to interdigital or hairy areas and may be used in conjunction with wet dressings in exudative dermatoses. They are less drying to the skin than tinctures or paints.

EMULSIONS AND CREAMS

Water-in-oil emulsions, such as cold cream, are much more occlusive than creams and may retain heat, increase hydration, and impede water loss. Creams are semisolid emulsions of oil-in-water made by complicated procedures utilizing emulsifying agents. Since the water content is higher, these agents may be drying, and because of lack of occlusiveness they should be applied frequently and the patient should be instructed to rub the cream in until it vanishes.

It is important to decide exactly what the objectives of treatment are and why the application is being used. The base which penetrates the skin most effectively should be used when carrying medication into the site of the problem. If, however, soothing and protecting of the skin is important, then a preparation which stays on the surface may be more useful.

GELS

Gels are colorless and transparent semisolid emulsions that can be rubbed in to disappear completely. The agent liquifies on contact with the skin, leaving a nonocclusive, thin, greaseless film. Gels are very useful in hairy areas because they leave the skin without a sticky sensation.

OINTMENTS

Ointments are semisolid vehicles which are thicker than lotions or creams and have a higher oil content. Ointment bases tend to produce a more complete cover over the skin surface and serve to relieve scaliness, dryness, and fissures through their lubricating effect, as well as by the prevention of water loss from the skin. Ointments are excellent carriers of chemically active agents. The solubility of the active agents varies with the base used, and the chemical's clinical effect may be different from one ointment to another. There are essentially three types of ointments: those that are insoluble in water, those that will emulsify in water, and those that are soluble in water.

The water-repellant (insoluble) ointments (petrolatum (USP) and liquid petrolatum, (USP)) are difficult to wash off and will not dry out. Because the melting point is close to the skin temperature, these ointments may stain clothing, and patients should be so warned. The greasy ointments can be made more acceptable to patients by having them lightly powder the ointment with baby talc after it has been applied to the skin.

The emulsifiable ointments (lanolin and hydrophilic petrolatum (USP)) are insoluble in water. However, they are capable of absorbing large amounts of water and become water-in-oil emulsions.

The water-soluble ointments (polyethylene glycol (USP)) are completely soluble in water and are frequently used as lubricants. Since they can be thoroughly rubbed into the skin, they are excellent vehicles for allowing absorption of medications into the skin.

POWDERS

Powders may be applied directly to the skin surface and are drying, cooling, and lubricating in nature. Dusting powders have a very superficial effect on the skin and also provide antipruritic sensations. In general, powders are best used in intertriginous areas and between the toes because these sites are normally moistened by perspiration and can become macerated and irritated. The powder will absorb the moisture and lubricate the opposing skin surfaces, minimizing the frictional effect.

Talcum powder, magnesium stearate, zinc oxide or stearate, and cornstarch are the most common types of powders. Talcum powder is the most lubricating and the least absorbent, and cornstarch is the least lubricating but most absorbent of these powders.

FIXED DRESSINGS

Fixed dressing are designed to provide maximum protection to the skin from external sources. They are usually bandages impregnated with vehicles or agents which dry and fix the covering in a firm or castlike fashion. The most commonly used fixed dressing is the Unna paste boot. There are several commercial types available, and they are used to cover and protect skin problems on the feet, ankles, or legs. When properly applied, they provide a great deal of support to the lower extremeity vascular system and are ideal for treating stasis dermatitis and ulcerations.

Medicated Topical Agents

TOPICAL ANTIBIOTICS

There is considerable controversy regarding topical antibiotics in the treatment of skin diseases. Although there is no firm documentation of the clinical value of topically applied antibiotics, there are those (3) who firmly believe that they are efficacious and that their hazards have been greatly exaggerated.

Skin infections are termed pyodermas, and they are classified as primary or secondary. The primary infections are seen in normal skin or skin that has suffered an injury, cut, or minor abrasion, which has then been invaded by a pathogen. The most common causative organisms in primary pyodermas are *Streptococcus pyogenes* and *Staphylococcus aureus* (4).

Secondary pyodermas usually appear in conjunction with other skin disorders, such as ulcerations, burns, contact dermatitis, atopic dermatitis, or preexisting fungal infections. In these cases, the preceding inflammatory condition becomes invaded and colonized by a pathogen.

One of the problems in the proper management of skin infections is the overall interpretation of the isolates from the wound. The agents associated with these infections may be normal skin bacteria. Therefore, the isolates could represent the causative bacteria or simply a contaminant. The most effective approach to the problem usually requires an overall assessment by the podiatrist of the case, including a gram stain and the observation for the presence of pus.

There are many antibiotic agents available for topical use and, in general, the most beneficial appear to be the poorly absorbed topical antibiotics such as bacitracin, gramicidin, neomycin, and polymyxin B. Bacitracin is particularly useful against streptococci, and staphylococci are particularly susceptible to neomycin. Polymyxin B is effective against many gram-negative organisms, except *Proteus* and *Serratia*, and gramicidin is very useful against many gram-positive organisms. Since culturing of uncomplicated superficial infections may delay treatment time and increase cost to the patient, and because multiple organism are frequently reported, combinations of the nonabsorbable antibiotics are used frequently.

The use of combinations or mixtures of topical antibiotics may be beneficial: They can treat a wide range of pathogens in a mixed infection, and they can allow use of drugs that are potentially toxic when given systemically. Moreover, they can be used in relatively small amounts, and since many are predominantly synergistic, they increase the potential rate of bactericidal action and, thus, probably increase their spectrum of action.

Topical erythromycin is also very effective and may be the drug of choice when sensitivity occurs to the poorly absorbed antibiotics or when contact irritation occurs. I have found that topical erythromycin solution (A/T/S, Hoechst-Roussel) is extremely effective in treating pitted keratolysis of the soles caused by *Corynebacterium.*

Gentamycin is useful in treating infections caused by gram-negative organisms, especially *Pseudomonas.* Topical resistant strains do not appear to be a major problem in outpatient use; however, they are not recommended for general topical care in hospital cases, except in the treatment of burns.

Systemic toxicity from topical antibiotics has occurred when large quantities were used, or after application to large areas of denuded skin. No systemic toxicity has been reported from topical usage for minor wounds or even with prolonged use on chronically inflammed skin (3).

Neomycin is the only potential allergen, and the reported incidence of hypersensitivity to a 20% concentration of topically applied neomycin is between 3.7 and 60% in individuals with contact dermatitis or chronic dermatoses. The incidence of sensitization of the general population is around 1% (5).

The choice of a topical antibiotic agent is dependent upon its efficacy, safety, and cost. In determining the efficacy of topical vs. systemic antibiotics in infective dermatitis, it seems that the approach would require a thorough assessment of the clinical picture, appropriate bacteriologic examination, including gram stain, and antibiotic selection from the sensitivity studies. The final decision on the route of administration should include the extent of the lesions, with topical therapy being shown to be as effective as systemic therapy in minor or localized lesions (6), and the clinical and immunologic state of the host.

Topical antibiotics have a definite place in the practice of podiatric medicine, and in appropriate situations they are a safe and effective means of controlling the bacteria usually found in superficial wounds. These antibiotics may also be effective in preventing infections in clean wounds and may reduce the systemic effects of infection and speed healing in infected wounds such as lacerations, incisions, or burns.

TOPICAL ANTIFUNGALS

For most practical purposes, fungal infections are divided into three main categories: dermatophytic, systemic, and candidal. The dermatophytic group is the most common type of fungal infection and usually involves the skin, hair, and nails. The dermatophyte fungi are a unique and distinct class of fungi which survive in the superficial layers of the epidermis, nails, and hair. They do not penetrate below the keratin layers because there is a serum fungal inhibitory factor in the deep intravascular space which prevents deep penetration of fungal elements (7).

Approximately 20 different species of *Epidermophyton, Trichophyton,* and *Microsporin* cause these infections. Essentially, there are four topical agents available for the treatment of fungal infections: a synthetic alkylaryl ether, haloprogin (Halotex); tolnaftate (Tinactin); and two synthetic imidazole compounds, clotrimazole (Lotrimin, Mycelex) and miconazole nitrate (Monistat-Derm). Other forms of topical antifungal agents also include nystatin and undecylenic acid. New topical antifungal medications such as econazole nitrate (Spectazole) are entering the market on a regular basis. Many of these will have to be tested, and clinical trials must be run before their total efficacy will be known (see Table 24.1).

Haloprogin (Halotex) is a synthetic topical antifungal agent used primarily in treatment of superficial fungal infections of the skin. It is also active against cutaneous candidal infections and may also be useful against certain bacterial infections caused by staphylococci and streptococci. Haloprogin may increase pruritus and maceration and exacerbate some preexisting lesions. Adverse reactions also include burning sensation, increased local irritation to the skin, and vesicle formation. The cure rate with haloprogin may be slightly

Table 24.1
Topical Antifungal Drugs

Drug	Recommended for *Candida*	Recommended for Tinea	Formulations
Econazole (Spectazole—Ortho)	X	X	Cream
Miconazole (Monistat-Derm—Ortho)	X	X	Lotion, cream
Clotrimazole	X	X	
(Mycelex—Miles)			Solution, cream
(Lotrimin—Schering)			Solution, cream
Ticonazole (tz-3—Leeming, Div. of Pfizer)		X	
Ciclopirox (Loprox—Hoechst-Roussel)	X	X	
Haloprogin (Halotex—Westwood)		X	Solution, cream
Tolnaftate		X	
(Tinactin—Schering)			Solution, powder, aerosol, cream
(Aftate—Plough)			Gel, aerosol, powder
Undecylenic acid and salts		X	
(Desenex—Pharmacraft)			Ointment, soap, powder, aerosol
(Cruex—Pharmacraft)			Cream
(Verdefam—Owen)			Solution
(Quinsana Plus—Mennen)			Powder
(Daliderm—Dalin)			Lotion
(Deso-creme—Columbia Medical)			Cream
Nystatin	X		
(Mycostatin—Squibb)			Ointment, powder, cream
(Nilstat—Lederle)			Ointment, cream
Amphotericin B (Fungizone—Squibb)	X		Lotion, ointment, cream

higher than that with tolnaftate, and the chances of recurrence may be less with haloprogin than with tolnaftate (8). Another important clinical study compared haloprogin and miconazole, with the results showing no significant superiority for either compound when the cure rate of topical infection was assessed by negative culture results (9).

Tolnaftate (Tinactin) was one of the first synthetic chemical topical antifungal agents developed. It is relatively effective against the skin infections, and only a few toxic reactions have been reported. It is not effective against candidal or bacterial infections. Fungal infections of the scalp, nails, soles, and palms usually do not respond well to tolnaftate. This agent is frequently used adjunctively with oral antifungal agents for its local benefit. Relapses are common with this particular agent, and newer agents appear to be much more effective.

Miconazole nitrate (Monistat-Derm) is a synthetic imidazole antifungal agent which is effective against most dermatophyte species, including candidal infections. It is similar in nature to clotrimazole and has a similar efficacy. In a double-blind study comparing miconazole and clotrimazole after 4 weeks of topical treatment, 83% of those patients treated with miconazole were found to be mycologically free from infection, as compared with 79% of patients treated with clotrimazole (10).

Clotrimazole (Lotrimin, Mycelex) is a synthetic imidazole agent which is closely related chemically to miconazole and has a broad antifungal spectrum which also includes candidal infections. It also inhibits growth of some gram-positive bacteria and in high concentrations is active against *Trichomonas* species. In a double blind trial comparing Whitfield's ointment with Clotrimazole cream following 4 weeks of topical therapy, the patients in each treatment group showed 88% of cure rate as evaluated by negative culture results (11).

Nystatin (Candex, Mycostatin) is a polyene antibiotic derived from *Streptomyces.*

It is a fungistatic or fungicidal, depending upon the concentration, route of administration, and infecting organism. It is effective against all forms of *Candida* species that cause infection in skin of man. Clinically, its use is limited to the treatment of candidal infections of the skin and mucous membranes.

Undecylenic acid (Desenex) appears to be a relatively useful proprietary agent for the treatment of dermatophytic infections. It is well tolerated and may be worth a trial in localized and mild infections. The initial cure rate may be very high, but recurrence is also relatively high.

The vast majority of topically applied antifungal agents now in use are odorless and nonstaining. Overall, the imidazole compounds appear to be the most consistent as far as cure rates are concerned, and reports of sensitization to these compounds are very uncommon.

Although there are many effective antifungal drugs for topical therapy, recurrence or relapse of dermatophyte infections still remains a chronic problem. The follow-up period in most studies is far too short to determine whether one antifungal drug is superior to another in effectively eliminating the causative fungus.

The search for new and more effective antifungal topical agents will continue because these infections are still among the most common diseases encountered in podiatric and medical dermatology practice. The one area where new agents are needed is in the topical treatment of toenail fungal infections. All of the above-mentioned topical drugs have decreased activity when treating onychomycosis and have never been found to be consistently effective.

Finally, the patient's acceptance of the length of time needed for accurate treatment and the form in which the drug is applied may, however, ultimately decide which of the available or new drugs is most successful in the future.

ANTIPERSPIRANTS AND ASTRINGENTS

The use of topically applied antiperspirants and astringents for the lower extremities is very common in the practice of podiatric medicine. The primary reason for using these agents is in acute inflammatory states and in the treatment of hyperhidrosis of the feet and soles. These agents are generally applied by topical mechanisms through wet dressings, baths, or astringent applicators. The most common of the topically applied astringents and antiperspirant drugs will be discussed.

Aldehydes induce a decrease in perspiration by blockage within the stratum corneum. Formaldehyde is a potent wide spectrum antiseptic and germicide that has been used as a solution in water to decrease perspiration. The main disadvantage of this particular agent is that it is very irritative to skin at concentrations required to achieve the desired response. Consequently, it is seldom used in podiatry for anhidrotic action of the soles.

Glutaraldehyde solution is a potent dialdehyde with a wide range of germicidal activity which is also rapidly sporicidal and actively decreases hyperhidrosis with regular use. Glutaraldehyde solution is generally applied threee times per week for 1 to 2 weeks until the excessive perspiration is under control. A 10% solution is recommended for soaking of the feet and may cause a temporary brown discoloration to appear. A 2% solution will not cause the discoloration and may be used for regular application; however, this concentration may not reduce excessive sweating. This glutaryl 2% solution has a pH 7.5 (Cidex) and is available as a nonprescription product for general use. It may cause some irritation to the skin with chronic application (12).

Methenamine is an antiseptic available as the free compound or as one of several salts that, when applied topically, hydrolyzes to form formaldehyde and ammonium chloride. Methenamine in a 5% applicator or in a 10% solution may be used to control moderate hyperhidrosis of the soles (13).

Aluminum compounds are frequently used in podiatry for antiperspirant and astringent effects. These astringents precipitate protein and decrease oozing. They also decrease perspiration directly. Aluminum acetates (Burow's solution) contains approximately 5% of aluminum acetate and is diluted 1:10 to 1:40 for use as a wet dressing astringent for the feet. This may be one of the most commonly used astringents for wet dressings which, unlike the aldehyde group, does not stain the skin and allows drying and soothing of hyperhidrotic or inflamed tissue. Aluminum chloride hexahydrate (Alu-Wets) may provide a much better compress type of dressing. Aluminum sulfate and calcium acetate combinations (Domeboro or Bluboro) are dispensed in powder or tablet form and quickly dissolve in warm water to create an aluminum diacetate combination. The liquid form of aluminum chloride hexahydrate (Drysol or Xerac-AC) may be applied directly to the skin as an antiperspirant solution. These agents are effective astringents and may be antibacterial in nature as well (14).

Biofeedback techniques may also be very effective in decreasing excessive palmoplantar hyperhidrosis and the chronic symptoms of plantar sole sweating (15). These relaxation techniques may also be added to the other antiperspirant and astringent topical agents for more effective and longlasting results in the treatment of a sometimes embarrassing and problematic condition of severe hyperhidrosis.

Iontophoresis utilizing tap water or combinations of anticholinergic drugs such as glycopyrrolate may effectively reduce hyperhidrosis of the soles for many weeks (16). The use of iontophoresis with tap water only is a very safe and effective way of inducing hypohidrosis (17).

Magnesium subsulfate (Epsom salt) is used frequently in our practice as an astringent foot soak. The patients are instructed to mix 2 tbsp per quart of warm water and soak for approximately 20 min. The combined effect is to reduce the skin surface of bacteria, and the astringent effect will cause drying of oozing lesions and will effectively reduce hyperhidrosis as well. If used on a routine basis, the soaking of all astringents may cause excessive drying of the skin which can be countered by the use of topical emollients or skin creams.

Normal saline (0.9% sodium chloride) may be utilized for the drying effect which results after soaking for approximately 20 min and then allowing the solution to evaporate from the skin while air drying the lower extremity. This solution may be approximated by adding 1 tsp of table salt to 480 ml of water.

ANTIPRURITICS

Pruritus is a symptom complex and not a dermatology condition. The intense discomfort produced by itching is probably the primary reason that patients come into the office for treatment. Pruritus may be noted only in certain phases of the dermatoses and may be the predominant feature and may precede all other symptoms. Mechanical injury to the skin may follow pruritus and result in excoriations and lichen simplex chronicus (18). Pruritus is a very common symptom with many skin diseases, and the primary treatment is relief of the itching in the early stages of the condition. Topical antipruritic and emollient drugs are often useful in relieving the severe itching. Many of the traditional antipruritic agents are currently used more frequently by dermatologists than podiatrists. The agents may be topical corticosteroids, antihistaminic agents, or simply soothing vehicles.

Cool water baths may alleviate itching and inflammation and are easily applied by most patients. Lubrication of wet skin with additives or the application of topical emulsion can also provide comfort to the patient. Cool compresses are also significant for relief of itching from pruritic skin.

Concentrations of 0.5 to 2% menthol, 0.5 to 1.5 phenol, and 1 to 3% camphor in various formulations may have very strong antipruritic action. The menthol action appears to be primarily that of a cooling sensation with evaporation. The phenol and camphor may cause an alteration of the cutaneous nerve transmission and may decrease the conceptualization of pruritis. Calamine lotion and phenolated calamine, USP lotions, are also effective in treating this particular condition.

Local anesthetic agents may also be applied to relieve pruritus by blocking nerve impulses at the sensory nerve ending level. One of the most commonly used nonprescription topical anesthetics is ethyl aminobenzoate (Benzocaine). The main problem with the use of topical Benzocaine is its short duration of anesthetic action. Another very effective topical agent is diphenhydramine hydrochloride (Benadryl).

Other topically applied over-the-counter products usually contain methylsalicylate, triethanolamine salicylate, thymol, eucalyptus oil, or other mild agents which act as irritants to the skin and thereby reduce the perception of pruritus.

Salicylic acid in 1 to 2% and tar solutions of 3 to 10% are also occasionally useful in the overall treatment of localized and less extensive pruritic lesions.

Topical steroid preparations are considered by many to be the most effective remedies for the treatment of pruritus. The fluorinated preparations appear to be most desirable for use on the soles of the feet. Nonfluorinated steroid preparations are much more effective and desirable for prolonged use on the upper surface of the foot and the ankle and leg regions. Cost may be a major consideration in using topical corticosteroid preparations: Other remedies may also aid in controlling the pruritus without the potential side effects (19).

ANTISEPTICS

Antiseptic agents are utilized on human skin primarily to inhibit or destroy microorganisms or to reduce the metabolic activities of these organisms. The major use of antiseptics by health care personnel are as hand scrubs, cleansers, irrigant flushes, and for protective dressings. They are also used for generalized hand washing to reduce the risk of cross contamination. In some cases they may be used preoperatively as a skin preparation.

The antiseptic agents most commonly used by health care professionals include ethyl and isopropyl alcohols, cationic surfactants (benzalkonium), chlorhexidine, iodine solutions, tincture or iodophors (povidone-iodine), and the phenolic compound hexachlorophene. Most of these agents, with the exception of hexachlorophene, are incorporated in over-the-counter products for use by the general public.

Disinfectants are frequently listed as antiseptic agents: However, these products are used primarily on inanimate objects to destroy microorganisms and prevent infections. Some disinfectants may also be used as antiseptics if the solutions are diluted sufficiently to avoid injury to living tissues. The principal disinfectants available were discussed earlier and are the aldehydes (formaldehyde and glutaraldehyde) and the products chlorine and cresol. Sterilization is the complete and total destruction of all microorganisms, including spores, fungi, and viruses. Ethylene oxide is the only chemical agent available that is approved for sterilization of objects that cannot be treated in the regular heated or physical methods of sterilization.

Alcohols

Ethyl alcohol is widely used for disinfection of skin and is a good bactericidal agent because it acts rapidly by coagulating protein. The 70% aqueous solution is most effective and is commonly used in hospitals. Isopropyl alcohol has a slightly greater bactericidal activity than ethyl alcohol due to its greater depression of surface tension. It kills vegitative forms of most bacteria when used at full strength or in the 70% aqueous mixture. Alcohols are listed as irritating to the skin and may cause increased inflammation when applied to denuded skin or after repeated use. It also is not recommended to disinfect wounds because of wound irritation resulting in burning and stinging and possible tissue necrosis.

Iodine compounds are excellent degerming agents available in a wide range of products including soaps, scrubs, and ointments (Betadine and Efodine). The iodophors have a broad spectrum of antimicrobial activity. They are used extensively as hand washes for health personnel and for presurgical hand scrubbing. Many institutions prepare the skin prior to surgery and prior to injection with these compounds. Povidone-iodine is also used for pyodermas and extensively damaged skin, such as occurs with infected burns.

Aluminum acetate (Burow's solution) is a very mild antiseptic and astringent agent and is frequently used in the clinical and office setting for these purposes. Hexachlorophene is a good degerming agent which requires multiple applications to be effective. This agent is no longer available over the counter and is used by hospital personnel as a hand washing and presurgical hand scrub agent. It is also used preoperatively to prepare the skin. Cleansing with alcohol or washing the skin with water or soap will remove the antibacterial residue of hexachlorophene. This agent is absorbed through intact skin and may cause a neurotoxic effect, and for this reason, care should be taken to avoid extensive application to broken or denuded skin.

Chlorhexidine is a topical antiseptic product which acts rapidly. However, it has characteristics similar to those of hexachlorophene in that it must be used repeatedly to have a cumulative antibacterial effect. It is frequently used as the antiseptic of choice for skin cleansing and surgical scrubs in surgicenters and hospitals (Hibiclens and Hibistat).

TOPICAL CORTICOSTEROIDS

Corticosteroids are the most effective and potent form of local antiinflammatory medications available and are widely used by physicians in the treatment of inflammatory and pruritic eruptions. Currently there are a large number of preparations available both over-the-counter and by prescription. The wide usage of the drug has been encouraged because of its desirable qualities and its broad application for treating a wide variety of common dermatology conditions. The primary action of corticosteroids accomplishes its antiinflammatory effect without production of pain or odor during application. Side effects are relatively few and minor (Table 24.2).

The indications for the use of topical corticosteroids are many. They primarily center around control of inflammatory changes and the symptoms associated with these conditions. In most cases they are useful where imflammation is the primary manifestation of the dermatosis and where the etiological factors are dealt with concurrently by the application of the corticosteroid. The anti-inflammatory activity of

Table 24.2
Common Topical Corticosteroids

I	(most potent)	Amcinonide ointment 0.1% (Cyclocort) Betamethasone dipropionate ointment 0.05% (Diprosone) Desoximethasone cream 0.25% (Topicort) Diflorasone diacetate ointment 0.05% (Lidex and Topsyn Gel) Halcinonide cream 0.1% (Halog)
II		Betamethasone benzoate gel 0.025% (Benisone) Betamethasone dipropionate cream 0.05% (Diprosone) Betamethasone valerate ointment 0.1% (Valisone) Diflorasone diacetate cream 0.05% (Florone) Triamcinolone acetonide cream 0.5% (Aristocort)
III		Amcinonide cream 0.1% (Cyclocort) Betamethasone valerate lotion 0.1% (Valisone) Fluocinolone acetonide cream 0.2%, ointment 0.025% (Fluonid, Synalar) Flurandrenolide ointment 0.05% (Cordran) Hydrocortisone valerate ointment 0.2% (Westcort) Triamcinolone acetonide ointment 0.1% (Aristocort, Kenalog)
IV		Betamethasone valerate cream 0.1% (Valisone) Clocortolone pivalate cream 0.1% (Cloderm) Fluocinolone acetonide cream 0.025% (Fluonid, Synalar) Hydrocortisone valerate cream 0.2% (Westcort) Triamcinolone acetonide cream 0.01%, lotion 0.025% (Kenalog, Aristocort)
V		Desonide cream 0.05% (Tridesilon) Flumethasone pivalate 0.03% (Locorten)
VI	(least potent)	Prednisolone 0.5% (Meti-Derm) Methylprednisolone 1% (Medrol) Fluorometholone 0.025% (Oxylone) Dexamethasone 0.1% (Decadron Phosphate) Hydrocortisone 0.25, 0.5, 1.0, 2.5% (Hytone, Nutraderm, Synacort)

corticosteroids is based on the properties of vasoconstriction, suppression of membrane permeability and the immune response, and antimycotic activity. This is expressed by the inhibition of the connective tissue response as well as by the control of reactive epidermal hyperplasia. The vasoconstrictor action of the corticosteroids decreases extravasation of serum into the skin and inhibits swelling and discomfort. These pharmacological effects produce many of the desired therapeutic effects and also produce many of the undesirable adverse reactions.

The total effectiveness of topical corticosteroids is related to the potency of the medications and the penetration ability of the drug through the cutaneous layers. There is a wide variation in the corticosteroid percutaneous penetration factor. A 1% hydrocortisone solution will easily penetrate normal skin on the forearm. The same solution may be absorbed 0.14 times faster through the plantar foot arch skin and 0.83 times faster through the palm, 1.7 times faster through the back, 3.5 times faster through the scalp, 6 times faster through the forehead, 13 times faster through the cheek of the jaw and 42 times faster through the skin of the scrotal area. This absorption rate can further be increased four to fivefold by complete hydration of the skin (7). Hydration is enhanced by occlusion with a plastic covering by as much as tenfold. The choice of vehicle is important in the overall desired absorption penetration of the medication (20). Ointments are more effective when hydrated than creams or lotions.

The most potent forms of topical corticosteroids are the fluorinated types. These agents may be more effective in areas where penetration is an especial problem such as the soles and palms and the adverse reactions from these drugs may also be increased. Some authors recommend that the less potent corticosteroids be utilized along with measures to increase their absorption (such as occlusive vehicles or dressings) rather than to begin with the more potent steroid groups. They further recommend that the less potent steroids be used to maintain therapy after the initial dermatosis has been reduced or controlled, especially in those chronic skin diseases such as psoriasis (21).

The most common side effects and adverse reactions of topical corticosteroids include itching, irritation of the skin, burning, and excessive dryness. These problems are commonly related to the vehicle of the preparation and the state of the skin prior to treatment. Other reactions which result from excessive occlusion are miliaria, foliculitis, and maceration. Prolonged use of corticosteroids also cause a well-demarcated cutaneous atrophy and telangiectasia. This adverse effect is also increased dramatically with the use of occlusive techniques. Areas of atrophic change may also demonstrate purpura and cutaneous thinning with striae after prolonged use. This is especially true for these areas of the feet and legs where the skin is already much thinner. As discussed earlier, the more potent the corticosteroid, the more severe and more rapid the side effects will be. Additional side effects and adverse reactions include a contact dermatitis to the vehicle or, in some cases, to the corticosteroid itself, hypopigmentary changes of the darker complected skin and hyperpigmentary changes in the light complexioned skin, hypertrichosis, and a rosacea-like dermatitis. *Candida* or bacterial infections may also fulminate with corticosteroid applications. All side effects, with the exception of striae (especially in the intertriginous areas), will reverse after stopping the corticosteroid application.

CYTOTOXICS, KERATOLYTICS, AND CAUSTICS

The cytotoxic drugs are not used frequently in podiatry; however, they may be useful for certain types of hyperplastic skin disorders, such as psoriasis, and may be used in the treatment of warts and porokeratotic lesions. The keratolytic agents are primarily used in the treatment of these disorders and will be discussed in the following section. The primary cytotoxic agents are anthralin, cantharidin, fluorouracil, and podophyllin.

Anthralin, sometimes listed as a cytostatic agent, may be very useful when combined with zinc oxide paste to treat psoriatic plaques on the lower extremities. The commercial forms of anthralin frequently are dispensed in ointment form. This agent may be staining to the skin and acts as an irritant and should not be used in the treatment of acute inflammatory reactions or the interdigital areas. This particular agent has very little use in current podiatric dermatology.

Cantharidin causes intraepidermal vesiculation and is used primarily in the treatment of benign cutaneous lesions and warts, especially the periungual variety. When applied under occlusive bandage, the skin will blister, and an obvious reaction will occur within 24 hr. The blister will break, crust, and fall off in about 1 week to 10 days. This particular agent is very active and should be used with care.

Fluorouracil is a cytotoxic drug used topically to remove multiple premalignant lesions, porokeratotic lesions, and warts. Fluorouracil acts primarily against atypical epidermal cells by inhibiting RNA synthesis. The degree of response is usually evaluated by limiting the area of application to the specific lesion; the effectiveness of treatment is dependent upon duration of the treatment and the visible reaction. If there is excessive inflammatory response on the normal skin, treatment should be discontinued. A 2% solution (Efudex) can be applied to resistant warts and even to porokeratotic lesions once or twice daily for 2 to 6 weeks until the acceptable inflammatory response is obtained. The excessive inflammatory reaction produced by this particular chemical places substantial limitation on the use of the product, and other agents may be more practical. It has also been implicated as a possible carcinogen.

Podophyllin is a toxic extract from the roots of the may apple or mandrake plant species and is useful in the treatment of warts. Podophyllin can induce severe and active erosive changes in the adjacent tissue, and the peripheral skin must therefore be protected prior to the use of this agent. A combination of podophyllin (5%) with salicylic acid and cantharidin is a commonly used product (Verrusol) for the treatment of plantar verrucae.

Dinitrochlorobenzene (DNCB), a known tissue sensitizer, may be used topically in the treatment of recalcitrant verrucae (those that have not responded to the routine treatment programs). The patient is sensitized to DNCB 1% in acetone, and once the reaction has occurred, the application is discontinued. After the sensitization site is clear, the topical treatment of the warts is begun with DNCB 1% in a vehicle such as collodion. The resultant cytotoxic reaction causes blisters and bulla formation and subsequent resolution of the verrucae (22).

KERATOLYTIC AGENTS

Benzoyl peroxide is a very potent oxidizing agent sometimes listed with the keratolytic agents. It has been used with good success in promoting debridement and early granulation tissue in the treatment of ulcers (23). A 5% or 10% benzoyl peroxide (Benoxyl, Desquam-X) may be applied to the ulceration, after the adjacent normal skin has been covered with an ointment and placed under occlusion for 8 to 12 hours. Regular dressing changes and routine wound care seem to accelerate the debridement and healing of ulcerations.

Propylene glycol is primarily used as a vehicle in other formulations. In concentrations of 40 to 60% it markedly increases hydration and softening of the skin and will cause desquamation of the upper layer of scales and hyperkeratotic tissue. This action is greatly increased by occlusive dressings. The keratolytic action of salicylic acid is enhanced by propylene glycol, and this combination is frequently used in conditions causing excessive scaling and dryness on the lower extremities. Overnight occlusion is used until improvement is seen. Thereafter, once or twice weekly applications will be sufficient for most conditions. Allergic contact dermatitis may occur with propylene glycol and when keratolytic agents containing this agent cause excessive irritation or reaction, the propylene glycol component should be suspected (24).

Resorcinol (Resorcin) is found in numerous nonprescription preparations in a 2 to 10% concentration. This phenolic derivative is a mild keratolytic agent which also has bactericidal and fungicidal activities. Today, more potent and specific keratolytic, antibacterial, and antifungal agents are available, and these newer agents may be much more efficient.

Retinoic acid and variations in formulation are used topically in the treatment of keratinizing disorders and hyperkeratotic conditions. A 0.05% tretinoin (vitamin A acid, Retin-A) has been used successfully in the local treatment of hypertrophic scars and keloids (25).

Salicylic acid is one of the most frequently used keratolytic agents by podiatrists. Salicylic acid (3 to 6% in an ointment base) is excellent for treating scaly conditions of the lower extremity and is relatively nonirritating. A 6% concentration is useful to remove superficial diffuse calluses. A popular agent (Keralyt) combines a 6% salicylic acid with a propylene glycol 60% in a gel base. This agent appears to be very effective in the treatment of plantar hyperkeratoses (26). Preparations containing greater than 6% salicylic acid are destructive and are very useful in the treatment of specific lesions such as warts and deep keratotic plugs. Combination agents include salicylic acid and lactic acid, each at 16.7% concentration in a flexible collodion mixture (Duo-Film). As plasters or paste, salicylic acid is usually in the concentration of 40 to 60% and is sometimes used to treat resistant warts and corns. In some cases of dry squamous-type fungal infections, salicylic acid may accelerate the improvement (27).

Sodium pyruvate, a keratolytic agent, may be used in severe congenital hyperkeratotic disorders and in treating generalized forms of plantar keratoderma. They used a 5% concentration of pyruvate acid in Eucerin to treat several different forms of severe ichthyosiform dermatoses and found the agent to be nonirritating and extremely effective.

Urea disrupts the normal hydrogen bonding of the keratinic protein, which allows hydration and keratolytic actions to occur. Urea compounds also have antipruritic effects, which appears to enhance its usefulness in treating dry scaly conditions such as atopic dermatitis and other hyperkeratotic diseases. Useful concentrations for treating anhydrous skin conditions topically are 2% (Aquacare), 10% (Aquacare/HP, Carmol-10), and 20% (Carmol-20). When urea is added in a concentration of 10% to topical steroid cream, it appears to be a much better agent in the treatment of subacute and atopic eczema (28). In concentrations greater than 20%, urea is destructive and is recommended primarily for the nonsurgical avulsion of dystrophic nails (29, 30).

CAUSTICS

Caustics are applied topically primarily for the destruction of superficial lesions and are also useful in producing hemostasis during limited surgical procedures. Ferric subsulfate (Monsel's solution) is a very effective hemostatic agent, but it is not strong enough to be used as a caustic in the treatment of plantar lesions. Mono-, di-, and trichloroacetic acids are the most effective and rapid local caustic agents. Because of the destructive keratolytic action of these agents, the surrounding normal skin should be protected with petrolatum prior to application. Less caustic agents are preferred in most cases. Silver nitrate 5% to 10% solution is useful as a caustic agent for the treatment of fissures or excessive granulation tissue. Silver nitrate sticks (94.5%) become a potent caustic agent once they are dipped in water.

ENZYMES

Enzymes degrade protein, aiding in the removal of necrotic tissue, prurulent exudates, clotted blood, infected wounds, and ulcers. These agents tend to promote healing by the facilitation of cleansing of the wound. The most important part about generalized wound care is the mechanical debridement and the selection of an appropriate topical enzyme. These agents may be completely inactivated by topical hexachlorophene, tincture of iodine, aluminum acetate soaks, benzalkonium chloride, and topical detergents. Common topical preparations include a mixture of fibrinolysin and desoxyribonuclease (Elase), collagenase (Santyl), sutilains (Travase), and streptokinase-streptodornase (Varidase). The collagenase enzyme appears to be most satisfactory in treating dermal ulcerations, and complete debridement usually occurs in 1 to 2 weeks followed by granulation and epithelialization of the wound.

INTRALESIONAL THERAPY

Corticosteroids

Intralesional corticosteroid injections are frequently used in lesions which are resistant to the topical application of corticosteroids. The mechanism of action of the intralesional injection is similar to that of topical agents and may provide a very rapid resolution of the problem. When topical agents are not potent enough or do not penetrate the epidermal barrier well enough to create a change in the disease process, intralesional corticosteroid injections are preferred. In some conditions, such as lichen planus and psoriasis, intralesional corticosteroid injections may be used as an adjunctive form of therapy. In most cases the intralesional injection is delivered with a tuberculin syringe with a 30-gauge needle or with an airpowered gun (Mada-Jet). The needle technique is preferred when exact location of the corticosteroid placement is important. Also, the air-powered apparatus may cause disruption of the underlying elastic fibers and subsequently may cause some scarring (31). Several precautions are necessary when utilizing intralesional injections to prevent hypopigmentation, hyperpigmentation, atrophy, or telangiectasia (32). Intralesional injections should not be performed where the skin is thin or already atrophic. For keloids, hypertrophic scars, and corticosteroid-responsive lesions, I tend to prefer triamcinolone diacetate, administered by the syringe with the 30-gauge needle technique. The lesions are injected, depending upon their size and shape, with a range of from 1/8 to 1/2 ml. Compression dressings applied to the lesions following intralesional injection appear to increase the desired results. Another form of treatment utilizing intralesional injections also includes the additional use of cryosurgery. Freezing with liquid nitrogen in the conventional manner of cryosurgery, followed by immediate injection of triamcinolone acetonide, has been found to be very effective in the treatment of hypertrophic scars and keloids (33). Several preparations of corticosteroids for intralesional injection are available (see Table 24.3).

SCLEROSING AGENTS

There are currently many different types of sclerosing agents available, and for the purposes of this section we will deal with three types which include sodium chloride (20%) injectable, sodium tetradecyl sulfate (1% and 3%), and a combination of absolute alcohol and local anesthetic agent. The sodium chloride (20%) sterile injectable solution is useful in lower extremity dermatology to eradicate small superficial lesions and unsightly vascular disorders such as small spider telangiectasia and small varicosities. This agent must be used with extreme care because of its sclerosing properties and, since it is injected very superficially, pigmentary changes and ulcerative changes may be induced. It is recommended that small amounts, ranging from 0.1 to 0.4 ml, be injected during any one visit. Sodium tetradecyl sulfate (Sotradecol) is a sterile solution containing, in each milliliter, sodium tetradecyl sulfate 10 mg (1%) or 30 mg (3%) in water for injection with 0.02 ml benzyl alcohol and a buffering solution. This solution is recommended for sclerosing of small varicose veins and other uncomplicated vascular disorders of the lower extremities. Any podiatric physician utilizing this technique should be familiar with the indications and contraindications, as well as the precautions, for this sclerosing agent. The dosage utilized should be less

Table 24.3
Corticosteroids for Intralesional Injection

Generic name	Trade name	Dosage (mg/ml)	Manufacturer
Betamethasone sodium phosphate	Celestone	3	Schering Corporation
Betamethasone acetate and betamethasone sodium phosphate	Celestone Soluspan	6	Schering Corporation
Dexamethasone sodium phosphate	Decadron	4	Merck Sharp & Dohme
Dexamethasone acetate phosphate	Decadron-LA	8	Merck Sharp & Dohme
Prednisolone acetate	Meticortelone Acetate	25	Schering Corporation
Triamcinolone acetonide	Kenalog	10 or 40	E.R. Squibb & Sons, Inc.
Triamcinolone diacetate	Aristocort	40	Lederle Laboratories
Triamcinolone hexacetonide	Aristospan	20	Lederle Laboratories

than 1 ml for each injection, and the initial injections should be 0.1 to 0.5 ml. It is important to observe the patient and the local reaction to rule out any possibility of anaphylactic shock prior to the injection of larger dosage. This agent may also be utilized to create underlying fibrosis and scarring deep subcutaneous layers for joint stability. However, there is no documentation of the safety and effectiveness of this method. Finally, a sclerosing solution prepared by mixing 2 ml of absolute ethyl alcohol with 48 ml of a 2% local anesthetic, such as lidocaine with epinephrine 1:100,000, has been used successfully in the treatment of many lower extremity conditions. This preparation is a 4% solution of absolute alcohol by volume. A 2% solution may be prepared by mixing 1 ml of absolute ethyl alcohol with 49 ml of 2% local anesthetic. The porokeratotic lesions described by Taub and Steinberg in 1970 respond extremely well to the injection of a small amount of 2% or 4% sclerosing solutions on a weekly interval (34). I usually use 0.5 to 1.0 ml of sclerosing solution injected at 45° to the lesion with a 25-gauge 5/8-inch needle, using a tuberculin syringe. The technique and further discussions of the lesions are outlined by Dribbon (35) in 1971 and Weisfeld in 1973 (35). I have found the 2% and 4% sclerosing solutions useful in treating other lesions, such as fibromas, hypertrophic scars, and keloids, and have used the 4% sclerosing solution with very high success in treating intermetatarsal neuromas.

Other intralesional injection techniques include the injections of small amounts of 5-fluorouracil (5-FU) in the treatment of plantar verrucae (36). This technique appears to be very successful; however, several cases in our series showed excessive hyperpigmentary changes in the area surrounding the infiltrative injections of 5-FU. These all resolved with time; however, the patient should be forewarned of the possibility for cosmetic reasons. Dinitrochlorobenzene has also been recommended as an intralesional injectable agent for the treatment of verrucae (37). Intralesional injections of bleomycin have also been reported to cause a high cure rate of warts. This is a cytotoxic, injectable drug with the major side effect of intralesional injection being pain. It is injected in a 0.1-ml volume of a 0.1% solution (38).

SYSTEMIC THERAPY

Antibiotics

The use of antibiotic oral and parenteral therapy in lower extremity dermatology is rather common. The primary conditions treated with antibiotics appear to be the secondary infection and ulceration infections. In mild infections and responsive conditions, orally administered agents are recommended. In suspected or proved severe bacterial infections, parenteral therapy with antimicrobial agents is more appropriate. During the critical period of about 48 hr from the initial stage of the infection, treatment is based entirely on clinical information obtained from the patient and physical examination. Simple laboratory evaluations such as the gram stain may also provide immediate information. Antibiotic therapy is usually initiated with agents that will broadly cover the microorganisms under consideration. The choice of the antibiotic, whether it be a penicillin, aminoglycoside, cephalosporin, or some other type, depends on the relative susceptibility pattern and degree of resistance seen. Many newer forms of aminoglycosides and cephalosporins are entering the market on a regular basis. Currently, it is not clear as to whether these newer agents will be active against a broader range of infective agents and whether the long-term cost and potential benefits outweigh the use of standard established agents. Once speciation of the microorganism and the minimal inhibitory concentration (MIC) of the various antibiotic agents has become available, definitive therapy should begin immediately. The therapeutic regimen may be changed from an aminoglycoside to a less toxic agent, such as ampicillin or cephalosporin, if the microorganism is susceptible. It is recommended that a change in the program be initiated even if the patient is responding satisfactorily to the initial therapy.

Antibiotic agents, such as the penicillins and the cephalosporins which have a wide margin of safety between the therapeutic and the toxic blood levels, are usually given in the standardized dosage recommended, independent of the patient's weight. For those antibiotic agents, such as aminoglycosides (amikacin, gentamicin, and tobramycin), in which there is a narrow margin between the therapeutic and the toxic blood levels, dosage should be based on the patient's weight and body weight per day (milligram per kilogram) divided into three equal doses given every 8 hr. Peak and trough blood levels should be monitored along with the serum creatinine concentration. Underdosing is a common problem with the aminoglycosides, based on the general concern for toxic side effects.

Many of the common bacterial infections can be managed with the use of the general group agents shown in Table 24.4. This list of agents constitutes the majority of the antibiotics necessary to treat most bacterial infections of the lower extremities.

As was mentioned earlier, new agents are entering the market on a regular basis. These new products can be classified into three groups: (*a*) derivatives of preexisting agents with altered pharmacological properties, such as increased half-life; (*b*) derivatives of preexisting agents with increased spectrum of activity or a change in the resistance to inactivating enzymes; and (*c*) entirely new classes of antibacterial agents. Erythromycin and its derivatives belong in the first category. The value of reducing the total number of daily doses is usually not great in antibiotic therapy. The increased cost of this adjustment probably is not warranted. Ampicillin, carbenicillin, amikacin, tobramycin, and piperacillin are in the second group, which has a more practical value. Many of the second and third generation cephalosporins also fit into group 2 and are valuable in treating infections due to microorganisms which are resistant to the original cephalosporins.

Table 24.4
Common Groups of Antibiotic Agents

Group	Oral form	Parenteral form
Aminoglycosides		Gentamycin
Cephalosporins	Cephalexin	Cephalothin
	Cephradine	Cefazolin
Clindamycin	Clindamycin	Clindamycin
Chloramphenicol	Chloramphenicol	Chloramphenicol
Erythromycin	Erythromycin	Erythromycin
Penicillins	Penicillin VK	Penicillin G
		Procaine penicillin G
	Amoxicillin	Ampicillin
		Carbenicillin
	Dicloxacillin	Oxacillin

It is important to be cautious in the use of antimicrobial agents which make new claims and counterclaims regarding the superiority of the new agent. It is better to be extremely familiar with a few, well-established antibiotic agents than to use every new agent without follow-up or good general understanding of the long-term effect. Finally, the increased cost of the newer antibiotics may be prohibitive and may also reduce patient compliance because of added expense (39).

ANTIFUNGAL AGENTS

The two primary antifungal agents used in the treatment of mycotic infections of the lower extremities are griseofulvin and ketoconazole. Other antifungal agents used for deep-seated mycotic infections will not be discussed in this section. Griseofulvin is an antifungal antibiotic effective against most dermatophytes. It is ineffective against *Candida* species. Griseofulvin may be used in severe fungal infections of the lower extremities that do not respond to topical therapy. Interdigital moist fungal infections appear to respond much faster with a combination of oral griseofulvin and topical antifungal agents. Treatment of onychomycosis usually takes from 9 to 15 months or longer, and reinfection of toenails is frequent. For this reason, the long-term cost and potential risk of this medication may far outweigh its potential benefits.

Ketoconazole (Nizoral) is a water-soluble imidazole derivative with a wide spectrum antifungal activity. Oral administration in 200-mg doses is well absorbed and has few adverse side effects. Because of abnormal liver function tests, hepatitis, and several cases of hepatic necrosis, liver function tests should be monitored in patients on ketoconazole therapy. Severe dermatophyte infection appears to respond favorably to ketoconazole and at a higher percentage cure rate with a lower recurrence rate (40). Ketoconazole spectrum of activity includes *Candida* species, *B. dermatitidis*, *C. immitis*, *H. capsulatum*, *P. brasilien-*

sis, and *P. boydii* (41). It is also effective in all the superficial fungal infections and is believed to be an effective and safe treatment for dermatophytosis, which is nonresponsive to the standard topical approach (42).

ANTI-INFLAMMATORY AGENTS

In this category we will discuss primarily the nonsteroidal anti-inflammatory agents which will be helpful in the overall treatment of lower extremity dermatology problems by reducing the inflammatory response. Aspirin is the baseline and is the usual initial agent; however, the newer nonsteroidal anti-inflammatory drugs are becoming much more popular and better understood. Most of these agents are primarily indicated in the treatment of arthritis or inflammatory pain syndromes; however, they may be very beneficial in relieving symptoms of a wide variety of dermatoses (see Table 24.5).

Fenoprofen calcium, is a phenylpropionic acid derivative which is chemically and pharmaceutically similar to ibuprofen. It has anti-inflammatory, analgesic, and antipyretic properties and is very useful as an alternative to aspirin or other nonsteroidal agents in the treatment of lower extremity symptoms secondary to dermatoses. Absorption and availability of this drug are reduced when this agent is given with food, but these factors are not affected by the administration of an antacid.

Ibuprofen is also a phenylpropionic acid derivative, and this agent is chemically and pharmacologically similar to fenoprofen. It also has analgestic, anti-inflammatory, and antipyretic action. However, the anti-inflammatory effect of this agent is clinically demonstrated only in doses of 1.6 or 2.4 g per day. When this drug is taken immediately after meals, the absorption and the peak plasma concentrations are lower.

Indomethacin is a powerful nonsteroidal anti-inflammatory agent with analgesic and antipyretic effects. There are multiple serious adverse reactions to this agent, and it is not recommended as a simple analgesic or antipyretic and has relatively few indications in the treatment of lower extremity dermatoses. This drug has not been recommended in pregnant women, nursing mothers, infants, and children under 15 years of age.

Naproxen is chemically related to the phenylpropionic acid group of agents, and it has analgesic, anti-inflammatory, and antipyretic actions. Absorption of the drug is not delayed by the presence of food, but it may be decreased by antacids such as magnesium and aluminum hydroxide. The most frequent adverse reactions are gastrointestinal disturbances. We have seen one case of lichen planus-like drug eruptions secondary to oral naproxen, and this phenomenon has recently been reported in the medical literature (43).

Phenylbutazone is a very potent anti-inflammatory, antipyretic, and analgesic agent which is also limited because of the potential serious adverse reactions. In almost all cases we recommend a very short treatment period ranging from 3 to 7 days. The most serious adverse reaction is bone marrow depression (i.e., leukopenia, pancytopenia, agranulocytosis, and aplastic anemia). These drugs are contraindicated in children 15 years of age or under.

Piroxicam is an anti-inflammatory, analgesic, and antipyretic agent which can rapidly reduce erythema, tissue proliferation, edema, and pain. Concurrent administration of aspirin may reduce the plasma levels of piroxicam to 80% of its normal

Table 24.5
Nonsteroidal Anti-inflammatory Agents

Generic name	Trade name	Manufacturer
Fenoprofen calcium	Nalfon	Dista Products Co.
Ibuprofen	Motrin	Upjohn Company
Indomethacin	Indocin	Merck Sharp & Dohme
Naproxen	Naprosyn	Syntex Laboratories
Phenylbutazone	Butazolidin	Geigy Pharmaceuticals
Piroxicam	Feldene	Pfizer Laboratories
Sulindac	Clinoril	Merck Sharp & Dohme
Tometin sodium	Tolectin	McNeil Pharmaceuticals

value. The concomitant administration of antacids appears to have no effect on the piroxicam plasma level. The most common reported side effect is gastrointestinal tract irritation. Interestingly enough, I have seen three cases of piroxicam-induced lichen planus-like dermatitis on the lower extremities. All three of these patients had been on the piroxicam (20 mg) for at least 10 days prior to the skin eruptions.

Sulindac is a substituted indene analog of indomethacin with similar anti-inflammatory property. Like aspirin and other nonsteroidal anti-inflammatory drugs, sulindac inhibits platelet aggregation and prolongs bleeding time. For this reason it should be used with caution in patients with bleeding disorders or gastric ulcers. The most common side effects of sulindac are abdominal pain, dyspepsia, nausea, and diarrhea. It usually has a lower incidence of gastrointestinal disturbances than aspirin and is in the same class as ibuprofen and fenoprofen in this category.

Tolmetin sodium is a pyrrole-acetic acid derivative which differs chemically from the other nonsteroidal anti-inflammatory agents, but the pharmacological factors are similar. The most frequently reported adverse reactions are gastrointestinal disturbances; however, the reports are less frequent and less severe than with aspirin. Unlike aspirin, this drug has a minimal effect on platelet aggregation. It is the only anti-inflammatory agent recommended in the treatment of children under the age of 15, and the general recommendation is for the treatment of children over 2 years of age with 20 mg/kg of body weight daily in divided doses to begin therapy.

ANTIPRURITICS AND ANTIHISTAMINES

Systemic antipruritics and antihistamines are usually in the same chemical categories and will be discussed as a general unit in this section. As discussed earlier in the section under topical antipruritics, the symptom complex of pruritus is a primary factor in many lower extremity skin problems. The antihistamines are rapidly absorbed after systemic administration, and relief is usually noted within 15 to 30 min and last up to 6 hours. The action of timed release preparations may persist from 8 to 12 hr. However, they may be less than effective when compared to conventional dosage forms because of lower total blood levels. The most common adverse side effect is sedation, and ambulatory patients must be warned of this effect. These agents may alleviate urticaria and pruritus induced by histamines, and these agents may be the drugs of choice in the treatment of acute urticarial reactions (see Table 24.6). Antipruritics and antihistamines are useful in the treatment of atopic dermatitis, contact dermatitis, dermatitis medicamentosa, and fixed drug eruptions. They are usually of little benefit in the treatment of erythema multiforme and exfoliative dermatitis. Systemic administration of antihistamines and antipruritics, when combined with appropriate topical therapy, will reduce the pruritus accompanying many lower extremity dermatoses.

SYSTEMIC CORTICOSTEROIDS

Systemic corticosteroids are used to treat a large number of responsive skin diseases. Because there are many well known and serious adverse reactions to the corticosteroids, the primary decision on their usage should center around the risk involved in each clinical situation, as well as the alternatives of treatment and the contraindications to this approach. In almost all situations involving lower extremity dermatoses, the short course of therapy is recommended. Use of systemic corticosteroids is contraindicated with acute infection and trauma and is not recommended in the treatment of patients with psychotic tendencies, peptic ulcers, diabetes mellitus, hypertension, and in pregnant females (44). Systemic corticosteroids are classified into three main groups according to the duration of activity (see Table 24.7).

ORAL ENZYMES

The oral enzymes are generally classified in the anti-inflammatory group. The proteolytic and other oral enzymes are said to be indicated in the reduction of edema and inflammation in postoperative tissue reactions and accidental trauma. Podiatrists tend to use these oral agents for elective reconstructive surgery and in the treatment of sprains, strains, and fractures of the lower extremities. An excellent review of the inflammatory process, the fibrinolytic

Table 24.6
Common Antipruritic-Antihistamines

Drug class	Generic name	Trade name	Manufacturer
Ethanolamines	Carbinoxamine maleate	Clistin	McNeil
	Dimenhydrinate	Dramamine	Searle
	Diphenhydramine HCl	Benadryl	Parke, Davis
Ethylenediamines	Tripelennamine citrate	PBZ Citrate	Geigy
	Tripelennamine HCl	PBZ HCl	Geigy
Alkylamines	Brompheniramine maleate	Dimetane	Robins
	Chlorpheniramine maleate	Chlor-Trimeton	Schering
	Dexchlorpheniramine maleate	Polaramine	Schering
Phenothiazines	Methdilazine	Tacaryl	Westwood
	Promethazine HCl	Phenergan	Wyeth
	Trimeprazine tartrate	Temaril	Smith Kline & French
Piperidines	Azatadine maleate	Optimine	Schering
	Cyproheptadine HCl	Periactin	Merck Sharp & Dohme
Miscellaneous	Cimetidine	Tagamet	Smith Kline & French
	Hydroxyzine HCl	Atarax	Roerig
	Hydroxyzine pamoate	Vistaril	Pfizer

Table 24.7
Systemic Corticosteroids

Activity	Generic name	Dosage
Short-acting		
Oral	Methylprednisolone	2, 4, 8, 16, 24, and 32 mg
	Prednisolone	5 mg
	Prednisone	1, 2.5, 5, 10, 20, and 50 mg
Injectable	Dexamethasone sodium phosphate	4 mg/ml
Intermediate-acting		
Oral	Triamcinolone	1, 2, 4, 8, and 16 mg
Injectable	Triamcinolone diactonide	25 and 40 mg/ml
	Dexamethasone acetate	8 mg/ml
	Betamethasone sodium phosphate	6 mg/ml
Long-acting		
Oral	Dexamethasone	0.75, 4, 5, 20, and 25 mg
	Betamethasone	0.6 mg
Injectable	Triamcinolone hexacetonide	5 and 40 mg/ml
	Triamcinolone acetonide	10 and 40 mg/ml

process, and the role of anti-inflammatory oral enzymes, along with a graph of enzyme preparations, was presented in 1976 by Rogers and Ransom (45) (see Table 24.8).

CONCLUSIONS

It can be noted from this very lengthy chapter and from the extensive references listed that the topic of "podiatric dermatological therapeutics" covers a wide variety of topics and issues dealing with the principles of treatment with topical, intralesional, and systemic medications, as well as the use of peripheral agents such as vehicles and carrying agents. It is very important to note that this paper does not deal with all of the possible areas and only deals with the most common and the most frequently used agents in general practice. Furthermore, all practitioners should be advised to refer to product information and specific sources for additional detailed instructions regarding the use of any medications or drugs within this section. Special attention should be given to systemic medication and the use of these agents in nursing mothers, pregnant women, infants and children, and in patients with other illnesses.

Table 24.8
Common Oral Anti-Inflammatory Enzymes[a]

Generic name	Trade name(s)	Action	Dose[b]
Streptokinase-streptodornase[c]	Varidase (10,000 U of SK[b] and at least 2500 U of SD)	Fibrinolytic Deoxyribonuclease	Tabs: 1 q.i.d.
Trypsin-chymotrypsin[d]	Chymoral (50,000 U of enzymatic activity)	Proteolytic	Tabs: 1 to 2 q.i.d.
	Chymoral (100,000 U of enzymatic activity)		
	Chymolase (50,000 U of enzymatic activity)		Tabs: 1 to 2 q.i.d.
Trypsin-chymotrypsin + 2% ribonuclease	Orenzyme (54,000 U of enzymatic activity)	Proteolytic	Tabs: 1 to 2 q.i.d.
	Orenzyme Bitabs (108,000 U of enzymatic activity)		Tabs: 1 q.i.d.
Chymotrypsin	Avazyme (50,000 U of enzymatic activity)	Proteolytic	Tabs: 1 to 2 q.i.d.
	Avazyme-100 (100,000 U of enzymatic activity)		Tabs: 1 q.i.d.
Carica papaya	Papase (10,000 Warner-Chilcott U of enzymatic activity)	Proteolytic	Tabs: 2 q.i.d.
Bromelains	Ananase (50,000 Rorer U of enzymatic activity)	Proteolytic	Tabs: 1 q.i.d.
	Ananase-100 (100,000 Rorer U of enzymatic activity)		Tabs: 1 q.i.d.

[a] From Rogers JE, Ransom RA: A review of the oral anti-inflammatory enzymes. *J Am Podiatry Assoc* 66:313–320, 1976.
[b] Dose to be given 1 to 2 hr before surgery, or immediately after accidental trauma, and continued for a period of 4 to 5 days.
[c] SK, streptokinase; SD, streptodornase.
[d] Ratio of trypsin to chymotrypsin varies with each manufacturer.

Newer agents are constantly arriving within each of the categories discussed within this secion. These agents all claim superiority in application, effectiveness, lack of adverse reactions, or some other advantageous reason for the patient or physician. Each of these agents must be evaluated and studied independently and in each given clinical situation before the long-term efficacy and benefits will be known. Further evaluation is needed within the study of podiatric dermatological preparations and, hopefully, publications such as this one will stimulate additional works in this field.

References

1. Schwarz RH, Crombleholme WR: Antibiotics in pregnancy. *Southern Med J* 72:1315, 1979.
2. Schwarz RH: On making the best of antibiotics in pregnancy. *Emerg Med*:66–77, 1980.
3. Leyden JJ, Kligman AM: Rationale for topical antibiotics. *Cutis* 26:515–527, 1978.
4. Rosen T, Rudolph AH: Identifying and treating bacterial and fungal infections of skin. *Geriatrics* 33:71–82, 1978.
5. Prystowsky SD, Allen AM, Smith RW et al: Allergic contact hypersensitivity to nickel, neomycin, ethylenediamine and benzocaine: Relationships between age, sex, history of exposure, and reactivity to standard patch tests and use tests in a general population. *Arch Dermatol* 115:959, 1979.
6. Leyden JJ, Kligman AM: The case for topical antibiotics. *Prog Dermatol* 10:13, 1976.
7. Arndt KA: *Manual of Dermatologic Therapeutics*, ed 3. Boston, Little, Brown, 1983.
8. Keczkes K, Leighton I, Good CS: Topical treatment of phytoses and conidioses. *Practitioner* 214:412, 1975.
9. Clayton YM: Dermatophyte infections. *Postgrad Med J* 55:605–607, 1979.

10. Clayton YM, Knight AG: A clinical double-blind trial of topical miconazole and clotrimazole against superficial fungal infections and erythrasma. *Clin Exp Dermatol* 1:225, 1976.
11. Clayton YM, Connor BL: Comparison of clotrimazole cream, Whitfield's ointment and nystatin ointment for the topical treatment of ringworm infections, pityriasis versicolor, erythrasma and candidiasis. *Br J Dermatol* 89:297, 1973.
12. Gordon HH: Hyperhidrosis: treatment with glutaraldehyde. *Cutis* 9:375–378, 1972.
13. Cullen SI: Topical methenamine therapy for hyperhidrosis. *Arch Dermatol* 111:1158–1160, 1975.
14. Holzle E, Kligman AM: Mechanism of antiperspirant action of aluminum salts. *J Soc Cosmet Chem* 30:279–295, 1979.
15. Duller P, Gentry WD: Use of biofeedback in treating chronic hyperhidrosis: a preliminary report. *Br J Dermatol* 103:143, 1980.
16. Levit F: Treatment of hyperhidrosis by tap water iontophoresis. *Cutis* 26:192–194, 1980.
17. Shrivastava SN, Singh G: Tap water iontophoresis in palmoplantar hyperhidrosis. *Br J Dermatol* 96:189–195, 1977.
18. Dockery GL: Psychocutaneous disorders: some lower extremity presentations. *J Am Podiatry Assoc* 80:388–395, 1982.
19. Bagatell FK, Augustine MA: Evaluation of corticosteroids intended for topical anti-inflammatory drugs. *Curr Ther Res* 16:748–756, 1974.
20. Roenigk HH: *Office Dermatology*. Baltimore, Williams & Wilkins, 1981.
21. Kligman AM, Kaidbey KH: Hydrocortisone revisted: historical and experimental evaluation. *Cutis* 22:232–244, 1978.
22. Carrel JM, Davidson DM: Topical immunotherapy of recalcitrant verrucae. *J Am Podiatry Assoc* 63:293–296, 1973.
23. Coleman GJ, Roenigk HH: Topical therapy of leg ulcers with 20 percent benzoyl peroxide lotion. *Cutis* 21:491, 1978.
24. Fisher AA: Propylene glycol dermatitis. *Cutis* 21:166–178, 1978.
25. Delimpens AM: The local treatment of hypertrophic scars and keloids with topical retinoic acid. *Br J Dermatol* 103:319–323, 1980.
26. Drucker M: Evaluation of a keratolytic gel in the treatment of plantar hyperkeratosis. *J Am Podiatry Assoc* 66:372–374, 1976.
27. Bade HP: Fungal infections: treatment with a keratolytic gel. *Cutis* 16:574–575, 1975.
28. Hindson TC: Urea in the topical treatment of atopic eczema. *Arch Dermatol J* 104:284, 1971.
29. South DA, Farber EM: Urea ointment in the nonsurgical avulsion of nail dystrophies: a reappraisal. *Cutis* 25:609–612, 1980.
30. Port M, Sanicola KF: Nonsurgical removal of dystrophic nails utilizing urea ointment occlusion. *J Am Podiatry Assoc* 70:521–523, 1980.
31. Callen JP: Intralesional corticosteroids. *J Am Acad Dermatol* 4:149–151, 1981.
32. Goldberg LC: An evaluation of sublesional injection treatment of local skin lesions with triamcinolone diacetate. *Antibiot Chemother* 11(9):560–565, 1961.
33. Ceilley RI, Babin RW: The combined use of cryosurgery and intralesional injections of suspensions of fluorinated adrenocorticosteroids for reducing keloids and hypertrophic scars. *J Dermatol Surg Oncol* 5:54–56, 1979.
34. Taub J, Steinberg M: Porokeratosis plantaris discreta. *Int J Dermatol* 9:83, 1970.
35. Dribbon B: The utilization of an alcohol-local anesthetic solution in the treatment of the plugged duct cyst. *J Am Podiatry Assoc* 61:203, 1971.
36. McCarthy DJ, Tate R, Rusin J: Intradermal use of 5-fluorouracil in human pedal verrucae. *J Am Podiatry Assoc* 69:587–595, 1979.
37. Buckner D, Price NM: Immunotherapy of verrucae vulgaris with dinitrochlorobenzene. *Br J Dermatol* 98:451–455, 1978.
38. Shumack PH, Haddock MJ: Bleomycin: an effective treatment of warts. *Aust J Dermatol* 20:41, 1979.
39. Wilkowske CJ, Hermans PE: General principles of antimicrobial therapy. *Mayo Clin Proc* 58:6–13, 1983.
40. Cox FW, Stiller RL, South DA, Stevens DA: Oral ketoconazole for dermatophyte infections. *J Am Acad Dermatol* 6:455–562, 1982.
41. Herman PE, Keys TF: Antifungal agents used for deep-seated mycotic infections. *Mayo Clin Proc* 58:223–231, 1983.
42. Jones HE, Simpson JG, Artis WM: Oral ketoconazole: an effective and safe treatment for dermatophytosis. *Arch Dermatol* 117:129–134, 1981.
43. Heyman WR, Lerman JS, Luftschein S: Naproxen-induced lichen planus (letter to the editor). *J Am Acad Dermatol* 10:299, 1984.
44. Storrs FJ: Use and abuse of systemic corticosteroid therapy. *J Am Acad Dermatol* 1:95–105, 1979.
45. Rogers JE, Ransom RA: A review of the oral anti-inflammatory enzymes. *J Am Podiatry Assoc* 66:313–320, 1976.

Suggested Readings

Bagatell FK: Topical therapy for onychomycosis. *Arch Dermatol* 11:378, 1977.

Baruch K: Injection method for treatment of porokeratosis. *J Podiatr Educ* 3:1, 1972.

Belcon MC: Topical versus systemic antibiotics in the treatment of acute superficial skin infections. *J Natl Med Assoc* 71:63, 1979.

Boeker MJ, Leu MM: A study of the effects of hydration and emollients on the feet of the aged. *J Am Podiatry Assoc* 68:402–418, 1968.

Clayton YM, Gange RW, MacDonald DM, Carruthers JG: A clinical double-blind trial of topical haloprogin and miconazole against superficial fungal infections. *Clin Exp Dermatol* 4:65, 1979.

Curin G, Cowin RM, Riegelhaupt RW: The incidence and antimicrobial treatment of infections of the foot. *J Am Podiatry Assoc* 71:209–214, 1981.

Dockery GL: *The Drug Formulary.* Cleveland, Ohio, Academy Press, 1975.

Dockery GL: Common skin conditions of the foot. *Today's Jogger* 2(8):54–56, 1978.

Dockery GL, Newell SG: Keratoderma climactericum. *J Am Podiatry Assoc* 68(8):595–597, 1978.

Dockery GL: Lower extremity skin problems related to sports. In: *Sports Medicine.* Mt. Kisco, NY, Futura, 1980.

Edson RS, Keys TF: The aminoglycosides. *Mayo Clin Proc* 58:99–102, 1983.

Farber EM, South DA: Urea ointment in the nonsurgical avulsion of nail dystrophies. *Cutis* 22:689, 1978.

Fisher AA: The antihistamines. *J Am Acad Dermatol* 3:303–306, 1980.

Fitzpatrick TB (ed): Oral ketoconazole: treatment of yeast and fungus—How well does it compare? *Dermatol Capsule Comment* 4(2): 1982.

Fitzpatrick TB, Eisen AZ, Wolff K et al (eds): Principles of topical therapy. In *Dermatology in General Medicine*, ed 2. New York, McGraw-Hill, 1979, pp 1753–1758.

Fitzpatrick TB, Polano MD, Suurmond D: *Color Atlas and Synopsis of Clinical Dermatology.* New York, McGraw-Hill, 1983.

Frost P, Gomez EC, Zaias N (eds): *Recent Advances in Dermatopharmacology.* New York, Spectrum Publications, 1978.

Helfand AD: A clinical study of methylprednisolone acetate (Depo-Medrol) in the treatment of pain and inflammation associated with various foot disorders. *J Am Podiatry Assoc* 63:287–292, 1973.

Hellier FF: Creams, ointments and lotions. *Practitioner* 202:23–26, 1969.

Lamid S, Wang RH: The range of local anesthetics. *Drug Ther* 5:103–113, 1975.

Legendre R, Steltz M: A multi-center, double-blind comparison of ketoconazole and griseofulvin in the treatment of infections due to dermatophytes. *Rev Infect Dis* 2:586–591, 1980.

Leyden JJ, Kligman AM: Criticism of "the case against topical antibiotics." *Prog Dermatol* 11:7, 1977.

Maddin SW (ed): *Current Dermatologic Therapy*, ed 3. Philadelphia, W.B. Saunders, 1982.

Mailbach HI, Stoughton RB: Topical corticosteroids. In Azarnoff DL (ed): *Steroid Therapy*, Philadelphia, W.B. Saunders, pp 174–190, 1975.

Marples RR, Kligman AM: Methods of evaluating topical antibacterial agents on human skin. *Antimicrob Agents Chemother* 5:323, 1974.

Noble WC: Choice of topical antibiotic—a microbiological view point. *Clin Exp Dermatol* 6:503–507, 1981.

Olmstead CB: Antibiotics in dermatology. *Cutis* 24:414–425, 1979.

Rassmussen JE: Topical antibiotics. *J Dermatol Surg* 2:69–71, 1976.

Rebora A, Marples RR, Kligman AM: Erosio interdigitalis blastomycetica. *Arch Dermatol.* 108:66–68, 1973.

Sauer GC: *Manual of Skin Disease*, ed. 3. Philadelphia, J.B. Lippincott, 1973, pp 31–44.

Savin JA: Do systemic antipruritic agents work? *Br J Dermatol* 102:113–118, 1980.

Scoggins RB, Klinman R: Percutaneous absorption of corticosteroids: systemic effects. *N Engl J Med* 273:831–840, 1965.

Sheard C: *Treatment of Skin Diseases: A Manual.* Chicago, Year Book Medical, 1978.

Spector R: Rational use of topical antibiotics. *J Iowa Med Soc* 70:262–263, 1980.

Stoughton RB: Evaluation of new potent steroids. In Frost P et al (eds): *Recent Advances in Dermatopharmacology.* Spectrum Publications, New York, pp 105–112, 1978.

Stoughton RB: Principles of topical steroid treatment in skin diseases. In *Topics in Internal Medicine.* Baltimore, Williams & Wilkins, 1980.

Thompson RL, Wright AJ: Cephalosporin antibiotics. *Mayo Clin Proc* 58:79–87, 1983.

Vance CE: Differential diagnosis of mycosis. *Arch Podiatry Med Foot Surg* 4:7–13, 1978.

Weisfeld M: Understanding porokeratosis plantaris descreta. *J Am Podiatry Assoc* 63:138–144, 1973.

Wilkinson DS: Dermatological dressings. *Practitioner* 202:27–36, 1969.

Wilson WR, Cockerill FR: Tetracyclines, chloramphenicol, erythromycin and clindamycin. *Mayo Clin Proc* 58:92–98, 1983.

Wright AJ, Wilkowske CJ: The penicillins. *Mayo Clin Proc* 58:21–32, 1983.

Index

Page numbers followed by *t* or *f* denote tables or figures respectively.